Stedman's
PATHOLOGY &
LAB MEDICINE
WORDS

SECOND EDITION

Stedman's

PATHOLOGY & LAB MEDICINE
WORDS

SECOND EDITION

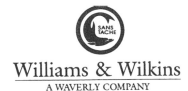

Williams & Wilkins
A WAVERLY COMPANY

BALTIMORE • PHILADELPHIA • LONDON • PARIS • BANGKOK
BUENOS AIRES • HONG KONG • MUNICH • SYDNEY • TOKYO • WROCLAW

Series Editor: Elizabeth B. Randolph
Managing Editor: Maureen Barlow Pugh
Editor: Christa Scott, CMT
Production Coordinator: Marette Magargle-Smith
Typesetter: Peirce Graphic Services, Inc.
Printer & Binder: Vicks Lithograph & Printing

Printed in the United States of America

First Edition, 1993

Library of Congress Cataloging-in-Publication Data

Stedman's pathology & lab medicine words / editor, Christa Scott. — 2nd ed.
    p.   cm.
  ISBN 0-683-40191-2
  1. Pathology—Terminology.   2. Diagnosis, Laboratory—Terminology.
I. Stedman's pathology, lab medicine words.
RB115.S73   1997
616.07′01′4—dc21

                        97-15929
                            CIP
                    97 98 99
        1 2 3 4 5 6 7 8 9 10

Contents

Acknowledgments

An important part of our editorial process is the involvement of medical transcriptionists—as advisors, reviewers and/or editors.

Special thanks are due Christa Scott, CMT for proofreading the first edition of the book, editing and proofing the manuscript, and helping with the appendices. We also would like to extend our thanks to Darla Haberer, CMT who edited all the new terms that were added to *Stedman's Pathology & Lab Medicine Words, Second Edition,* as well as the entire manuscript.

Thanks also to our *Stedman's Pathology & Lab Medicine Words* MT Editorial Advisory Board, consisting of Wendy Ryan, ART; Genny Smith, CMT; Karen L. Thomas, CMT; and Andrea Topolewski, CMT. These medical transcriptionists served as editors and advisors, and spent hours perusing texts, journals, and manufacturer's information to compile the latest terms in the specialties of pathology and laboratory medicine.

Other important contributors to this revised edition include: Melania Droppa, Laurie DiPaula, Diane Edgar, and Pamela Maykulsky, all of whom gathered new words and/or provided invaluable suggestions. Barb Ferretti played an integral role in the process by updating the database and providing a final quality check.

As with all our *Stedman's* word references, we have benefitted from the suggestions and expertise of our many contacts in the medical transcriptionist community. Thanks to all our advisory board participants, reviewers and editors, AAMT meeting attendees, and others who have written in with requests and comments—keep talking, and we'll keep listening.

Preface to the Second Edition

When asked to write a preface for the second edition of *Stedman's Pathology & Lab Medicine Words,* I began thinking about the reasons I was in the field of medical transcription. I realized it was my total obsession with medicine and words—absolutely insisting on correctness, punctuation, grammar, clarity—and then, enjoying the beauty of the printed page.

Having always wanted to be a physician or maybe a pharmacist, but not wanting to "get my hands dirty," transcription was the perfect fit—I could continue learning all I could about the medical field and still be involved in producing an accurate and "beautiful" document.

This second edition of *Stedman's Pathology & Lab Medicine Words* is the result of extensive cultivating of the first edition to ensure correct spelling, capitalization, diacritical marks, punctuation, timeliness and appropriateness to the field of pathology and laboratory medicine.

More important, it is also a compilation of the latest terms including laboratory tests and equipment, the ever-expanding branch of immunopathology, "bug" nomenclature such as bacteria, virus, fungi and parasites, microbiology, and of course, diseases and syndromes.

In closing, I would like to thank Darla Haberer, CMT, for her expertise in making this project a success, and the many others who spent their valuable time researching and submitting these new terms. A big thank-you also goes to Maureen Barlow Pugh and Williams & Wilkins for allowing me to participate in making this second edition the most accurate, up-to-date, beautifully-printed edition yet.

Christa L. Scott, CMT

Publisher's Preface

Stedman's Pathology & Lab Medicine Words, Second Edition offers an authoritative assurance of quality and exactness to the wordsmiths of the health care professions — medical transcriptionists, medical editors and copy editors, health information management personnel, court reporters, and the many other users and producers of medical documentation.

Users of the first edition of *Stedman's Pathology & Lab Medicine Words* will notice we have added more terms in the areas of lab equipment, microbiology, genetics, and immunopathology in this second edition.

Stedman's Pathology & Lab Medicine Words, Second Edition, can be used to validate both the spelling and the accuracy of terminology specific to clinical pathology, anatomical pathology, hematology, medical technology, blood banking, and clinical chemistry. The user will find listed thousands of lab test names, medical abbreviations, diseases and syndromes. Bacteria, fungi, parasites, and viruses are also well covered. Appendices of laboratory reference range values, lab test names, and culture media are featured at the back of the book.

Because our goal has been to provide a comprehensive yet streamlined reference tool, we have omitted terminology that is not specific to these specialties. Thus, some terms (such as anatomy and physiology terms) that are often dictated in these specialties are not included in this text, as they can be found in general medical dictionaries.

This compilation of over 69,000 entries, fully cross-indexed for quick access, was built from a base vocabulary of over 46,589 medical words, phrases, abbreviations and acronyms. The extensive A–Z list was developed from the database of *Stedman's Medical Dictionary* and supplemented by terminology found in current medical literature (please see list of References on page xvi).

We at Williams & Wilkins strive to provide you with the most up-to-date and accurate word references available. Your use of this word book will prompt new editions, which will be published as often as justified by updates and revisions. We welcome your suggestions for improvements, changes, corrections, and additions — whatever will make this *Stedman's* product more useful to you. Please use the postpaid card at the back of this book and send your recommendations care of "Stedmans" at Williams & Wilkins.

Explanatory Notes

Medical transcription is an art as well as a science. Both are needed to correctly interpret a physician's dictation, whose language is a product of education, training, and experience. This variety in medical language means that there are several acceptable ways to express certain terms, including jargon. This second edition of *Stedman's Pathology & Lab Medicine Words* provides variant spellings and phrasings for many terms. This, in addition to complete cross-indexing, makes *Stedman's Pathology & Lab Medicine Words, Second Edition* a valuable resource for determining the validity of terms as they are encountered.

Alphabetical Organization

Alphabetization of entries is letter by letter as spelled, ignoring punctuation, spaces, prefixed numbers, Greek letters, or other characters. For example:

acid-fast staining methods

acid formaldehyde hematin

α-acid glycoprotein

acid hematin

In subentries, the abbreviated singular form or the spelled-out plural form of the noun main entry word is ignored in alphabetization.

Format and Style

All main entries are in **boldface** to speed up location of a sought-after entry, to enhance distinction between main entries and subentries, and to relieve the textual density of the pages.

Irregular plurals and variant spellings are shown on the same line as the singular or preferred form of the word. For example:

scolex pl. **scoleces**

Selivanoff reagent, Seliwanow reagent

Hyphenation

As a rule of style, multiple eponyms (e.g., Recklinghausen-Applebaum syndrome) are hyphenated. Also, hyphens have been added between a manufacturer and one or more eponyms (e.g., Vital-Metzenbaum dissecting scissors). Please note that hyphenation is a question of style, not of accuracy, and thus is a matter of choice.

Possessives

Possessive forms have been dropped in this reference for the sake of consistency and to conform to the guidelines outlined by the American Association for Medical Transcription (AAMT) and other groups. Please note, however, that retaining the possessive is a question of style, not of accuracy, and thus is a matter of choice. To form the possessive of a word, simply add the apostrophe or apostrophe "s" to the end of the word.

Cross-indexing

The word list is in an index-like main entry-subentry format that contains two combined alphabetical listings:

(1) A *noun* main entry-subentry organization typical of the A-Z section of medical dictionaries like **Stedman's:**

agar
    ascitic a.
    bile salt a.
    birdseed a.
    bismuth sulfite a.

acidosis
    carbon dioxide a.
    compensated a.
    diabetic a.
    lactic a.

(2) An *adjective* main entry-subentry organization, which lists words and phrases as you hear them. The main entries are the adjectives or modifiers in a multi-word term. The subentries are the nouns around which the terms are constructed and to which the adjectives or modifiers pertain:

acetone
    a. body
    a. compound
    a. fixative
    a. test

endometrial
    e. curettage
    e. cyst
    e. hyperplasia
    e. polyp

This format provides the user with more than one way to locate and identify a multi-word term. For example:

reaction
    alkaline r.

alkaline
    a. reaction

amino acid
    glucogenic a.a.

glucogenic
    g. amino acid

It also allows the user to see together all terms that contain a particular descriptor as well as all types, kinds, or variations of a noun entity. For example:

eczema
    chronic e.
    e. erythematosum
    e. hypertrophicum
    lichenoid e.

enzyme
    activating e.
    allosteric e.
    e. analyzer
    e. assays

Wherever possible, abbreviations are separately defined and cross-referenced. For example:

CFP
    chronic false-positive

chronic
    c. false-positive (CFP)

false-positive
    chronic f.-p. (CFP)

References

In addition to the manufacturers' literature we gather at various medical meetings, scientific reports from hospitals, and our MT Editorial Advisory Board members' lists (from their daily transcription work), we used the following sources for new words for *Stedman's Pathology & Lab Medicine Words, Second Edition:*

Books

Pathology/Laboratory words & phrases, 2ed. Modesto: Health Professions Institute, 1996.

Lance LL. Quick look drug book. Baltimore: Williams & Wilkins, 1997.

Pyle V. Current medical terminology, 5th ed. Modesto: Health Professions Institute, 1994.

Stedman's medical dictionary. 26th ed. Baltimore: Williams & Wilkins, 1995.

Sloane SB. The medical word book, 3ed. Philadelphia: WB Saunders Company, 1991.

Sloane SB, Dusseau, A word book in pathology & laboratory medicine, Philadelphia: WB Saunders, 1995.

Journals

The American Journal of Clinical Pathology. Chicago: American Society of Clinical Pathologists, 1992–1997.

The American Journal of Surgical Pathology. Hagerstown, MD: Lippincott-Raven Publishers, 1992–1997.

Journal of the American Association for Medical Transcription. Modesto: American Association for Medical Transcription, 1995–1997.

The Latest Word. Philadelphia: WB Saunders Company, 1994–1996.

Perspectives on the Medical Transcription Profession. Modesto: Health Professions Institute, 1993–1997.

α (*var. of* alpha)
    α actinin
    α agglutinin
    α amino nitrogen test
    α hemolysin
    α hemolysis
    α metachromasia
    α-thalassemia intermedia
    α unit
α_2 (*var. of* alpha-2)
    α_2 globulins
α_1 (*var. of* alpha-1)
    α_1 antichymotrypsin
α_1PI
    α_1-protease inhibitor
A
    absolute temperature
    ampere
    Ångstrom unit
    mass number
    total acidity
        A band
        A cell
        A virus hepatitis
A_2
    hemoglobin A_2
    A_2 thalassemia
A_{1c}
    hemoglobin A_{1c}
A
    absorbance
a
    ampere
    area
    asymmetric
    total acidity
AA
    atomic absorption
        AA spectrophotometer
AAA
    abdominal aortic aneurysm
    androgenic anabolic agent
AAC
    antibiotic-associated colitis
AACC
    American Association for Clinical
    Chemistry
AAH
    atypical adenomatous hyperplasia
AAM
    American Academy of Microbiology
AAMI
    Association for the Advancement of
    Medical Instrumentation

AAN
    American Association of
    Neuropathologists
    amino acid nitrogen
        AAN test
AAP
    American Association of Pathologists
AAPA
    American Association of Pathologist
    Assistants
AAPB
    American Association of Pathologists and
    Bacteriologists
AAR
    antigen-antiglobulin reaction
Aarskog-Scott syndrome
Aarskog syndrome
AAS
    aortic arch syndrome
    atomic absorption spectrophotometry
A1AT
    α_1 antitrypsin
AAV
    adeno-associated virus
AB
    abnormal
    abortion
    Alcian blue
    asbestos body
    asthmatic bronchitis
A/B
    acid-base ratio
Ab
    antibody
abacterial thrombotic endocarditis
abarognosis
abarticular gout
ABB
    acute bronchitis/bronchiolitis
Abbé
    A. condenser
    A. test plate
Abbé-Zeiss
    A.-Z. apparatus
    A.-Z. counting chamber
Abbott
    A. Cell-Dyn hematology analyzer
    A. stain for spores
ABC
    avidin-biotin-peroxidase complex
    ABC Elite staining kit
    ABC technique
abdominal
    a. aneurysm
    a. aortic aneurysm (AAA)

abdominal *(continued)*
    a. dropsy
    a. fibromatosis
    a. fistula
    a. muscle deficiency syndrome
Abell-Kendall method
Abelson murine leukemia virus
Abercrombie syndrome
aberrant
    a. ductule
    a. ganglion
    a. goiter
    a. hemoglobin
    a. pancreas
    a. renal vessel
    a. rest
    a. tissue
aberration
    chromatic a.
    chromosomal a.
    chromosome a.
    heterosomal a.
    homosomal a.
    interchromosomal a.
    intrachromosomal a.
    karyotype a.
    penta-X chromosomal a.
    tetra-X chromosomal a.
    triple-X chromosomal a.
abetalipoproteinemia (ABL)
ABG
    arterial blood gas
abiotrophy
ABL
    abetalipoproteinemia
ablastin
ablate
ablatio
    a. placentae
    a. retinae
ablation
ablative chemotherapy
ablepharon
ABN, Abn, abn
    abnormal
abnormal (AB, ABN, Abn, abn)
    a. chorion
    a. chorionic villi
    a. endochondral ossification
    a. flow
    a. glucose tolerance test (AGTT)
    a. mucopolysacchariduria (AMPS)
    a. shortening
abnormality
    bone marrow a.
    cytologic a.
    fetal a.
    genetic a.

    morphologic a.
    nonspecific hepatocellular a. (NHA)
    no serious a. (NSA)
    no significant a. (NSA)
    traumatic a.
ABO
    A. antibodies
    A. antigen
    A. blood group
    A. compatibility
    A. factor
    A. hemolytic disease of the newborn
    A. incompatibility
    A. typing
Abopon
ABO-Rh typing
aborted ectopic pregnancy
abortion (AB)
    afebrile a.
    ampullar a.
    artificial a.
    cervical a.
    complete a.
    criminal a.
    equine virus a.
    habitual a.
    imminent a.
    incomplete a.
    induced a.
    inevitable a.
    infected a.
    justifiable a.
    missed a.
    septic a.
    spontaneous a.
    therapeutic a. (TA)
    threatened a.
    tubal a.
abortive
    a. infection
    a. neurofibromatosis
    a. transduction
    a. viral disease
abortus fever
abraded wound
Abrams test
abrasion
abruptio placentae
Abrus
ABS
    alkylbenzene sulfonate
abscess
    acute a.
    a. aerobic culture
    alveolar a.
    amebic a. of liver
    apical a.

appendiceal a.
Bartholin a.
Bezold a.
bicameral a.
bone a.
brain a.
Brodie a.
bursal a.
caseous a.
cerebral epidural a.
chronic a.
cold a.
collar-button a.
crypt a.
diffuse a.
Douglas a.
dry a.
Dubois a.
embolic a.
epidural a.
fecal a.
follicular a.
gas a.
gravitation a.
gummatous a.
hematogenous a.
hepatic a.
hot a.
hypostatic a.
ischiorectal a.
Kogoj a.
lacunar a.
lung a.
mastoid a.
metastatic a.
migrating a.
miliary a.
Munro a.
mycotic a.
orbital a.
otic a.
parafrenal a.
parametric a.
parametritic a.
paranephric a.
parotid a.
Pautrier a.
pelvic a.
perforating a.
periapical a.
periappendiceal a.
periarticular a.

perinephric a.
perirectal a.
peritonsillar a.
periureteral a.
periurethral a.
phlegmonous a.
Pott a.
premammary a.
psoas a.
pyemic a.
residual a.
retrobulbar a.
retrocecal a.
retropharyngeal a.
satellite a.
septicemic a.
shirt-stud a.
stellate a.
stercoral a.
sterile a.
stitch a.
subacute a.
subdiaphragmatic a.
subepidermal a.
subhepatic a.
subphrenic a.
subungual a.
sudoriparous a.
syphilitic a.
thecal a.
thymic a.
Tornwaldt a.
tropical a.
tuberculous a.
tubo-ovarian a. (TOA)
verminous a.
wandering a.
worm a.

abscissa
absence
    congenital a.
Absidia
    A. *corymbifera*
    A. *ramosa*
absolute
    a. alcohol
    atmosphere a.
    a. cell increase
    a. eosinophil count
    a. erythrocytosis
    a. iodine uptake (AIU)
    a. leukocytosis

NOTES

absolute *(continued)*
    a. retention time (ART)
    a. system of units
    a. temperature (A)
    a. temperature scale
    a. unit
    a. value
    a. viscosity
    a. zero
absorb
absorbance (*A*)
absorbed dose
absorbefacient
absorbency index
absorbent
    carbon dioxide a.
absorber
absorption
    atomic a. (AA)
    a. cavity
    a. cell
    a. coefficient
    a. constant
    disjunctive a.
    a. of erythrocyte antibody
    fat a.
    iron a.
    a. peak
    a. spectrum
absorption-equivalent thickness (AET)
absorptive
    a. cell
    a. lipemia
    a. state
absorptivity
    molar a.
    specific a.
abstinence
    alimentary a.
abstriction
AC
    anticoagulant
    anticomplementary
    anti-inflammatory corticoid
ac
    acute
ACA
    adenocarcinoma
Academy of Clinical Laboratory Physicians and Scientists (ACLPS)
acanthamebiasis
Acanthamoeba
    A. castellanii
    A. culbertsoni
    A. hartmannella
    A. hatchetti
    A. keratitis

    A. polyphaga
    A. rhysodes
acanthella
Acanthia lectularia
Acanthobdella
Acanthocephala
acanthocephaliasis
Acanthocheilonema
    A. perstans
    A. streptocerca
acanthocyte
acanthocytosis
acanthoid cell
acantholysis
acanthoma
    a. adenoides cysticum
    basal cell a.
    clear cell a.
    pilar sheath a.
    a. verrucosa seborrheica
acanthopodia
acanthor
acanthorrhexis
acanthosis
    glycogen a.
    glycogenic a.
    a. nigricans
acanthotic
acanthrocyte
acanthrocytosis
acapnia
acapnial alkalosis
acarbia
acardiacus
acardius
acariasis
acaricide
acarid
Acaridae
acaridan
acaridiasis
Acarina
acarine
acarinosis
acarodermatitis
acaroid
acarology
Acarus
    A. folliculorum
    A. gallinae
    A. hordei
    A. rhizoglypticus hyacinthi
    A. scabiei
    A. siro
acaryote
acatalasemia
acatalasia
acathectic

acathexia
Acaulium
ACC
    acinar cell carcinoma
    adenoid cystic carcinoma
accelerant
accelerated
    a. reaction
    a. rejection
acceleration
    growth a.
accelerator
    a. factor
    a. globulin (AcG, ac-g)
    proserum prothrombin conversion a.
      (PPCA)
    prothrombin a.
    serum a.
    serum prothrombin conversion a.
      (SPCA)
    serum thrombotic a. (STA)
accelerin
accentuator
acceptor
    hydrogen a.
    oxygen a.
    proton a.
access
    exit a.
    multiple a.
    sequential a.
    a. time
accessory
    a. adrenal
    a. atrium
    a. cell
    a. chromosome
    a. molecule
    a. organ
    a. pancreas
    a. spleen
accident
    cardiovascular a. (CVA)
    cerebrovascular a. (CVA)
    serum a.
accidental
    a. host
    a. parasite
acclimation
accolé forms
accommodation

account
    dose a.
accreta
    placenta a.
AccuData Easy glucose meter
accumulation
    a. of carbohydrates
    a. of complex lipids
    a. disease
    a. of glycogen
    intracellular a.
    a. of pigment
    a. of protein
accumulator
accuracy
    photometric a.
    wavelength a.
ACD
    acid-citrate-dextrose
ACE
    adrenocortical extract
acellular
acclom
acelomate
acentric
acephaline
acephalocyst
acephalous
acervulus
acestoma
acetabuli
    protrusio a.
acetal
acetaldehydase
acetaldehyde
acetamide
acetaminophen
    a. assay
    a. hepatic toxicity
acetate
    cresyl violet a.
    deoxycorticosterone a. (DOCA)
    ethyl a.
    methyl a.
Acetest
acetic
    a. acid-alcohol-formalin
    a. acid and potassium ferrocyanide
      test
    a. aldehyde
    a. anhydride
    a. orcein

NOTES

acetoacetic
 a. acid test
 a. aciduria
acetoacetyl
acetoacetyl-CoA
 a.-C. reductase
 a.-C. thiolase
Acetobacter
 A. aceti
 A. xylinum
acetocarmine
acetoin
 a. test
acetolysis
acetone
 a. body
 a. compound
 a. fixative
 a. test
acetone-insoluble antigen
acetonemia
acetonemic
acetonitrile
acetonuria
aceto-orcein stain
acetowhite test
aceturate
 diminazene a.
acetylation
acetylcholine receptor antibody
acetylcholinesterase
 a. assay
acetyl-CoA
 a.-C. acetyltransferase
 a.-C. acyltransferase
 a.-C. carboxylase
 a.-C. hydrolase
 a.-C. synthetase
acetylcoenzyme A
acetylene trichloride
N-**acetylgalactosamine**
N-**acetylglucosamine**
N-**acetylmannosamine**
acetylmethylcarbinol
N-**acetylneuraminic**
acetylsalicylic acid
acetyltransferase
 acetyl-CoA a.
acetyl value
AcG, ac-g
 accelerator globulin
ACH
 adrenocortical hormone
achalasia
 biliary a.
 esophageal a.
 pelvirectal a.
 sphincteral a.

Achard syndrome
Achard-Thiers syndrome
Achenbach syndrome
Achillea
achiral
achlorhydria
 watery diarrhea, hypokalemia, a.
 (WDHA)
achlorhydric anemia
achlorophyllous
Acholeplasma
 A. laidlawii
Acholeplasmataceae
acholic
 a. stool
acholuria
acholuric
 a. jaundice
achondrogenesis
achondroplasia
 homozygous a.
achondroplastic
 a. dwarf
 a. dwarfism
achondroplasty
Achorion
 A. violaceum
achrestic anemia
achroacytosis
achrodextrin (*var. of* achroodextrin)
achromacyte
achromasia
achromate
achromatic
 a. lens
 a. objective
 a. spindle
achromatism
achromatocyte
achromatolysis
achromatophil
achromatophilia
achromatosis
achromatous
achromaturia
achromia
 congenital a.
 cortical a.
 a. parasitica
 a. unguium
achromic
Achromobacter
Achromobacteraceae
achromocyte
achromophil
achromophilic
achromophilous
achroodextrin, achrodextrin

Achucárro stain
achylia
acid

N-acetylaspartate a.
N-acetylmuramic a.
acetylsalicylic a.
adenylic a.
a. agglutination
a. alcohol
aldaric a.
aldonic a.
alginic a.
aliphatic a.
allantoic a.
alpha amino a.'s
amino a.
aminoacetic a.
p-aminobenzoic a. (PAB, PABA)
γ-aminobutyric a. (GABA)
aminoglutaric a.
p-aminohippuric a. (PAH, PAHA)
aminolevulinic a. (ALA)
aminopenicillanic a. (APA)
6-aminopenicillanic a.
aminosuccinic a.
a. anhydride method
arachidonic a.
aromatic a.
ascorbic a.
asparaginic a.
aspartic a. (Asp)
aurin tricarboxylic a.
behenic a.
benzoic a.
benzoylaminoacetic a.
bile a.'s
binary a.
boric a.
Brönsted-Lowry a.
butanoic a.
butyric a.
cacodylic a.
carbolic a.
carbonic a.
carboxylic a.
carminic a.
catechinic a.
catechuic a.
cerebronic a.
a. challenge test
chenodeoxycholic a.
cholic a.

chromic a.
chromotropic a.
citric a.
a. clearance test (ACT)
conjugate a.
cytidylic a.
decanoic a.
dehydroascorbic a.
deoxyadenylic a.
deoxycholic a.
deoxycytidylic a.
deoxyguanylic a.
deoxyribonucleic a. (DNA)
deoxyuridylic a.
diacetic a.
dibasic a.
dicarboxylic a.
(2,4-dichlorophenoxy)acetic a.
diethylenetriaminepentaacetic a.
dihydrofolic a.
dihydroxymandelic a. (DHMA, DOMA)
3,4-dihydroxymandelic a.
2,5-dihydroxyphenylacetic a.
1-dimethylaminoaphthalene-5 sulfonic a. (DANS)
dipicolinic a.
a. dye
edetic a.
elaidic a.
a. elution test
epsilon a.
essential fatty a.'s (EFA)
ethacrynic a. (ECA)
ethanoic a.
ethylenediaminetetraacetic a. (EDTA)
ethylene tetraacetic a.
a. fast (AF)
fatty a. (FA)
flavianic a.
folic a.
folinic a.
a. formaldehyde hematin
formic a.
formiminoglutamic a. (FIGLU)
free a. (FA)
free fatty a.'s (FFA)
a. fuchsin
fumaric a.
gamma-aminobutyric a. (GABA)
glacial acetic a.

NOTES

acid *(continued)*
   ᴅ-glucaric a.
   glucuronic a.
   glutamic a. (Glu)
   glutaric a.
   glycochenodeoxycholic a.
   glycocholic a.
   glycodeoxycholic a.
   glycolithocholic a.
   a. glycoprotein
   guanidino-aminovaleric a.
   guanylic a.
   a. hemolysin test
   heparinic a.
   hexanoic a.
   hexuronic a.
   hippuric a.
   homogentisic a. (HGA)
   homovanillic a. (HVA)
   hyaluronic a.
   hydrochloric a.
   hydrocyanic a.
   hydrofluoric a.
   a. hydrolase
   p-hydroxybenzoic a.
   5-hydroxyindoleacetic a.
   o-hydroxyphenylacetic a.
   p-hydroxyphenyllactic a.
   p-hydroxyphenylpyruvic a.
   iduronic a.
   imidazolepyruvic a.
   imino a.
   indolacetic a.
   indolaceturic a.
   indollactic a.
   inorganic a.
   inosinic a.
   a. intoxication
   iodic a.
   a. ionization constant
   isobutyric a.
   isocitric a.
   isovaleric a.
   keto a.
   lactic a.
   lauric a.
   leukocyte ascorbic a. (LAA)
   Lewis a.
   lignoceric a.
   linoleic a.
   linolenic a.
   lipoic a.
   lithic a.
   lithocholic a.
   long-chain fatty a. (LCFA)
   a. magenta
   malic a.
   malonic a.

medium-chain fatty a. (MCFA)
mercaptoacetic a.
metaphosphoric a.
methoxyhydroxymandelic a.
  (MOMA)
methylmalonic a.
monoaminodicarboxylic a.
monoaminomonocarboxylic a.
monobasic a.
monoenoic fatty a.
a. mucopolysaccharide (AMP)
a. mucopolysaccharides (AMPS)
muramic a.
mycolic a.
myristic a.
neuraminic a.
nitrous a.
nonesterified fatty a.
a. number
octanoic a.
octulosonic a.
oleic a.
a. orcein
organic a.
orotic a.
orthophosphoric a.
osmic a.
oxalic a.
oxaloacetic a.
oxo a.
3-oxobutyric a.
2-oxoglutaric a.
oxolinic a.
palmitic a.
palmitoleic a.
pantothenic a.
para-aminobenzoic a.
para-aminohippuric a.
peracetic a.
perchloric a.
performic a.
a. perfusion test
periodic a.
phenaceturic a.
phenylacetic a.
phenyllactic a.
phenylpyruvic a.
a. phosphatase
a. phosphatase assay
a. phosphatase stain
a. phosphatase staining
a. phosphatase test
a. phosphatase test for semen
a. phosphate
phosphatidic a.
6-phosphogluconic a.
5-phosphomevalonic a.
phosphomolybdic a.

phosphonoacetic a.
phosphoric a.
phosphotungstic a. (PTA)
phthalic a.
phytanic a.
phytic a.
picramic a.
picric a.
polyadenylic a.
polybasic a.
polyenoic a.
polyphosphoric a.
polysialic a.
polyunsaturated fatty a. (PUFA)
polyuridylic a.
pristanic a.
propanoic a.
propionic a.
prostanoic a.
proton a.
prussic a.
pteroic a.
pteroylglutamic a.
4-pyridoxic a.
pyrophosphoric a.
pyroracemic a.
pyruvic a.
quinolinic a.
radioiodinated fatty a. (RIFA)
a. reaction
a. red 87
a. red 91
a. reflux test
retinoic a.
rhodanic a.
ribonucleic a. (RNA)
ribothymidylic a.
ricinoleic a.
p-rosolic a.
rubeanic a.
saccharic a.
salicylic a.
salicylsalicylic a.
salicylsulfonic a.
salicyluric a.
saturated fatty a.
a. seromucoid
serum uric a. (SUA)
sialic a.
silicic a.
soluble ribonucleic a. (SRNA)
stearic a.

succinic a.
sugar a.
sulfanilic a.
sulfindigotic a.
sulfinic a.
sulfonic a.
sulfosalicylic a. (SSA)
sulfuric a.
sulfurous a.
tannic a.
tartaric a.
taurochenodeoxycholic a.
taurocholic a.
taurodeoxycholic a.
taurolithocholic a.
^{99m}Tc pentetic a.
teichoic a.
ternary a.
n-tetracosanoic a.
tetrahydrofolic a.
thio a.
thioctic a.
thioglycolic a.
thiolaminopropionic a.
thymidylic a.
a. tide
titratable a. (TA)
toluic a.
total fatty a.'s (TFA)
tribasic a.
tricarboxylic a.
trichloroacetic a. (TCA)
(2,4,5-trichlorophenoxy)acetic a.
tuberculostearic a.
tungstic a.
UDP-glucuronic a.
UDP-iduronic a.
unesterified fatty a. (UFA)
uridylic a.
urobenzoic a.
urocanic a.
uronic a.
ursodeoxycholic a.
vaccenic a.
valeric a.
valproic a.
a. value
vanillic a.
vanillylmandelic a. (VMA)
vinegar a.
a. wave

NOTES

acid *(continued)*
    xanthurenic a.
    xanthylic a.
acid-alcohol-formalin
    acetic a.
Acidaminococcus
    A. fermentans
acidaminuria
acid-base
    a.-b. balance
    a.-b. diagram
    a.-b. indicator
    a.-b. nomogram
    a.-b. ratio (A/B)
acid-citrate-dextrose (ACD)
acidemia
    argininosuccinic a.
    lactic a.
    methylmalonic a.
    propionic a.
acid-fast
    a.-f. bacillus (AFB)
    a.-f. bacterium
    a.-f. stain
    a.-f. staining method
α-acid glycoprotein
α$_1$-acid glycoprotein
acidic
    a. dye
acidifiable
acidified serum test
acidifier
acidify
acidimetry
acidity
    a. reduction test
    total a. (A, a)
acid-lability test
acidocyte
acidocytopenia
acidocytosis
acidogenic
acidophil, acidophile
    a. adenoma
    alpha a.
    a. cell
    a. granule
acidophilic
    a. adenoma
    a. body
    a. index
    a. leukocyte
    a. necrosis
    a. normoblast
acidophilus milk
acidosis
    carbon dioxide a.
    compensated a.

    diabetic a.
    hypercapnic a.
    lactic a.
    metabolic a.
    potassium a.
    primary renal tubular a.
    renal tubular a. (RTA)
    respiratory a.
    secondary renal tubular a.
    a. test
    uncompensated a.
acidotic
acid-Schiff
    periodic a.-S. (PAS)
    a.-S. stain
acid-secretion rate
aciduria
    acetoacetic a.
    β-aminoisobutyric a.
    argininosuccinic a.
    beta aminoisobutyric a.
    L-glyceric a.
    glycolic a.
    methylmalonic a.
    orotic a.
    paroxysmal a.
    propionic a.
    xanthurenic a.
aciduric
acinar
    a. cell
    a. cell carcinoma (ACC)
    a. cell tumor
Acinetobacter
    A. anitratus
    A. calcoaceticus
    A. calcoaceticus anitratus
    A. calcoaceticus lwoffi
    A. parapertussis
acinic
    a. cell adenocarcinoma
    a. cell carcinoma
    a. cell tumor
    a. cell tumor of lung
    a. cell tumor of salivary gland
aciniform
acinitis
acinose carcinoma
acinotubular
acinous carcinoma
acinus
ACLA
    American Clinical Laboratory
      Association
Acladium
aclasis
    diaphysial a.
    tarsoepiphyseal a.

ACLPS
  Academy of Clinical Laboratory
    Physicians and Scientists
ACM
  albumin-calcium-magnesium
acne
  a. atrophia
  a. conglobata
  a. rosacea
  a. rosacea keratitis
  a. vulgaris
acneiform
aconitase
aconitate hydratase
Aconitum
Acosta disease
acoustic
  a. coupler
  a. neurilemoma
  a. neurinoma
  a. neuroma
  a. schwannoma
ACP
  American College of Pathologists
ACPA
  anticytoplasmic antibody
  ACPA test
acquired
  a. agammaglobulinemia
  a. atrophy
  a. character
  a. defect
  a. deformity
  a. dysplasia
  a. hemolytic anemia (AHA)
  a. hemolytic icterus
  a. hypogammaglobulinemia
  a. ichthyosis
  a. immunity
  a. immunodeficiency syndrome
    (AIDS)
  a. leukoderma
  a. leukopathia
  a. methemoglobinemia
  a. nevus
  a. sensitivity
  a. toxoplasmosis in adults
acquista
  epidermolysis bullosa a.
acral lentiginous melanoma
acrania
Acrel ganglion

Acremonium
acridine
  a. dye
  a. hydrochloride
  a. orange (AO)
  a. orange method
  a. orange stain
  tetramethyl a.
  a. yellow
acriflavine
acroasphyxia
acrobrachycephaly
acrobystitis
acrocentric
acrocephalia
acrocephalic
acrocephalosyndactyly
acrocephalous
acrocephaly
acrochordon
acrocyanosis
acrodermatitis
  a. chronica atrophicans
  a. continua
  a. perstans
acrodolichomelia
acroedema
acrofacial
  a. dysostosis
  a. syndrome
acrogenous
acrokeratoelastoidosis
acrokeratosis
  paraneoplastic a.
  a. verruciformis
acrolein
acromegalia
acromegalic
acromegalogigantism
acromegaloidism
acromegaly
acromelia
acromelic
  a. dwarfism
acromesomelia
acromicria
acro-osteolysis
acropachy
acropachyderma
acropathy
acropetal
acropleurogenous

NOTES

acroposthitis
acroscleroderma
acrosclerosis
acrosomal
    a. granule
    a. vesicle
acrosome reaction
acrospiroma
    eccrine a.
acrostealgia
Acrotheca
    A. pedrosoi
acrotheca
Acrothesium
    A. floccosum
acrotrophoneurosis
acrylamide gel electrophoresis
acrylonitrile
ACS
    American Chemical Society
    antireticular cytotoxic serum
    Association of Clinical Scientists
        ACS grade
ACT
    acid clearance test
    activated coagulation time
    anticoagulant therapy
Actaea
ACTH
    adrenocorticotropic hormone
        ACTH stimulation test
ACTH-producing adenoma
ACTH-RF
    adrenocorticotropic hormone-releasing
    factor
actin
    anti-sarcomeric a.
    anti-smooth muscle a.
    muscle-specific a. (HHF-35)
    sarcomeric a.
    smooth-muscle a. (SMA)
    α-smooth-muscle a.
actinic
    a. dermatitis
    a. keratosis
    a. porokeratosis
    a. reticuloid
actinide
actinin
    α a.
    alpha a.
actinium
Actinobacillus
    A. actinomycetemcomitans
    A. equuli
    A. lignieresii
    A. mallei
    A. pseudomallei

actinohematin
actinoides
    Thysanosoma a.
Actinomadura
    A. africana
    A. madurae
    A. pelletieri
Actinomyces
    A. bovis
    A. congolensis
    A. eriksonii
    A. israelii
    A. muris
    A. muris-ratti
    A. naeslundii
    A. necrophorus
    A. odontolyticus
    A. rhusiopathiae
    A. vinaceus
    A. viscosus
Actinomycetaceae
Actinomycetales
actinomycete
    thermophilic a.
actinomycetic
actinomycetoma
actinomycin
actinomycosis
actinomycotic
    a. appendicitis
    a. mycetoma
actinomyoma
Actinomyxidia
actinophage
actinophytosis
Actinoplanaceae
Actinoplanes
Actinopoda
action
    buffer a.
    calorigenic a.
    capillary a.
    cumulative a.
    diastasic a.
    law of mass a.
    opsonic a.
    specific dynamic a.
    thermogenic a.
    vitaminoid a.
activated
    a. charcoal
    a. coagulation time (ACT)
    a. complex
    a. lymphocyte
    a. macrophage
    a. partial thromboplastin substitution
    test

a. partial thromboplastin time (APTT, aPTT)

activating
    a. agent
    a. enzyme

activation
    allosteric a.
    a. analysis
    complement a.
    cross a.
    a. energy
    lymphocyte a.
    plasma a.
    trans a.
    very late a. (VLA)

activator
    plasminogen a.
    polyclonal a.

active
    a. anaphylaxis
    a. chronic hepatitis
    a. chronic inflammation
    a. electrode
    a. immunity
    a. immunization
    a. prophylaxis
    a. rosette test
    a. sensitization
    a. transport

activity
    blood granulocyte-specific a. (BGSA)
    chemotactic a.
    colony-stimulating a. (CSA)
    a. determination
    general gonadotropic a. (GGA)
    insulin-like a. (ILA)
    nonsuppressible insulin-like a. (NSILA)
    optical a.
    plasma insulin a. (PIA)
    plasma renin a. (PRA)
    postheparin lipolytic a. (PHLA)
    a. ratio
    relative specific a. (RSA)
    renal vein renin a. (RVRA)
    rheumatoid factor-like a. (RFLA)
    surface-oriented pinocytic a.
    thyroxine-specific a. (T_4SA)
    total antitryptic a. (TAT)
    tryptic a.

actomyosin
    platelet a.

Actonia

ACTP
    adrenocorticotropic polypeptide

actuate

Acuaria spiralis

aculeate

acuta
    pityriasis lichenoides et varioliformis a. (PLEVA)

acute (ac)
    a. abscess
    a. anterior poliomyelitis
    a. atrophic paralysis
    a. bacterial endocarditis
    a. bronchitis
    a. bronchitis/bronchiolitis (ABB)
    a. bulbar poliomyelitis
    a. cardiovascular disease (ACVD)
    a. cellular rejection
    a. and chronic inflammation
    a. compression triad
    a. contagious conjunctivitis
    a. crescentic glomerulonephritis
    a. diffuse peritonitis
    a. disseminated encephalomyelitis (ADEM)
    a. disseminated myositis
    a. dissseminated lupus erythematosus
    a. epidemic conjunctivitis
    a. epidemic infectious adenitis
    a. epidemic leukoencephalitis
    a. exudative glomerulonephritis
    a. febrile jaundice
    a. fibrinous pleuritis
    a. focal hepatitis
    a. follicular conjunctivitis
    a. fulminating meningococcal septicemia
    a. gangrenous appendicitis
    a. gastritis
    a. gelatinous pneumonia
    a. glomerulonephritis (AGN)
    a. goiter
    a. granulocytic leukemia (AGL)
    a. hemolytic transfusion reaction
    a. hemorrhagic bronchopneumonia
    a. hemorrhagic cholecystitis
    a. hemorrhagic cystitis
    a. hemorrhagic encephalitis

NOTES

acute *(continued)*
a. hemorrhagic glomerulonephritis
a. hemorrhagic inflammation
a. hemorrhagic leukoencephalitis (AHLE)
a. hemorrhagic pancreatitis
a. hemorrhagic ulcer
a. hemorrhagic ulceration
a. idiopathic polyneuritis
a. infarct
a. infectious disease (AID)
a. infectious nonbacterial gastroenteritis
a. infective endocarditis
a. inflammatory exudate
a. inflammatory infiltrate
a. inflammatory membrane
a. inflammatory necrosis
a. inflammatory transudate
a. intermittent porphyria (AIP)
a. interstitial nephritis (AIN)
a. isolated myocarditis
a. lymphoblastic leukemia (ALL)
a. lymphocytic leukemia (ALL)
a. mastitis
a. megakaryoblastic leukemia
a. miliary tuberculosis
a. monoblastic leukemia (AML, AMoL)
a. monocytic leukemia (AML, AMoL, MLa)
a. myelocytic leukemia (AML)
a. myelogenous leukemia
a. myelomonocytic leukemia (AMML)
a. myocardial infarction (AMI)
a. necrotizing encephalitis
a. necrotizing enterocolitis
a. necrotizing hemorrhagic encephalomyelitis
a. necrotizing myelitis
a. nephritis
a. nephrosis
a. nonlymphocytic leukemia (ANLL)
otitis media, purulent, a. (OMPA)
a. parenchymatous hepatitis
a. paroxysmal myoglobinuria
a. phase protein
a. phase reactant
a. phase reaction
a. posthemorrhagic anemia
a. post-streptococcal glomerulonephritis
a. primary hemorrhagic meningoencephalitis
a. proliferative (AP)

a. promyelocytic leukemia (APL)
a. pulmonary alveolitis
a. pyelonephritis
a. pyogenic membrane
a. recurrent rhabdomyolysis
a. renal failure (ARF)
a. respiratory disease (ARD)
a. respiratory distress syndrome (ARDS)
a. respiratory failure (ARF)
a. rheumatic arthritis
a. rhinitis
a. rickets
a. salivary adenitis
a. serous synovitis
a. splenic tumor
a. splenitis
a. suppurative appendicitis
a. thyroiditis
a. transverse myelitis
a. tubular necrosis (ATN)
a. ulcerative colitis
a. undifferentiated leukemia (AUL)
a. uric acid nephropathy
a. viral hepatitis (AVH)
a. yellow atrophy
a. yellow atrophy of liver

ACVD
acute cardiovascular disease

acyl
a. carrier protein
a. peroxide

acylation

acyl-CoA
a. dehydrogenase
a. synthetase

acyloxy group

N-acylsphingosine

acylsphingosine deacylase

acyltransferase
acetyl-CoA a.
lecithin-cholesterol a. (LCAT)
phosphatidylcholine-cholesterol a.

AD
Aleutian disease
average deviation

ADA
adenosine deaminase

adactyly

Adair-Dighton syndrome

1-adamantanamine

adamantine prism

adamantinoma
a. of long bones
pituitary a.

adamantoblast

Adamkiewicz test

A

Adams-Stokes
    A.-S. attack (ASA)
    A.-S. disease (AS)
Adansonia
adaptation
    cellular a.
    enzymatic a.
    genetic a.
    phenotypic a.
adapter
adaptive
    a. enzyme
    a. hormone
    a. hypertrophy
ADCC
    antibody-dependent cell-mediated
    cytotoxicity
addict
addiction
    alcohol a.
    drug a.
Addis
    A. count
    A. test
Addison
    A. anemia
    A. disease
    A. keloid
Addison-Biermer disease
addisonian
    a. anemia
    a. crisis
    a. syndrome
addisonism
addition
    binary a.
    a. polymer
    a. reaction
addition-deletion mutation
additive
address
addressin
addressing
    indirect a.
    a. ligand
adduct
adduction
ADEM
    acute disseminated encephalomyelitis
adenectopia
Aden fever
adenine arabinoside

adenitis
    acute epidemic infectious a.
    acute salivary a.
    cervical a.
    mesenteric a.
    phlegmonous a.
    a. tropicalis
adenoacanthoma
adenoameloblastoma
adeno-associated virus (AAV)
adenocarcinoma (ACA)
    acinic cell a.
    alveolar a.
    anaplastic a.
    bronchiolar a.
    bronchioloalveolar a.
    clear cell a.
    colloid a.
    endometrial a.
    follicular a.
    gelatinous a.
    infiltrating duct a.
    inflammatory a.
    lobular a.
    Lucké a.
    medullary a.
    mesonephric a.
    mixed squamous cell carcinoma
      and a.
    a. of Moll
    mucinous a.
    mucoid a.
    oxyphilic endometrioid a.
    papillary a.
    renal a.
    sebaceous a.
    signet ring a.
    a. in situ
    sweat gland a.
    trabecular a.
    undifferentiated a.
adenocellulitis
adenochondroma
adenocystic carcinoma
adenocystoma
adenodiastasis
adenoepithelioma
adenofibroma
adenofibromyoma
adenofibrosis
adenohypophyseal hormone
adenohypophysis

NOTES

adenohypophysitis
    lymphocytic a.
adenoid
    a. cystic carcinoma (ACC)
    a. face
    a. facies
    a. squamous cell carcinoma
    a. tumor
adenoidal-pharyngeal-conjunctival (APC)
adenoleiomyofibroma
adenolipoma
adenolipomatosis
    symmetric a.
adenolymphocele
adenolymphoma
adenolysis
adenoma
    acidophil a.
    acidophilic a.
    ACTH-producing a.
    adnexal a.
    adrenocortical a.
    aldosterone-producing a. (APA)
    angioinvasive a.
    apocrine a.
    basal cell a.
    basophil a.
    bile duct a.
    bronchial a.
    carcinoma ex pleomorphic a.
    ceruminous a.
    chief cell a.
    chromophil a.
    chromophobe a.
    clear cell a.
    colloid a.
    depressed a.
    embryonal a.
    eosinophil a.
    fetal a.
    fibroid a.
    a. fibrosum
    follicular a.
    Fuchs a.
    gonadotropin-producing a.
    growth hormone-producing a.
    hepatic a.
    hepatocellular a.
    Hürthle cell a.
    islet cell a.
    lactating a.
    Leydig cell a.
    macrofollicular a.
    malignant a.
    mammosomatotropic a.
    microfollicular a.
    monomorphic a.
    multiple a.

    nephrogenic a. (na)
    a. of nipple
    null-cell a.
    oncocytic a.
    ovarian tubular a.
    oxyphil a.
    papillary cystic a.
    papillary a. of large intestine
    Pick tubular a.
    pituitary a.
    pleomorphic a.
    polypoid a.
    prolactin-producing a.
    prostatic a.
    renal cortical a.
    sebaceous a.
    a. sebaceum
    somatotroph a.
    sweat duct a.
    sweat gland a.
    testicular tubular a.
    thyrotropin-producing a.
    toxic a.
    trabecular a.
    tubovillous a.
    tubular a.
    undifferentiated cell a.
    villous a.
adenomatoid
    a. odontogenic tumor
adenomatosis
    endocrine a.
    erosive a. of nipple
    familial multiple endocrine a., type
      1, 2
    fibrosing a.
    multiple endocrine a. (MEA)
    pluriglandular a.
    polyendocrine a.
    pulmonary a.
adenomatous
    a. crypt
    a. goiter
    a. hyperplasia
    a. polyp
adenomyoepithelial adenosis
adenomyoepithelioma
adenomyofibroma
    atypical polypoid a. (APA)
adenomyoma
    atypical polypoid a. (APA)
adenomyosarcoma
adenomyosis
    a. uteri
adenopathy
adenophlegmon
Adenophorasida
Adenophorea

adenophyma
adenosalpingitis
adenosarcoma
    müllerian a.
adenosatellite virus
adenosine
    a. 3′,5′-cyclic monophosphate
    a. 3′,5′-cyclic phosphate (cyclic
      AMP) (cAMP)
    a. deaminase (ADA)
    a. deaminase assay
    a. deaminase deficiency
    a. diphosphate
    a. 5′-diphosphate (ADP)
    a. monophosphate (AMP)
    a. triphosphatase (ATPase)
    a. triphosphate (ATP)
    vaginal a.
adenosis
    adenomyoepithelial a.
    apocrine a.
    blunt duct a.
    fibrosing a.
    microglandular a.
    sclerosing a. ˙
    secretory a.
    simple a.
    vaginal a.
adenosquamous carcinoma
***S*-adenosyl-L-homocysteine**
***S*-adenosyl-L-methionine**
Adenoviridae
adenovirus
    canine a. 1
    a. immunofluorescence
    porcine a.
adenylate
    a. cyclase
    a. kinase
adenyl cyclase
adenylic acid
adenylosuccinate
adenylpyrophosphatase
adenylyl
adenylylation
ADH
    alcohol dehydrogenase
    antidiuretic hormone
      ADH assay
      ADH deficiency
adherence
    bacterial a.

    immune a.
    Treponema pallidum immobilization
      (immune) a. (TPIA)
adherens
    zonula a.
adherent
    a. pericarditis
    a. pericardium
adhesins
adhesion
    amniotic a.
    fibrinous a.
    fibrous a.
    a. molecule
    a. phenomenon
    sublabial a.
    a. test
adhesive
    albumin slide a.
    a. arachnoiditis
    a. capsulitis
    a. chronic pachymeningitis
    gelatin slide a.
    a. inflammation
    a. pericarditis
    a. peritonitis
    a. phlebitis
    a. pleurisy
    a. vaginitis
adiadochokinesia
Adiantum
adiaspiromycosis
adiaspore
adiasporosis
Adie
    A. pupil
    A. syndrome
Adinida
adiphenine hydrochloride
adipic
adipocele
adipoceratous
adipocere
adipocyte
adipocytic neoplasm
adipokinesis
adipokinetic hormone
adipolysis
adipolytic
adiponecrosis
adipose
    a. degeneration

NOTES

adipose *(continued)*
 a. infiltration
 a. tissue
 a. tissue extract (ATE)
 a. tumor
adiposis
 a. cardiaca
 a. cerebralis
 a. dolorosa
 a. hepatica
 a. orchica
 a. tuberosa simplex
 a. universalis
adiposity
adiposogenital dystrophy
adiposuria
aditus
adjusted rate
adjuvant
 Freund complete a.
 Freund incomplete a.
 mycobacterial a.
 a. vaccine
Adler test
admittance
ADN-B assay
adnexa
adnexal
 a. adenoma
 a. carcinoma
 a. neoplasm
adnexitis
adolescent
 a. albuminuria
 a. round back
adoptive
 a. immunity
 a. immunotherapy
ADP
 adenosine 5′-diphosphate
ADP/ATP ratio
adrenal
 accessory a.
 a. antibody
 a. ascorbic acid depletion test
 a. cortex
 a. cortical carcinoma
 a. cortical hyperplasia
 a. crisis
 a. disease
 a. epithelioid angiosarcoma (AEA)
 a. feminizing syndrome
 a. function test
 a. gland
 a. gland virilizing syndrome
 a. insufficiency
 Marchand a.'s
 a. medulla

 a. neoplasm
 a. rest
 a. tumor
 a. virilism
 a. virilization
adrenaline
adrenalin test
adrenalitis
adrenalopathy
adrenarche
 delayed a.
 precocious a.
adrenergic
 a. blocking
 a. blocking agent
 a. neuron blockade
 a. neuron blocking agent
α-adrenergic
 α-a. blockade
 α-a. receptor
β-adrenergic
 β-a. antagonist
 β-a. blockade
 β-a. blocking agent
adrenochrome
adrenocortical
 a. adenoma
 a. extract (ACE)
 a. hormone (ACH)
 a. inhibition test
 a. insufficiency
 a. rest tumor
adrenocorticosteroid
adrenocorticotropic
 a. cell
 a. hormone (ACTH)
 a. hormone assay
 a. hormone-releasing factor (ACTH-RF)
 a. hormone stimulation test
 a. hormone suppression test
 a. polypeptide (ACTP)
adrenocorticotropin
adrenodoxin
adrenogenital syndrome (AGS)
adrenomedullary
 a. hormone
 a. triad
adrenomegaly
adrenopathy
Adriamycin
 A. cardiomyopathy
ADS
 antibody deficiency syndrome
 antidiuretic substance
adsorb
adsorbate
adsorbed plasma

adsorbent
gastrointestinal a.
adsorption
agglutinin a.
chemical a.
a. chromatography
immune a.
physical a.
adult
a. celiac disease
a. cystic teratoma
a. gonococcal conjunctivitis
a. granulosa cell tumor (AGCT)
a. hemoglobin
a. medulloepithelioma
a. polycystic disease
a. respiratory distress syndrome (ARDS)
a. T-cell leukemia (ATL)
a. T-cell lymphoma (ATL)
a. tuberculosis
adulteration
adult-onset diabetes
adultorum
blennorrhea a.
adult-type xanthogranuloma (AXG)
adventitia
aortic tunica a.
adventitial neuritis
adventitious
a. albuminuria
a. cyst
adynamia
hereditary a.
adynamic ileus
AE
antitoxic unit
AE1
antikeratin
AE1 immunoperoxidase stain
AE1 plus CAM
AE1/3 antibody
AE1/AE3 antibody
AEA
adrenal epithelioid angiosarcoma
AEC detection system
Aedes
A. *aegypti*
A. *albopictus*
A. *cinereus*
A. *flavescens*
A. *leucocelaenus*

A. *sollicitans*
A. *spencerii*
A. *taeniorhynchus*
Aelurostrongylus
AEM
analytical electron microscope
AEq
age equivalent
AER
aldosterone excretion rate
aerated
aeration
aerial mycelium
Aerobacter
A. *aerogenes*
A. *cloacae*
A. *liquefaciens*
A. subgroup A, B, C
aerobe
obligate a.
aerobic
a. and anaerobic blood culture
a. bacterium
a. diphtheroid
a. metabolism
aerobiology
aerobiosis
aerobiotic
aerocele
Aerococcus
A. *viridans*
aerodermectasia
aeroembolism
aerogen
aerogenesis
aerogenic
aerogenous
Aeromonas
A. *hydrophila*
A. *liquefaciens*
A. *punctata*
A. *salmonicida*
aerophil, aerophile
aerophilic
aerophilous
aeroplankton
aerosis
aerosol generator
aerotaxis
aerotitis media
aerotolerant
aerotonometer

NOTES

aerotropism
aestivoautumnal fever
AET
    absorption-equivalent thickness
AF
    acid fast
    aldehyde fuchsin
    antibody-forming
AFB
    acid-fast bacillus
        AFB smear
        AFB stain
AFC
    antibody-forming cell
afebrile
    a. abortion
affected
    part a. (Par. aff.)
affinity
    a. antibody
    a. chromatography
    a. constant
    a. label
    testosterone-binding a. (TBA)
afibrinogenemia
    congenital a.
AFIP
    Armed Forces Institute of Pathology
Afipia felis
aflatoxicosis
aflatoxin
AFP
    α-fetoprotein
African
    A. hemorrhagic fever
    A. histoplasmosis
    A. horse sickness
    A. horse sickness virus
    A. sleeping sickness
    A. swine fever
    A. swine fever virus
    A. tick-borne fever
    A. trypanosomiasis
afterchroming
aftergilding
aftosa
AG
    antiglobulin
    atrial gallop
A/G
    albumin-globulin
        A/G ratio
        A/G ratio test
Ag
    antigen
    silver
AGA
    appropriate for gestational age

agamete
agamic
agammaglobulinemia
    acquired a.
    Bruton type a.
    congenital a.
    primary a.
    secondary a.
    Swiss-type a. (SAG)
    transient a.
    X-linked a.
agamocytogeny
Agamodistomum
    A. ophthalmobium
Agamofilaria
agamogenesis
agamogenetic
agamogony
Agamomermis culicis
Agamonema
Agamonematodum
    A. migrans
agamont
agamous
aganglionic
    a. megacolon
aganglionosis
    congenital a.
agar
    ascitic a.
    bile esculin a.
    bile salt a.
    birdseed a.
    bismuth-sulfite a. (BSA)
    blood a.
    Bordet-Gengou potato blood a.
    brain-heart infusion a.
    brilliant green bile salt a.
    casein a.
    CB a.
    chocolate blood a.
    Christensen urea a.
    citrate a.
    Columbia blood a.
    cornmeal a.
    a. cutter
    cystine trypticase a.
    Czapek-Dox a.
    Czapek solution a.
    deep a.
    deoxycholate-citrate a. (DCA)
    deoxyribonuclease a.
    a. diffusion method
    DNase a.
    egg-yolk a.
    EMB a.
    Emmon modification of Sabouraud
        dextrose a.

eosin-methylene blue a.
French proof a.
Hektoen enteric a.
inhibitory mold a.
Kliger iron a. (KIA)
laked blood a.
lysine-iron a.
MacConkey a.
malt a.
Martin-Lester a.
Middlebrook a.
Mueller-Hinton a.
mycobiotic a.
nitrate a.
nutrient a.
oatmeal-tomato paste a.
Pfeiffer blood a.
phenylalanine a.
phenylethyl alcohol blood a.
a. plate count
potato dextrose a.
rabbit blood a.
rice-Tween a.
Sabhi a.
Sabouraud dextrose and brain heart
  infusion a.
Salmonella-Shigella a.
Schaedler blood a.
serum a.
sheep blood a.
Simmons citrate a.
TCBS a.
Thayer-Martin a.
triple sugar iron a.
trypticase soy a. (TSA)
tryptic soy a.
TSI a.
urea a.
Wilkins-Chilgren a.
XLD a.
xylose-lysine-deoxycholate a.
yeast extract a.
Agarbacterium
agaric
deadly a.
fly a.
Agaricus
agarose gel electrophoresis
Ag-AS
silver-ammoniacal silver
  Ag-AS stain

AGCT
adult granulosa cell tumor
age
appropriate for gestational a.
  (AGA)
chronological a. (CA)
a. equivalent (AEq)
gestational a. (GA)
age-adjusted rate
aged serum
agenesis
cerebellar a.
gonadal a.
pure red cell a. (PRCA)
renal a.
testicular a.
thymic a.
agent
activating a.
adrenergic blocking a.
β-adrenergic blocking a.
adrenergic neuron blocking a.
alkylating a.
androgenic anabolic a. (AAA)
antibacterial a.
antifungal a.
antiviral a.
bacteriostatic a.
beta-adrenergic blocking a.
biological alkylating a.
Bittner a.
caudalizing a.
chelating a.
chimpanzee coryza a. (CCA)
cholinergic blocking a.
δ a.
delta a.
drying a.
Eaton a.
embedding a.'s
etiologic a.
F a.
fertility a.
foamy a.
ganglionic blocking a. (GBA)
gonadotropin-releasing a. (GRA)
Gordon a.
Hawaii a.
infectious a.
initiating a.
LDH a.
lysing a.

NOTES

agent *(continued)*
    Marburg a.
    Marcy a.
    MS-1, -2 a.
    nitrosourea a.
    Norwalk a.
    A. Orange
    oxidizing a.
    PANTA antimicrobial a.
    Pittsburgh pneumonia a.
    progestational a.
    promoting a.
    reducing a.
    reovirus-like a.
    surface-active a.
    thrombolytic a.
    transforming a.
    vacuolating a.
    virus-inactivating a. (VIA)
    wetting a.
age-specific rate
agglutinate
agglutinating antibody
agglutination
    acid a.
    bacterial a. (BA)
    bacteriogenic a.
    chick-cell a. (CCA)
    cold a.
    cross a.
    direct a. (DA)
    false a.
    group a.
    H a.
    immune a.
    indirect a.
    intravascular a.
    latex a. (LA)
    macroscopic a.
    mediate a.
    microscopic a.
    mixed a.
    nonimmune a.
    O a.
    passive a.
    platelet a.
    reverse a.
    salt a.
    slide latex a. (SLA)
    spontaneous a.
    T a.
    a. test
    a. titer
    Treponema pallidum a. (TPA)
    tube a. (TA)
    Vi a.
agglutinative thrombus

agglutinator
    rheumatoid a.
agglutinin
    α a.
    a. adsorption
    alpha a.
    anti-Rh a.
    β a.
    beta a.
    blood group a.'s
    chief a.
    cold a.
    cross-reacting a.
    febrile a.'s
    flagellar a.
    group a.
    H a.
    heterophil a.
    immune a.
    incomplete a.
    latex a.
    leukocyte a.
    major a.
    Mg a.
    minor a.
    O a.
    partial a.
    plant a.
    platelet a.
    Rh a.
    saline a.
    salmonella a.
    serum a.
    somatic a.
    warm a.
    wheat germ a. (WGA)
agglutinogen
    blood group a.'s
    T a.
agglutinogenic
agglutinophilic
agglutinoscope
agglutogen
agglutogenic
aggregate
    a. anaphylaxis
    cytoplasmic crystalline a.
    cytoplasmic lipid a.
    cytoplasmic macromolecule a.
    nuclear crystalline a.
    nuclear lipid a.
aggregated
    a. albumin
    a. microsphere
aggregation
aggregometer
aggressin
aggressive infantile fibromatosis

A

aging
agitation
AGL
    acute granulocytic leukemia
aglobulia
aglobuliosis
aglobulism
aglomerular
aglutition
aglycemia
aglycogenosis
aglycone
aglycosuria
aglycosuric
AGN
    acute glomerulonephritis
agnathus
agnogenic myeloid metaplasia
agonadal
agonadism
agonal
    a. leukocytosis
    a. thrombosis
    a. thrombus
agonist
agouti
agranular
    a. endoplasmic reticulum
    a. leukocyte
agranulocyte
agranulocytic angina
agranulocytosis
    feline a.
agranuloplasia
agranuloplastic
agretope
Agrobacterium
AGS
    adrenogenital syndrome
AGT
    antiglobulin test
AGTT
    abnormal glucose tolerance test
ague
AGV
    aniline gentian violet
agyria
AH
    amenorrhea and hirsutism
    antihyaluronidase
    Arachis hypogaea
    arterial hypertension

    AH assay
    AH titer
AHA
    acquired hemolytic anemia
    autoimmune hemolytic anemia
ahaptoglobinemia
ahaustral
AHD
    arteriosclerotic heart disease
    atherosclerotic heart disease
AHF
    antihemophilic factor A
AHG
    antihemophilic globulin
    antihuman globulin
        AHG factor
AHH
    analog of histidine
AHLE
    acute hemorrhagic leukoencephalitis
AHLS
    antihuman lymphocyte serum
AHT
    antihyaluronidase titer
    augmented histamine test
Ahumada-Del Castillo syndrome
AI
    angiotensin I
    aortic incompetence
    aortic insufficiency
Aicardi syndrome
AID
    acute infectious disease
Aid
        Cryostat Frozen Sectioning A.
AIDS
    acquired immunodeficiency syndrome
        AIDS serology
AIDS-related
        A.-r. complex (ARC)
        A.-r. virus (ARV)
AIEP
    amount of insulin extractable from
        pancreas
AIH
    homologous artificial insemination
AIHA
    autoimmune hemolytic anemia
AII
    angiotensin II
AIII
    angiotensin III

NOTES

AIL
angiocentric immunoproliferative lesion
AILD
angioimmunoblastic lymphadenopathy with dysproteinemia
AIN
acute interstitial nephritis
ainhum
AIO
amyloid of immunoglobulin origin
AIP
acute intermittent porphyria
automated immunoprecipitation
air
alveolar a.
a. core
a. dose
a. embolism
a. embolus
a. foil
a. monitor
a. quality standard
a. thermometer
airborne infection
air-dried smear
AITT
arginine insulin tolerance test
AIU
absolute iodine uptake
AJCCS
American Joint Committee on Cancer Staging
Ajellomyces
A. capsulatum
A. dermatitidis
A. dermatitis
Akabane virus
akamushi disease
akeratosis
AKT1 virus
AKT8 retrovirus
Akureyri disease
ALA
aminolevulinic acid
ALA test
ALAD
aminolevulinic acid dehydrase
alaninemia
hyper-β-a.
hyperbeta-a.
alaninuria
alanyl
alanyl-RNA synthetase
alar chest
alarm
fuse a.
AlaSTAT latex allergy test
alastrim

alba
pityriasis a.
Albarrán disease
Albers-Schönberg disease
Albert
A. disease
A. stain
Albert-Linder bone sectioning
albicans
albiduria
albinism
albino
albinuria
Albright
A. disease
A. hereditary osteodystrophy
A. syndrome
Albright-McCune-Sternberg syndrome
albuginea
tunica a.
albumin
a. A
aggregated a.
a. assay
a. B
Bence Jones a.
blood a.
bovine serum a. (BSA)
chromated Cr 51 serum a.
a. clearance (C/alb/)
coagulated a.
crystalline egg a. (CEA)
derived a.
a. Ghent
hematin a.
human serum a. (HSA)
iodinated human serum a. (IHSA)
iodinated I-125 serum a. (human)
iodinated I-131 serum a. (human)
iodinated macroaggregated a. (IMAA)
macroaggregated a. (MAA)
a. Mexico
a. Naskapi
native a.
normal human serum a.
Patein a.
a. quotient
radioactive iodinated human serum a. (RIHSA)
radioactive iodinated serum a. (RISA)
radioiodinated serum a.
a. Reading
serum a. (SA)
a. slide adhesive
a. suspension test
^{99m}Tc serum a.

thyroxine-binding a.
a. X
a. X_1
albuminaturia
albumin-calcium-magnesium (ACM)
albumin-globulin (A/G)
albuminiferous
albuminiparous
albuminocholia
albuminocytological
albuminocytologic dissociation
albuminogenous
albuminoid degeneration
albuminoptysis
albuminorrhea
albuminous
a. degeneration
a. swelling
albuminuria
adolescent a.
adventitious a.
a. of athletes
Bamberger a.
Bence Jones a.
benign a.
cardiac a.
colliquative a.
cyclic a.
dietetic a.
digestive a.
essential a.
false a.
febrile a.
functional a.
intermittent a.
lordotic a.
march a.
neuropathic a.
orthostatic a.
physiologic a.
postrenal a.
postural a.
prerenal a.
recurrent a.
regulatory a.
transient a.
albuminuric
albumose-free tuberculin (TAF)
ALC
approximate lethal concentration
Alcaligenes
A. *bookeri*

A. *bronchisepticus*
A. *denitrificans*
A. *faecalis*
A. *marshalli*
A. *odorans*
A. *recti*
alcaptonuria
Alcian
A. blue (AB)
A. blue stain
ALCL
anaplastic large cell lymphoma
alcohol
absolute a.
acid a.
a. addiction
aliphatic a.
allyl a.
anhydrous a.
a. assay
benzyl a.
blood a.
butyl a.
dehydrated a.
a. dehydrogenase (ADH)
dihydric a.
ethyl a.
a. fixation
isobutyl a.
monohydric a.
polyhydric a.
polyvinyl a. (PVA)
propyl a.
a. thermometer
alcoholic
a. cardiomyopathy
a. cirrhosis
a. coma
a. formalin
a. hepatitis
a. hyalin
a. hyaline
a. hyaline body
a. myopathy
alcohol-soluble eosin
aldaric acid
aldehyde
acetic a.
a. dehydrogenase
a. fixative
formic a.

NOTES

25

aldehyde *(continued)*
    a. fuchsin (AF)
    a. oxidase
Alder-Reilly
    A.-R. anomaly
    A.-R. body
aldicarb
aldimine
aldofuranose
aldohexose
aldolase
    a. assay
    fructose-bisphosphate a.
    a. test
aldonic acid
aldopentose
aldopyranose
aldose
aldosterone
    a. assay
    a. excretion rate (AER)
    a. secretion defect (ASD)
    a. secretion rate (ASR)
    a. secretory rate (ASR)
    a. stimulation test
    a. suppression test
aldosterone-producing adenoma (APA)
aldosteronism
aldotransferase
aldotriose
Aldrich syndrome
aldrin
Alectorobius talaje
alert check
Aletris
aleukemia
aleukemic
    a. granulocytic leukemia
    a. lymphocytic leukemia
    a. monocytic leukemia
    a. myelosis
aleukemoid
aleukia
aleukocytic
aleukocytosis
aleurioconidium
aleuriospore
Aleutian
    A. disease (AD)
    A. mink disease
    A. mink disease virus
Alexander
    A. disease
    A. leukodystrophy
alexin
    a. unit
aleydigism
Alezzandrini syndrome

ALG
    antilymphocyte globulin
algae
algebra
    Boolean a.
algesidystrophy
algid
    a. malaria
    a. stage
algin
alginate
alginic acid
Alginomonas
algodystrophy
algoid cell
ALGOL
    algorithm-oriented language
algorithm
algorithm-oriented language (ALGOL)
algoscopy
Aliber disease
alicyclic
    a. hydrocarbon
alienia
aliesterase
align
aligned grid
alignment chart
alimentary
    a. abstinence
    a. diabetes
    a. glycosuria
    a. lipemia
    a. osteopathy
    a. pentosuria
    a. tract smear
aliphatic
    a. acid
    a. alcohol
    a. saturated hydrocarbon
    a. unsaturated hydrocarbon
aliquant
aliquot
alizarin
    a. cyanin
    a. indicator
    a. purpurin
    a. red
    a. red S
    a. test
    a. yellow
alkalemia
alkalescence
alkali
    a. denaturation test
    a. metal
    olatile a.
    a. tolerance test

alkalimetry
alkaline
    a. earth metal
    a. intoxication
    a. phosphatase (alk phos, alk phos)
    a. phosphatase activity of granular leukocyte (APGL)
    a. phosphatase assay
    a. phosphatase isoenzyme
    a. phosphatase isoenzyme electrophoresis
    a. phosphatase method
    a. phosphatase stain
    a. phosphatase staining
    a. phosphatase test
    a. reaction
    a. RNase
    a. tide
    a. toluidine blue O
    a. tuberculin (TA)
    a. wave
alkalinuria
alkali-soluble nitrogen (ASN)
alkaloid test
alkalosis
    acapnial a.
    compensated a.
    hypokalemic a.
    metabolic a.
    nonrespiratory a.
    potassium a.
    respiratory a.
    uncompensated a.
alkalotic
alkaluria
alkane
alkanet
alkannan
alkannin
    a. paper
alkapton body
alkaptonuria test
alkene
alkenyl
alkoxide ion
alkoxy
alk phos
    alkaline phosphatase
alkyl
    a. group
    a. peroxide
alkylate

alkylating agent
alkylation
alkylbenzene sulfonate (ABS)
alkyne
ALL
    acute lymphoblastic leukemia
    acute lymphocytic leukemia
allantoic
    a. acid
    a. cyst
allantoin
allantoinuria
allele
    multiple a.
allele-specific
    a.-s. loss
    a.-s. oligonucleotide (ASO)
    a.-s. oligonucleotide probe
    a.-s. PCR (A-PCR)
allelic
    a. exclusion
    a. gene
Allen
    A. correction
    A. test
Allen-Doisy
    A.-D. test
    A.-D. unit
Allen-Masters syndrome
allergen
    atopic a.
allergenic
    a. extract
    a. protein preparations
allergen-specific IgE antibody
allergic
    a. asthma
    a. conjunctivitis
    a. coryza
    a. dermatitis
    a. eczema
    a. encephalitis
    a. encephalomyelitis
    a. extract
    a. granulomatosis
    a. granulomatous angiitis
    a. inflammation
    a. neuritis
    a. purpura
    a. reaction
    a. rhinitis
    a. transfusion reaction

NOTES

allergin
allergist
allergization
allergized
allergoid
allergosis
allergy
> atopic a.
> bacterial a.
> cold a.
> contact a.
> delayed a.
> drug a.
> immediate a.
> latent a.
> physical a.
> polyvalent a.

Allescheria boydii
allescheriosis
alligator
> a. clip
> a. skin

alloagglutinin
alloalbuminemia
alloantibody
alloantigen
alloantin-D antibody
allocation
> dynamic storage a.
> static storage a.
> storage a.

allochezia, allochetia
allochroic
allochroism
Allodermanyssus
> *A. sanguineus*

allogenic, allogeneic
> a. antigen
> a. graft
> a. inhibition
> a. transplantation

allograft
> a. rejection

allogroup
alloimmune
alloimmunization
allometric
allometry
allophanamide
allophenic
alloplasia
alloplast
alloploidy
allopolyploidy
allopurinol
allosensitization
allosteric
> a. activation

> a. effector
> a. enzyme
> a. inhibition
> a. site

allostery
allothreonine
allotope
allotopia
allotransplantation
allotrope
allotropic
allotropy
allotype
> Gm a.
> InV a.
> Km a.

allotypic
> a. determinant
> a. marker

alloxan
alloxan-Schiff reaction
alloxuremia
alloxuria
alloy
allyl alcohol
Almeida disease
Almén test for blood
ALMI
> anterior lateral myocardial infarct

Alocinma
alopecia
> a. areatus
> congenital sutural a.
> a. mucinosa
> a. universalis

ALP
> antilymphocyte plasma

AL patch test
Alpers disease
alpha, α
> a. acid glycoprotein
> a. acidophil
> a. actinin
> a. adrenergic blockade
> a. adrenergic receptor
> a. agglutinin
> a. amino acids
> a. blockade
> a. cell
> a. cell of hypophysis
> a. cell of pancreas
> a. chain
> a. decay
> a. fetoprotein
> a. globulin antibody
> a. globulins
> 1,4-a. glucan branching enzyme

A

a. glucan-branching
glycosyltransferase
a. granule
a. heavy-chain disease
a. helix
a. hemolysin
a. hemolysis
17 a. hydroxyprogesterone
a. interferon therapy
a. lipoprotein
a. metachromasia
a. motor neuron
a. naphthol
a. particle
a. staphylolysin
a. streptococcus
a. substance
a. thalassemia
a. thalassemia intermedia
a. units
alpha-1, α_1
a. antichymotrypsin
a. antitrypsin
a. antitrypsin assay
a. antitrypsin deficiency
a. antitrypsin phenotyping
a. band
a. fetoglobulin
a. fetoprotein
a. fetoprotein assay
a. globulin
a. inhibitor
a. protease inhibitor
a. seromucoid
a. trypsin inhibitor
alpha-2, α_2
a. antiplasmin
a. globulin
a. macroglobulin
a. macroglobulin inhibitor
a. neuraminoglycoprotein
alpha-1-acid glycoprotein
alphabet
alpha cell
alpha-chain disease
alphameric
alphanumeric
alpha-particle detector
Alphavirus
alphavirus
Alport syndrome

ALS
amyotrophic lateral sclerosis
antilymphocyte serum
Alstonia
Alström syndrome
ALT
alanine aminotransferase
ALT test
ALT:AST ratio
alteration
bone matrix a.
cartilage matrix a.
chromosome a.
crystalline macromolecule a.
cyclic tissue a.
cytologic a.
cytoplasmic fiber a.
cytoplasmic fibril a.
cytoplasmic filament a.
cytoplasmic lipid droplet a.
cytoplasmic matrix a.
decidual a.
extracellular fibril a.
extracellular matrix a.
fibrocartilage matrix a.
Golgi cavity a.
Golgi membrane a.
Golgi vacuole a.
Golgi vesicle a.
hematopoietic maturation a.
keratohyaline a.
leukocytic maturation a.
mitochondrian cristae a.
mitochondrian matrix a.
mitochondrian membrane a.
Nissl substance a.
nuclear-cytoplasmic ratio a.
nuclear membrane a.
nuclear pore a.
nuclear sap a.
nuclear shape a.
nuclear size a.
pH a.
predecidual a.
syncytial a.
verrucopapillary a.
alterative inflammation
alternant
trace a.
Alternaria
A. *tenuis*
alternate host

NOTES

alternating current
alternation of generations
alternative
    a. complement pathway
    a. hypothesis
    a. inheritance
    one-side a.
    two-sided a.
altitude
    a. anoxia
    a. disease
Altmann
    A. anilin-acid fuchsin stain
    A. fixative
    A. granule
Altmann-Gersh method
alum
    a. carmine
    chrome a.
alum-hematoxylin
alumina
    hydrated a.
aluminosis
aluminum
    a. hydroxide
    a. hydroxide gel
    a. oxide
alum-precipitated
    a.-p. pyridine (APP)
    a.-p. toxoid (APT)
alveolar
    a. abscess
    a. adenocarcinoma
    a. air
    a. air equation
    a. asthma
    a. cell
    a. cell carcinoma
    a. fenestra
    a. hydatid
    a. hydatid cyst
    a. hydatid disease
    a. macrophage
    a. phagocyte
    a. pneumocyte hyperplasia
    a. pore
    a. proteinosis
    a. rhabdomyosarcoma
    a. soft part sarcoma
alveolar-arterial
    a.-a. carbon dioxide difference
    a.-a. oxygen difference
alveolitis
    acute pulmonary a.
    extrinsic allergic a.
alveoloclasia
alveolus
    pulmonary a.

alvinolith
ALW
    arch-loop-whorl
alymphia
alymphocytosis
alymphoplasia
    Nezelof type of thymic a.
    thymic a. (TAL)
Alzheimer
    A. disease
    A. fibrillary degeneration
    A. sclerosis
    A. type I, II astrocyte
AM
    amperemeter
amacrine cell
Amanita
    A. muscaria
    A. phalloides
    A. virosa
amanitin
amantadine
Am antigen
amaranth
amaranthum
amarillic typhus
amastia
amastigote
amaurotic familial idiocy
amazia
Ambard
    A. constant
    A. laws
Amberlite
amber mutation
ambient
    a. temperature
    a. temperature and pressure,
    saturated (ATPS)
ambiguous external genitalia
ambiguus
    Passalurus a.
Amblyomma
amblyopia neuropathy
amboceptor
    bacteriolytic a.
    Bordet a.
    hemolytic a.
    a. unit
Ambrosia
ameba
    coprozoic a.
amebacide
amebiasis
amebic
    a. abscess of liver
    a. colitis
    a. dysentery

a. granuloma
a. meningitis
a. meningoencephalitis
a. prevalence rate (APR)
a. ulcer
amebicidal
amebicide
amebiform
amebiosis
amebism
amebocyte
ameboflagellate
ameboid
a. cell
a. movement
ameboma
amebula
amebule
ameburia
amegakaryocytosis
amelanotic
a. melanoma
amelia
ameloblast
ameloblastic
a. adenomatoid tumor
a. fibroma
a. hcmangioma
a. neurilemoma
a. odontoma
a. sarcoma
ameloblastoma
calcifying a.
pigmented a.
pituitary a.
ameloblastomatous craniopharyngioma
amelogenesis imperfecta
amenorrhea
a. and hirsutism (AH)
primary a.
secondary a. (SA)
amenorrhea-galactorrhea syndrome
amentia
phenylpyruvic a.
American
A. Academy of Microbiology (AAM)
A. Association of Bioanalysts
A. Association of Blood Banks
A. Association for Clinical Chemistry (AACC)

A. Association of Neuropathologists (AAN)
A. Association of Pathologist Assistants (AAPA)
A. Association of Pathologists (AAP)
A. Association of Pathologists and Bacteriologists (AAPB)
A. Blood Commission
A. Board of Bioanalysis
A. Chemical Society (ACS)
A. Clinical Laboratory Association (ACLA)
A. College of Pathologists (ACP)
A. hookworm
A. Hospital Association
A. Joint Committee on Cancer Staging (AJCCS)
A. leishmaniasis
A. Medical Technologists (AMT)
A. National Standards Institute (ANSI)
A. rat flea
A. Society of Bacteriologists (ASB)
A. Society for Clinical Investigation (ASCI)
A. Society of Clinical Laboratory Technicians (ASCLT)
A. Society of Clinical Pathologists (ASCP)
A. Society of Cytology
A. Society for Experimental Pathology (ASEP)
A. Society of Hematology (ASH)
A. Society for Medical Technology (ASMT)
A. Society for Microbiology (ASM)
A. Society of Pathologists (ASP)
A. trypanosomiasis
A. Type Culture Collection (ATCC)
A. Urological System cancer staging classification
americium
amerism
ameristic
Ames
A. assay
A. test
amethyst violet

NOTES

AMEX processing and embedding
   method
AMF
   automated motility factor
AMG
   antimacrophage globulin
AMH
   anti-müllerian hormone
AMI
   . acute myocardial infarction
amiantacea
amianthoid
amicrobic
amidase
amide
amidobenzene
amido black 10B
amidonaphthol red
Amidostomum anseris
amikacin
amine
   aromatic a.
   a. precursor uptake and
     decarboxylation (APUD)
   pressor a.
amino
   3-a.-9-ethyl carbazole
   3-a.-9-ethylcarbazole stain
   a. terminal
aminoacetic acid
amino acid
   a. a.-activating enzyme
   a. a. analyzer
   a. a. assay
   a. a. fractionation assay
   glucogenic a. a.
   ketogenic a. a.
   modified a. a.
   a. a. nitrogen (AAN)
   a. a. screen
   a. a. screen
   a. a. sequencer
aminoacidemia
aminoacidopathy
aminoaciduria
   branched-chain a.
9-aminoacridine
5-aminoacridine hydrochloride
9-aminoacridine hydrochloride
aminoacyl-histidine dipeptidase
aminoacyl-tRNA hydrolase
aminoanthraquinone dye
aminobenzene
aminobutyrate aminotransferase
γ-aminobutyric acid (GABA)
p-aminodimethylaniline
aminoglutaric acid
aminoglycoside

p-aminohippurate
   p-a. clearance (C/pah/)
   p-a. clearance test
β-aminoisobutyric aciduria
aminoketone dye
aminolevulinic
   a. acid (ALA)
   a. acid dehydrase (ALAD)
aminomethane
   tris(hydroxymethyl) a.
aminopenicillanic
   a. acid (APA)
   6-a. acid
aminopeptidase (AP)
   a. cytosol
   leucine a. (LAP)
aminophenol
aminopropyltriethyloxysilane-coated glass
   slide
aminopurine
aminopyrine breath test
aminosuccinic acid
aminotransferase
   alanine a. (ALT)
   aminobutyrate a.
   aspartate a. (AST)
   ornithine a.
   ornithine-oxo-acid a.
   valine a.
aminuria
amiodarone
amitosis
amitotic
amitriptyline
   a. and nortriptyline assays
AML
   acute monoblastic leukemia
   acute monocytic leukemia
   acute myelocytic leukemia
AMLS
   anti-mouse lymphocyte serum
AMM
   ammonia
ammeter
AMML
   acute myelomonocytic leukemia
ammonemia
ammonia (AMM)
   a. assay
ammoniacal
   a. silver nitrate test
   a. silver solutions
   a. urine
ammonia-lyase
   L-histidine a.
ammoniemia
ammonium
   a. chloride loading test

a. magnesium phosphate
a. molybdate
a. oxalate
a. peroxysulfide
a. silver carbonate stain
a. sulfate
ammoniuria
amniocentesis
amnioma
amnion
a. nodosum
amnionitis
amniorrhea
amniotic
a. adhesion
a. corpuscle
a. fluid
a. fluid analysis
a. fluid bilirubin
a. fluid creatinine
a. fluid embolism
a. fluid embolus
a. fluid lecithin/sphingomyelin ratio
a. fluid pulmonary surfactant
a. infection syndrome of Blane
Amoeba
A. *buccalis*
A. *coli*
A. *coli mitis*
A. *dentalis*
A. *dysenteriae*
A. *histolytica*
A. *meleagridis*
A. *urogenitalis*
A. *verrucosa*
Amoebotaenia
AMoL
acute monoblastic leukemia
acute monocytic leukemia
amorph
amorphic
amorphous fraction of adrenal cortex
amorphus
amount (amt)
a. of insulin extractable from pancreas (AIEP)
a. of substance
amoxapine
AMP
acid mucopolysaccharide
adenosine monophosphate
cyclic AMP

amp
ampere
amperage
ampere (A, a, amp)
kilovolt a. (kVa)
amperemeter (AM)
ampere-second
amperometry
amphetamine assay
amphibolic
a. fistula
a. pathway
amphibolous fistula
amphichroic
amphichromatic
amphicrine
a. cell
a. differentiation
amphicyte
amphigonous inheritance
amphileukemic
Amphimerus
amphimicrobe
amphipath
amphipathic
amphiphile
amphiphilic
amphiprotic
amphistome
amphitrichate
amphitrichous
amphixenoses
amphixenosis
amphochromatophil, amphochromatophile
amphochromophil, amphochromophile
amphocyte
ampholyte
amphophil, amphophile
a. cell
a. granule
amphophilic
a. cytoplasm
amphophilous
amphoteric
a. dye
a. electrolyte
a. reaction
Amphotericin B
amphotropic virus
amplification
Chelex DNA a.
a. factor

NOTES

amplification (*continued*)
  gas a.
  gene a.
amplifier
  audio a.
  buffer a.
  complementary symmetry a.
  Darlington a.
  difference a.
  direct-coupled a.
  electrometer a.
  a. host
  linear a.
  lock-in a.
  logarithmic a.
  operational a.
  power a.
  push-pull a.
amplitude
  peak a.
  peak-to-peak a.
  wave a.
AMPS
  abnormal mucopolysacchariduria
  acid mucopolysaccharides
ampule
ampullar abortion
ampullary aneurysm
ampullitis
amputating ulcer
amputation
  a. neuroma
  spontaneous a.
AMS
  antimacrophage serum
  automated multiphasic screening
Amsterdam syndrome
AMT
  American Medical Technologists
amt
  amount
amu
  atomic mass unit
AMV2
  avian myelocytomatosis virus
amyctic
amyelia
amyeloic
amyelonic
amygdalase
amyl
amylacea
  corpora a.
amylaceous corpuscle
amylase
  a. assay
  a. clearance (C/am/)
  pancreatic a.

  salivary a.
  serum a.
  a. test
  urinary a.
amylase-creatinine clearance ratio
amylasuria
amylemia
amyloclast
amylo-1,6-glucosidase
amyloid
  a. angiopathy
  a. bodies of prostate
  a. corpuscle
  a. degeneration
  Highman method for a.
  a. of immunoglobulin origin (AIO)
  a. kidney
  a. nephrosis
  a. neuropathy
  a. stain
  a. staining
  a. tumor
  a. of unknown origin (AUO)
amyloidosis
  a. cutis
  diffuse a.
  familial primary systemic a.
  focal a.
  lichen a.
  macular a.
  a. of multiple myeloma
  nodular a.
  primary a.
  renal a.
  secondary a.
  senile a.
  systemic familial primary a.
amylolytic enzyme
amylopectin
amylopectinosis
amylorrhea
amylose
  crystalline a.
amylosuria
amyluria
amyoplasia
  a. congenita
amyotonia congenita
amyotrophia
amyotrophic
  a. lateral sclerosis (ALS)
amyotrophy
  diabetic a.
  neuralgic a.
amyous
ANA
  antinuclear antibody
anabiotic cell

anabolic
    a. steroid
anabolism
anabolism-promoting factor (APF)
anabolite
anacidity
anacmesis
anacrotism
anadenia
    a. ventriculi
anaerobe
    facultative a.
    obligate a.
anaerobia
anaerobian
anaerobiase
anaerobic
    a. bacteria culture
    a. bacterium
    a. chamber
    a. diphtheroid
    a. jar
    a. metabolism
    a. neisseria
    a. streptococcus
anaerobiosis
anaerogenic
anákhré
anakmesis
anal
    a. atresia
    a. fistula
    a. papillitis
    a. skin tag
anal.
    analysis
analbuminemia
analeptic
analgesic
    a. nephritis
    a. nephropathy
anallergenic serum
anallergic
analog, analogue
    a. data
    a. of histidine (AHH)
    a. signal
analogous structure
analog-to-digital converter
analogue (*var. of* analog)
analysis, pl. **analyses (anal.)**
    activation a.

amniotic fluid a.
automated cell image a.
blood gas a.
body fluid a.
breakpoint a.
cerebrospinal fluid a.
clinicopathologic a.
compartmental a.
critical path a.
cytometric image a.
cytospin a.
discriminant a.
displacement a.
electroblot a.
flow cytometric reticulocyte a.
Fourier a.
gastric a. (GA)
genetic abnormality a.
genetic linkage a.
graphic a.
hair a.
head space a.
image a.
image display and a. (IDA)
kidney stone a.
microdiffusion a.
Northern blot a.
qualitative a.
quantitative a.
saturation a.
semiquantitative a.
sequential a.
Southern blot a.
univariate a.
a. of variance (ANOVA)
Western blot a.
analyte
analytic
    a. cytology
    a. method
    a. ultracentrifuge
analytical
    a. balance
    a. chemistry
    a. electron microscope (AEM)
    a. immunofiltration
    a. reagent grade (AR)
    a. sensitivity
    a. specificity
    a. toxicology
analyzer, analyzor
    Abbott Cell-Dyn hematology a.

NOTES

analyzer *(continued)*
    amino acid a.
    APEC glucose a.
    Bactalert a.
    centrifugal fast a.
    Cobas Fara H centrifugal a.
    Cobas Helios differential a.
    Coulter STKS hematology a.
    enzyme a.
    Hitachi 704 a.
    infrared CO_2 a.
    kinetic a.
    multichannel a. (MCA)
    NOVA Celltrak 12 hematology a.
    oxygen a.
    pulse height a. (PHA)
    spectrum a.
    Sysmex NE-8000 CBC a.
    wave a.
    YSI 2300 STAT glucose and
      lactate a.
anamnesis
anamnestic
    a. reaction
    a. response
anamorph
ananaphylaxis
anangioplasia
anangioplastic
ANAP
    anionic neutrophil activating peptide
anaphase lag
anaphoresis
anaphylactic
    a. antibody
    a. intoxication
    a. reaction
    a. shock
    a. transfusion reaction
anaphylactogen
anaphylactogenesis
anaphylactogenic
anaphylactoid
    a. crisis
    a. purpura
    a. reaction
    a. shock
anaphylatoxin
    a. inactivator
anaphylaxis
    active a.
    aggregate a.
    antiserum a.
    chronic a.
    eosinophil chemotactic factor of a.
      (ECF-A)
    generalized a.
    inverse a.

    local a.
    passive cutaneous a. (PCA)
    reversed passive a.
    slow-reacting substance of a. (SRS-
      A, SRSA)
    systemic a.
anaphylotoxin
anaplasia
Anaplasma
Anaplasmataceae
anaplasmosis
anaplastic
    a. adenocarcinoma
    a. astrocytoma
    a. carcinoma
    a. cell
    a. large cell lymphoma (ALCL)
    a. large cell malignant lymphoma
    a. oligodendroglioma
anaplerotic
anapophysis
anarchic phenomenon
anasarca
    fetoplacental a.
anasarcous
anastomosis, pl. **anastomoses**
    ileal pouch-anal a. (IPAA)
anatomical
    a. pathology
    a. tubercle
    a. wart
anatomically
    a. patent foramen ovale
anatomicopathological
anatomic pathology
anatomy
    pathologic a.
anatoxic
anatoxin
Anatrichosoma
anazoturia
ANCA
    antineutrophil cytoplasmic antibody
    antineutrophil cytoplasmic autoantibody
anchorage
    a. dependence
    a. independence
anchusin
anconitis
ancrod
Ancylidae
Ancylostoma
    A. braziliense
    A. caninum
    A. duodenale
ancylostomatic
ancylostomiasis
Anders disease

A

Andersen
 A. syndrome
 A. triad
Anderson-Collip test
Anderson and Goldberger test
Andes disease
AND gate
androblastoma
androgen
 a. receptor
 a. unit
androgenesis
androgenic
 a. anabolic agent (AAA)
 a. hormone
androgenization
andropathy
androstanediol
androstene
androstenediol
androstenedione
 a. test
androsterone
anectasis
anemia
 achlorhydric a.
 achrestic a.
 acquired hemolytic a. (AHA)
 acute posthemorrhagic a.
 Addison a.
 addisonian a.
 angiopathic hemolytic a.
 aplastic a.
 aregenerative a.
 asiderotic a.
 autoallergic hemolytic a.
 autoimmune hemolytic a. (AHA, AIHA)
 Belgian Congo a.
 Biermer a.
 blood loss a.
 brickmaker's a.
 cameloid a.
 chlorotic a.
 chronic a.
 a. of chronic disease
 a. of chronic renal failure
 congenital aplastic a.
 congenital aregenerative a.
 congenital atransferrinemia
 congenital dyserythropoietic a. (types I–III) (CDA)

congenital hemolytic a.
congenital hypoplastic a. (CHA)
congenital nonregenerative a.
congenital nonspherocytic hemolytic a.
Cooley a.
crescent cell a.
deficiency a.
Diamond-Blackfan a.
dilution a.
dimorphic a.
Diphyllobothrium a.
Dresbach a.
dyserythropoietic congenital a.
dyshemopoietic a.
Ehrlich a.
elliptocytic a.
equine infectious a.
erythroblastic a.
Estren-Dameshek a.
Faber a.
factor deficiency a.
false a.
familial erythroblastic a.
familial hemolytic a.
familial hypoplastic a.
familial microcytic a.
familial pyridoxine-responsive a.
familial splenic a.
Fanconi a.
fish tapeworm a.
folic acid a.
genetic a.
globe cell a.
glucose-6-phosphate dehydrogenase deficiency a.
goat's milk a.
a. gravis
ground itch a.
Hayem-Widal a.
Heinz-body hemolytic a.
hemolytic a.
hemolytic a. of newborn
hemorrhagic a.
hemotoxic a.
hereditary hemolytic a. (HHA)
hereditary nonspherocytic hemolytic a. (HNSHA)
hereditary spherocytosis (HS)
hookworm a.
hyperchromatic a.
hyperchromic a.

NOTES

anemia *(continued)*
    hypochromic microcytic a.
    hypoferric a.
    hypoplastic a.
    iatrogenic a.
    icterohemolytic a.
    a. infantum pseudoleukemica
    infectious a.
    intertropical a.
    iron deficiency a. (IDA)
    isochromic a.
    isoimmune hemolytic a.
    lead a.
    Lederer a.
    leukoerythroblastic a.
    local a.
    a. lymphatica
    macrocytic achylic a.
    macrocytic a. of pregnancy
    malignant a.
    Marchiafava-Micheli a.
    Mediterranean a.
    megaloblastic a.
    megalocytic a.
    metaplastic a.
    microangiopathic hemolytic a.
      (MHA)
    microcytic hypochromic a.
    microdrepanocytic a.
    milk a.
    molecular a.
    myelopathic a.
    myelophthisic a.
    neonatal a.
    a. neonatorum
    normochromic a.
    normocytic a.
    nosocomial a.
    nutritional a.
    osteosclerotic a.
    ovalocytic a.
    pernicious a. (PA)
    physiologic a.
    polar a.
    posthemorrhagic a.
    primaquine-sensitive a.
    primary a. (PA)
    primary erythroblastic a.
    primary refractory a.
    production-defect a.
    protein deficiency a.
    pure red cell a.
    radiation a.
    refractory sideroblastic a.
    secondary a. (SA)
    secondary refractory a.
    sickle cell a.
    sideroachrestic a.

    sideroblastic a.
    sideropenic a.
    slaty a.
    spastic a.
    spherocytic a.
    splenic a.
    target cell a.
    thrombopenic a.
    toxic a.
    traumatic a.
    tropical a.
    unstable hemoglobin hemolytic a.
    vitamin deficiency a.
anemic
    a. anoxia
    a. halo
    a. hypoxia
    a. infarct
anemotrophy
anencephalia
anencephalic
anencephalous
anencephaly
anenterous
anenzymia
    a. catalasia
anephric
anergic
    a. leishmaniasis
anergy
    cachectic a.
    negative a.
    nonspecific a.
    positive a.
    specific a.
anerythroplasia
anerythroplastic
anerythroregenerative
anesthetic leprosy
anetoderma
    a. erythematosum
    Schweninger-Buzzi a.
aneucentric
aneuploid cell
aneuploidy
    DNA a.
aneurysm
    abdominal a.
    abdominal aortic a. (AAA)
    ampullary a.
    a. by anastomosis
    aortic arch a.
    arteriosclerotic aortic a.
    arteriosclerotic thrombosed a.
    arteriovenous a.
    atherosclerotic a.
    axial a.
    bacterial a.

benign bone a.
Bérard a.
berry a.
cardiac a.
cirsoid a.
compound a.
congenital ruptured a.
consecutive a.
cylindroid a.
cystogenic a.
diffuse a.
dissecting a.
ectatic a.
embolic a.
embolomycotic a.
endogenous a.
erosive a.
exogenous a.
false a.
fusiform a.
hernial a.
intracavernous a.
intracranial a. (ICA)
luetic a.
miliary a.
mural a.
mycotic a.
Park a.
peripheral a.
popliteal a.
Poll a.
racemose a.
Rasmussen a.
Richet a.
Rodrigues a.
ruptured a.
saccular a.
sacculated a.
serpentine a.
syphilitic a.
thoracic a.
thrombosed arteriosclerotic a.
traction a.
traumatic a.
true a.
tubular a.
varicose a.
ventricular a.
aneurysmal
    a. bone cyst
    a. dilatation

a. sac
a. varix
aneurysmatic
aneusomatic
aneusomy
ANF
    antinuclear factor
Angelucci syndrome
Anger camera
angiectasia
    congenital dysplastic a.
angiectasis
angiectatic
angiectopia
angiitic granulomatosis
angiitis, angitis
    allergic granulomatous a.
    Churg-Strauss a.
    consecutive a.
    cutaneous systemic a.
    hypersensitivity a.
    leukocytoclastic a.
    a. livedo reticularis
    necrotizing a.
angileucitis
angina
    agranulocytic a.
    Ludwig a.
    lymphatic a.
    a. lymphomatosa
    monocytic a.
    neutropenic a.
    a. pectoris (AP)
    Prinzmetal a.
    Vincent a.
anginal
anginose scarlatina
angioblastoma
angiocentric
    a. immunoproliferative lesion (AIL)
    a. lymphoproliferative lesion
    a. pattern
angiocentricity
angiocholecystitis
angiocholitis
angiodermatitis
angiodestruction
angiodestructive pattern
angiodysgenetic myelomalacia
angiodystrophia
angiodystrophy
angioedema

NOTES

angioelephantiasis
angioendothelioma
angioendotheliomatosis
    proliferating systematized a.
angiofibrolipoma
angiofibroma
    juvenile a.
angiofibrosis
angiofollicular mediastinal lymph node hyperplasia
angiogenesis
    a. factor
    tumor a.
angioglioma
angiogliomatosis
angiogliosis
angiohemophilia
angiohyalinosis
angiohypertonia
angiohypotonia
angioimmunoblastic
    a. lymphadenopathy
    a. lymphadenopathy with dysproteinemia (AILD)
angioinvasion
angioinvasive
    a. adenoma
angiokeratoma
    a. corporis diffusum
    diffuse a.
    Fordyce a.
    Mibelli a.
angiokeratosis
angioleiomyoma
angioleiomyomata
angiolipofibroma
angiolipoma
angiolith
angiolithic
    a. degeneration
    a. sarcoma
angiolymphatic invasion
angiolymphoid hyperplasia with eosinophilia
angioma
    cavernous a.
    cherry a.
    littoral-cell a.
    a. lymphaticum
    petechial a.
    a. serpiginosum
    spider a.
    telangiectatic a.
    a. venosum racemosum
angiomatoid
    a. tumor
angiomatosis
    cephalotrigeminal a.

    congenital dysplastic a.
    cutaneomeningospinal a.
    encephalotrigeminal a.
    oculoencephalic a.
    telangiectatic a.
angiomatous
    a. meningioma
angiomegaly
angiomyofibroma
angiomyolipoma
    pulmonary a.
angiomyoma
angiomyoneuroma
angiomyopathy
angiomyosarcoma
angiomyxoma
angioneuromyoma
angioneurotic edema
angio-osteohypertrophy syndrome
angioparalysis
angioparesis
angiopathic
    a. hemolytic anemia
angiopathy
    amyloid a.
    cerebral amyloid a.
    congenital dysplastic a.
    congophilic a.
    diabetic a.
angiophacomatosis
angioplany
angiorrhexis
angiosarcoma
    adrenal epithelioid a. (AEA)
angiosis
angiospasm
angiospastic
angiostaxis
angiostenosis
angiostrongylosis
Angiostrongylus
    A. cantonensis
angiotelectasia
angiotelectasis
angiotensin
    a. I (AI)
    a. I-converting enzyme
    a. II (AII)
    a. III (AIII)
    a. I, II test
angiotensin-converting enzyme
angiotensinogen
angitis (*var. of* angiitis)
angle
    a. closure glaucoma
    critical a.
    a. head
    a. of incidence

a. of reflection
a. of refraction
solid a.
Angstrom
Å. law
Å. unit (A)
angstrom
Anguillula
angular
a. conjunctivitis
a. frequency
angulation
anhemolytic streptococcus
anhidrosis
anhidrotic ectodermal dysplasia
anhydrase
carbonic a.
anhydration
anhydride
acetic a.
basic a.
anhydrous alcohol
ani (*pl. of* anus)
anicteric virus hepatitis
aniline
a. blue
a. dye
a. fuchsin
a. gentian violet (AGV)
anilinism
anilinophil, anilinophile
anilinophilous
animal
a. cell culture
control a.
conventional a.
Houssay a.
normal a.
a. protein factor (APF)
sentinel a.
a. toxin
a. virus
animalcule
animatum
contagium a.
virus a.
anion
cyanide a.
a. gap
a. gap test
a. interference

anion-exchange
a.-e. chromatography
a.-e. resin
anionic
a. detergent
a. dye
a. neutrophil activating peptide
(ANAP)
anionotropy
aniridia
anisakiasis
anisakid
Anisakidae
Anisakis
A. marina
anise oil
anisochromasia
anisochromia
anisocytosis
anisohypercytosis
anisohypocytosis
anisokaryosis
anisoleukocytosis
anisonucleolinosis
anisonucleosis
anisotropic
anisotropy
Anitschkow
A. cell
A. myocyte
ankylocolpos
ankyloglossia
ankyloproctia
ankylosing spondylitis
ankylosis
bony a.
extracapsular a.
fibrous a.
intracapsular a.
osseous a.
Ankylostoma
ankylostomiasis
ankyrin
anlage
ANLL
acute nonlymphocytic leukemia
Ann Arbor
A. A. staging classification
A. A. staging system
A. A. tumor classification
anneal
annelid

NOTES

Annelida
annellide
annelloconidium
annellophore
annexitis
annihilation
    positron a.
annotto
annular pancreas
annulate lamellae
annulus
anochromasia
anodal
anode voltage
anodontia
anogenital wart
anomalad
anomalous
    a. muscle band
    a. origin
    a. vascular distribution
    a. venous connection
    a. venous drainage
anomalus
    Hoplopsyllus a.
anomaly
    Alder-Reilly a.
    Chédiak-Steinbrinck-Higashi a.
    congenital a.
    Ebstein a.
    Freund a.
    Hegglin a.
    May-Hegglin a.
    Pelger-Huët nuclear a.
    Shone a.
    Uhl a.
    Undritz a.
    vascular a.
anomer
anomeric
Anopheles
    A. maculipennis
anophelicide
anophelifuge
Anophelinae
anopheline
Anophelini
anophelism
anophthalmia
Anoplocephala
Anoplocephalidae
Anoplura
anorectic
anorexia
    a. nervosa
anosmia
anosteoplasia
anostosis

ANOVA
    analysis of variance
anovular
anovulation
anovulatory
anoxemia
anoxemic
anoxia
    altitude a.
    anemic a.
    anoxic a.
    fulminating a.
    histotoxic a.
    hypoxic a.
    myocardial a.
    a. neonatorum
    oxygen affinity a.
    a. reaction
    stagnant a.
anoxic
    a. anoxia
    a. encephalopathy
ANS
    antineutrophilic serum
    arteriolonephrosclerosis
ansa
anserina
    cutis a.
anserine
anseris
    Amidostomum a.
ANSI
    American National Standards Institute
ant
    fire a.
antagonism
    bacterial a.
    metabolic a.
    microbial a.
    protein induced by vitamin K a.
      (PIVKA)
    salt a.
antagonist
    β-adrenergic a.
    competitive a.
    enzyme a.
    insulin a.
    metabolic a.
    narcotic a.
    sulfonamide a.
antecedent
    plasma thromboplastin a. (PTA)
antegrade
antemortem
    a. clot
    a. thrombus
antenatal
antepartum hemorrhage (APH)

anterior
  a. acute poliomyelitis
  a. complete dislocation
  a. displacement
  a. horn cell
  a. lateral myocardial infarct
    (ALMI)
  a. pituitary extract (APE)
  a. pituitary hormone (APH)
  a. pituitary-like (APL)
  a. wall (AW)
  a. wall infarction (AWI)
  a. wall myocardial infarction
    (AWMI)
anterofacial dysplasia
anterograde
anteroposterior facial dysplasia
anteroseptal myocardial infarct (ASMI)
anteverted/anteflexed (AV/AF)
anthelminthic
anthelmintic
anthelmycin
antheridium
anthocyanidin
anthocyanin
Anthomyia
  A. canicularis
  A. incisura
Anthomyiidae
anthracemia
anthracene
  a. blue
anthracic
anthracin
anthracoid
anthracometer
anthracosilicosis
anthracosis
  a. linguae
anthracotic
  a. pigment
  a. tuberculosis
anthracycline cardiotoxicity
anthramucin
anthrapurpurin
anthraquinone dye
anthrax
  a. bacillus
  cutaneous a.
  a. septicemia
  a. toxin
anthrone

anthropoid
anthroponosis, pl. **anthroponoses**
anthropophilic
anthropozoonosis
antiagglutinin
antialexin
antialkaline phosphatase method
antiallergic
antiallotype
antialopecia factor
antianaphylaxis
antiandrogen
  pure a.
antianemic
  a. factor
  a. principle
antiantibody
antiantitoxin
antiarachnolysin
antiautolysin
antibacterial
  a. agent
  a. agent susceptibility testing
anti-basement
  a.-b. membrane antibody
  a.-b. membrane glomerulonephritis
  a.-b. membrane nephritis
antibiogram
antibiont
antibiosis
antibiotic
  a. antitumor drug
  bactericidal a.
  bacteriostatic a.
  broad-spectrum a.
  a. enterocolitis
  a. level
  macrolide a.
  oral a.
  polyene a.
  a. sensitivity
  a. sensitivity test
antibiotic-associated colitis (AAC)
antibiotic-resistant
antibody (Ab)
  ABO a.'s
  absorption of erythrocyte a.
  acetylcholine receptor a.
  adrenal a.
  AE1/3 a.
  AE1/AE3 a.
  affinity a.

NOTES

43

antibody *(continued)*
    agglutinating a.
    allergen-specific IgE a.
    alloantin-D a.
    alpha globulin a.
    anaphylactic a.
    anti-basement membrane a.
    anticardiolipin a.
    anticentromere a.
    anticytokeratin a.
    anticytoplasmic a. (ACPA)
    anti-fas/APO-1 a.
    anti-idiotype a.
    antimetallothionein a. (MT)
    antimicrosomal a.
    antimitochondrial a.
    antineutrophil cytoplasmic a.
      (ANCA, C-ANCA)
    antinuclear a. (ANA)
    antiphospholipid a.
    antiplatelet a.
    anti-smooth muscle a.
    anti-*Toxoplasma* a.'s (ATA)
    antitubular basement membrane a.
    avidity a.
    B72.3 a.
    basal cell carcinoma specific a.
    bcl-2 a.
    34BE12 a.
    Ber-EP4 a.
    Ber-H2 a.
    35BH11 a.
    bivalent a.
    BLA 36 monoclonal a.
    blocking a. (BA)
    blood group a.'s
    C8/144 a.
    CAM 5.2 a.
    a. catabolism
    cathepsin D a.
    CD8 a.
    CD20 a.
    CD21 a.
    CD31 a.
    CD35 a.
    CD43 a.
    CD45 a.
    CD74 a.
    CD1a a.
    CD45RO a.
    cell-bound a.
    CF a.
    chimeric a.
    Clonad monoclonal a.
    cold a.
    cold-reacting a.
    cold-reactive a.
    a. combining site

complement-fixing a. (CFA)
complete a.
cross-reacting a.
cytomegalovirus a.
cytophilic a.
cytotropic a.
a. deficiency disease
a. deficiency syndrome (ADS)
desmin a.
a. detection
direct fluorescent a. (DFA)
Donath-Landsteiner a. (D-L Ab)
dystrophin a.
EMA a.
a. excess
a. excess zone
ferritin-conjugated a. (FCA)
ferritin-coupled a.
fluorescent a. (FA)
fluorescent antinuclear a. (FANA)
fluorescent treponemal a. (FTA)
Forssman a.
α-globulin a.
glomerular basement membrane a.
HAM-56 a.
hemagglutinating a. (HA)
hemagglutinating anti-penicillin a.
  (HAPA)
hemagglutination-inhibition a. (HIA)
a. to the hepatitis B core antigen
  (HB$_c$Ab)
a. to the hepatitis B surface
  antigen (HB$_s$Ab)
herpes simplex a.
heterocytotropic a.
heterogenetic a.
heterophil a.
HMB-45 a.
homocytotropic a.
HTLV-I a.
a. identification
idiotype a.
IgA a.'s
IgA endomysial a.
IgG desmoplakin a.
immobilizing a.
incomplete a.
inhibiting a.
islet cell a. (ICA)
Ki-67 a.
kidney-fixing a. (KFAb)
Ki-FDC1p a.
KIM1P a.
Ki-M4p a.
KP1 a.
KP1/CD68 monoclonal a.
L26 a.
LCA a.

Legionnaire's disease a.
Leu 2 a.
Leu 3 a.
Leu 4 a.
Leu 7 a.
Leu 8 a.
Leu 12 a.
Leu 14 a.
Leu 22 a.
Leu M1 a.
Lewis a. (Le^b, Le^a)
LN1 a.
LN2 a.
LN3 monoclonal a.
lymphocytotoxic a.
lymphoid monoclonal a.
MAb 12C3 monoclonal a.
Mac387 a.
measles a.
MIC2 a.
microsomal thyroid a.
mitochondrial a.
monoclonal a. (MAb, MAB, MoAb)
MSA a.
MTI a.
natural a.
NCL-ARm monoclonal a.
NCL-ARp polyclonal a.
NCL-ER-LH2 monoclonal a.
NCL-PCR monoclonal a.
nephrotoxic a. (NTAB)
neutralizing a. (NA)
no demonstrable a.'s (NDA)
nonprecipitable a.
nonprecipitating a.
normal a.
OPD4 a.
P-K a.
polyclonal a.
Prausnitz-Küstner a.
precipitating a.
reaginic a.
S-100 a.
Sjögren a.
skeletal muscle a.
skin-sensitizing a. (SSA)
SMA a.
smooth muscle a.
a. stain
thyroid microsomal a.
a. titer

treponema-immobilizing a.
treponemal a.
TSH-displacing a. (TDA)
UCHL1 a.
UCHL1^a a.
UCL3D3 a.
ULCL4D12 a.
univalent a.
Vi a.
vimentin a.
warm a.
Wassermann a.
Yersinia enterocolitica a.
Yersinia pestis a.
antibody-absorption
    fluorescent treponemal a. (FTA-ABS, FTA-AB)
antibody-conjugate
    antidigoxigenin alkaline phosphatase a.-c.
antibody-dependent cell-mediated cytotoxicity (ADCC)
antibody-forming (AF)
    a.-f. cell (AFC)
anticardiolipin antibody
anticentromere antibody
anti-c-*erb*B-2
anti-*Chlamydia* antibody test
anticholera serum
anticholinergic
anticholinesterase
antichromogranin
antichymotrypsin
    α_1 a.
    alpha 1 a.
    a. test
anticoagulant (AC)
    a. heparin solution
    a. therapy (ACT)
anticoagulant-citrate-dextrose
anticoagulant-citrate-phosphate-dextrose
anticoagulated blood
anticoagulative
anticoagulin
anticodon
anticolibacillary
anticollagenase
anticolloidoclastic
anti-common leukocyte antigen
anticomplement
anticomplementary (AC)

NOTES

anticomplementary *(continued)*
    a. factor
    a. serum
anticontagious
anticonvulsant
anticytokeratin
    a. antibody
anticytoplasmic
    a. antibody (ACPA)
    a. autoantibodies
anticytotoxin
antideoxyribonuclease
    a. B titer
    a. B titer test
antidepressant
    tricyclic a.
antidesmin
antidigoxigenin alkaline phosphatase
  antibody-conjugate
anti-D immunoglobulin
antidiphtheric serum
antidiphtheritic globulin
antidiuretic
    a. hormone (ADH)
    a. hormone deficiency
    a. substance (ADS)
anti-DNA
    a.-D. antibody assay
anti-DNase
    a.-D. B assay
antidote
antidromic
antienzyme
antiepithelial serum
antiestrogen
    a. receptor
antifactor
    a. I–IX disorder
    a. Xa
anti-fas/APO-1 antibody
antifibrinogen
antifibrinolysin
antifibrinolytic
antifol
antifolic
antifungal
    a. agent
anti-GBM disease
antigen (Ag)
    ABO a.
    acetone-insoluble a.
    allogenic a.
    Am a.
    antibody to the hepatitis B core a.
      (HB$_c$Ab)
    antibody to the hepatitis B
      surface a. (HB$_s$Ab)
    anti-common leukocyte a.

anti-sialosyl-Tn a.
Aus a.
Australia a. (AU, Au Ag)
Be^a a.
Becker a.
Bi a.
Bile a.
blood group a.
By a.
capsular a.
carbohydrate a.
carcinoembryonic a. (CEA)
C carbohydrate a.
CD1 a.
CD15 a.
CD20 a.
CD22 a.
CD31 a.
CD43 a.
CD45 a.
CD57 a.
CD68 a.
CD74 a.
CDE a.
CD45RO a.
CDw75 a.
Chlamydia a.
cholesterinized a.
Chr^a a.
class I, II, III a.'s
common a. (CA)
complete a.
conjugated a.
core a.
cross-reacting a.
cryptococcal a.
cytokeratin 19 a.
δ a.
D a.
D10 a.
delta a.
Dharmendra a.
Di a.
Diego a.
Duffy a.
E a.
early a. (EA)
epithelial membrane a. (EMA)
Epstein-Barr nuclear a. (EBNA)
erythrocyte a.
a. excess
extractable nuclear a. (ENA)
1F6 a.
fetal a.
flagellar a.
Forssman a.
Fy a.
G a.

a. gain
Ge a.
Gm a.
Good a.
Gr a.
Gross virus a. (GSA)
group a.'s
H a.
H-2 a.
HBA71 a.
He a.
heart a.
hepatitis a.
hepatitis-associated a. (HAA)
hepatitis B$_e$ a. (HBe)
hepatitis B core a. (HB$_c$Ag)
hepatitis B surface a. (HB$_s$Ag)
heterogeneic a.
heterogenetic a.
heterogenic enterobacterial a.
heterophil a.
hexon a.
histocompatibility a.
HLA a.
HLA-D a.
HLA-DR a.
HLA-type II a.
HMB-45 a.
Ho a.
homologous a.
Hu a.'s
human leukemia-associated a.
human leukocyte a. (HLA)
human lymphocyte a.
H-Y a.
I a.
Ia a.
incomplete a.
a. interferon
InV group a.
Jk a.
Jobbins a.
Js a.
K a.
36KD a.
Kell a.'s
Ki-1 a.
Ki-67 a.
Km a.
Kveim a.
Kveim-Stilzbach a.
Lan a.

Le a.
Leu 1 a.
leukocyte a.
leukocyte common a. (LCA)
Leu-M1 a.
Levay a.
Lu a.
lymphocyte function associated a.
lymphogranuloma venereum a.
Lyt a.
M a.
M$_1$ a.
merozoite a.
MIB-1 a.
Mitsuda a.
MNSs a.
monoclonal antiepithelial
  membrane a.
mouse-specific lymphocyte a.
  (MSLA)
Mu a.
mumps skin test a.
O a.
oncofetal a.
oncoprotein a.
organ-specific a.
Ot a.
P a.
partial a.
penton a.
pollen a.
polyclonal anti-carcinoembryonic a.
a. presentation
private a.
a. processing
proliferating cell nuclear a.
  (PCNA)
prostate-specific a. (PSA)
public a.
R a.
a. recognition
Rh a.
Rhus toxicodendron a.
Rhus venenata a.
rose bengal a. (RBA)
S a.
SD a.
sensitized a.
sequestered a.
serologically defined a.
shock a.
Sialosyl-Tn a.

NOTES

antigen *(continued)*
    Sm a.
    soluble a.
    somatic a.
    species-specific a.
    specific a.
    S-100 protein a.
    Stobo a.
    Streptococcus M a.
    Sw^a a.
    Swann a.
    T a.
        tumor antigen
    Tac a.
    TAG-72 a.
    T-dependent a.
    theta a.
    Thy-1 a.
    thymus-dependent a.
    thymus-independent a.
    thymus-leukemia a.
    tissue-specific a.
    Tj a.
    TL a.
    Tr^a a.
    transplantation a.
    tumor a. (T antigen)
    tumor-associated a.
    tumor-associated rejection a.
      (TARA)
    tumor-specific a.
    tumor-specific transplantation a.
      (TSTA)
    a. unit
    V a.
    Vel a.
    Ven a.
    Vi a.
    viral capsid a. (VCA)
    VLA a.
    von Willebrand a.
    Vw a.
    Wassermann a.
    Webb a.
    Wr^a a.
    Wright a. (Wr^a)
    Xg a.
    Yt^a a.
antigen-antibody
    a.-a. complex
    a.-a. reaction
antigen-antiglobulin reaction (AAR)
antigen-binding
    a.-b. region
    a.-b. site
antigen-combining site
antigenemia

antigenic
    a. assay
    a. competition
    a. complex
    a. deletion
    a. determinant
    a. drift
    a. modulation
    a. shift
    a. structural grouping
antigenicity
antigen-presenting cell
antigen-responsive cell
antigen-sensitive cell
antigen-specific
    a.-s. helper factor
    a.-s. suppressor factor
anti-GFAP staining
antiglobulin (AG)
antiglobulin test (AGT)
anti-HB$_c$
anti-HB$_e$
anti-HB$_s$
antihemagglutinin
antihemolysin
antihemolytic
antihemophilic
    a. factor
    a. factor A (AHF)
    a. factor B
    a. globulin (AHG)
    a. globulin A
    a. globulin B
    a. plasma
    a. plasma human
antihemorrhagic
antiheparin factor
antihepatic serum
antiheterolysin
antihistamine
antihistaminic
antihormones
antihuman
    a. globulin (AHG)
    a. globulin test
    a. lymphocyte serum (AHLS)
antihyaluronidase (AH)
    a. assay
    a. titer (AHT)
antihypercholesterolemic
antihypertensive
anti-idiotype
    a.-i. antibody
    a.-i. autoantibody
anti-infective
anti-inflammatory
    a.-f. corticoid (AC)

anti-isolysin
antikeratin (AE1)
anti-kidney serum nephritis
anti-LA/SS-B test
antileukocidin
antileukotoxin
antilewisite
    British a.
antilymphocyte
    a. globulin (ALG)
    a. plasma (ALP)
    a. serum (ALS)
antilymphocytic globulin
antilysin
antimacrophage
    a. globulin (AMG)
    a. serum (AMS)
antimalarial
antimeningococcus serum
antimetabolite
antimetallothionein antibody (MT)
antimicrobial
    a. spectrum
    a. therapy
antimicrosomal antibody
antimitochondrial
    a. antibody
    a. antibody assay
antimode
antimony
    a. assay
    a. chloride
    a. hydride
    a. poisoning
    a. stain
    a. trichloride
antimorph
antimorphic
anti-mouse lymphocyte serum (AMLS)
anti-müllerian hormone (AMH)
antimutagen
antimycotic
antimyoglobin
antineoplastic
antineurotoxin
antineutrophil
    a. cytoplasmic antibody (ANCA, C-ANCA)
    a. cytoplasmic autoantibody (ANCA)
antineutrophilic serum (ANS)

antinuclear
    a. antibody (ANA)
    a. antibody assay
    a. factor (ANF)
antioxidant
anti-p53
antiparallel
antiparasitic
antiparietal cell antibody assay
antiparticle
antipedicular
antipediculotic
antiperiodic
antipernicious anemia factor (APA)
antipertussis serum
antiphagocytic
antiphospholipid
    a. antibody
    a. syndrome
antiplague serum
antiplasmin
    α_2-a.
    alpha-2 a.
antiplatelet
    a. antibody
    a. serum
antipneumococcic
antipneumococcus serum
antiport
anti-Pr cold autoagglutinin
antiprecipitin
antiproaccelerin
antiprogesterone receptor
antiprothrombin
anti-*Pseudomonas* human plasma (APHP)
antipyogenic
antirabies serum (ARS)
antireticular cytotoxic serum (ACS)
anti-Rh
    a.-R. agglutinin
    a.-R. titer
antiricin
anti-Ro/SS-A test
anti-S
anti-S-100
    a.-S-100 protein
anti-sarcomeric actin
antiscarlatinal serum
antisense
antisepsis
antiseptic

NOTES

antiserum
  a. anaphylaxis
  blood group a.s
  heterologous a.
  homologous a.
  human thymus a. (HUTHAS)
  monovalent a.
  nerve growth factor a.
  NGF a.
  polyvalent a.
  rat thymus a. (RATHAS)
  specific a.
anti-sialosyl-Tn antigen
anti-smooth
  a.-s. muscle actin
  a.-s. muscle antibody
  a.-s. muscle antibody assay
anti-Sm test
antisnake venom (ASV)
antistaphylococcic
antistaphylococcus serum
antistaphylolysin
antistatic spray
antisteapsin
antistreptococcic
antistreptococcin
antistreptococcus serum
antistreptokinase
antistreptolysin
antistreptolysin-O (ASO)
  a. test
  a. titer
antisubstance
anti-tac
antitetanic serum (ATS)
antithrombin
  a. III (AT III, AT-III)
  a. III test
  normal a.
antithromboplastin
antithymocyte
  a. serum (ATS)
antithyroglobulin (ATG)
antitoxic
  a. serum
antitoxic unit (AE)
antitoxigen
antitoxin
  bivalent gas gangrene a.
  bothropic a.
  Bothrops a.
  botulinum a.
  botulism a.
  bovine a.
  Crotalus a.
  despeciated a.
  diphtheria a. (DAT)
  dysentery a.

  gas gangrene a.
  normal a.
  pentavalent gas gangrene a.
  plant a.
  a. rash
  scarlet fever a.
  staphylococcus a.
  tetanus a. (TAT)
  tetanus and gas gangrene a.'s
  tetanus-perfringens a.
  a. unit (AU)
antitoxinogen
anti-*Toxoplasma* antibodies (ATA)
antitoxoplasma antibody test
antitrypsin
  α_1 a. (A1AT)
  alpha-1 a.
  a. deficiency
  a. test
α_1-antitrypsin
  α_1-a. assay
  α_1-a. deficiency
  α_1-a. phenotyping
antitryptic index
antitubular basement membrane antibody
antitumor enzyme
antitumorigenesis
antityphoid
antivenene unit
antivenin
antivenomous serum
antivimentin
antiviral
  a. agent
  a. immunity
  a. protein
antiyphoid serum
Anton
  A. syndrome
  A. test
Antoni
  A. type A neurilemoma
  A. type B neurilemoma
antral gastritis
anuclear
anucleated
anulus fibrosus of aorta
anuresis
anuria
anus, pl. ani
  imperforate a.
  melanocarcinoma of a.
  a. vesicalis
  vestibular a.
  vulvovaginal a.
AO
  acridine orange

AOD
    arterial occlusive disease
aorta, pl. **aortae**
    anulus fibrosus of a.
    coarctation of a.
    cystic medial necrosis of
      ascending a. (CMN-AA)
    medial necrosis of a.
    postductal coarctation of a.
    preductal coarctation of a.
aortic
    a. arch aneurysm
    a. arch syndrome (AAS)
    a. atresia
    a. body
    a. body tumor
    a. dissection
    a. incompetence (AI)
    a. insufficiency (AI)
    a. septal defect
    a. stenosis (AS)
    a. tunica adventitia
    a. tunica intima
    a. tunica media
    a. valve replacement (AVR)
aortica
    glomera a.
aortitis
    bacterial a.
    Döhle-Heller a.
    giant cell a.
    luetic a.
    rheumatoid a.
    syphilitic a.
aortoiliac occlusive disease
aortosclerosis
AP
    acute proliferative
    aminopeptidase
    angina pectoris
APA
    aldosterone-producing adenoma
    aminopenicillanic acid
    antipernicious anemia factor
    atypical polypoid adenomyofibroma
    atypical polypoid adenomyoma
apallic
    a. syndrome
APA-LMP
    atypical polypoid adenomyofibroma of
      low malignant potential
Apathy gum syrup medium

apatite calculus
APC
    adenoidal-pharyngeal-conjunctival
      APC virus
A-PCR
    allele-specific PCR
APE
    anterior pituitary extract
APEC glucose analyzer
apeidosis
Apert-Crouzon disease
Apert disease
aperture
    numerical a.
apeu virus
APF
    anabolism-promoting factor
    animal protein factor
APGL
    alkaline phosphatase activity of granular
      leukocyte
APH
    antepartum hemorrhage
    anterior pituitary hormone
aphakia
aphasmid
Aphasmidia
apheresis
APHP
    anti-*Pseudomonas* human plasma
aphthous
    a. fever
    a. stomatitis
    a. ulcer
    a. ulceration
aphthovirus
aphylactic
aphylaxis
apiamine
apical
    a. abscess
    a. granuloma
apicitis
Apicomplexa
apiculate
apiculus
apiospermum
    Monosporium a.
    Scedosporium a.
API 20 Strep System
Apium

NOTES

APL
  acute promyelocytic leukemia
  anterior pituitary-like
aplanatic
  a. lens
  a. objective
aplasia
  congenital thymic a.
  congenital a. of thymus
  erythroid a.
  germinal a.
  gonadal a.
  granulocytic a.
  hematopoietic a.
  megakaryocytic a.
  nuclear a.
  pure red cell a. (PRCA)
  red cell a.
  retinal a.
  thymic-parathyroid a.
aplasmic
aplastic
  a. anemia
  a. anemia syndrome
  a. bone marrow
  a. crisis
  a. lymph
apobiosis
apochromatic objective
apocrine
  a. adenoma
  a. adenosis
  a. carcinoma
  a. hidrocystoma
  a. metaplasia
  a. miliaria
  a. nevus
Apocynum
apoenzyme
apoferritin
apogamia
apolipoprotein
apomixia
aponeurosis
aponeurositis
aponeurotic fibroma
apophylaxis
apophyseal
apophysis
apophysitis
  a. tibialis adolescentium
apoplasmatic
apoplasmia
apoplectic
  a. coma
  a. cyst
apoplexy
apoprotein

apoptosis
apoptotic body
aposiderin
apothecium
APP
  alum-precipitated pyridine
apparatus, pl. apparatus
  Abbé-Zeiss a.
  Beckman Paragon SPE-II Gel A.
  Golgi a.
  juxtaglomerular a.
  Roughton-Scholander a.
  Van Slyke a.
apparent power
appearance
  cotton-wool a.
  withering crypt a.
appendiceal abscess
appendicitis
  actinomycotic a.
  acute gangrenous a.
  acute suppurative a.
  catarrhal a.
  chronic a.
  focal a.
  gangrenous a.
  healed a.
  healing a.
  lumbar a.
  obstructive a.
  stercoral a.
  subperitoneal a.
  suppurative acute a.
appendiclausis
appendicolithiasis
apple jelly nodule
appliqué form
apposition
appositional growth
appropriate for gestational age (AGA)
approximate lethal concentration (ALC)
APR
  amebic prevalence rate
apraxia
apron
  lead a.
aprotic solvent
APT
  alum-precipitated toxoid
APTT, aPTT
  activated partial thromboplastin time
  APTT test
Apt test
aptyalism
APUD
  amine precursor uptake and
    decarboxylation
apyknomorphous

A

aquagenic urticaria
aqua regia
aquatic
aqueduct veil
aqueous
    a. humor
    a. mounting media
    a. solution
    a. vaccine
aquocobalamin
aquosa
    polyemia a.
AR
    analytical reagent grade
    Argyll Robertson
    AR grade
arabinose operon
arabinoside
    adenine a.
    cytosine a. (CA)
arabinosuria
arachidonate
arachidonic acid
Arachis hypogaea (AH)
Arachnia
    A. propionica
Arachnida
arachnidism
arachnodactyly
arachnoid
    a. cyst
    a. granulation
arachnoidism
arachnoiditis
    adhesive a.
    neoplastic a.
    obliterative a.
arachnolysin
Araldite
Aran-Duchenne disease
araneism
arborescence
arborescent
arborization
arborizing pattern
arboroid
arborvirus (*var. of* arbovirus)
arbor viruses A, B, and C
arboviral virus disease
arbovirus, arborvirus
    a. group A
    a. group unclassified

ARC
    AIDS-related complex
archil
architecture
    loculated a.
    papillary/verrucous a.
arch-loop-whorl (ALW)
arctation
arcus senilis
arc-welder's disease
ARD
    acute respiratory disease
ARDS
    acute respiratory distress syndrome
    adult respiratory distress syndrome
area, pl. **areae (a)**
    body surface a. (BSA)
    Broca a.
    a. cribrosa
    paucicellular a.
    peak a.
    a. postrema
    regulated a.
    skip areae
    a. striata
arcata
areatus
    alopecia a.
arecoline
areflexia
aregenerative anemia
arenaceous
Arenaviridae
Arenavirus
arenavirus
arene
areola, pl. **areolae**
    Chaussier a.
areolar
    a. connective tissue
ARF
    acute renal failure
    acute respiratory failure
arg
    argentum
Argas
    A. persicus
    A. reflexus
argasid
Argasidae
argentaffin
    a. cell

NOTES

argentaffin *(continued)*
  a. granule
  a. reaction
  a. stain
argentaffine
argentaffinoma
argentation
Argentinean hemorrhagic fever
Argentine hemorrhagic fever virus
argentophil, argentophile
argentum (arg)
arginase
arginine
  a. deiminase
  a. glutamate
  a. hydrochloride
  a. insulin tolerance test (AITT)
  a. monohydrochloride
  suberyl a.
  a. test
  a. vasopressin (AVP)
argininemia
argininosuccinate
  a. lyase
  a. lyase assay
  a. synthetase
  a. synthetase deficiency
argininosuccinic
  a. acidemia
  a. aciduria
arginyl
Argo corn starch test
argon
Argonz-Del Castillo syndrome
Argyll Robertson (AR)
  A. R. pupil
argyremia
argyria
argyrophil, argyrophile
argyrophilic
  a. cell
  a. fiber
argyrosis
arhinencephaly
Arias-Stella
  A.-S. cell
  A.-S. effect
  A.-S. phenomenon
  A.-S. reaction
Arias syndrome
ariboflavinosis
Arizona
  A. hinshawii
  A. organism
Arlex gelatin
ARM
  artificial rupture of membranes
arm

Armanni-Ebstein
  A.-E. cell
  A.-E. change
  A.-E. disease
  A.-E. kidney
armed
  A. Forces Institute of Pathology (AFIP)
  a. macrophage
Armigeres
  A. obturbans
Armillifer
  A. armillatus
  A. moniliformis
armored heart
Armstrong disease
Arndt-Gottron syndrome
Arneth
  A. classification
  A. count
  A. formula
  A. index
  A. stage
Arnold
  A. body
  A. nerve reflex cough syndrome
Arnold-Chiari
  A.-C. deformity
  A.-C. malformation
  A.-C. syndrome
aromatic
  a. acid
  a. amine
  a. compound
  a. hydrocarbon
  a. ring
aromaticity
arrangement
  bcl-2 gene a.
array
arrest
  cardiac a. (CA)
  developmental a.
  epiphyseal a.
  hematopoietic maturation a.
  maturation a.
  mitotic a.
  spermatogenic maturation a.
arrested tuberculosis
arrhaphia
Arrhenius-Madsen theory
arrhenoblastoma
arrhinencephaly
ARS
  antirabies serum
arsenate
arsenic
  a. assay

a. keratosis
a. pigmentation
a. poisoning
a. stain
arsenical keratosis
arsenic-fast
arsine
ART
absolute retention time
automated reagin test
ART test
arterial
a. blood
a. blood collection
a. blood gas (ABG)
a. embolism
a. hemangioma
a. hypertension (AH)
a. line culture
a. nephrosclerosis
a. occlusive disease (AOD)
a. Pco$_2$
a. Po$_2$
a. pressure
a. sclerosis
a. spider
arterialized blood
arterioatony
arteriocapillary sclerosis
arteriolar
a. nephrosclerosis
a. sclerosis
a. thrombonecrosis
arteriolith
arteriolitis
necrotizing a.
arteriolonecrosis
arteriolonephrosclerosis (ANS)
arteriolosclerosis
hyaline a.
arteriolosclerotic kidney
arteriomalacia
arteriomyomatosis
arterionephrosclerosis
arteriopathy
hypertensive a.
plexogenic pulmonary a.
arterioplania
arteriosclerosis (AS, ATS)
hyperplastic a.
hypertensive a.
medial a.

Mönckeberg a.
nodular a.
a. obliterans (ASO)
senile a.
arteriosclerotic
a. aortic aneurysm
a. cardiovascular disease (ASCVD)
a. gangrene
a. heart disease (AHD)
a. kidney
a. thrombosed aneurysm
arteriostenosis
arteriosus
persistent truncus a. (PTA)
pseudotruncus a.
arteriovenous (A-V)
a. aneurysm
a. carbon dioxide difference
a. fistula (AVF)
a. malformation (AVM)
a. oxygen difference
arteritis
cranial a.
equine viral a.
giant cell a.
a. nodosa
a. obliterans
obliterating a.
rheumatic a.
rheumatoid a.
Takayasu a.
temporal a.
Arterivirus
artery
dolichoectatic a.
end a.
pipestem a.
transposition of great a.'s (TGA)
arthragra
arthralgia
rheumatic a.
a. saturnina
arthritic
a. calculus
arthritis, pl. arthritides
acute rheumatic a.
atrophic a.
chronic absorptive a.
chronic proliferative a.
chronic villous a.
chylous a.
a. deformans

NOTES

arthritis *(continued)*
    degenerative a. (DA)
    exudative a.
    filarial a.
    gouty a.
    hypertrophic a.
    Jaccoud a.
    juvenile rheumatoid a. (JRA)
    a. mutilans
    navicular a.
    neuropathic a.
    a. nodosa
    ochronotic a.
    proliferative chronic a.
    psoriatic a.
    rheumatoid a. (RA)
    suppurative a.
    a. uratica
    vertebral a.
arthritis-dermatitis syndrome
arthrochondritis
arthroconidium
Arthroderma
Arthrographis
    A. langeroni
arthrokatadysis
arthrolith
arthrolithiasis
arthro-onychodysplasia
arthro-ophthalmopathy
    hereditary progressive a.
arthropathy
    Charcot a.
    Jaccoud a.
    neurogenic a.
    osteopulmonary a.
arthrophyma
arthropod
    a. identification
Arthropoda
arthropod-borne
    a.-b. viral disease
    a.-b. virus encephalitis
arthropodiasis
arthropodic
arthrosis
arthrospore
arthrosynovitis
arthrotropic
Arthus
    A. phenomenon
    A. reaction
articular
    a. calculus
    a. chondrocalcinosis
    a. gout
    a. leprosy
    a. rheumatism

articulated
artifact
    electrical a.
    fixation a.
    movement a.
    shock a.
artificial
    a. abortion
    a. active immunity
    a. kidney
    a. language
    a. melanin
    a. passive immunity
    a. rupture of membranes (ARM)
Artyfechinostomum
ARV
    AIDS-related virus
arylaminopeptidase
arylesterase
aryl-ester hydrolase
aryl group
arylsulfatase
    a. test
arytenoiditis
AS
    Adams-Stokes disease
    aortic stenosis
    arteriosclerosis
    atherosclerosis
ASA
    Adams-Stokes attack
ASAP Biopsy System
ASB
    American Society of Bacteriologists
asbestoid
asbestos
    a. body (AB)
    a. transformation
asbestosis
ascariasis
    a. serological test
ascaricidal
ascaricide
ascarid
Ascaridae
Ascaridata
ascarides
Ascaridia
ascaridiasis
Ascaridida
Ascarididae
Ascarididea
Ascaridoidea
Ascaridorida
Ascaris
    A. alata
    A. canis
    A. lumbricoides

A

A. *mystax*
A. *pneumonitis*
A. *suum*
Ascaroidea
ascaron
Ascarops strongylina
ascending
a. chromatography
a. degeneration
a. myelitis
a. pyelonephritis
Aschelminthes
Ascher syndrome
Aschheim-Zondek (A-Z)
A.-Z. hormone
A.-Z. test (AZT)
Aschoff
A. body
A. cell
A. nodule
Aschoff-Rokitansky sinus
ASCI
American Society for Clinical
Investigation
asci (*pl. of* ascus)
ascites
a. adiposus
chyliform a.
a. chylosus
chylous a.
fatty a.
gelatinous a.
hemorrhagic a.
milky a.
pseudochylous a.
ascitic
a. agar
a. fluid
ascitogenous
ASCLT
American Society of Clinical Laboratory
Technicians
ascocarp
ascogenous
ascogonium
Ascoli
A. reaction
A. test
ascomycete
Ascomycetes
ascomycetous
Ascomycota

Ascomycotina
ascorbate
ascorbate-cyanide test
ascorbic
a. acid
a. acid assay
a. acid test
ascospore
ascospore-forming fungus
ASCP
American Society of Clinical Pathologists
ASCUS
atypical squamous cells of undetermined
significance
ascus, pl. asci
ASCVD
arteriosclerotic cardiovascular disease
atherosclerotic cardiovascular disease
ASD
aldosterone secretion defect
atrial septal defect
ASEP
American Society for Experimental
Pathology
asepsis
aseptate
aseptic
a. meningitis
a. necrosis
asexual
a. reproduction
ASH
American Society of Hematology
asymmetrical septal hypertrophy
Ashby differential agglutination method
Asherman syndrome
asialoglycoprotein
Asiatic cholera
asiderosis
asiderotic anemia
Askanazy cell
Askin tumor
Ask-Upmark kidney
ASM
American Society for Microbiology
ASMI
anteroseptal myocardial infarct
ASMT
American Society for Medical
Technology
ASN
alkali-soluble nitrogen

NOTES

Asn
    asparagine
ASO
    allele-specific oligonucleotide
    antistreptolysin-O
    arteriosclerosis obliterans
        ASO probe
        ASO test
        ASO titer
ASP
    American Society of Pathologists
Asp
    aspartic acid
asparaginase
asparagine (Asn)
asparaginic acid
asparaginyl
aspartate
    a. aminotransferase (AST)
    a. aminotransferase assay
    a. kinase
    a. transaminase
aspartic acid (Asp)
aspartokinase
aspartyl
aspect
aspergillina
    otomycosis a.
aspergilloma
aspergillosis
    bronchopulmonary a.
    disseminated a.
    invasive a.
    pulmonary a.
Aspergillus
    A. antibody test
    A. *auricularis*
    A. *barbae*
    A. *bouffardi*
    A. *candidus*
    A. *clavatus*
    A. *concentricus*
    A. *fisherii*
    A. *flavus*
    A. *fumigatus*
    A. *giganteus*
    A. *glaucus*
    A. *gliocladium*
    A. *mucoroides*
    A. *nidulans*
    A. *niger*
    A. *ochraceus*
    A. *parasiticus*
    A. *pictor*
    A. *repens*
    A. serology
    A. *terreus*
    A. *versicolor*

aspermatism
aspermatogenesis
    induced a.
aspermia
aspheric
asphyxia
asphyxial
asphyxiant
    chemical a.
    simple a.
asphyxiating
    a. thoracic chondrodystrophy
    a. thoracic dysplasia
    a. thoracic dystrophy (ATD)
asphyxiation
Aspiculuris tetraptera
aspidium oleoresin
aspirate
    bronchotracheal a.
aspiration
    a. biopsy
    bone marrow a.
    a. cytology
    foreign body a.
    meconium a.
    a. pneumonia
    a. pneumonitis
    suprapubic needle a.
    tracheal a.
    uterine a. (UA)
    vacuum a. (VA)
aspiration-biopsy cytology
aspirator
    water a.
aspirin
    a. tolerance test
    a. toxicity
asplenia
asplenic
asporogenic
asporogenous
asporous
asporulate
ASR
    aldosterone secretion rate
    aldosterone secretory rate
assassin bug
assay
    acetaminophen a.
    acetylcholinesterase a.
    acid phosphatase a.
    adenosine deaminase a.
    ADH a.
    ADN-B a.
    adrenocorticotropic hormone a.
    AH a.
    alanine aminotransferase a.
    albumin a.

alcohol a.
aldolase a.
aldosterone a.
alkaline phosphatase a.
alpha-1 antitrypsin a.
alpha-1 fetoprotein a.
Ames a.
amino acid a.
amino acid fractionation a.
amitriptyline and nortriptyline a.'s
ammonia a.
amphetamine a.
amylase a.
anti-DNA antibody a.
anti-DNase B a.
antigenic a.
antihyaluronidase a.
antimitochondrial antibody a.
antimony a.
antinuclear antibody a.
antiparietal cell antibody a.
anti-smooth muscle antibody a.
α_1-antitrypsin a.
argininosuccinate lyase a.
arsenic a.
ascorbic acid a.
aspartate aminotransferase a.
bacterial killing a.
barbiturate a.
Beckman a.
benzene a.
benzodiazepine a.
bile acids a.
bilirubin a.
biologic a.
biological a.
biotin a.
bismuth a.
blastogenesis a.
boron a.
Breslow malignant melanoma a.
bromide a.
butanol extractable iodine a.
CA-125 a.
CA 19-9 a.
cadmium a.
caffeine a.
calcitonin a.
calcium a.
calcium ionized a.
camphor a.
carbamazepine a.

carbaryl a.
carbon dioxide concentration a.
carbon disulfide a.
carbon monoxide a.
carbon tetrachloride a.
carboxyhemoglobin a.
Cardiac T Rapid a.
carotene a.
catecholamine a.
CD31 quantitative
    immunohistochemical a.
CEA a.
cell-mediated lympholysis a.
cerebrospinal fluid a.
ceruloplasmin a.
chemiluminescence a.
chemotaxis a.
Chlamydiazyme EIA a.
chloral hydrate a.
chloranil a.
chlorate a.
chlordiazepoxide a.
chlorinated hydrocarbon pesticide a.
chloroform a.
chlorohydrocarbon a.
chlorpromazine a.
cholesterol a.
cholinesterase a.
chorionic gonadotropin a.
chromium a.
citric acid a.
clonogenic a.
coagulation factor a.
cobalt a.
cocaine metabolite a.
codeine a.
competitive protein-binding a.
complement binding a.
compressed spectral a. (CSA)
copper a.
coproporphyrin a.
cortisol a.
CPB a.
C-reactive protein a.
creatine kinase a.
creatinine a.
cresol a.
cyanide a.
cytochrome b_5 reductase a.
D-dimer a.
DDT a.
DeBakey aortic a.

NOTES

assay *(continued)*
    depramine a.
    desipramine a.
    diazepam a.
    1,25-dihydroxycholecalciferol a.
    diquat a.
    direct fluorescent a. (DFA)
    disulfiram a.
    double antibody sandwich a.
    doxepin hydrochloride a.
    drug screening a.
    EAC rosette a.
    E erythrocyte rosette a.
    ELISA titer a.
    endorphin a.
    enzyme a.
    enzyme-linked immunosorbent a.
      (ELISA)
    epinephrine and norepinephrine a.'s
    Epstein-Barr virus antibody a.
    Erlanger and Gasser peripheral
      nerve a.
    erythrocyte, antibody, complement
      rosette a.
    ESR a.
    estradiol a.
    estriol a.
    estrogen receptor a. (ERA)
    ethanol a.
    ethchlorvynol a.
    ethosuximide a.
    ethylene glycol a.
    factor a.
    fat a.
    fatty acid a.
    ferritin a.
    α_1-fetoprotein a.
    fluorescent cytoprint a.
    fluoride a.
    fluoroacetate a.
    fluorocarbon a.
    folic acid a.
    follicle-stimulating hormone a.
    fructose a.
    FSH a.
    FSH-RH a.
    galactose a.
    gastrin a.
    GGT a.
    glucose a.
    glucosephosphate isomerase a.
    glucosylceramidase a.
    glutathione reductase a.
    glutethimide a.
    glycine a.
    gold a.
    guanine deaminase a.

Guthrie bacterial inhibition a.
  (GBIA)
halogenated hydrocarbon a.
haloperidol a.
halothane a.
hamster egg penetration a.
haptoglobin a.
HDL cholesterol a.
HDRA a.
    histoculture drug response assay
hemagglutination inhibition a.
hemoglobin F a.
hemoglobin H a.
hemolytic plaque a.
hexachlorophene a.
histoculture drug response a.
  (HDRA assay)
Histoplasma antibody a.
17-hydroxycorticosteroid a.
5-hydroxyindoleacetic acid a.
hydroxyproline a.
25-hydroxyvitamin D a.
iditol dehydrogenase a.
imipramine and desipramine a.'s
immune adherence
  hemagglutination a.
immunochemical a.
immunoconcentration a.
immunoenzymometric a.
immunofluorescent a.
immunoradiometric a. (IRMA)
indirect a.
inhibitor a.
iodide a.
ionized calcium a.
iron a.
isocitrate dehydrogenase a.
isoniazid a.
isopropanol a.
Jaffe a.
Jerne plaque a.
17-ketogenic steroids a.
17-ketosteroid a.
lactate dehydrogenase a.
lactic acid a.
LDL cholesterol a.
lead a.
leukotactic a.
lidocaine a.
limulus amebocyte lysate a.
lipase a.
lipid a.
lipoprotein a.
lithium a.
long-acting thyroid-stimulator
  hormone a.
luteinizing hormone a.
lymphocyte microcytotoxicity a.

lysergic acid diethylamide a.
lysozyme a.
macroglobulin a.
magnesium a.
manganese a.
meprobamate a.
mercury a.
metanephrine a.
methadone a.
methanol a.
methaqualone a.
methemalbumin a.
p-methoxyamphetamine a.
3,4-methylenedioxyamphetamine a.'s
methylphenidate
methyprylon a.
metronidazole a.
microbiologic a.
microbiological a. (MB)
microhemagglutination a.
microlymphocytotoxicity a.
microtoxicity a.
morphine a.
mucoprotein a.
nephelometric inhibition a. (NIA)
opiate a.
organothiophosphate compound a.
ornithine carbamoyl transferase a.
oxalic acid a.
pantothenic acid a.
paraldehyde a.
paraquat a.
pentose a.
pepsinogen a.
phencyclidine a.
phenobarbital a.
phenol a.
phenothiazine tranquilizers a.'s
phenylalanine a.
phenylbutazone a.
phenytoin a.
phosphate a.
6-phosphogluconate
  dehydrogenase a.
phospholipid a.
phosphorus a.
phytohemagglutinin a.
plaque-forming cell a.
plasminogen activator inhibitor a.
  (PHA)
polychlorinated biphenyl a.
polyethylene glycol precipitation a.

porphobilinogen synthase a.
porphyrin a.
potassium a.
pregnanediol a.
primidone a.
procainamide a.
progesterone a. (PRA)
properdin a.
propoxyphene a.
propranolol a.
protein a.
protein-bound iodine a.
protoporphyrin a.
protriptyline a.
PSFR a.
PTH a.
pyrimethamine a.
pyruvate kinase a.
pyruvic acid a.
quinidine a.
quinine a.
radioenzymatic a. (REA)
radioimmunoprecipitation a.
radioligand a.
radioreceptor a. (RRA)
Raji cell radioimmune a.
renal venous renin a. (RVRA)
renin a.
riboflavin a.
Rio-rad protein a.
salicylate a.
selenium a.
serial cardiac isoenzyme a.
serotonin a.
sodium and potassium a.'s
spectrophotometric a.
sperm penetration a.
stem cell a.
strychnine a.
sulfonamide a.
sulfonylurea a.
superoxide a.
Syva EMIT-II a.
TBG a.
T and B lymphocyte subset a.
tellurium a.
thallium a.
theophylline a.
thiamine a.
thiamphenicol a.
thioridazine a.
thyroid-stimulating hormone a.

NOTES

assay *(continued)*
    thyroxine a.
    thyroxine-binding globulin a.
    thyroxine-binding globulin a.
    total calcium a.
    TPI a.
    transferrin a.
    transketolase a.
    Treponema pallidum
      immobilization a.
    triglyceride a.
    triiodothyronine a.
    triosephosphate isomerase a.
    trypsin a.
    tyrosine a.
    UDP-glucose-hexose-1-phosphate
      uridylyl-transferase a.
    urea nitrogen a.
    uric acid a.
    urobilin a.
    urobilinogen a.
    uromucoid a.
    uropepsinogen a.
    uroporphyrin a.
    vitamin A and carotene a.'s
    vitamin B_{12} a.
    vitamin B_6 a.
    vitamin D a.
    vitamin E a.
    vitamin K a.
    volatile organic substances a.
    von Kossa calcium a.
    warfarin a.
    zinc a.
assembler
assembly
    a. language
assignment statement
assimilation limit
Assmann tuberculous infiltrate
associated macrophage
associates
    microbial a.
association
    A. for the Advancement of
      Medical Instrumentation (AAMI)
    A. of Clinical Scientists (ACS)
    a. constant
associative reaction
assortative mating
assortment
    independent a.
AST
    aspartate aminotransferase
    AST test
astacoid rash
astasia
astatine

asteatosis
aster
asterixis
Asterococcus
asteroid body
asthma
    allergic a.
    alveolar a.
    atopic a.
    bronchial a. (BA)
    chronic bronchitis with a. (CBA)
    cotton dust a.
    a. crystal
    emphysematous a.
    essential a.
    extrinsic a.
    grinders' a.
    hay a.
    intrinsic a.
    miller's a.
    miner's a.
    potters' a.
    steam-fitter's a.
    stone-strippers' a.
    summer a.
asthmatic
    a. bronchitis (AB)
asthmaticus
    status a.
asthmogenic
Astler-Coller modification of Dukes
    classification
astomatous
Astra
    A. Blue
    A. profile test
astringent
astroblastoma
astrocyte
    Alzheimer type I, II a.
    fibrillar a.
    fibrillary a.
    fibrous a.
    gemistocytic a.
    protoplasmic a.
    reactive a.
    a. stain
    a. staining
astrocytic tumor
astrocytoma
    anaplastic a.
    cerebellar a.
    desmoplastic cerebral a.
    fibrillary a.
    fibrous a.
    gemistocytic a.
    grade I, II, III, IV a.
    juvenile cerebellar a.

low grade a.
pigmented pilocytic a.
pilocytic a.
piloid a.
protoplasmic a.
subependymal giant cell a.
astrocytosis
a. cerebri
astroependymoma
astroglia
Astwood test
ASV
antisnake venom
asymmetric (a)
a. carbon atom
a. septal hypertrophy
a. unit membrane
asymmetrical
a. chondrodystrophy
a. septal hypertrophy (ASH)
asymmetry
asymptomatic coccidioidomycosis
asymptote
asynapsis
asynchronism
asynchronous data transmission
asynchrony
asynechia
asystematic
ATA
anti-*Toxoplasma* antibodies
Atabrine
atavistic phenomenon
ataxia
a. telangiectasia
a. telangiectasia syndrome
ATCC
American Type Culture Collection
ATD
asphyxiating thoracic dystrophy
ATE
adipose tissue extract
atelectasis
a. neonatorum
obstructive a.
primary a.
round a.
secondary a.
atelia
ateliosis
ateliotic
Atelosaccharomyces

ATG
antithyroglobulin
AT/GC ratio
atheroembolism
atherogenesis
atherogenic
atherogenicity
atheroma
a. embolism
atheromatosis
atheromatous
a. degeneration
a. embolus
a. plaque
atherosclerosis (AS)
atherosclerotic
a. aneurysm
a. cardiovascular disease (ASCVD)
a. heart disease (AHD)
atherosis
atherothrombosis
atherothrombotic
athetoid
athetosis
athetotic
athlete's foot
athletic heart
athrepsia
athrombia
AT III, AT-III
antithrombin III
ATL
adult T-cell leukemia
adult T-cell lymphoma
atmosphere
a. absolute
explosive a.
atmospheric monitoring
ATN
acute tubular necrosis
atom
asymmetric carbon a.
atomic
a. absorption (AA)
a. absorption spectrophotometer
a. absorption spectrophotometry
(AAS)
a. mass
a. mass unit (amu)
a. number
a. spectrum

NOTES

atomic *(continued)*
    a. weight
    a. weight unit (awu)
atomization
atomizer
atony
atopen
atopic
    a. allergen
    a. allergy
    a. asthma
    a. dermatitis
    a. disease
    a. reagin
atopy
ATP
    adenosine triphosphate
    ATP pyrophosphohydrolase
ATPase
    adenosine triphosphatase
    calcium-activated A.
    magnesium-activated A.
    Padykula-Herman stain for
      myosin A.
    A. stain
ATPS
    ambient temperature and pressure,
    saturated
atransferrinemia
Atrax
    A. *robustus*
atrepsy
atresia
    anal a.
    a. ani
    aortic a.
    biliary a.
    choanal a.
    congenital a.
    duodenal a.
    esophageal a.
    follicular a.
    intestinal a.
    mitral a.
    prepyloric a.
    pulmonary a.
    tricuspid a.
    vaginal a.
    valvular a.
atresic
atretic
    a. follicle
atretocystia
atretogastria
atria *(pl. of* atrium)
atrial
    a. gallop (AG)
    a. infarction

    a. myxoma
    a. septal defect (ASD)
    a. septum
atrichous
atriodigital dysplasia
atriomegaly
atrioventricular (A-V)
    a. block
atrium, pl. **atria**
    accessory a.
Atropa
atrophedema
atrophia
    acne a.
    a. maculosa varioliformis cutis
atrophic
    a. arthritis
    a. chronic gastritis
    a. endometrium
    a. fenestration
    a. glossitis
    a. inflammation
    a. kidney
    a. lichen planus
    a. pharyngitis
    a. rhinitis
    a. rhinitis of swine
    a. thrombosis
atrophicans
    acrodermatitis chronica a.
atrophied
atrophoderma
    a. albidum
    a. maculatum
    a. neuriticum
    a. pigmentosum
    a. reticulatum
atrophy
    acquired a.
    acute yellow a.
    acute yellow a. of liver
    brown a.
    cerebral a.
    Charcot-Marie-Tooth muscular a.
    circumscribed a.
    compensatory a.
    cyanotic a.
    cyanotic a. of liver
    cystic a.
    disuse a.
    essential a.
    exhaustion a.
    fatty a.
    focal a.
    gelatinous a.
    granular a.
    hypertropic polyneuritic-type
      muscular a.

infantile muscular a.
ischemic muscular a.
Kienböck a.
Leber optic a.
lobar cerebral a.
macular a.
marantic a.
mucinous a.
muscular a.
neuritic a.
neurogenic muscular a. (NMA)
neurotrophic a.
olivocerebellar a.
olivopontocerebellar a.
optic a.
peroneal muscular a.
Pick a.
polyneuritic-type hypertrophic
    muscular a.
postmenopausal a.
pressure a.
progressive muscular a. (PMA)
progressive spinal muscular a.
red a.
senile a.
serous a.
simple a.
subtotal villose a. (STVA)
Sudeck a.
traction a.
traumatic a.
villous a.
yellow a. of liver

atropine suppression test
ATS
antitetanic serum
antithymocyte serum
arteriosclerosis

attached cranial section
attachment
a. plaque
spindle a.

attack
Adams-Stokes a. (ASA)
a. rate
transient ischemic a. (TIA)

attenuant
attenuate
attenuated
a. culture
a. tuberculosis

a. vaccine
a. virus

attenuation
attenuator
attraction sphere
attribute
atypia
cellular a.
koilocytotic a.

atypical
a. adenomatous hyperplasia (AAH)
a. fibrous histiocytoma
a. fibroxanthoma
a. insulin
a. lipoma
a. lymphocyte
a. measles
a. melanocytic hyperplasia
a. mycobacteria
a. polypoid adenomyofibroma
    (APA)
a. polypoid adenomyofibroma of
    low malignant potential (APA-
    LMP)
a. polypoid adenomyoma (APA)
a. primary pneumonia
a. regeneration
a. squamous cells of undetermined
    significance (ASCUS)
a. verrucous endocarditis

atypism
AU
antitoxin unit
Australia antigen

Au Ag
Australia antigen

Auchmeromyia
A. luteola

audio amplifier
Auer
A. body
A. rod

Auger
A. effect
A. electron

augmented histamine test (AHT)
Aujeszky
A. disease
A. disease virus

AUL
acute undifferentiated leukemia

NOTES

AUO
amyloid of unknown origin
aural polyp
auramine
a. O fluorescent stain
auramine-rhodamine stain
aurantiasis
Aureobasidium
A. pullulans
aureus
methicillin-resistant
Staphylococcus a. (MRSA)
Staphylococcus a.
auricular docimasia
auriculoventricular (A-V)
aurin
a. tricarboxylic acid
aurochromoderma
Aurococcus
Aus antigen
auscultatory gap
Australia antigen (AU, Au Ag)
Australian
A. X disease
A. X disease virus
A. X encephalitis
A. X encephalitis virus
autecic
autoadsorption
autoagglutination
autoagglutinin
anti-Pr cold a.
cold a.
autoallergic hemolytic anemia
autoallergization
autoallergy
AutoAnalyzer
autoanalyzer
sequential multichannel a. (SMA)
autoanaphylaxis
autoantibody
anticytoplasmic a.'s
anti-idiotype a.
antineutrophil cytoplasmic a.
(ANCA)
cold a.
Donath-Landsteiner cold a.
hemagglutinating cold a.
idiotype a.
platelet a.
thymocytotoxic a.
warm a.
autoanticomplement
autoantigen
autoantitoxin
autoassay
autoblast
autocatalysis

autochthonous
autoclasia
autoclasis
autoclave
autocorrelation function
autocrine
a. growth factor
a. hypothesis
a. motility factor
autocytolysin
autocytolysis
autocytotoxin
autodigestion
autoerythrocyte
a. sensitization
a. sensitization syndrome
autoerythrophagocytosis
autofluorescence
autofluoroscope
autogamous
autogamy
autogeneic graft
autogenesis
autogenetic
autogenic
a. graft
autogenous
a. vaccine
autograft
autografting
autohemagglutination
autohemagglutinin
autohemolysin
autohemolysis
a. test
autohemotherapy
autoimmune
a. disease
a. encephalomyelitis
a. hemolytic anemia (AHA, AIHA)
a. hepatitis
a. leukopenia
a. neonatal thrombocytopenia
a. orchitis
a. pancytopenia
a. reaction
a. thrombocytopenic purpura
a. thyroiditis
autoimmunity
autoimmunization
autoimmunocytopenia
autoinfection
autoinoculable
autoinoculation
autoisolysin
autokine
Autolet blood glucose test

autologous
- a. graft
- a. hemagglutinin
- a. transfusion
- a. transplantation

autolyse

autolysin

autolysis

autolysosome

autolytic
- a. enzyme

autolyze

automated
- a. activated partial thromboplastin
- a. bacteriology
- a. cell image analysis
- a. differential leukocyte counter
- a. immunoprecipitation (AIP)
- a. motility factor (AMF)
- a. multiphasic screening (AMS)
- a. reagin
- a. reagin test (ART)
- a. reticulocyte counting
- a. slide staining

automatic
- a. hone
- a. tissue processing

automation
- blood cell count a.
- clinical chemistry a.
- differential leukocyte count a.
- microbiology a.
- radioimmunoassay a.

automixis

automutagen

auto-oxidation

auto-oxidative

autoparenchymatous metaplasia

Autopath QC test

autophagia

autophagic
- a. vacuole

autophagosome

autophagy

autoplast

autoplastic
- a. graft

autoplasty

autoploidy

autoprothrombin

autopsy

autoradiograph

autoradiography
- contact a.
- dip-coating a.
- film stripping a.
- thick-layer a.
- two-emulsion a.

autoradiolysis

autoreinfection

autoreproduction

autosensitization

autosensitize

autosepticemia

autoserotherapy

autoserum
- a. therapy

autosomal
- a. dominant disorder
- a. dominant inheritance
- a. heredity
- a. recessive disorder
- a. recessive inheritance

autosome
- a. translocation

Autostainer
- Jung A. XL

autotherapy

autotomy

autotoxemia

autotoxicus
- horror a.

autotransformer
- variable a.

autotransfusion

autotransplant

autotransplantation

autotroph
- facultative a.
- obligate a.

autotrophic
- a. bacterium
- a. fixation

autovaccination

auxanography

auxesis

auxilytic

auxochrome

auxocyte

auxotroph

auxotrophic
- a. mutation

A-V
- arteriovenous

NOTES

A-V *(continued)*
    atrioventricular
    auriculoventricular
       A-V block
Av
    avoirdupois
AV/AF
    anteverted/anteflexed
available
       no data a. (NDA)
avalanche ionization
avascular
       a. necrosis
Avellis syndrome
average
       a. deviation (AD)
       a. gradient
       a. life
       Walsh a.
       weighted a.
averaging
       signal a.
AVF
    arteriovenous fistula
AVH
    acute viral hepatitis
Aviadenovirus
aviadenovirus
avian
       a. diphtheria
       a. encephalomyelitis virus
       a. erythroblastosis virus
       a. infectious encephalomyelitis
       a. infectious laryngotracheitis
       a. infectious laryngotracheitis virus
       a. influenza
       a. influenza virus
       a. leukosis
       a. leukosis-sarcoma complex
       a. leukosis-sarcoma virus
       a. lymphomatosis
       a. lymphomatosis virus
       a. monocytosis
       a. myeloblastosis
       a. myeloblastosis virus
       a. myelocytomatosis virus (AMV2)
       a. neurolymphomatosis virus
       a. pneumoencephalitis virus
       a. reticuloendotheliosis
       a. sarcoma
       a. sarcoma virus
       a. tubercle bacillus
       a. viral arthritis virus
avidin
avidin-biotin
       a.-b. complex

       a.-b. detection system
       a.-b. immunoperoxidase technique
avidin-biotin-peroxidase complex (ABC)
avidity
       a. antibody
       a. testing
Avipoxvirus
avipoxvirus
avirulence
avirulent
avitaminosis
avium-intracellulare
       Mycobacterium a.-i. (MAC, MAI)
AVM
    arteriovenous malformation
Avogadro number
avoirdupois (Av)
AVP
    arginine vasopressin
AVR
    aortic valve replacement
avulsed wound
avulsion
AW
    anterior wall
AWI
    anterior wall infarction
AWMI
    anterior wall myocardial infarction
awu
    atomic weight unit
Axenfeld syndrome
axenic
axes (*pl. of* axis)
AXG
    adult-type xanthogranuloma
axial aneurysm
axiopodium
axis, pl. axes
       cell a.
       renin-aldosterone a.
       a. of rotation
       a. of symmetry
axonal
       a. degeneration
       a. demyelination
axoneme
axonotmesis
axon staining method
axoplasm
axopodium
axostyle
Ayerza
       A. disease
       A. syndrome
Ayoub-Shklar method
Ayre spatula

A-Z
    Aschheim-Zondek
    A-Z test
azan stain
azar
    kala a.
azathioprine
azeotrope
azeotropic solution
azeotropy
azide
azidothymidine (AZT)
azin dye
azinphosmethyl
azo
    a. coupling reaction
    a. dye
azobenzene
azobilirubin
azocarmine
    a. B
    a. dye
    a. G
azoic
    a. dye
azolitmin
    a. paper
azoospermia
azophloxin
azoprotein

azote
azotemia
    chloropenic a.
    extrarenal a.
    hypochloremic a.
    nonrenal a.
    postrenal a.
    prerenal a.
    renal a.
azotemic
Azotobacter
azotorrhea
azoturia
azovan blue
AZT
    Aschheim-Zondek test
    azidothymidine
azure
    a. A, B, C
    a. I, II
    methylene a.
azure-eosin stain
azuresin
azurophil, azurophile
    a. granule
azurophilia
azurophilic granule
azymia
Azzopardi criteria

NOTES

β (*var. of* beta)
    β agglutinin
    β hemolysin
    β hemolysis
    β metachromasia
    β radiation
    β ray
B
    bacillus
    Baumé scale
    Benoist scale
    whole blood
        B cell
        B cell antigen receptor
        B lymphocyte
        B virus
        B virus hepatitis
b
    bis
    blood
4B
B5 fixative
B-5 sodium acetate-sublimate formalin
10B
B19 virus
B72.3
    B. antibody
    B. stain
BA
    bacterial agglutination
    blocking antibody
    bronchial asthma
Baastrup syndrome
Babcock tube
Babes-Ernst granule
Babesia
    B. microti
Babesiella
Babesiidae
babesiosis
    b. serological test
Babès node
Babinski-Fröhlich syndrome
Babinski-Nageotte syndrome
Babinski syndrome
Babinski-Vaquez syndrome
baby
    blue b.
    collodion b.
    giant b.
BAC
    blood alcohol concentration
Bachman-Pettit test
Bachman test
Bacillaceae

bacillary
    b. dysentery
    b. embolism
    b. emulsion (tuberculin) (BE)
    b. hemoglobinuria
Bacille
    B. bilié de Calmette-Guérin (BCG)
bacillemia
bacilli (*pl. of* bacillus)
bacilliform
bacillosis
bacilluria
Bacillus
    B. aerogenes capsulatus
    B. aertrycke
    B. alvei
    B. ambiguus
    B. anthracis
    B. anthracis toxin
    B. botulinus
    B. brevis
    B. bronchisepticus
    B. cereus
    B. circulans
    B. coli
    B. diphtheriae
    B. dysenteriae
    B. enteritidis
    B. faecalis alcaligenes
    B. influenzae
    B. larvae
    B. leprae
    B. licheniformis
    B. mallei
    B. megaterium
    B. necrophorus
    B. oedematiens
    B. oedematis maligni
    B. oedematis maligni No. II
    B. pertussis
    B. pestis
    B. pneumoniae
    B. polymyxa
    B. proteus
    B. pseudomallei
    B. pumilus
    B. pyocyaneus
    B. sphaericus
    B. stearothermophilus
    B. subtilis
    B. suipestifer
    B. tetani
    B. tuberculosis
    B. tularense
    B. typhi

Bacillus (continued)
    B. *typhosus*
    B. *welchii*
    B. *whitmori*
bacillus, pl. bacilli (B)
    acid-fast b. (AFB)
    anthrax b.
    avian tubercle b.
    Bang b.
    Battey b.
    Boas-Oppler b.
    Bordet-Gengou b.
    bovine tubercle b.
    Calmette-Guérin B.
    B. Calmette-Guérin vaccine
    cholera b.
    coliform b.
    colon b.
    comma b.
    diphtheria b.
    diphtheroid bacilli
    Döderlein b.
    Ducrey b.
    dysentery bacilli
    enteric b.
    Escherich b.
    Fick b.
    Flexner-Strong b.
    Friedländer b.
    fusiform b.
    Gärtner b.
    Ghon-Sachs b.
    glanders b.
    Gram-negative bacilli
    Gram-positive bacilli
    Hansen b.
    Hofmann b.
    human tubercle b.
    Johne b.
    Klebs-Löffler b.
    Klein b.
    Koch-Weeks b.
    leprosy b.
    Morax-Axenfeld b.
    Morgan b.
    Newcastle-Manchester b.
    Nocard b.
    paracolon b.
    Park-Williams b.
    Pfeiffer b.
    plague b.
    Preisz-Nocard b.
    pseudotuberculosis b.
    rhinoscleroma b.
    Schmitz b.
    Schmorl b.
    Shiga b.
    smegma b.

    Sonne-Duval b.
    Strong b.
    tetanus b.
    timothy b.
    tubercle b. (TB)
    typhoid b.
    vole b.
    Welch b.
    Whitmore b.
bacitracin disk test
back
    adolescent round b.
backbone
backcross
background
    b. count
    flame b.
    b. interference
    pathoanatomic b.
    smear b.
backlash
backwash ileitis
bact
    bacterium
Bactalert
    B. analyzer
    B. FAN culture medium
    B. system
BACTEC blood culture system
bacteremia
bacteria (*pl. of* bacterium)
bacteria-free stage of bacterial
    endocarditis
bacterial
    b. adherence
    b. agar method
    b. agglutination (BA)
    b. allergy
    b. aneurysm
    b. antagonism
    b. antigen detection method
    b. aortitis
    b. capsule
    b. culture
    b. culturing
    b. dissociation
    b. encephalitis
    b. endaortitis
    b. endarteritis
    b. endocarditis (BE)
    b. enzyme
    b. filter
    b. genetics
    b. hemolysin
    b. interference
    b. killing assay
    b. meningitis
    b. nephritis

B

b. opsonin
b. overgrowth syndrome
b. pathogenicity
b. pericarditis
b. plaque
b. serology
b. spore
b. stain
b. staining
b. susceptibility testing
b. toxin
b. transformation
b. transfusion reaction
b. urinary cast
b. vegetation
b. virus
bactericholia
bactericidal
b. antibiotic
b. concentration (BC)
bactericide
specific b.
bacterid
pustular b.
bacteriemia
bacterioagglutinin
bacteriocide
bacteriocidin
bacteriocin factor
bacteriocinogen
bacteriocinogenic plasmid
bacterioclasis
bacteriogenic agglutination
bacterioid
bacteriological index (BI)
bacteriologic specimen
bacteriologist
bacteriology
automated b.
clinical diagnostic b.
medical b.
public health b.
sanitary b.
systematic b.
bacteriolysin
bacteriolysis
bacteriolytic
b. amboceptor
b. serum
bacteriolyze
bacterio-opsonin
bacteriopexy

bacteriophage
defective b.
filamentous b.
b. genetics
b. immunity
mature b.
b. resistance
temperate b.
typhoid b.
b. typing
vegetative b.
virulent b.
bacteriophagia
bacteriophagology
bacteriopsonic
bacteriopsonin
bacteriosis
bacteriostasis
bacteriostat
bacteriostatic
b. agent
b. antibiotic
bacteriotoxic
bacteriotropic
b. substance
bacteriotropin
Bacterium
bacterium, pl. **bacteria (bact)**
acid-fast b.
aerobic b.
anaerobic b.
autotrophic b.
beaded b.
bifid b.
chemoautotrophic b.
chemoheterotrophic b.
chromogenic b.
denitrifying b.
endogenous b.
exogenous b.
facultative b.
Gram-negative b.
Gram-positive b.
heterotrophic b.
higher bacteria
hydrogen b.
indigenous b.
intermediate coliform bacteria
lactic acid bacteria
lysogenic b.
mesophilic b.
monocytogenes bacteria

NOTES

73

bacterium (*continued*)
    nitrifying b.
    organotropic b.
    psychrophilic b.
    pyogenic b.
    rough b.
    smooth b.
    sulfur b.
    thermophilic b.
    toxigenic b.
    water b.
bacteriuria
    significant asymptomatic b. (SAB)
bacteroid
Bacteroidaceae
Bacteroides
    B. corrodens
    B. fragilis
    B. funduliformis
    B. fusiformis
    B. melaninogenicus
    B. ochraceus
    B. oralis
    B. pneumosintes
    B. ruminicola
    B. serpens
bacteruria
Bactometer
Baculoviridae
Baehr-Lohlein lesion
Baelz disease
Bäfverstedt syndrome
bagassosis
Baggenstoss
    B. change
    B. change in pancreas
Baker
    B. acid hematein
    B. acid hematein test
    B. cyst
    B. formol calcium
    B. pyridine extraction
    B. pyridine extraction test
    B. Sudan black method
baker's eczema
bakers' yeast
BAL
    bronchoalveolar lavage
Balamuth
    B. buffer solution
    B. culture medium
balance
    acid-base b.
    analytical b.
    calcium b.
    enzyme b.
    fluid b.
    genic b.

    microchemical b.
    nitrogen b.
    b. translocation
balanced
    b. polymorphism
    b. salt solution (BSS)
balanitis
    b. xerotica obliterans
balanoposthitis
balantidial
    b. colitis
    b. dysentery
balantidiasis
Balantidium
    B. coli
Balbiani
    B. body
    B. chromosome
    B. ring
Balfour disease
Balint syndrome
Balkan nephropathy
ball
    chondrin b.
    food b.
    fungus b.
    hair b.
    pleural fibrin b.
    b. thrombus
Baller-Gerold syndrome
Ballet disease
Ballingall disease
balloon
    b. cell
    b. cell nevus
    b. dilatation
ballooning
    b. colliquation
    b. degeneration
ball-valve
    b.-v. obstruction
    b.-v. thrombus
Baló disease
balsam
    Canada b.
Bamberger
    B. albuminuria
    B. disease
Bamberger-Marie
    B.-M. disease
    B.-M. syndrome
BamH1 enzyme
Bamle disease
Bancroft
    B. filarial worm
    B. filariasis
bancroftiasis

B

band
  α_1-b.
  A b.
  alpha-1 b.
  anomalous muscle b.
  b. cell
  centromeric b.
  chromosomal b.
  chromosome b.
  contraction b.
  b. form
  H b.
  I b.
  b. keratopathy
  Ladd b.
  M b.
  moderator b.
  monoclonal b.
  b. neutrophil
  oligoclonal b.
  Soret b.
  b. spectrum
  theta b.
band-form granulocyte
banding
  BrDu-b.
  C-b.
  chromosome b.
  G-b.
  high-resolution b.
  NOR-b.
  oligoclonal b.
  prometaphase b.
  Q-b.
  quinacrine b.
  R-b.
  reverse b.
  T b.
  telomere b.
  terminal b.
Bandl ring
bandpass
bandwidth
Bang
  B. bacillus
  B. disease
bank
  blood b. (BB)
Bannister disease
Banti
  B. disease

  B. spleen
  B. syndrome
BAO
  basal acid output
BAP
  blood agar plate
bar
  median b. of Mercier
  terminal b.
baragnosis
Barany caloric test
Barbados leg
barbae
barber's itch
barbiero
barbital
barbiturate
  b. assay
  b. level
  b. spindle
Barclay-Baron disease
Barcoo disease
Bardet-Biedl syndrome
Bard needle
bare lymphocyte syndrome
Bargen streptococcus
barium test
Barlow
  B. disease
  B. syndrome
Barnett-Bourne acetic alcohol-silver nitrate method
barometer
barometric pressure
barosinusitis
Barr
  B. body
  B. body test
Barraquer disease
Barré-Guillain syndrome
barrel chest
barreling distortion
Barrett
  B. epithelium
  B. esophagus
  B. syndrome
  B. ulcer
barrier
  blood-air b.
  blood-brain b. (BBB)
  blood-cerebral b.
  b. filter

NOTES

barrier-layer cell
Barrnett-Seligman
    B.-S. dihydroxydinaphthyl disulfide
      method
    B.-S. indoxyl esterase method
Barroso-Moguel and Costero silver
    method
Bartholin
    B. abscess
    B. cyst
bartholinitis
Bartholin, urethral, Skene glands (BUS)
Bartonella
    B. *bacilliformis*
    B. *elizabethae*
    B. *henselae*
    B. *quintana*
Bartonellaceae
bartonellosis
Bart syndrome
Bartter syndrome
baruria
basal
    b. acid output (BAO)
    b. body
    b. cell
    b. cell acanthoma
    b. cell adenoma
    b. cell carcinoma
    b. cell carcinoma specific antibody
    b. cell epithelioma
    b. cell hyperplasia
    b. cell nevus
    b. cell nevus syndrome
    b. cell papilloma
    b. feet
    b. granule
    b. lamina
    b. metabolic rate (BMR)
    b. metabolism
    b. secretory flow rate (BSFR)
    b. squamous cell carcinoma
    b. striation
    b. tuberculosis
basalioma
basaloid carcinoma
basaloma
base
    blood buffer b. (BB)
    Brönsted-Lowry b.
    buffer b. (BB)
    complementary b.
    conjugate b.
    b. deficit (BD)
    b. excess (BE)
    b. ionization constant
    Lewis b.
    b. pair (bp)

    b. pairing
    pressor b.
    purine and pyrimidine b.'s
    pyrimidine b.
    b. ratio
    Schiff b.
    b. units
Basedow disease
baseline steady state
basement membrane
basic
    b. anhydride
    b. dye
    b. fuchsin
    b. fuchsin-methylene blue stain
    b. magenta
Basidiobolus
    B. *haptosporus*
Basidiomycetes
Basidiomycota
basidiospore
basidium
basilar
    b. leptomeningitis
    b. meningitis
basipetal
basisquamous (*var. of* basosquamous)
basket cell
baso
    basophil
basocyte
basocytopenia
basocytosis
basoerythrocyte
basoerythrocytosis
basometachromophil,
    basometachromophile
basopenia
basophil, basophile (baso)
    b. adenoma
    beta b.
    b. cell
    b. chemotactic factor (BCF)
    b. degranulation test
    b. granule
    polymorphonuclear b. (PMB)
basophilia
    Grawitz b.
    pituitary b.
    punctate b.
basophilic
    b. erythroblast
    b. granular degeneration
    b. granule
    b. hyperplasia
    b. leukemia
    b. leukocyte
    b. leukocytosis

b. leukopenia
b. marrow
b. megakaryocyte
b. metamyelocyte
b. myelocyte
b. normoblast
b. promyelocyte
b. stippling
basophilism
Cushing b.
pituitary b.
basophilocyte
basophilocytic leukemia
basoplasm
basosquamous, basisquamous
basosquamous carcinoma
Bassen-Kornzweig syndrome
bat
Bateman syndrome
bath
flotation b.
water b.
bathing trunk nevus
bathochromic shift
bathophenanthroline
bathycardia
bathygastry
Batten disease
Batten-Mayou syndrome
Battey
B. bacillus
Battey-type mycobacterium
battledore placenta
Bauer
B. chromic acid leucofuchsin stain
B. reaction
Baumé scale (B)
Baumgartner method
bauxite workers' disease
**Bayer/Technicon H1 automated flow
cytometer**
Bayes theorem
Bayle disease
Baylisascaris
Bazex syndrome
Bazin disease
Bazolyze reagent
BB
blood bank
blood buffer base
blue bloater

breakthrough bleeding
breast biopsy
buffer base
orseillin BB
BBB
blood-brain barrier
bundle-branch block
BC
bactericidal concentration
BCB
brilliant cresyl blue
B-cell
B.-c. differentiating factor
B.-c. differentiation/growth factor
B.-c. growth factor I, II
B.-c. lymphoma (BCL)
B.-c. malignancy
B.-c. marker
B.-c. stimulating factor
BCF
basophil chemotactic factor
BCG
Bacille bilié de Calmette-Guérin
bicolor guaiac (test)
bromocresol green
BCG vaccine
BCL
B-cell lymphoma
bcl-2
bcl-2 antibody
bcl-2 gene arrangement
bcl-2 oncogene
bcl-2 protein
bcl-2 proto-oncogene
bcl-1/PRAD1 gene rearrangement
BCNU
bischloroethylnitrosourea
bischloronitrosourea
BCP-D
bromocresol purple desoxycholate
BD
base deficit
Bdellonyssus
B. bacoti
BDG
buffered desoxycholate glucose
BE
bacillary emulsion (tuberculin)
bacterial endocarditis
base excess
bovine enteritis

NOTES

beaded
  b. bacterium
  b. hair
beading
  b. of the ribs
beaked pelvis
beaker
beam
  electron b.
  b. splitting
bean
  castor b.
Be^a antigen
Beard
  B. disease
  B. test
Beau
  B. disease
  B. line
  B. syndrome
Beauvais disease
Beauvaria
beauvariosis
Beaver direct smear method
Bechterew disease
Beck
  B. disease
  B. triad
Becker
  B. antigen
  B. disease
  B. dystrophy
  B. nevus
  B. stain for spirochetes
Beckman
  B. assay
  B. Paragon SPE-II Gel Apparatus
Beckmann thermometer
Beckwith syndrome
Beckwith-Wiedemann syndrome
becquerel (Bq)
Becton-Dickinson needle
bedbug
Bednar tumor
Bedsonia
beef tapeworm
Beer law
beeturia
bee venom toxin
Begbie disease
Béguez César disease
behavior genetics
Behçet
  B. disease
  B. syndrome
behenic acid
Behnken unit (R)
Behr disease

Behring law
BEI
  butanol-extractable iodine
  BEI test
Beigel disease
bejel
Bekhterev disease
bel
Belascaris
Belgian Congo anemia
Belke-Kleihauer stain
belladonna
  opium and b. (O&B)
  b. and opium (B&O)
Bell disease
Bell-Magendie law
belly
  prune b.
Bence
  B. Jones (BJ)
  B. Jones albumin
  B. Jones albuminuria
  B. Jones cylinder
  B. Jones myeloma
  B. Jones protein (BJP)
  B. Jones protein test
  B. Jones proteinuria
  B. Jones reaction
Benditt hypothesis
Benedict
  B. solution
  B. test
  B. test for glucose
Benedict-Hopkins-Cole reagent
Benedikt syndrome
bengal
  rose b.
Bengston method
benign
  b. albuminuria
  b. bone aneurysm
  b. chronic bullous dermatosis of
    childhood
  b. dry pleurisy
  b. dyskeratosis
  b. epithelial breast tumor
  b. epithelioma
  b. familial icterus
  b. giant lymph node hyperplasia
  b. glycosuria
  b. inoculation lymphoreticulosis
  b. inoculation reticulosis
  b. intracranial hypertension (BIH)
  b. juvenile melanoma
  b. lymphadenosis
  b. lymphocytoma cutis
  b. lymphoepithelial lesion
  b. lymphoma

b. lymphoma of the rectum
b. mediastinal lymph node
    hyperplasia
b. mesenchymoma
b. mesothelioma
b. mesothelioma of genital tract
b. monoclonal gammopathy (BMG)
b. mucosal pemphigoid
b. mucous membrane pemphigus
b. myalgic encephalomyelitis
b. neoplasm
b. nephrosclerosis (BNS)
b. paroxysmal peritonitis
b. prostatic hyperplasia
b. prostatic hypertrophy (BPH)
b. teratoma
b. tertian malaria
Bennett
    B. disease
    B. sulfhydryl method
Bennhold
    B. Congo red method
    B. Congo red stain
Benoist scale (B)
Bensley
    B. aniline-acid fuchsin-methyl green
        method
    B. osmic dichromate fluid
    B. safranin acid violet
Benson disease
bentiromide
    b. test
bentonite flocculation test (BFT)
benzalkonium chloride
benzene
    b. assay
    b. hexachloride (BHC)
benzeneamine
benzidine
    b. method for myoglobin
        peroxidase
    b. test
benzo[a]pyrene
benzoate
    caffeine sodium b.
    estradiol b. (EB)
benzodiazepine assay
benzoflavine
benzoic acid
benzol
benzopurpurin 4B
benzo sky blue method

benzoylaminoacetic acid
benzoylation
benzoylecgonine
benzoylglycine
3,4-benzpyrene
benzyl alcohol
benzylamine
Beradinelli syndrome
Bérard aneurysm
Ber-EP4
    B.-E. antibody
    B.-E. immunoperoxidase stain
Berg
    B. chelate removal method
    B. stain
bergamot oil
Berger
    B. disease
    B. focal glomerulonephritis
Bergeron
    B. chorea
    B. disease
Bergey classification
Ber-H2 antibody
beriberi
Berkefeld filter
berkelium
Berlin
    B. blue
    B. disease
Bernard-Horner syndrome
Bernard-Sergent syndrome
Bernard-Soulier syndrome
Bernard syndrome
Bernhardt disease
Bernhardt-Roth syndrome
Bernheim syndrome
Bernstein test
Bernthsen methylene violet
berry
    b. aneurysm
    b. cell
Berson test
Berthelot reaction
Bertiella
    B. studeri
bertiellosis
Bertolotti syndrome
berylliosis
beryllium granuloma
Besnier-Boeck disease

NOTES

Besnier-Boeck-Schaumann
B.-B.-S. disease
B.-B.-S. syndrome
Besnoitia
besnoitiasis
Besnoitiidae
besnoitiosis
Bessey-Lowry-Brock (BLB)
Bessey-Lowry unit (BLU)
Bessman anemia classification
Best
B. carmine stain
B. disease
beta, β
b. adrenergic blockade
b. adrenergic receptor
b. agglutinin
b. aminoisobutyric aciduria
b. basophil
beta lipoprotein
b. blocker
b. cell
b. cell of hypophysis
b. cell of pancreas
b. corynebacteriophage
b. decay
b. emitter
b. endorphin
17 b. estradiol
b. fetoprotein
b. galactosidase
b. galactosylhydrolase
b. globulin
b. glucosidase
b. glycoprotein
b. glycoproteinase
b. granule
b. hemolysin
b. hemolysis
b. hemolytic streptococcus
b. hydroxybutyrate
b. lactoglobulin
b. lysin
b. metachromasia
b. microglobulin
b. monooxygenase
b. naphthol
b. particle
b. phage
b. ray
b. staphylolysin
b. streptococcus
b. substance
b. thalassemia
b. thromboglobulin
b. tubulin
beta-1A globulin
beta-1C globulin

beta-1E globulin
beta-2 microglobulin
beta-adrenergic blocking agent
betacyaninuria
beta-*d*-glucuronidase deficiency
beta-1F globulin
betaglobulin
steroid-binding b.
betaine
betel cancer
Bethesda
B. Pap smear
B. System
B. unit
Bethesda-Ballerup Group of *Citrobacter*
Bethe stain
Betke-Kleihauer test
Betke stain
Bettendorff test
Betula
Betz cell
Beutler test
BeWo choriocarcinoma cell line
bezoar
Bezold abscess
BF
blastogenic factor
B/F
bound-free ratio
bf
bouillon filtrate (tuberculin)
BFP
biologic false-positive
BFR
biologic false-positive reactor
bone formation rate
BFT
bentonite flocculation test
BFU-E
burst-forming unit-erythroid
BG
blood glucose
bone graft
BGG
bovine gamma globulin
BGH
bovine growth hormone
BGSA
blood granulocyte-specific activity
BGTT
borderline glucose tolerance test
BHBA
β-hydroxybutyrate
BHC
benzene hexachloride
BHI
brain-heart infusion

BHS
β-hemolytic streptococcus
BHTU microscope
BH/VH
body hematocrit-venous hematocrit ratio
BI
bacteriological index
burn index
Bial
B. reagent
B. test
Bianchi syndrome
Bi antigen
bias
forward b.
reverse b.
biased estimate
biatriatum
cor pseudotriloculare b.
cor triloculare b.
bibulous
bicameral abscess
bicarbonate
blood b.
b. buffer
b. buffer system
plasma b.
standard b.
b. titration test
biciliate
biclonal
b. gammopathy
b. peak
biclonality
bicolor guaiac (test) (BCG)
biconcave
biconvex
BIDLB
block in posteroinferior division of left branch
Biebrich
B. scarlet
B. scarlet-picroaniline blue
B. scarlet red
Biedl disease
Bielschowsky
B. disease
B. method
B. stain
Bielschowsky-Jansky disease
Biemond syndrome

bieneusi
Enterocytozoon b.
Biermer
B. anemia
B. disease
bifid
b. bacterium
b. tongue
b. ureter
b. uterus
bifida
spina b.
Bifidobacterium
B. *bifidum*
B. *eriksonii*
B. *infantis*
bifurcation
bigeminal
bigeminy
ventricular b.
BIH
benign intracranial hypertension
bilat
bilateral
bilateral (bilat)
b. left-sidedness
b. otitis media (BOM)
b., symmetrical, and equal (BSE)
b. symmetry
Bilderbeck disease
bile
b. acids
b. acids assay
b. acid tolerance test
B. antigen
b. canaliculi
b. cast
b. duct adenoma
b. duct canaliculus
b. duct carcinoma
b. esculin agar
b. esculin hydrolysis test
b. esculin test
b. extravasation
b. fluid examination
b. infarct
b. lake
b. nephrosis
b. peritonitis
b. pigment
b. pigment demonstration in tissue
b. pigment hemoglobin

NOTES

81

bile *(continued)*
    b. pigment test
    b. salt agar
    b. salt breath test
    b. salt deficiency syndrome
    b. salts
    b. solubility test
    b. stasis
    b. thrombus
    white b.
Bilharzia
bilharzial
    b. deposition pigment
    b. dysentery
    b. granuloma
    b. pigment deposition
bilharziasis
bilharziosis
biliary
    b. achalasia
    b. atresia
    b. calculus
    b. cirrhosis
    b. colic
    b. fistula
    b. obstruction
    b. tract disease
    b. xanthomatosis
biliousness
bilious remittent malaria
bilirubin
    amniotic fluid b.
    b. assay
    conjugated b.
    b. demonstration in tissues
    direct reacting b.
    b. encephalopathy
    indirect reacting b.
    minimum concentration of b.
      (MCBR)
    neonatal b.
    serum b. (SB)
    b. tolerance test
    unconjugated b.
    volume of distribution of b.
      (VDBR)
bilirubinemia
    hereditary nonhemolytic b.
bilirubinuria
biliuria
biliverdin
biliverdinglobin
Billheimer method
Billroth disease
bilobate placenta
bilobed right lung
biloculare
    cor b.

bilocular stomach
Bilopaque
bimetal thermometer
bimodal
bimolecular
bimorphic
binary
    b. acid
    b. addition
    b. fission
    b. nomenclature
    b. variate
binasal hemianopsia
binding
    b. constant
    b. energy
    protein b. (PB)
binocular microscope
binomial
    b. coefficient
    b. distribution
    b. nomenclature
Binswanger
    B. disease
    B. encephalopathy
binuclear
binucleate
binucleated
Binz test
bioaccumulation
bioassay
bioavailability
biocenosis
biochemical
    b. energetics
    b. genetics
    b. metastasis
    b. profile
biochemistry
biochemorphology
biocidal
bioclimatology
biodegradability
biodegradable
bioenergetics
bioequivalence
biogenesis
biogenetic
biogenic amine hypothesis
biohazard
biologic
    b. assay
    b. false-positive (BFP)
    b. false-positive reactor (BFR)
    b. half-life
biological
    b. alkylating agent
    b. assay

b. clock
b. immunotherapy
B. Matrix Reference Materials
B. Stain Commission
b. standard unit
b. vector
biologicals
biology
cellular b.
molecular b.
population b.
bioluminescence
biomass
biomechanical preparation
biomechanics
biomedical engineering
biometrician
biometry
Biomphalaria
B. glabrata
Biondi-Heidenhain stain
Biondi ring
bionics
biophage
biophagism
biophagous
biophagy
biophylactic
biophylaxis
biophysics
biopsy
aspiration b.
bone marrow b.
cone b.
CT-guided stereotactic b.
excisional b.
fine-needle aspiration b. (FNAB)
incisional b.
muscle b.
punch b.
scalene node b. (SNB)
stereotactic brain b.
thin-needle b.
biopterin
biopyoculture
biosafety
biospectrometry
biospectroscopy
biospelcology
biosynthesis
biosynthetic pathway

biotin
b. assay
b. streptavidin detection method
biotope
biotoxin
biotransformation
biotype
BIP
bismuth iodoform paraffin
biparasitism
biparental
b. inheritance
biphasic response
biphenotypic
b. differentiation
b. lymphoma
biphenotypy
biphenyl
polychlorinated b. (PCB)
bipolar
b. cell
b. needle electrode
b. neuron
b. spindle
b. stain
b. staining
bipyridyl
Birbeck granule
Birch-Hirschfeld stain
bird
B. disease
b. nest lesion
b. unit
bird-breeder's
b.-b. disease
b.-b. lung
birdseed agar
birefringence
crystalline b.
flow b.
form b.
strain b.
birefringent crystal
Birnaviridae
Birnavirus
birth injury
birthmark (bmk)
strawberry b.
vascular b.
bis (b)
bisalbuminemia
bischloroethylnitrosourea (BCNU)

NOTES

bis(2-chloroethyl)sulfide
bischloronitrosourea (BCNU)
bisection
Bismarck
    B. brown
    B. brown R
    B. brown Y
bismuth
    b. assay
    b. iodide
    b. iodoform paraffin (BIP)
    b. pigmentation
    b. subnitrate
    b. triiodide
bismuth-sulfite agar (BSA)
bisphosphate
    fructose b.
bisphosphatidylglycerol
2,3-bisphosphoglycerate
bisphosphoglycerate phosphatase
bisphosphoglyceromutase
bis-trimethylsilylacetamide
bis-trimethylsilyltrifluoroacetamide
  (BSTFA)
bisulfate
bisulfide
    carbon b.
bisulfite
bit
    check b.
    parity b.
bitartrate
    levarterenol b.
bitemporal hemianopsia
Bithynia
Bitot spot
bitropic
bitten colony
Bittner
    B. agent
    B. milk factor
    B. virus
biundulant
    b. meningoencephalitis
    b. milk fever virus
biuret
    b. reaction
    b. test
biuret-reactive material (BRM)
bivalent
    b. antibody
    b. gas gangrene antitoxin
    heteromorphic b.
    homomorphic b.
biventriculare
    cor triloculare b.
bixin

Bizzozero
    B. corpuscle
    B. red cell
BJ
    Bence Jones
Björnstad syndrome
BJP
    Bence Jones protein
BK virus
BL
    bleeding
    blood loss
    Burkitt lymphoma
black
    amido b. 10B
    b. box
    b. currant rash
    b. fly
    b. hairy tongue
    b. jaundice
    b. lead
    b. light
    b. lung
    b. lung disease
    b. periodic acid method
    b. piedra
    b. plague
    Sudan b. B
    b. urine
    b. widow spider
black-dot ringworm
Blackfan-Diamond syndrome
blackhead
bladder
    fasciculate b.
    low-compliance b.
    b. neck obstruction (BNO)
    neurogenic b.
    poorly compliant b.
    b. tumor (BT)
bladderworm
BLA 36 monoclonal antibody
blanch
bland
    b. embolism
    b. embolus
    b. infarct
Blane
    amniotic infection syndrome of B.
blank
blast
    b. cell
    b. cell leukemia
    b. chest
    b. crisis
    b. injury
blastema
blastic

Blastoconidium
Blastocystis
    B. hominis
blastocyte
blastocytoma
blastogenesis
    b. assay
blastogenetic
blastogenic factor (BF)
blastoma
    pleuropulmonary b.
    pluricentric b.
    pulmonary b.
    unicentric b.
blastomere
blastomogenic
Blastomyces
    B. brasiliensis
    B. coccidioides
    B. dermatitidis
blastomycin
blastomycosis
    European b.
    North American b.
    b. serology
    South American b.
blastophore
blastospore
blastula, pl. **blastulae**
blastulation
Blatin syndrome
Blatta
Blattella
Blattidae
BLB
    Bessey-Lowry-Brock
    Boothby, Lovelace, Bulbulian
    BLB mask
    BLB unit
bleach
bleaching
bleb
    emphysematous b.
bleeder
bleeding (BL)
    breakthrough b. (BB, BTB)
    estrogen withdrawal b. (EWB)
    functional b.
    implantation b.
    occult b.
    placentation b.

    b. polyp
    b. time (BT)
blennadenitis
blennorrhagia
blennorrhagic
    b. inflammation
blennorrhea
    b. adultorum
    inclusion b.
    b. inclusion
    b. neonatorum
blennorrheal conjunctivitis
blennuria
bleomycin
    doxorubicin (Adriamycin),
      cyclophosphamide, etoposide,
      ifosfamide, vincristine (Oncovin),
      methotrexate, b. (CAMBO-VIP)
    VEPA and b. (VEPA-B)
    vindesine, etoposide, procarbazine,
      prednisone, b. (FEPP-B)
bleomycin, prednisone
blepharitis
    b. ulcerosa
blepharoplast
blepharoptosis
BLG
    β-lactoglobulin
blighted ovum
blind
    b. fistula
    b. passage
    b. test
blister
    blood b.
    fever b.
bloater
    blue b. (BB)
bloc
    en b.
Bloch reaction
Bloch-Sulzberger
    B.-S. disease
    B.-S. syndrome
block
    b. in anterosuperior division of left
      branch (BSDLB)
    atrioventricular b.
    A-V b.
    bundle-branch b. (BBB)
    complete heart b. (CHB)

NOTES

block *(continued)*

    complete left bundle-branch b. (CLBBB)

    complete right bundle-branch b. (CRBBB)

    b. diagram

    incomplete right bundle-branch b. (IRBBB)

    left bundle-branch b. (LBBB)

    paraffin b.

    b. in posteroinferior division of left branch (BIDLB)

    second degree heart b.

    third degree heart b.

blockade

    α-b.

    α-adrenergic b.

    β-adrenergic b.

    adrenergic neuron b.

    alpha b.

    alpha adrenergic b.

    beta adrenergic b.

    cholinergic b.

    combined androgen b.

    narcotic b.

    renal b.

    virus b.

blocker

    β-b.

    beta b.

blocking

    adrenergic b.

    b. antibody (BA)

    b. antibody reaction

    b. filter

Blocq disease

blood (b)

    b. agar

    b. agar plate (BAP)

    b. albumin

    b. alcohol

    b. alcohol concentration (BAC)

    anticoagulated b.

    arterial b.

    arterialized b.

    b. bank (BB)

    b. bank technology specialist

    b. bicarbonate

    b. blister

    b. buffer base (BB)

    b. buffering capacity

    b. calculus

    b. cast

    b. cell

    b. cell count

    b. cell count automation

    chocolate b. (CB)

    citrated b.

    b. clot

    b. coagulation disorder

    b. component

    cord b.

    b. corpuscle

    b. count

    b. crisis

    b. crystal

    b. culture

    b. cyst

    b. cytolysate

    defibrinated b.

    b. disk

    b. donation

    b. dust

    b. dyscrasia

    b. extravasation

    b. factor

    b. film

    b. filter

    b. fluke

    b. gas

    b. gas analysis

    b. ghost

    b. glucose (BG)

    b. granulocyte-specific activity (BGSA)

    b. group

    b. group agglutinins

    b. group agglutinogens

    b. group antibodies

    b. group antigen

    b. group antiserums

    b. group chimera

    b. grouping

    b. group-specific substances A and B

    b. group systems

    b. indices

    b. island

    laky b.

    b. loss (BL)

    b. loss anemia

    b. lymph

    mixed venous b.

    b. mole

    b. mote

    occult b.

    oxygen capacity of b.

    oxygen content of b.

    peripheral b.

    b. plasma

    b. plasma fraction

    b. plastid

    b. plate

    platelet-poor b. (PPB)

    b. poisoning

    b. pressure (BP)

B

b. puzzles
b. quotient
red venous b. (RVB)
b. serum
sludged b.
b. smear
b. smear morphology
b. spot
strawberry-cream b.
b. substitute
b. sugar (BS)
b. tumor
b. type
b. typing
b. urea clearance
b. urea nitrogen (BUN)
b. urea nitrogen test
venous b.
b. vessel
b. volume
b. volume measurement
b. volume nomogram
b. warming
whole b. (B, WB)
blood-air barrier
blood-brain barrier (BBB)
blood-cerebral barrier
blood-clot lysis time (BLT)
Bloodgood disease
bloodless
bloodworm
bloom
Bloom syndrome
Bloor test
blot
b. test
Western b.
Blount
B. disease
B. test
Blount-Barber disease
blowback
blowfly
blowout pipette
Bloxam test
BLT
blood-clot lysis time
BLU
Bessey-Lowry unit
blue
Alcian b. (AB)
aniline b.

anthracene b.
Astra B.
azovan b.
b. baby
Berlin b.
Biebrich scarlet-picroaniline b.
b. bloater (BB)
b. bloater emphysema
brilliant cresyl b. (BCB)
bromophenol b.
bromothymol b.
bromphenol b.
bromthymol b.
carbolic methylene b. (CMB)
cresyl b.
dextran b. (DB)
Diagnex B.
b. diaper syndrome
b. dome cyst
b. edema
Evans b.
indigo b.
Isamine b.
isosulfan b.
lactophenol cotton b.
leucomethylene b.
leuco patent b.
Luxol fast b.
methyl b.
methylene b. (MB)
Prussian b.
b. pus
pyrrol b.
rhodanile b.
b. rubber-bleb nevi
sky b.
b. spot
thymol b.
toluidine b. (TB)
trypan b.
Turnbull b.
victoria b.
bluecomb
b. disease of chickens
b. disease of turkeys
b. virus
blueing
bluetongue
b. virus
Blumenthal disease
Blum syndrome

NOTES

blunt
    b. duct adenosis
    b. end
BLV
    bovine leukemia virus
B-lymphocyte stimulatory factor (BSF)
BM
    body mass
BMG
    benign monoclonal gammopathy
bmk
    birthmark
B-mode
BMR
    basal metabolic rate
BMT
    bone marrow transplantation
BN
    branchial neuritis
BNO
    bladder neck obstruction
BNS
    benign nephrosclerosis
B&O
    belladonna and opium
Boas-Oppler bacillus
Boas test
Bodansky unit (BU)
Bodian
    B. copper-PROTARGOL stain
    B. method
Bodo
    B. caudatus
    B. saltans
    B. urinaria
body
    acetone b.
    acidophilic b.
    alcoholic hyaline b.
    Alder-Reilly b.
    alkapton b.
    amyloid b.'s of prostate
    aortic b.
    apoptotic b.
    Arnold b.
    asbestos b. (AB)
    Aschoff b.
    asteroid b.
    Auer b.
    Balbiani b.
    Barr b.
    basal b.
    Bollinger b.
    Borrel b.
    brassy b.
    Cabot ring b.
    Call-Exner b.
    cancer b.

    carotid b.
    b. cavity
    cell b.
    chromaffin b.
    chromatin b.
    chromatinic b.
    Civatte b.
    colloid b.
    conchoidal b.
    Councilman hyaline b.
    Cowdry type A inclusion b.
    Cowdry type B inclusion b.
    creola b.
    cytoid b.
    cytoplasmic inclusion b.
    Deetjen b.
    demilune b.
    dense b.
    Döhle inclusion b.
    Donné b.
    Donovan b.
    Dutcher b.
    Ehrlich inner b.
    elementary b.
    F b.
    ferruginous b.
    fibrin b.
    fibrous b.
    b. fluid analysis
    b. fluids
    foreign b. (FB)
    fruiting b.
    fuchsin b.
    Gall b.
    Gamna-Favre b.
    Gandy-Gamna b.
    glass b.
    Gordon b.
    Guarnieri b.
    Halberstaedter-Prowazek b.
    Heinz-Ehrlich b.
    b. hematocrit-venous hematocrit
      ratio (BH/VH)
    hematoxylin b.
    Herring b.
    Howell-Jolly b. (HJ)
    hyaline b.
    inclusion b. (IB)
    intraocular foreign b. (IOFB)
    intrauterine foreign b. (IUFB)
    Joest b.
    ketone b. (KB)
    Lafora b.
    Lallemand b.
    LE b.
    Leishman-Donovan b. (L-D)
    Lewy b.
    Lindner b.

b. louse
Luse b.
b. of Luys syndrome
Mallory b.
Maragiliano b.
b. mass (BM)
May-Hegglin b.
melon seed b.
membranous cytoplasmic b. (MCB)
metachromatic b.
metallic foreign b. (MFB)
Michaelis-Gutmann b. (MG)
mineral foreign b.
mineral oil foreign b.
Miyagawa b.
molluscum b.
multilamellar b.
multivesicular b.
Negri b.
Nissl b.
nodular b.
nuclear inclusion b.
onion b.
oxyphil inclusion b.
Pappenheimer b.
Paschen b.
pectinate b.
Pick b.
Plimmer b.
polar b.
polyhedral b.
Prowazek-Greeff b.
psammoma b.
psittacosis inclusion b.
Renaut b.
residual b.
retained foreign b. (RFB)
rice b.
Rushton b.
Russell b.
sand b.
Schaumann b.
sclerotic b.
selenoid b.
spiculated b.
b. surface area (BSA)
b. surface burned (BSB)
b. temperature
b. temperature, ambient pressure,
  saturated (BTPS)
thermostable b.
threshold b.

Todd b.
trachoma b.
Trousseau-Lallemand b.
tuffstone b.
ultimobranchial b.
Verocay b.
Weibel-Palade b.
Wesenberg-Hamazaki b.
Wolf-Orton b.
X chromatin b.
Y b.
yellow b.
zebra b.
body-section radiography
Boeck
 B. disease
 B. sarcoid
**Boeck-Drbohlav-Locke egg-serum
  medium**
Boehmer hematoxylin
Boerhaave syndrome
Boettcher cell
Bogaert disease
Bohr
 B. effect
 B. equation
boil
 Madura b.
boiling point (bp)
Boletus
Boling burner
Bolivian hemorrhagic fever
Bollinger
 B. body
 B. granule
Boltzmann constant
BOM
 bilateral otitis media
bombardment
Bombay
 B. blood group
 B. phenotype
Bombidae
Bonanno test
bond
 chemical b.
 coordinate covalent b.
 covalent b.
 disulfide b.
 electron pair b.
 b. energy
 high-energy b.

NOTES

bond *(continued)*
   hydrogen b.
   ionic b.
   metallic b.
   π-b.
   peptide b.
   pi b.
   σ-b.
   sigma b.
   triple b.
bonding
bone
   b. abscess
   brittle b.
   cancellous b.
   cartilage b.
   b. cell
   b. chip
   compact b.
   cortical b.
   creeping substitution of b.
   b. cyst
   dermal b.
   epihyal b.
   b. formation rate (BFR)
   b. graft (BG)
   heterologous b.
   b. infarct
   malignant giant cell tumor of b.
   marble b.
   b. marrow
   b. marrow abnormality
   b. marrow aspiration
   b. marrow aspiration and biopsy
   b. marrow biopsy
   b. marrow depression
   b. marrow differential count
   b. marrow embolism
   b. marrow embolus
   b. marrow scan
   b. marrow transplantation (BMT)
   b. matrix alteration
   ping-pong b.
   b. resorption
   b. sclerosis
   trabeculae of b.
   b. tumor
   woven b.
Bonnet-Dechaume-Blanc syndrome
Bonnevie-Ullrich syndrome
Bonnier syndrome
bony
   b. ankylosis
   b. callus
   b. heart
Böök syndrome

Boolean
   B. algebra
   B. function
BOOP
   bronchiolitis obliterans with organizing
   pneumonia
Boophilus
   B. annulatus
booster
   b. dose
   b. response
Boothby, Lovelace, Bulbulian (BLB)
borate
borax
Borchgrevink method
border
   brush b.
borderline
   b. glucose tolerance test (BGTT)
   b. leprosy
   b. tumor
Bordet
   B. amboceptor
   B. and Gengou reaction
Bordetella
   B. bronchiseptica
   B. parapertussis
   B. pertussis
   B. pertussis indirect fluorescent
Bordet-Gengou
   B.-G. bacillus
   B.-G. phenomenon
   B.-G. potato blood agar
boric
   b. acid
   b. acid broth
borism
Börjeson-Forssman-Lehmann syndrome
Börjeson syndrome
Borna
   B. disease
   B. disease virus
Bornholm
   B. disease
   B. disease virus
boron
   b. assay
   b. trifluoride-methanol
Borrel
   B. blue stain
   B. body
Borrelia
   B. burgdorferi
   B. duttonii
   B. hermsii
   B. hispanica
   B. parkeri
   B. persica

B. *recurrentis*
B. *turicatae*
B. *venezuelensis*
borreliosis
Lyme b.
Borrmann classification
Borst-Jadassohn type intraepidermal epithelioma
boss
bosselated
bosselation
Bostock disease
Boston
B. exanthem
B. exanthema
botfly
bothria
bothridium
bothriocephaliasis
Bothriocephalus
bothrium
bothropic antitoxin
Bothrops
B. antitoxin
B. *atrox* serine proteinase
botryoid
b. rhabdomyosarcoma
b. sarcoma
botryoides
sarcoma b.
Botryomyces
botryomycosis
botryomycotic
bots
Böttcher crystal
bottle
Roux b.
botulin
botulinum
b. antitoxin
b. toxin
botulinus toxin
botulism
b. antitoxin
wound b.
botulismotoxin (*var. of* botulinus toxin)
Bouchard
B. disease
B. node
Bouffardi
B. black mycetoma
B. white mycetoma

Bouguer law
Bouillaud
B. disease
B. syndrome
bouillon filtrate (tuberculin) (bf)
Bouin
B. fluid
B. picroformol-acetic fixative
B. solution
bound-free ratio (B/F)
bound serum iron (BSI)
bouquet fever
Bourneville disease
Bourneville-Pringle disease
boutonneuse fever
Bouveret
B. disease
B. syndrome
Bovicola
bovine
b. antitoxin
b. colloid
b. enteritis (BE)
b. ephemeral fever
b. gamma globulin (BGG)
b. growth hormone (BGH)
b. herpes mammillitis
b. leukemia virus (BLV)
b. leukosis virus
b. malaria
b. mastitis
b. papular stomatitis
b. papular stomatitis virus
b. red blood cell (BRBC)
b. rhinovirus
b. serum albumin (BSA)
b. spongiform encephalopathy
b. tubercle bacillus
b. ulcerative mammillitis
b. vaccinia mammillitis
b. virus diarrhea
b. virus diarrhea virus
bovinum
cor b.
bowel bypass syndrome
Bowen
B. disease
B. precancerous dermatosis
bowenoid papulosis
Bowers-McComb unit
Bowie stain

NOTES

box
    black b.
Boyden
    B. chamber
    B. chamber assay device
boydii
    Allescheria b.
    Pseudallescheria b.
Boyle law
BP
    blood pressure
    bypass
bp
    base pair
    boiling point
BPD
    bronchopulmonary dysplasia
BPH
    benign prostatic hypertrophy
Bq
    becquerel
Brachmann-de Lange syndrome
Bracht-Wachter lesion
brachycephalic
brachydactyly
Bradley disease
Bradshaw test
bradykinin
bradyzoite
Brailsford-Morquio disease
brain
    b. abscess
    b. cicatrix
    b. concussion
    b. congestion
    b. contusion
    b. death
    b. death syndrome
    b. edema
    primary Ki-1 lymphoma of b.
    respirator b.
    b. sand
    b. swelling
    b. tumor (BT)
Brainerd diarrhea
brain-heart
    b.-h. infusion (BHI)
    b.-h. infusion agar
    b.-h. infusion broth medium
brainstem glioma
braking radiation
branch
branched
    b. calculus
    b. chain
branched-chain
    b.-c. alpha ketoacid decarboxylase
    b.-c. alpha ketoacid dehydrogenase

    b.-c. aminoaciduria
    b.-c. α-ketoacid decarboxylase
    b.-c. α-ketoacid dehydrogenase
    b.-c. ketoaciduria
    b.-c. ketonuria
brancher
    b. deficiency
    b. enzyme
branchial
    b. cleft cyst
    b. fistula
    b. neuritis (BN)
branching
    b. decay
    b. enzyme
    b. fraction
    b. glycogen storage disease
    b. ratio
branchioma
Branhamella
    B. catarrhalis
Brasil fixative
brasiliensis
    Paracoccidioides b.
brassy body
brazilein
Brazilian trypanosomiasis
brazilin
BRBC
    bovine red blood cell
BrDu
    bromodeoxyuridine
bread-and-butter pericardium
break
    isochromatid b.
breakbone fever
breakdown
    protein b.
    starvation-induced protein b.
breaker
    circuit b.
    vacuum b.
breakpoint
    b. analysis
    b. cluster region rearrangement
breakthrough bleeding (BB, BTB)
breast
    b. biopsy (BB)
    cystic disease of the b.
    fibrocystic disease of the b.
    funnel b.
    papillomatosis of b.
    pigeon b.
    shotty b.
    b. specimen radiography
    tension cyst of b.
    b. tumor
breath analysis test

B

Brecher-Cronkite method
Brecher new methylene blue technique
Breda disease
Breed smear
bregma
Breisky disease
bremsstrahlung
Brennemann syndrome
Brenner tumor
Breslow
    B. malignant melanoma assay
    B. thickness
Bretonneau disease
Breus mole
Brewer infarct
brickdust deposit
brickmaker's anemia
bridge
    conjugation b.
    intercellular b.
    myocardial b.
    b. rectifier
    salt b.
    Wheatstone b.
bridging
    b. fibrosis
    b. hepatic necrosis
bridle
bright
    b. contrast
Bright disease
Brill disease
brilliant
    b. cresyl blue (BCB)
    b. crocein
    b. green
    b. green bile salt agar
    b. vital red
    b. yellow
Brill-Symmers disease
Brill-Zinsser disease
Brinton disease
Brion-Kayser disease
Briquet syndrome
Brissaud disease
Brissaud-Marie syndrome
Brissaud-Sicard syndrome
Bristowe syndrome
British
    B. antilewisite
    B. thermal unit (BTU)
brittle bone

BRM
    biuret-reactive material
broad
    b. fish tapeworm
    b. spectrum
    b. urinary cast
broad-beta disease
broadening
    peak b.
broad-spectrum
    b.-s. antibiotic
Broca area
Brock syndrome
Brocq disease
Broders
    B. classification
    B. tumor index
Brodie
    B. abscess
    B. disease
    B. knee
broken
    b. cell preparation
    b. compensation
bromate
bromcresol
    b. green
    b. purple
bromelain
bromide
    b. assay
    cetyltrimethylammonium b.
    ethidium b.
    glycopyrronium b.
    hexamethonium b.
    methyl b.
bromination
bromine
brominism
bromism
bromocresol
    b. green (BCG)
    b. purple
    b. purple desoxycholate (BCP-D)
bromocriptine suppression test
bromodeoxyuridine (BrDu)
5-bromodeoxyuridine
bromoderma
bromoiodism
bromomethane
bromophenol blue
bromothymol blue

NOTES

bromphenol
    b. blue
    b. test
bromphenol blue
bromsulfophthalein
bromsulphalein test
bromthymol blue
bronchial
    b. adenoma
    b. aspirate anaerobic culture
    b. asthma (BA)
    b. calculus
    b. carcinoid
    b. carcinoma
    b. cyst
    b. pneumonia
    b. polyp
    b. washing
    b. washings cytology
bronchiectasia
    b. sicca
bronchiectasic
bronchiectasis
    cylindrical b.
    cystic b.
    dry b.
    fusiform b.
    saccular b.
bronchiectatic
bronchiolar
    b. adenocarcinoma
    b. carcinoma
    b. cell
bronchiolectasia
bronchiolectasis
bronchiolitis
    exudative b.
    b. fibrosa obliterans
    b. obliterans
    b. obliterans syndrome
    b. obliterans with organizing
      pneumonia (BOOP)
    proliferative b.
bronchioloalveolar
    b. adenocarcinoma
    b. carcinoma
bronchiostenosis
bronchitic
bronchitis
    acute b.
    asthmatic b. (AB)
    chronic b. (CB)
    croupous b.
    fibrinous b.
    infectious avian b.
    b. obliterans
    obliterative b.

    plastic b.
    pseudomembranous b.
bronchitis/bronchiolitis
    acute b. (ABB)
bronchoalveolar lavage (BAL)
bronchoaspergillosis
bronchoblastomycosis
bronchocandidiasis
bronchocavernous
bronchocentric granulomatosis
bronchoconstriction
bronchoconstrictor
bronchodilatation
bronchodilator
bronchoedema
bronchoesophageal fistula
bronchogenic
    b. carcinoma
    b. cyst
bronchography
    Cope method of b.
broncholith
broncholithiasis
bronchomalacia
bronchomycosis
bronchopathy
bronchopleural fistula
bronchopneumonia
    acute hemorrhagic b.
    confluent b.
    diffuse b.
    focal b.
    hemorrhagic b.
    necrotizing b.
    sequestration b.
    subacute b.
    tuberculous b.
    virus b.
bronchopneumopathy
bronchopulmonary
    b. aspergillosis
    b. dysplasia (BPD)
    b. lavage
    b. sequestration
bronchoscopic smear
bronchostenosis
bronchotracheal
    b. aspirate
bronchus
    mucous gland adenoma of b.
      (MGAB)
Brönsted-Lowry
    B.-L. acid
    B.-L. base
bronzed disease
bronze diabetes

Brooke
    B. disease
    B. tumor
broth
    boric acid b.
    carbohydrate b.
    Casman b.
    chopped meat b.
    decarboxylase b.
    Eijkman lactose b.
    ethyl violet azide b.
    glucose-format b.
    glycerin b.
    glycerin-potato b.
    GN b.
    Gram-negative b.
    haricot b.
    hippurate b.
    indole-nitrate b.
    inosite-free b.
    iron b.
    Kitasato b.
    Koser citrate b.
    lactose-litmus b.
    lauryl sulfate b.
    lead b.
    MacConkey b.
    malachite green b.
    malt extract b.
    Martin b.
    Middlebrook b.
    MR-VP b.
    Mueller-Hinton b.
    nitrate b.
    nutrient b.
    Parietti b.
    Pike streptococcal b.
    Roscnow veal-brain b.
    selenite b.
    selenite-cystine b.
    serum b.
    sodium chloride (6.5 %) b.
    Spirolate b.
    sterility test b.
    Stuart b.
    sugar b.
    tetrathionate enrichment b.
    thioglycollate b.
    thioglycollate-135C b.
    Todd-Hewitt b.
    trypticase soy b. (TSB)
    trypticase soy with agar b.

    urease test b.
    Voges-Proskauer b.
    wheat b.
    wort b.
brown
    b. adipose tissue
    b. atrophy
    Bismarck b.
    Bismarck b. R
    Bismarck b. Y
    b. edema
    b. fat
    b. induration of the lung
    b. recluse spider
    Sudan b.
    b. tumor
Brown-Brenn
    B.-B. stain
    B.-B. technique
Brown-Hopp tissue Gram stain
brownian
    b. motion
    b. movement
Brown-Symmers disease
Brucella
    B. abortus
    B. bronchiseptica
    B. canis
    B. melitensis
    B. suis
brucella
    b. agglutination test
    b. strain 19 vaccine
Brucellaceae
brucellergin
brucellin
brucellosis
    b. agglutinins
Bruch membrane
Bruck disease
Brugia
    B. malayi
    B. microfilariae
Brugsch syndrome
bruise
bruising
Brumpt white mycetoma
Brunhilde virus
Brunn epithelial nest
Brunner gland
brunneroma
brunnerosis

NOTES

Bruns syndrome
Brunsting syndrome
brush
    b. border
    endometrial b.
    b. specimen
brushings cytology
Bruton
    B. disease
    B. type agammaglobulinemia
BS
    blood sugar
BSA
    bismuth-sulfite agar
    body surface area
    bovine serum albumin
BSB
    body surface burned
BSDLB
    block in anterosuperior division of left
    branch
BSE
    bilateral, symmetrical, and equal
BSF
    B-lymphocyte stimulatory factor
BSFR
    basal secretory flow rate
        BSFR test
BSI
    bound serum iron
BSP excretion test
BSS
    balanced salt solution
    buffered saline solution
BSTFA
    bis-trimethylsilyltrifluoroacetamide
BT
    bladder tumor
    bleeding time
    brain tumor
BTB
    breakthrough bleeding
BTPS
    body temperature, ambient pressure,
    saturated
        BTPS conditions of gas
BTU
    British thermal unit
BU
    Bodansky unit
bubas
bubo
    climatic b.
    malignant b.
    primary b.
    tropical b.
bubonic
    b. plague

bubonulus
buccal
    b. smear
    b. smear for sex chromatin
    evaluation
Buckley syndrome
Bucky grid
bud
Budd
    B. cirrhosis
    B. disease
    B. syndrome
Budd-Chiari syndrome
budding
Buerger disease
buffalo neck
buffer
    b. action
    b. amplifier
    b. base (BB)
    bicarbonate b.
    cacodylate b.
    b. capacity
    Holmes alkaline b.
    Krebs-Ringer bicarbonate b. (KRB)
    Millonig phosphate b.
    phosphate b.
    protein b.
    secondary b.
    b. system
    b. value
    b. value of the blood
    veronal b.
buffered
    b. desoxycholate glucose (BDG)
    b. formalin fixative
    b. neutral formalin
    b. saline solution (BSS)
buffy
    b. coat
    b. coat micromethod
    b. coat smear
    b. coat smear study
    b. coat smear test
buffy-coated cell
bug
    assassin b.
    cone-nose b.
    harvest b.
Buhl disease
bulbar
    b. conjunctiva
    b. myelitis
bulbitis
bulimia
Bulimus
    B. fuchsianus

Bulinus
bulla, pl. **bullae**
    intraepidermic b.
    pulmonary b.
    subepidermic b.
bulldog head
Bullis fever
bull neck
bullosa
    Pseudostertagia b.
bullosis
    b. diabeticorum
bullous
    b. disease
    b. edema
    b. edema vesicae
    b. emphysema
    b. eruption
    b. granulomatous inflammation
    b. impetigo
    b. impetigo of newborn
    b. lichen planus
    b. myringitis
    b. pemphigoid
bull's-cye lesion
BUN
    blood urea nitrogen
BUN/creatinine ratio
bundle
    collagen b.
bundle-branch block (BBB)
bungpagga
bunion
Bunoslomum
Bunsen
    B. burner
    B. coefficient
Bunyamwera
    B. fever
    B. virus
Bunyaviridae
Bunyavirus
bunyavirus encephalitis
buoyant density
buphthalmos
Burchard-Liebermann reaction
Bureau of Radiologic Health
buret, burette
Bürger-Grütz syndrome
Burkitt
    B. lymphoma (BL)
    B. tumor

burn
    b. culture
    first degree b.
    fourth degree b.
    full-thickness b.
    b. index (BI)
    partial-thickness b.
    screen b.
    second degree b.
    superficial b.
    third degree b.
    ultraviolet b.
burned
    body surface b. (BSB)
burner
    Boling b.
    Bunsen b.
    laminar flow b.
Burnett syndrome
burn-in
Burow solution
burr cell
burrow
"bursa-equivalent" tissue
bursal
    b. abscess
    b. cyst
bursitis
    xanthogranulomatous b.
burst
    respiratory b.
burst-forming unit-erythroid (BFU-E)
Buruli ulcer
Bury disease
BUS
    Bartholin, urethral, Skene glands
Buschke disease
Buschke-Löwenstein
    B.-L. giant condyloma
    B.-L. tumor
Buschke-Ollendorf syndrome
Busquet disease
Buss disease
Busse-Buschke disease
Busse saccaromyces
busulfan, busulphan
    b. lung
butane
butanoic acid
butanol-extractable
    b.-e. iodine (BEI)
    b.-e. iodine test

NOTES

butanol extractable iodine assay
butanone
Butchart tumor staging
butter
    b. of antimony
    b. yellow
butterfly lung
buttonhole stenosis
butyl
    b. alcohol
    b. methacrylate
butyraceous
butyrate esterase stain
butyric acid

butyrous
    b. colony
buyo cheek cancer
Bwamba
    B. fever
    B. fever virus
By antigen
Byler disease
bypass (BP)
    b. capacitor
    cardiopulmonary b. (CPB)
byssinosis
Bywaters syndrome

C

calculus
Celsius
Celsius temperature scale
centigrade
centigrade temperature scale
curie
large calorie
 C carbohydrate antigen
 C cell
 C group virus
 C lactose test
 C peptide
 C region
 C virus

c

contact
curie
small calorie

C1

 C. esterase
 C. esterase inhibitor

C1q radioassay

C3

 C. proactivator
 C. proactivator convertase

CA

cancer
carcinoma
cardiac arrest
chronological age
common antigen
cytosine arabinoside
 CA 19-9 assay
 CA virus

Ca

calcium
cancer

CA-125, CA125

 CA-125 assay

CABG

coronary artery bypass graft

cabinet

Cabot ring body

Cacchi-Ricci syndrome

cache

 c. memory
 C. Valley virus

cachectic

 c. anergy
 c. endocarditis

cachectin

cachexia

 cancerous c.
 c. exophthalmica

c. hypophysiopriva
malarial c.
c. strumipriva
c. suprarenalis
thyroid c.
uremic c.

cacocholia

cacodylate

 c. buffer
 sodium c.

cacodylic acid

cactinomycin

cacumen

CAD

coronary artery disease

cadaver donor (CD)

cadaveric spasm

cadaverine

cadence

counting c.

cadmium

 c. assay
 c. telluride detector

café au lait spot

caffeine

 c. assay
 c. sodium benzoate

Caffey

 C. disease
 C. syndrome

Caffey-Silverman syndrome

CAG

chronic atrophic gastritis

CAH

chronic active hepatitis
congenital adrenal hyperplasia

CAHD

coronary atherosclerotic heart disease

CAHM

complex atypical hyperplasia/metaplasia

caisson disease

Cajal

 C. astrocyte stain
 C. formol ammonium bromide
  solution
 C. gold sublimate method
 C. gold sublimate stain
 C. uranium silver method

cake kidney

Cal

large calorie

cal

small calorie

Calabar swelling

C/alb/
albumin clearance
calcar
calcareous
c. degeneration
c. infiltration
c. metastasis
calcarine
calcariuria
calcemia
calcergy
calcicosis
calcific
c. concretion
c. nodular aortic stenosis
calcification
dystrophic c.
focal c.
medial c.
metastatic c.
mitral valve c.
Mönckeberg medial c.
pathologic c.
soft tissue c. (STC)
calcified
c. cartilage
c. granuloma
c. granulomatous inflammation
calcifying
c. ameloblastoma
c. epithelial odontogenic tumor
(CEOT)
c. epithelioma of Malherbe
c. pancreatitis
calcigerous
calcinosis
c. circumscripta
c. cutis
c. cutis, Raynaud phenomenon,
sclerodactyly, and telangiectasia
(CRST)
dystrophic c.
c. intervertebralis
c., Raynaud phenomenon,
esophageal motility disorders,
sclerodactyly, and telangiectasia
(CREST)
reversible c.
tumoral c.
c. universalis
calcinuric diabetes
calciokinesis
calciokinetic
calciorrhachia
calciotropism
calcipenia
calcipexic
calcipexis

calcipexy
calciphilia
calciphylaxis
systemic c.
topical c.
calcite
calcitonin
c. assay
c. gene-related peptide (CGRP)
c. testing
calcitrans
Stomoxys c.
calcium (Ca)
c. acetate formalin
c. assay
Baker formol c.
c. balance
c. deposit demonstration
c. deposition
c. disodium edetate
endogenous fecal c. (EFC)
c. gout
c. ionized assay
c. oxalate
c. oxalate calculus
c. oxalate test
c. phosphate
c. phosphate calculus
c. pyrophosphate deposition disease
(CPPD)
c. red
c. time
calcium-45
calcium-activated ATPase
calciuria
calcofluor white stain
calcospherite
calculated
c. mean organism (CMO)
c. serum osmolality
calculi (*pl. of* calculus)
calculosis
calculous pigment
calculus, pl. calculi (C)
apatite c.
arthritic c.
articular c.
biliary c.
blood c.
branched c.
bronchial c.
calcium oxalate c.
calcium phosphate c.
cardiac c.
cerebral c.
cholesterol c.
combination c.
coral c.

cystine c.
decubitus c.
dendritic c.
dental c.
encysted c.
fibrin c.
fusible c.
gastric c.
hemic c.
indigo c.
intestinal c.
joint c.
lacrimal c.
mammary c.
matrix c.
mixed c.
mulberry c.
nephritic c.
oxalate c.
pancreatic c.
pharyngeal c.
pigment c.
pleural c.
pocketed c.
preputial c.
primary renal c.
prostatic c.
renal c.
salivary c.
secondary renal c.
staghorn c.
struvite c.
urate c.
uric acid c.
urinary c.
uterine c.
vesical c.
weddellite c.
whewellite c.
Caldwell-Moloy
    C.-M. classification
    C.-M. method
calefacient
caliber
calibrate
calibration
    c. curve
    film density c.
    c. material
calibrator
    dose c.
calicectasis

Caliciviridae
Calicivirus
calicivirus
caliculus
caliectasis
California
    C. encephalitis (CE)
    C. encephalitis virus
    C. encephalitis virus titer
    C. virus
californium
Call-Exner body
Calliphora
    C. vomitoria
Calliphoridae
Callison fluid
Callitroga
callosity
callus
    bony c.
    central c.
    definitive c.
    ensheathing c.
    myelogenous c.
    provisional c.
Calmette-Guérin
    Bacille bilié de C.-G. (BCG)
    C.-G. Bacillus
    C.-G. vaccine
Calmette test
calmodulin
calomel electrode
calor
    c. febrilis
    c. fervens
    c. innatus
    c. mordicans
caloric
    c. disease
    c. quotient
calorie
    large c. (C, Cal)
    small c. (c, cal)
calorigenesis
calorigenic
    c. action
calorimeter
calorimetry
calretinin
calsequestrin
Calvatia
    C. gigantea

C

NOTES

Calvé-Perthes disease
Calvé-Perthes-Legg disease
calycectasis
calyectasis
Calymmatobacterium
    C. donovania
    C. granulomatis
CAM
    contralateral axillary metastasis
    AE1 plus CAM
    CAM 5.2 antibody
C/am/
    amylase clearance
cambium
    c. layer
CAMBO-VIP
    doxorubicin (Adriamycin),
    cyclophosphamide, etoposide,
    ifosfamide, vincristine (Oncovin),
    methotrexate, bleomycin
Cameco Syringe Pistol
cameloid anemia
camera
    Anger c.
    gamma c.
    Nikon microprocessor-controlled c.
    scintillation c.
camerostome
CAMP
    Christie-Atkins-Munch-Petersen
    CAMP factor
    CAMP test
cAMP
    adenosine 3',5'-cyclic phosphate (cyclic
    AMP)
camp
    c. fever
Campanacci
    osteofibrous dysplasia of C.
Camp-Gianturco method
camphor assay
camphorism
camptocormia
Campylobacter
    C. fetus
    C. fetus intestinalis
    C. fetus jejuni
    C. pylori
    C. sputorum
Camurati-Engelmann disease
Canada balsam
Canada-Cronkhite syndrome
canal
    interfacial c.
    Lambert c.
canaliculus, pl. canaliculi
    bile canaliculi

    bile duct c.
    intercellular c.
    Thiersch canaliculi
canalized thrombus
canarypox virus
Canavalia
Canavan
    C. disease
    C. sclerosis
C-ANCA
    antineutrophil cytoplasmic antibody
cancellous
    c. bone
    c. tissue
cancer (CA, Ca)
    betel c.
    c. body
    buyo cheek c.
    chimney sweep's c.
    colloid c.
    conjugal c.
    c. à deux
    encephaloid c.
    c. en cuirasse
    epidermoid c.
    epithelial c.
    familial c.
    c. family
    glandular c.
    green c.
    c. juice
    kang c.
    kangri c.
    c. management therapy
    mouse c.
    mule-spinner's c.
    paraffin c.
    peritoneal c.
    pipe-smoker's c.
    pitch-worker's c.
    c. promoter
    scar c.
    spider c.
    c. staging
    stump c.
    telangiectatic c.
canceration
cancer-free white mouse (CFWM)
cancericidal
cancerigenic
cancerocidal
cancerous
    c. cachexia
cancra (*pl. of* cancrum)
cancriform
cancroid
cancrum, pl. cancra

c. nasi
c. oris
candela (cd)
Candida
    C. albicans
    C. albidus
    C. glabrata
    C. guilliermondi
    C. klebsiella
    C. krusei
    C. meningitis
    C. parapsilosis
    C. pseudotropicalis
    C. stellatoidea
    C. tropicalis
candidal
candida precipitin test
candidemia
candidiasis
    c. serologic test
candidid
candidosis
canine
    c. adenovirus 1
    c. distemper virus
    c. herpesvirus
    c. herpetovirus
    c. oral papilloma
caninum
    Dipylidium c.
Canis
canities
canium
    Neospora c.
canker
    c. sore
cannabinoids
Cannabis
cannabism
cantharidin
C8/144 antibody
CAO
    chronic airway obstruction
caoutchouc pelvis
CAP
    College of American Pathologists
cap
    c. cell
    cradle c.
    phrygian c.
    TBG c.

capacitance
    membrane c.
capacitation
capacitive reactance
capacitor
    bypass c.
    ceramic c.
    coupling c.
    disk c.
    electrolytic c.
    filter c.
    junction c.
    Mylar c.
    output c.
    paper c.
    variable c.
capacity
    blood buffering c.
    buffer c.
    dye-binding c. (DBC)
    iron-binding c. (IBC)
    latent iron-binding c. (LIBC)
    storage c.
    total iron-binding c. (TIBC)
    trypsin-inhibitory c. (TIC)
    unsaturated vitamin B_{12}-binding c. (UBBC)
Capdepont disease
Capella
    tumor of C.
Capgras syndrome
capillarectasia
Capillaria
    C. hepatica
    C. philippinensis
capillariasis
capillaris
    Muellerius c.
capillaritis
capillarity
capillaropathy
capillary
    c. action
    c. embolism
    c. flame
    c. fragility
    c. fragility test
    c. hemangioma
    c. loop
    c. nevus
capillatus
    Solenopotes c.

C

NOTES

Capim virus
capistration
capita (*pl. of* caput)
capitis (*gen. of* caput)
capitular
capitulum
Caplan
    C. nodule
    C. syndrome
capneic
Capnocytophaga
capnohepatography
capon-comb-growth test
capping
caprate
    cellulose c.
caprine
    c. herpesvirus
    c. herpetovirus
Capripoxvirus
capsid
capsomer
    c. capsular space
    c. capsule
capsular
    c. antigen
    c. cell
    c. cirrhosis of liver
    c. lipochondral degeneration
    c. precipitation reaction
    c. synovial-like hyperplasia (CSH)
capsulata
    Emmonsiella c.
capsulatum
    Ajellomyces c.
    Histoplasma c.
capsule
    bacterial c.
    capsomer c.
    c. cell
    hyaline c.
    sooty c.
capsulitis
    adhesive c.
    hepatic c.
capture
    c. cross section
    electron c. (EC)
    K c.
    radiative c.
caput, gen. capitis, pl. capita
    c. medusae
    pityriasis capitis
    c. quadratum
Caraparu virus
Carazzi hematoxylin
carbamate

carbamazepine
    c. assay
carbamide
carbamino-carbon dioxide
carbamino compound
carbaminohemoglobin
carbamoyl phosphate synthetase I
    deficiency
carbamoyltransferase
    ornithine c. (OCT)
carbamyl phosphate
carbamylurea
carbanion
carbaryl assay
carbazole
    3-amino-9-ethyl c.
carbenicillin
    c. indanyl sodium
carbhemoglobin
carbinol
Carbitol
carbohemoglobin
carbohydrate (CHO)
    accumulation of c.'s
    c. antigen
    c. broth
    c. fermentation test
    c. identification test
    c. inversion
    c. metabolism index (CMI)
    c. utilization test
carbohydrate-induced hyperlipidemia
carbohydraturia
carbol-fuchsin (CF)
    c.-f. stain
carbol-fuchsin-methylene blue staining
    method
carbolic
    c. acid
    c. methylene blue (CMB)
carbolism
carbol-thionin stain
carboluria
carbolxylene
carbomycin
carbon
    c. bisulfide
    c. dioxide (CO_2)
    c. dioxide absorbent
    c. dioxide acidosis
    c. dioxide combining power
    c. dioxide combining power
      measurement
    c. dioxide combining power test
    c. dioxide concentration
    c. dioxide concentration assay
    c. dioxide content
    c. dioxide dissociation curve

c. dioxide electrode
c. dioxide fixation
c. dioxide narcosis
c. dioxide output ($\mathring{V}_{CO_2}$)
c. dioxide pressure ($P\mathring{C}O_2$, pCO_2)
c. dioxide production
c. dioxide response curve
c. dioxide tension
c. disulfide
c. disulfide assay
c. disulfide poisoning
c. gelatin mass
c. inorganic compound
c. 13-labeled ketoisocaproate breath test
c. monoxide
c. monoxide assay
c. monoxide hemoglobin
c. monoxide poisoning
c. resistor
c. tetrachloride
c. tetrachloride assay
c. tetrachloride poisoning
carbon-11, -12, -13, -14
carbonate dehydratase
carbon-film resistor
carbonic
    c. acid
    c. anhydrase
    c. anhydrase inhibitor
carbonium ion
carbon monoxide
    fractional uptake of c. m.
carbonuria
    dysoxidative c.
carbonyl
carbonylhemoglobin
carbophenothion
Carborundum
Carbowax
carboxyhemoglobin (COHB, HbCO)
    c. assay
carboxyhemoglobinemia
carboxyhemoglobinuria
carboxylase
    acetyl-CoA c.
    propionate c.
    propionyl-CoA c.
    pyruvate c.
carboxylate
    c. ion
    pyrrolidone c.

carboxylesterase
carboxylic acid
carboxyl terminal
carboxymethylcellulose
carboxymethyl cellulose (CM-cellulose)
carboxypeptidase
carbuncle
    kidney c.
    malignant c.
    renal c.
carbuncular
carbunculosis
carcinelcosis
carcinemia
carcinoembryonic
    c. antigen (CEA)
carcinogen
    complete c.
carcinogenesis
carcinogenic
    c. hydrocarbon
carcinoid
    bronchial c.
    c. heart disease
    c. syndrome
    c. tumor
carcinolytic
carcinoma, pl. **carcinomas, carcinomata (CA)**
    acinar cell c. (ACC)
    acinic cell c.
    acinose c.
    acinous c.
    adenocystic c.
    adenoid cystic c. (ACC)
    adenoid squamous cell c.
    adenosquamous c.
    adnexal c.
    adrenal cortical c.
    alveolar cell c.
    anaplastic c.
    apocrine c.
    basal cell c.
    basaloid c.
    basal squamous cell c.
    basosquamous c.
    bile duct c.
    bronchial c.
    bronchiolar c.
    bronchioloalveolar c.
    bronchogenic c.
    ceruminous c.

C

NOTES

carcinoma *(continued)*
    chorionic c.
    clear cell c. (CCC)
    clear cell c. of kidney
    cloacogenic c.
    colloid c.
    contralateral infiltrating duct c.
    cribriform c.
    c. cutaneum
    cylindromatous c.
    cystic c.
    duct c.
    ductal c.
    Ehrlich ascites c. (EAC)
    embryonal cell c.
    endometrial c.
    endometrioid c.
    epidermoid c.
    epidermoid c. in situ
    epimyoepithelial c.
    c. ex pleomorphic adenoma
    fibrolamellar liver cell c.
    follicular c.
    gelatinous c.
    giant cell c.
    giant cell c. of thyroid gland
    glandular c.
    glassy cell c.
    glycogen-rich squamous cell c.
    granulosa cell c.
    hepatocellular c. (HCC)
    hepatocellular bile duct c.
    histiocytoid c.
    Hürthle cell c.
    hyalinizing clear cell c. (HCCC)
    infiltrating duct c.
    infiltrating ductal c. (IDC)
    infiltrating lobular c. (ILC)
    inflammatory c.
    intermediate c.
    intraductal c. (IDC)
    intraductal papillary c. (IPC)
    intraepidermal c.
    intraepidermal squamous cell c.
    intraepithelial c.
    invasive c.
    ipsilateral intraductal c.
    islet cell c.
    Jewett bladder c.
    juvenile c.
    kangri burn c.
    large cell c.
    latent c.
    lateral aberrant thyroid c.
    leptomeningeal c.
    liver cell c.
    lobular c.
    lobular c. in situ (LCIS)

    Lucké c.
    medullary c.
    melanotic c.
    meningeal c.
    mesometanephric c.
    metaplastic c.
    metastatic c.
    metatypical c.
    microinvasive c.
    mixed hepatocellular c.
    mucin-depleted mucoepidermoid c.
    mucinous c.
    mucoepidermoid c.
    myoblastomatoid c.
    c. myxomatodes
    noninfiltrating lobular c.
    non-small-cell c. (NSCLC)
    oat cell c.
    occult c.
    oncoplastic c.
    oxyphilic papillary c.
    papillary transitional cell c.
    pleomorphic c.
    primary c.
    pseudovascular adenoid squamous
      cell c. (PASCC)
    recurrent c.
    renal cell c. (RCC)
    reserve cell c.
    residual c.
    Robson stage I, II renal c.
    Sakamoto poorly differentiated c.
    sarcomatoid c.
    scar c.
    scirrhous c.
    sebaceous c.
    secondary c.
    secretory c.
    signet-ring cell c.
    c. simplex
    sinonasal undifferentiated c.
      (SNUC)
    c. in situ (CIS)
    small cell lung c. (SCLC)
    solid c.
    spindle cell c.
    squamous cell c. (SCC)
    superficial multicentric basal cell c.
    sweat gland c.
    thymic c.
    trabecular c.
    transitional cell c.
    tubular c.
    tubulopapillary c.
    undifferentiated epidermoid c.
    undifferentiated squamous cell c.
    V-2 c.
    verrucous c.

villous c.
Walker c.
well-differentiated c. (WDCA)
Wolfe breast c.
wolffian duct c.
yolk sac c.
carcinomatosis
leptomeningeal c.
meningeal c.
carcinomatous
c. encephalomyelopathy
c. implant
c. meningoencephalopathy
c. myelopathy
c. myopathy
c. neuromyopathy
c. pericarditis
carcinosarcoma
embryonal c.
renal c.
Walker c.
carcinosis
carcinostatic
carcoma
cardiac
c. albuminuria
c. aneurysm
c. arrest (CA)
c. calculus
c. cirrhosis
c. decompensation
c. dilation
c. disease (CD)
c. diuretic
c. edema
c. enlargement (CE)
c. enzymes/isoenzymes
c. failure (CF)
c. glycoside
c. hemoptysis
c. heterotaxia
c. histiocyte
c. index
c. liver
c. myxoma
c. polyp
c. sclerosis
c. shunt detection
c. silhouette
c. standstill
c. tamponade
c. thrombosis

C. T Rapid assay
c. valve myxomatosis
c. valvular malformation
c. valvular regurgitation
cardiasthenia
cardiectasis
Cardiobacterium
    C. hominis
cardiocentesis
cardiochalasia
cardiogenic shock
Cardio-Green (CG)
cardiolipin
cardiolith
cardiomalacia
cardiomegaly
cardiomyoliposis
cardiomyopathy (CMP)
Adriamycin c.
alcoholic c.
cardiotoxic
hypertrophic obstructive c. (HOCM)
idiopathic c.
periportal c.
primary c.
cardionecrosis
cardionector hypothesis
cardiopathy
cardioplegia
cardioptosia
cardiopulmonary bypass (CPB)
cardiotoxicity
anthracycline c.
cardiotoxic myolysis
cardiovascular
c. accident (CVA)
c. disease (CD, CVD)
c. malformation
c. renal disease (CVRD)
cardiovascular-renal (CVR)
cardioversion
cardioverter
Cardiovirus
carditis
rheumatic c.
streptococcal c.
verrucous c.
Carey Ranvier technique
CA15-3 RIA test
Carica
    C. papaya

NOTES

C

caries
   dental c.
carinate
carinatum
   pectus c.
carinii
   Pneumocystis c.
cariogenesis
carious
carmalum
carmine
   alum c.
   chrome alum c.
   indigo c.
   lithium c.
   Schneider c.
carminic acid
carminophil, carminophile
carminophilous
carneous
   c. degeneration
   c. mole
Carney complex
carnification
carnitine
carnosinase
carnosine
carnosinemia
carnosinuria
carnosity
Carnoy fixative
Caroli disease
carotene
   c. assay
carotenemia
carotenoid
carotid
   c. body
   c. body tumor
   c. sinus syndrome
carotid-cavernous fistula
carotinemia
carpal tunnel decompression (CTD)
Carpenter syndrome
Carpoglyphus
   C. passularum
carrier
   c. cell
   convalescent c.
   female c.
   c. gas
   incubatory c.
   c. protein
   c. state
   c. strain
carrier-free (CF)
carrier-mediated transport
Carrión disease

Carr-Price
   C.-P. reaction
   C.-P. test
Carter black mycetoma
cartesian
   c. coordinates
   c. nomogram
cartilage
   c. bone
   calcified c.
   c. matrix alteration
cartilage-hair hypoplasia (CHH)
cartilaginous
   c. metaplasia
   c. rest
caruncle
   urethral c.
cascade
   metastatic c.
case
   c. fatality rate
   c. history
   index c.
caseating
   c. granuloma
   c. granulomatous inflammation
caseation
   c. necrosis
case-control study
casei
   Philopia c.
   Piophila c.
casein
   c. agar
   c. hydrolysate
caseous
   c. abscess
   c. degeneration
   c. inflammation
   c. necrosis
   c. osteitis
   c. pneumonia
   c. tubercle
Casman broth
Casoni intradermal test
cassette
cast
   bacterial urinary c.
   bile c.
   blood c.
   broad urinary c.
   coma c.
   corrosion c.
   crystal urinary c.
   decidual c.
   endometrial c.
   epithelial c.
   epithelial cell urinary c.

false c.
fatty c.
fatty urinary c.
fibrinous c.
granular c. (GC)
granular urinary c.
hemoglobin c.
hyaline c. (HC)
hyaline urinary c.
mucous c.
red blood cell c.
red blood cell urinary c.
red cell c. (RC)
renal c.
spurious c.
tube c.
urinary c.
waxy c.
waxy urinary c.
white blood cell c.
white blood cell urinary c.
white (cell) c. (WC)

Castellanella
    C. *castellani*

Castellani
    C. disease
    C. test

Castellania
casting
Castle factor
Castleman
    C. disease
    C. syndrome
castor bean
castration
    c. cell
    female c.
    male c.
    parasitic c.
CAT
    chlormerodrin accumulation test
cat
    c. distemper virus
    c. liver fluke
    c. unit
catabolic
catabolism
    antibody c.
catabolite
    c. activator protein
    c. repression
cataclysm

catagenesis
catalase
    c. test
Catalpa
catalysis
    contact c.
catalyst
    negative c.
catalytic
catalyze
catalyzer
catanella
    Gonyaulax c.
cataphoresis
cataphoretic
cataphylaxis
cataract
    posterior subcapsular c. (PSC)
catarrh
    malignant c. of cattle
catarrhal
    c. appendicitis
    c. conjunctivitis
    c. dysentery
    c. gastritis
    c. inflammation
    c. jaundice
catatorulin test
catatrichy
cat-bite fever
cat-cry syndrome
catechin
catechinic acid
catechol
catecholamine
    c. assay
    c. test
catechuic acid
categorical data
Catenabacterium
catenating
catenoid
catenulate
caterpillar
    c. cell
    urticating c.
cathemoglobin
cathepsin D
    c. D antibody
catheptic enzyme
catheter
catheterization

NOTES

cathode
  c. ray tube (CRT)
cati
  Notoedres c.
cation
  c. channel
  c. interference
cation-anion difference
cation-exchange resin
cationic dye
cat-scratch disease
cat's-eye syndrome
cattle
  c. plague
  c. plague virus
  c. wart
Cattoretti technique
Catu virus
caudal dipygus duplication
caudalizing agent
cauliflower ear
Caulobacter
causative
cause
  constitutional c.
  c. of death (COD)
  predisposing c.
  proximate c.
cause-specific death rate
caustic
cauterant
cauterization
cautery
CAV
  congenital absence of vagina
  congenital adrenal virilism
Cavare disease
cave
  Meckel c.
cave-in
caveola, pl. caveolae
cavernitis
  fibrous c.
cavernositis
cavernous
  c. angioma
  c. hemangioma
  c. lymphangiectasis
cavitary
cavitating inflammation
cavitation
cavity
  absorption c.
  body c.
  chorionic c.
  idiopathic bone c.
  inflammatory c.
Cazenave disease

CB
  chocolate blood
  chronic bronchitis
    CB agar
CBA
  chronic bronchitis with asthma
C-banding
  C.-b. stain
CBC
  complete blood count
CBF
  cerebral blood flow
  coronary blood flow
CBG
  corticosteroid-binding globulin
  cortisol-binding globulin
CBS
  chronic brain syndrome
CBV
  central blood volume
  circulating blood volume
  corrected blood volume
CC
  cord compression
  creatinine clearance
CCA
  chick-cell agglutination
  chimpanzee coryza agent
CCAT
  conglutinating complement absorption
    test
CCC
  chronic calculous cholecystitis
  clear cell carcinoma
C cell
C-cell hyperplasia
CCF
  cephalin-cholesterol flocculation
  compound comminuted fracture
  congestive cardiac failure
CC/MCL
  centrocytic/mantle-cell lymphoma
C_4 complement
C_3 complement
CCP
  ciliocytophthoria
C/cr/
  creatinine clearance
CCV
  conductivity cell volume
CCW
  counterclockwise
CD
  cadaver donor
  cardiac disease
  cardiovascular disease
  consanguineous donor
  curative dose

cd
  candela
CD1 antigen
CD1a antibody
CD2
CD3
  cytoplasmic C.
CD4
CD4/CD8 count
CD8
  C. antibody
CD15 antigen
CD20
  C. antibody
  C. antigen
CD21 antibody
CD22 antigen
CD30
CD31
  C. antibody
  C. antigen
  C. quantitative immunohistochemical
    assay
CD35 antibody
CD43
  C. antibody
  C. antigen
CD45
  C. antibody
  C. antigen
CD45RO
  CD45RO antibody
  CD45RO antigen
CD$_{50}$
  median curative dose
CD 54
CD57 antigen
CD68 antigen
CD74
  C. antibody
  C. antigen
CD79a stain
CDA
  congenital dyserythropoietic anemia
    (types I–III)
CDC
  Centers for Disease Control
CDE antigen
CDH
  congenital dislocation of hip
cDNA
  complementary DNA

  cDNA clone
  cDNA library
CDP
  continuous distending pressure
CDP-choline
CDP-diglyceride
CDP-ethanolamine
CDw75 antigen
CE
  California encephalitis
  cardiac enlargement
CEA
  carcinoembryonic antigen
  crystalline egg albumin
    CEA assay
    CEA immunoperoxidase stain
CEA-M stain
ceanothus extract
CEA-P stain
cebocephalus
cebocephaly
cecitis
cedar oil
Ceelen-Gellerstadt syndrome
CEEV
  Central European encephalitis virus
CEF
  chick embryo fibroblast
cefaclor
cefamandole
cefoperazone
cefotaxime
cefoxitin
Celebes vibrio
celestine blue B
celiac
    c. crisis
    c. disease
    c. rickets
    c. sprue
celiocentesis
celioma
celiomyositis
celioparacentesis
celiopathy
celitis
cell
    A c.
    absorption c.
    absorptive c.
    acanthoid c.
    accessory c.

C

NOTES

cell *(continued)*
  acidophil c.
  acinar c.
  adrenocorticotropic c.
  algoid c.
  alpha c.
  alveolar c.
  amacrine c.
  ameboid c.
  amphicrine c.
  amphophil c.
  anabiotic c.
  anaplastic c.
  aneuploid c.
  Anitschkow c.
  anterior horn c.
  antibody-forming c. (AFC)
  antigen-presenting c.
  antigen-responsive c.
  antigen-sensitive c.
  argentaffin c.
  argyrophilic c.
  Arias-Stella c.
  Armanni-Ebstein c.
  Aschoff c.
  Askanazy c.
  c. axis
  B c.
  balloon c.
  band c.
  barrier-layer c.
  basal c.
  basket c.
  basophil c.
  berry c.
  beta c.
  beta c. of hypophysis
  beta c. of pancreas
  Betz c.
  BeWo choriocarcinoma c. line
  bipolar c.
  Bizzozero red c.
  blast c.
  c. block preparation
  blood c.
  c. body
  Boettcher c.
  bone c.
  bovine red blood c. (BRBC)
  bronchiolar c.
  buffy-coated c.
  burr c.
  C c.
  cap c.
  capsular c.
  capsule c.
  carrier c.
  castration c.

  caterpillar c.
  centroacinar c.
  centrofollicular c.
  chief c.
  chromaffin c.
  chromophobe c.
  chronic cell leukemia
  chronic lymphosarcoma c.
  circulating reticuloendothelial c.
  Clara c.
  clear c.
  cleavage c.
  cleaved c.
  c. coat
  columnar c.
  comet c.
  contrasuppressor c.
  Conway c.
  c. count
  c. counter
  crenated c.
  crescent c.
  crystal c.
  c. cycle
  c. cycle time
  cytomegalic c.
  cytotoxic T c.
  δ-c.
  c. death
  decidual c.
  decoy c.
  delta c.
  dendritic c.
  dermal dendritic c.
  c. differentiation
  c. division
  Dorothy Reed c.
  Downey c.
  dust c.
  effector c.
  electrochemical c.
  electrolytic c.
  elongated c.
  end c.
  endothelial c.
  enterochromaffin c.
  c. envelope
  ependymal c.
  epithelial c.
  epithelioid c.
  erythrocytic blood c.
  erythroid c.
  erythropoietin-responsive c. (ERC)
  established c. line
  exudation c.
  fat c.
  Ferrata c.
  flame c.

foam c.
follicular dendritic c. (FDC)
foreign body giant c.
foreign body giant c.
frozen red c. (FRC)
frozen red blood c.'s
fuchsinophil c.
c. fusion
galvanic c.
gamma c.
ganglion c. (GC)
Gaucher c.
gemistocytic c.
germ c.
ghost c.
giant c.
gitter c.
glioblastoma c. line
glitter c.
globoid c.
goblet c.
granulocytic blood c.
granulosa c.
granulosa-lutein c.
hair c. (HC)
hairy c.
Hargraves c.
heart failure c.
HeLa c.
helmet c.
helper c.
hematopoietic progenitor c.
hematopoietic stem c.
HEMPAS c.
hilar c.
hilus c.
H-2^b mouse c.
hobnail c.
Hofbauer c.
horse red blood c. (HRBC)
Hürthle c.
hyaline c.
hybrid c.
I c.
immunocompetent c. (ICC)
immunologically activated c.
immunologically competent c.
c. inclusion
inclusion c.
inducer c.
innocent bystander c.
interdigitating reticulum c.

interstitial c.
intimal c.
irreversibly sickled c. (ISC)
irritation c.
islet β c.
islet beta c.
islet delta c.
c. junction
juvenile c.
juxtaglomerular c. (JG)
K c.
killer c.
c. kinetics
Kupffer c.
lacunar c.
Langerhans c.
Langhans c.
Langhans giant c.
LE c.
Leishman chrome c.
lepra c.
leukocyte-poor red blood c.
Leydig interstitial c.
L/H c.
    lymphocytic-histiocytic
c. line
Lipschütz c.
littoral c.
Loevit c.
lupus erythematosus c.
lutein c.
lymph c.
lymphocytic blood c.
lymphoid stem c.
lymphokine-activated killer c.
  (LAK)
malignant giant c. tumor of soft
  parts
c. marker
mast c.
megakaryocytic blood c.
c. membrane
Merkel c.
mesenchymal c.
mesothelial c.
metallophil c.
metaphase c.
Mexican hat c.
migratory c.
migratory c.
Mikulicz c.
mirror-image c.

NOTES

C

cell *(continued)*

monocytic blood c.
monocytoid c.
monosomic c.
Mott c.
multinucleated giant c.
myeloid c.
myoepithelial c.
natural killer c.
navicular c.
c. nest
neuroendocrine c.
nevus c.
Niemann-Pick c.
NK c.
nucleated red blood c. (NRBC)
null c.
oat c.
OKT c.
olfactory c.
Opalski c.
osteoclast-like giant c. (OLGC)
oxyntic c.
oxyphil c.
π-c.
packed human blood c.'s
packed red c.'s (PRC)
packed red blood c.'s
Paget c.
Paneth c.
parafollicular c.
paraimmunoblast c.
parathyroid chief c.
parathyroid oxyphil c.
parathyroid transitional c.
parathyroid wasserhelle c.
parietal c.
pathologic c.
peptic c.
perineurial c.
perineuronal satellite c.
perivenular c.
pessary c.
pheochrome c.
photoconductive c.
photovoltaic c.
physaliphorous c.
pi-c.
Pick c.
picket c.
plaque-forming c. (PFC)
plasma blood c.
plasmacytic blood c.
plump c.
pluripotential stem c.
pluripotent myeloid stem c.
polychromatic c.
polychromatophil c.

polyhedral c.
popcorn c.
pre-B c.
primitive neuroblastic c.
primordial germ c.
primordial sex c.
principal c.
progenitor c.
c. proliferation
prolymphocyte c.
pseudo-Gaucher c.
pseudoxanthoma c.
pulmonary neuroendocrine c. (PNEC)
pulpar c.
Purkinje c.
pus c.
pyrrol c.
RA c.
Raji c.
reactive c.
red c. (RC)
red blood c. (rbc, RBC)
Reed-Sternberg c. (RS)
Renshaw c.
reserve c.
resting c.
reticular c.
reticulum c.
Rieder c.
Rindfleisch c.
rosette-forming c.
Rouget c.
Russell-Crooke c.
c. salvage
c. sap
sarcogenic c.
scavenger c.
Schwann c.
sedimented red c. (SRC)
segmented c.
sensitized c.
c. separation method
serous c.
Sertoli c.
sex c.
Sézary c.
shadow c.
sheep red c. (SRC)
sheep red blood c. (SRBC)
sickle c. (SC)
sickled c.
sickle c. β-thalassemia
signet-ring c.
silver c.
skein c.
small cleaved c.
small non-cleaved c. (SNCC)

smudge c.
somatic c.
somatostatin-producing small c.
spider c.
spindle c.
spindly squamoid c.
spur c.
squamous c.
stem c.
Sternberg-Reed c.
stichochrome c.
stipple c.
c. strain
strap c.
suppressor c.
c. surface marker
c. surface receptor
sustentacular c.
syncytiotrophoblastic c.
T c.
tadpole c.
tanned red c. (TRC)
target c.
tart c.
^{99m}Tc red blood c.
T cytotoxic c.
TDTH c.
teardrop c.
tennis racket c.
tetracarcinoma c.
Tg c.
theca c.
T helper c.
thymic reticulum c.
Tm c.
totipotential c.
Touton giant c.
c. transformation
trisomic c.
T-suppressor c.
tumor c.
Türk c.
tympanic c.
Type I, II c.'s
Tzanck c.
umbrella c.
unit c.
veiled c.
virus-transformed c.
c. volume (CV)
volume of packed red c.'s (VPRC)
c. volume profile (CVP)

c. wall
c. wall defective bacteria culture
c. wall-deficient bacterial forms
  (CWDF)
wandering c.
Warthin-Finkeldey-type giant c.
washed red c.'s (WRC)
washed red blood c.'s
wasserhelle c.
water-clear c.
c. web
white c. (WC)
white blood c. (WBC)
xanthoma c.
zymogenic c.
cell-bound antibody
cell-cycle inhibitor
Cellfalcicula
cell-free system
cell-mediated
  c.-m. immunity (CMI)
  c.-m. lympholysis assay
  c.-m. reaction
cellobiase
cellobiose
celloidin
cellophane
  c. tape method
Cellosolve
cellular
  c. adaptation
  c. atypia
  c. biology
  c. blue nevus
  c. cloning
  c. degeneration
  c. embolism
  c. hybridization
  c. immune theory
  c. immunity
  c. immunity deficiency syndrome
    (CIDS)
  c. immunodeficiency with abnormal
    immunoglobulin synthesis
  c. infiltration
  c. kinetic
  c. pathology
  c. polyp
  c. schwannoma
  c. spill
  c. swelling
  c. tumor

NOTES

C

cellulase
cellulite
cellulitic phlegmasia
cellulitis
    eosinophilic c.
    epizootic c.
    pelvic c.
    phlegmonous c.
    streptococcal c.
cellulocutaneous plague
cellulose
    c. acetate
    c. caprate
    carboxymethyl c. (CM-cellulose)
    c. tape technique
cellulosity
Cellvibrio
    C. mixtus
celom
celoschisis
celosomia
CELO virus
celozoic
Celsius (C)
    Celsius temperature scale (C)
    Celsius thermometer
Celsus kerion
cement
    intercellular c.
    c. line
    c. substance
cementification
cementifying fibroma
cementoblast
cementoblastoma
cementoma
cemento-ossifying fibroma (COF)
cementum
cenobium
cenocyte
cenocytic
censored observation
center
    chiral c.
    C.'s for Disease Control (CDC)
    follicular c.
    germinal c.
    progressive transformation of
      germinal c.'s (PTGC)
    pseudofollicular proliferation c.
centigrade (C)
    centigrade scale

centigrade temperature scale (C)
    centigrade thermometer
centigram (cg)
centiliter (cL, cl)
centimeter (cm)
    cubic c. (cu cm)
centimeter-gram-second (CGS, cgs)
    c. system
    c. unit
centimorgan (cMo)
centipede
centipoise (cP)
centistoke (cSt)
central
    c. blood volume (CBV)
    c. callus
    c. chemoreceptor
    c. chromatolysis
    c. core disease
    C. European encephalitis virus
      (CEEV)
    C. European tick-borne encephalitis
      virus
    C. European tick-borne fever
    c. excitatory state (CES)
    c. ganglioneuroma
    c. hemorrhagic necrosis (CHN)
    c. inhibitory state (CIS)
    c. lesion
    c. limit theorem
    c. necrosis
    c. nervous system tuberculosis
    c. nervous system tumor
    c. neurocytoma
    c. osteitis
    c. pneumonia
    c. pontine myelinolysis
    c. processing unit
    c. Recklinghausen disease type II
    c. tendency
    c. type neurofibromatosis
    c. venous pressure
centri-acinar emphysema
centric fusion
Centriflo filter
centrifugal
    c. fast analyzer
    c. flotation
    c. force
centrifugalization
centrifugalize
centrifugation
    density gradient c.
centrifuge
    Eppendorf c.
centrilobular
    c. emphysema
    c. necrosis

centriole
centripetal force
centroacinar cell
Centrocestus
centrocyte
centrocytic lymphoma
centrocytic/mantle-cell lymphoma
 (CC/MCL)
centrofollicular cell
centromere
    c. banding stain
    c. enumeration probe (CEP)
    c. interference
centromere/kinetochore antibody
centromeric band
centronuclear myopathy
centroplasm
centrosome
centrosphere
Centruroides
cenuris
cenurosis
cenurus
CEOT
    calcifying epithelial odontogenic tumor
CEP
    centromere enumeration probe
    congenital erythropoietic porphyria
Cephaelis
cephalad
cephaledema
cephalemia
cephalexin
cephalhematocele
cephalhematoma
cephalhydrocele
cephalic
    c. index
cephalin
    c. flocculation
    c. flocculation test
cephalin-cholesterol
    c.-c. flocculation (CCF)
    c.-c. flocculation test
cephaline
cephalitis
cephalocele
cephalocentesis
cephaloglycin
cephalohematocele
cephalohematoma
cephalohemometer

cephalomegaly
cephalomeningitis
Cephalomyia
cephalont
cephalo-oculocutaneous telangiectasia
cephalopathy
cephalopelvic disproportion (CPD)
Cephalopoda
cephaloridine
cephalosporin
Cephalosporium
    C. falciforme
    C. granulomatis
cephalothin
cephalothoracopagus
cephalotrigeminal angiomatosis
cephamycins
cephapirin
cephradine
cera
ceramic capacitor
ceramidase
ceramide
    glycosyl c.
    c. hexoside
    c. lactoside
    c. lactosidosis
    lactosyl c.
    c. trihexosidase
Ceratophyllidae
Ceratophyllus
Ceratopogonidae
cercaria
cercarien-hullen-reaktion test
cerci
cercocystis
cercomer
cercomonad
Cercomonas
Cercopithecus
cercosporamycosis
cercus
cerebellar
    c. agenesis
    c. astrocytoma
    c. cyst
    c. sarcoma
cerebellitis
cerebellomedullary malformation
 syndrome
cerebellopontine angle tumor
cerebellum

C

NOTES

cerebral
   c. amyloid angiopathy
   c. atrophy
   c. blood flow (CBF)
   c. calculus
   c. cladosporiosis
   c. compression
   c. cortex perfusion rate (CPR)
   c. death
   c. dysplasia
   c. edema
   c. embolism
   c. epidural abscess
   c. glucose oxygen quotient (CG/OQ)
   c. hemorrhage
   c. hernia
   c. herniation
   c. infarct
   c. infarction (CI)
   c. metabolic rate (CMR)
   c. metabolic rate of glucose (CMRG)
   c. metabolic rate of oxygen (CMRO)
   c. palsy (CP)
   c. porosis
   c. sphingolipidosis
   c. thrombosis (CT)
   c. tuberculosis
cerebralis
   adiposis c.
cerebriform
cerebris
   mycetismus c.
cerebritis
   suppurative c.
cerebrocuprein
cerebrohepatorenal syndrome
cerebromalacia
cerebromeningitis
cerebronic acid
cerebropathia
cerebropathy
cerebrosclerosis
cerebroside
   c. β-galactosidase
   c. β-glucosidase
   c. lipidosis
   c. sulfatide
cerebrosidosis
cerebrospinal
   c. fever
   c. fluid (CSF)
   c. fluid analysis
   c. fluid assay
   c. fluid culture
   c. fluid cytology

   c. fluid electrophoresis
   c. fluid IgG synthesis rate
   c. fluid myelin basic protein
   c. fluid oligoclonal bands
   c. fluid pressure
   c. fluid protein electrophoresis
   c. meningitis (CSM)
cerebrospinant
cerebrotendinous
   c. cholesterinosis
   c. xanthomatosis
cerebrovascular
   c. accident (CVA)
   c. obstructive disease (CVOD)
   c. resistance (CVR)
Cerithidea
cerium
ceroid
   c. pigment
   c. storage disease
ceroplasty
certified
   C. Laboratory Assistant (CLA)
   c. stain
   c. standard
cerulea
   macula c.
cerulein
ceruleus
   locus c.
ceruloplasmin
   c. assay
   c. test
cerumen
ceruminoma
ceruminous
   c. adenoma
   c. carcinoma
cervical
   c. abortion
   c. adenitis
   c. culture
   c. diverticulum
   c. dysplasia
   c. fistula
   c. hygroma
   c. intraepithelial neoplasia (CIN)
   c. mucus sperm penetration test
   c. polyp
   c. rib syndrome
   c. scraper
   c. secretion
   c. smear
   c. somatosensory evoked potential
   c. spondylosis
cervical/vaginal cytology
cervices (*pl. of* cervix)

cervicitis
    cystic chronic c.
cervicovaginal lavage
cervix, pl. **cervices**
    incompetent c.
CES
    central excitatory state
cesarean-obtained barrier-sustained (COBS)
cesarean section
cesium
Cestan-Chenais syndrome
Cestan-Raymond syndrome
Cestan syndrome
C$_1$ esterase inhibitor
Cestoda
Cestodaria
cestode
cestodiasis
Cestoidea
Cetraria
cetyl
cetylpyridium chloride test
cetyltrimethylammonium bromide
ceylonica
    Haemadipsa c.
CF
    carbol-fuchsin
    cardiac failure
    carrier-free
    chemotactic factor
    Chiari-Frommel syndrome
    citrovorum factor
    complement fixation
    complement-fixing
    cystic fibrosis
        CF antibody
        CF antibody titer
        CF test
CFA
    complement-fixing antibody
CFF
    critical flicker fusion
        CFF test
c-fos oncogene
CFP
    chronic false-positive
    cystic fibrosis of pancreas
CFT
    complement-fixation test
CFU-C
    colony-forming unit-culture

CFU-E
    colony-forming unit-erythroid
CFU/mL
    colony-forming units/mL
CFU-S
    colony-forming unit-spleen
CFWM
    cancer-free white mouse
CG
    Cardio-Green
    chorionic gonadotropin
    chronic glomerulonephritis
    colloidal gold
    phosgene (choking gas)
        chrome violet CG
cg
    centigram
CGD
    chronic granulomatous disease
CGL
    chronic granulocytic leukemia
C-glycoholic acid breath test
CGN
    chronic glomerulonephritis
CG/OQ
    cerebral glucose oxygen quotient
CGP
    chorionic growth hormone prolactin
    circulating granulocyte pool
CGRP
    calcitonin gene-related peptide
CGS, cgs
    centimeter-gram-second
        CGS system
        CGS unit
CGT
    chorionic gonadotropin
CGTT
    cortisone-glucose tolerance test
CH
    cholesterol
    crown-heel
CHA
    congenital hypoplastic anemia
Chabert disease
Chabertia
Chaetoconidium
Chaetomium
Chagas
    C. disease
    C. disease serological test
Chagas-Cruz disease

NOTES

C

chagoma
Chagres virus
chain
    α-c.
    alpha c.
    branched c.
    γ-c. disease
    μ-c. disease
    electron transport c.
    H c.
    heavy c.
    hemolytic c.
    c. isomerism
    J c.
    κ-c.
    kappa c.
    λ-c.
    L c.
    lambda c.
    light c.
    nuclear c.
    c. reaction
    respiratory c.
    sympathetic c.
chaining
chalasia
chalaza
chalazion, pl. chalazia
chalcogen
chalcogenide
chalcone
chalcosis
chalicosis
challenge
chalone
chamber
    Abbé-Zeiss counting c.
    anaerobic c.
    Boyden c.
    counting c.
    hyperbaric c.
    ionization c.
    multiwire proportional c.
    Shandon cytospin c.
    Thoma counting c.
    Zappert counting c.
Chamberland filter
chamecephaly
Championnière disease
Champy fixative
chancre
    hard c.
    mixed c.
    monorecidive c.
    c. redux
    soft c.
    sporotrichositic c.
    tularemic c.

chancriform
    c. pyoderma
    c. syndrome
chancroid
chancroidal
    c. ulcer
chancrous
chandeliers
    favic c.
Chang aniline-acid fuchsin method
change
    Armanni-Ebstein c.
    Baggenstoss c.
    Crooke hyaline c.
    decidual c.
    degenerative c.
    fatty c.
    harlequin color c.
    onionskin c.'s
    Paneth cell-like c. (PCLC)
    polycystic c.
    pseudocarcinomatous c.
    Tenney c.'s
channel
    cation c.
Chantemesse reaction
character
    acquired c.
    c. density
    dominant c.
    mendelian c.
    monogenic c.
    primary sex c.
    recessive c.
    secondary sex c.
    sex-conditioned c.
    sex-limited c.
    sex-linked c.
    X-linked c.
    Y-linked c.
characteristic
    c. curve
    receiver operating c.
charcoal
    activated c.
Charcot
    C. arthropathy
    C. disease
    C. syndrome
Charcot-Böttcher crystalloid
Charcot-Leyden crystal
Charcot-Marie-Tooth
    C.-M.-T. disease
    C.-M.-T. muscular atrophy
Charcot-Neumann crystal
Charcot-Robin crystal
Charcot-Weiss-Barker syndrome

charge
    elementary c.
    ionic c.
    space c.
charged particle
charge-transfer complex
Charles law
Charlin syndrome
Charlouis disease
chart
    alignment c.
    flow c.
    Levey-Jennings c.'s
    pedigree c.
    quality control c.
Chauffard-Still syndrome
Chauffard syndrome
Chaussier areola
CHB
    complete heart block
CHD
    congestive heart disease
    coronary heart disease
ChE
    cholesterol ester
    cholinesterase
Cheadle disease
check
    alert c.
    c. bit
    Δ c.
    δ c.
    c. digit
    limit c.
    linearity c.
    parity c.
    previous value c.
Chédiak-Higashi
    C.-H. disease
    C.-H. syndrome (CHS)
Chédiak-Steinbrinck-Higashi
    C.-S.-H. anomaly
    C.-S.-H. syndrome
Chédiak test
cheek
    cleft c.
cheese
    c. washer's disease
    c. worker's lung
cheesy pus
cheilitis
cheilosis

cheiragra
cheirarthritis
chelate
chelating agent
chelation
Chelex DNA amplification
chelicera
cheloid
chemical
    c. adsorption
    c. asphyxiant
    c. bond
    c. equation
    c. equilibrium
    c. incompatibility
    incompatible c.'s
    c. inhibition isoamylase test
    c. interference
    c. mediator
    c. peritonitis
    c. pneumonia
    c. pneumonitis
    c. prophylaxis
    c. reaction
    c. shift
    c. styptic
    c. waste
chemically pure (CP)
chemiluminescence
    c. assay
    electrogenerated c. (ECL)
    c. test
cheminosis
chemiosmotic
    c. hypothesis
chemisorption
chemistry
    analytical c.
    clinical c.
    inorganic c.
    organic c.
    physical c.
    physiologic c.
    c. profile
chemoattractant
chemoautotroph
chemoautotrophic bacterium
chemocoagulation
chemodectoma
chemodectomatosis
chemoheterotroph
chemoheterotrophic bacterium

C

NOTES

chemoimmunology
chemoimmunotherapy (CI)
chemokines
chemokinesis
chemolithotroph
chemoluminescence
chemoorganotroph
chemoreceptor
  central c.
  peripheral c.
  c. tumor
chemoresistance
chemosensitive
chemostat
chemosterilant
chemosynthesis
chemotactic
  c. activity
  c. factor (CF)
chemotactin
chemotaxin
chemotaxis assay
chemotherapeutic index (CI)
chemotherapy
  ablative c.
chemotransmitter
chemotroph
chemotropism
Chemstrip BG test
ChemTRAK liquid chemistry control
Cheney syndrome
chenodeoxycholate
chenodeoxycholic
  c. acid
  c. acid test
Chenopodium
chenopodium oil
Chen test
Cherchevski disease
Cherchewski disease
cherry
  c. angioma
  c. red spot
Cherry-Crandall procedure
cherubic facies
cherubism
chest
  alar c.
  barrel c.
  blast c.
  cobbler's c.
  foveated c.
  pterygoid c.
  tetrahedron c.
Chester disease
Cheyletiella
  C. parasitovorax

CHF
  congestive heart failure
CHH
  cartilage-hair hypoplasia
chi
Chiari
  C. disease
  C. II syndrome
  C. net
Chiari-Arnold syndrome
Chiari-Budd syndrome
Chiari-Frommel syndrome (CF)
chiasma
chick-cell agglutination (CCA)
chick embryo fibroblast (CEF)
chicken
  c. embryo lethal orphan virus
  c. fat clot
  c. louse
chickenpox
  c. immune globulin (human)
  c. immunoglobulin
  c. virus
Chick-Martin test
chief
  c. agglutinin
  c. cell
  c. cell adenoma
Chiffelle and Putt method
chigger
chigoe
chikungunya
  c. fever
  c. fever virus
Chilaiditi syndrome
chilblain
CHILD
  congenital hemidysplasia with
  ichthyosiform erythroderma and limb
  defects
  CHILD syndrome
Child
  C. hepatic risk criteria
childbed fever
childhood
  c. hemolytic uremic syndrome
  c. type tuberculosis
chilomastigiasis
Chilomastix
  C. mesnili
chilomastosis
chilopod
Chilopoda
chilopodiasis
chimera
  blood group c.
  dispermic c.
  heterologous c.

homologous c.
isologous c.
radiation c.
chimeric
    c. antibody
chimerism
    hematolymphoid c.
chimney sweep's cancer
chimpanzee coryza agent (CCA)
chin
    galoche c.
Chinese
    C. liver fluke
    C. restaurant syndrome (CRS)
chip
    bone c.
    c. fracture
chiral
    c. center
    c. crystal
chirality
Chiroptera
chi-squared
    c.-s. distribution
    c.-s. test
chitin
Chlamydia
    C. antigen
    C. culture
    C. group titer
    C. oculogenitalis
    C. pneumoniae
    C. psittaci
    C. trachomatis
    C. trachomatis direct FA test
Chlamydiaceae
chlamydial disease
Chlamydiazyme
    C. EIA assay
    C. test
chlamydiosis
Chlamydobacteriaceae
Chlamydobacteriales
chlamydoconidium
Chlamydophrys
chlamydospore
Chlamydozoon
chloasma
    c. bronzinum
chloracne

chloral
    c. hydrate
    c. hydrate assay
chloramine-T
chloramphenicol
chloranil assay
chloranilate method
chlorate
    c. assay
    potassium c.
chlorazol
    c. black E stain
chlorbenside
chlordane
chlordiazepoxide
    c. assay
chloremia
chloride
    benzalkonium c.
    cobaltous c.
    dansyl c.
    edrophonium c.
    gold c.
    hydrogen c.
    c. method
    methylrosaniline c.
    palladium c.
    polyvinyl c.
    pralidoxime c.
    Schales and Schales method for c.
    c. shield
    c. shift
    sodium c.
    vinyl c.
chloridimetry
chloridometer
chloriduria
chlorinated
    c. hydrocarbon pesticide
    c. hydrocarbon pesticide assay
chlorine
chlormerodrin accumulation test (CAT)
chloroanemia
Chlorobacteriaceae
Chlorobacterium
chlorobenzilate
Chlorobium
Chlorochromatium
chlorofluorocarbon
chloroform
    c. assay

C

NOTES

chloroform *(continued)*
  methyl c.
  c. poisoning
chloroform-methanol
chloroguanide hydrochloride
chlorohydrin
  ethylene c.
chlorohydrocarbon assay
chloroleukemia
chlorolymphosarcoma
chloroma
Chloromycetin
chloromyeloma
chloropenia
chloropenic azotemia
chlorophenol red
chlorophenoxy herbicide
chlorophyll unit
chloropicrin
Chloropidae
chloroplast
chloropsia
chloroquine
chlorosis
Chlorothion
chlorotic
  c. anemia
chlorous acid reagent
chlorpalladium fixative
chlorphenol red
chlorpromazine assay
chlortetracycline
chloruresis
chloruria
CHN
  central hemorrhagic necrosis
CHO
  carbohydrate
choanal
  c. atresia
  c. polyp
choanoflagellate
choanomastigote
Choanotaenia infundibulum
chocolate
  c. blood (CB)
  c. blood agar
  c. cyst
choke
  ophthalmovascular c.
chol.
  cholesterol
cholagogue
cholaneresis
cholangeitis
cholangiectasis
cholangiocarcinoma
cholangiofibrosis

cholangiolar proliferation
cholangiolitic
  c. cirrhosis
  c. hepatitis
cholangiolitis
cholangioma
cholangiostomy
cholangitis
  primary sclerosing c.
  sclerosing c.
  suppurative c.
cholate
cholecalciferol
cholecyst
cholecystagogue
cholecystectasia
cholecystenterostomy
cholecystitis
  acute hemorrhagic c.
  chronic c.
  chronic calculous c. (CCC)
  emphysematous c.
  follicular c.
  glandularis proliferans c.
  xanthogranulomatous c.
cholecystocolostomy
cholecystoduodenal fistula
cholecystoduodenostomy
cholecystogastrostomy
cholecystogram
  oral c. (OCG)
cholecystoileostomy
cholecystojejunostomy
cholecystokinin-pancreozymin
cholecystokinin test
cholecystolithiasis
cholecystosis
  hyperplastic c.
choledochal cyst
choledochitis
choledochoduodenostomy
choledochoenterostomy
choledocholith
choledocholithiasis
choledochostomy
choleglobin
cholehemia
cholelith
cholelithiasis
cholemia
cholemic
  c. nephrosis
cholepathia
choleperitoneum
choleperitonitis
cholera
  Asiatic c.
  c. bacillus

hog c.
pancreatic c.
c. sicca
c. toxin
typhoid c.
c. vaccine
c. vibrio
Choleraesuis
choleragen
choleraic
choleraphage
cholera-red reaction
cholestasia
cholestasis
cholestatic
c. hepatitis
c. jaundice
cholesteatoma
cholesteatomatous
cholesteremia
cholesterinemia
cholesterinized antigen
cholesterinosis
cerebrotendinous c.
cholesterinuria
cholesterohistechia
cholesterol (CH, chol.)
c. assay
c. calculus
c. deposition
c. embolism
c. ester (ChE)
c. ester storage disease
c. polyp
c. staining method
c. test
total c. (TC)
cholesterolemia
cholesterolestersturz
cholesterol-lecithin flocculation test
cholesterolosis
extracellular c.
cholesterol-phospholipid ratio (C/P)
cholesteroluria
cholestyramine resin
choleuria
cholic acid
cholicele
choline
lysophosphatidyl c.
cholinergic
c. blockade

c. blocking agent
c. urticaria
cholinesterase (ChE)
c. assay
c. inhibitor
c. test
chololith
chololithiasis
chololithic
choloplania
cholothorax
choluria
cholylglycine
Chondodendron
chondralloplasia
chondrification
chondrify
chondrin ball
chondritis
chondroblast
chondroblastoma
chondrocalcinosis
articular c.
chondrocyte
isogenous c.'s
c. lacuna
chondrodermatitis
c. nodularis chronica helicis
chondrodysplasia
hereditary deforming c.
c. punctata
chondrodystrophia
c. calcificans congenita
c. congenita punctata
chondrodystrophic dwarfism
chondrodystrophy
asphyxiating thoracic c.
asymmetrical c.
hereditary deforming c.
chondroectodermal dysplasia
chondrofibroma
chondrohypoplasia
chondroid
c. chordoma
c. metaplasia
c. syringoma
chondroitin
c. sulfate
c. sulfate stain
c. sulfate staining
chondroma
extraskeletal c.

C

NOTES

chondroma *(continued)*
    juxtacortical c.
    periosteal c.
chondromalacia
    c. fetalis
    generalized c.
    c. of larynx
    systemic c.
chondromatosis
    synovial c.
chondromatous
    c. exostosis
    c. giant cell tumor
chondrometaplasia
chondromucoprotein
chondromyxoid fibroma (CMF)
chondromyxoma
chondro-osteodystrophy
chondropathy
chondrophyte
chondroporosis
chondrosarcoma
chondrosis
chondrotropic hormone
CHOP
    cyclophosphamide, doxorubicin
      hydrochloride, vincristine (Oncovin),
      prednisone
chopped
    c. meat broth
    c. meat medium
chopper
chordee
chorditis
chordoblastoma
chordoma
    chondroid c.
chorea
    Bergeron c.
    Huntington c. (HC)
    Sydenham c.
choreic
choreiform
choreoathetosis
chorioadenoma
    c. destruens
chorioallantoic culture
chorioamnionitis
chorioangioma
chorioangiomatosis
chorioangiosis
choriocarcinoma
chorioepithelioma
chorioma
choriomeningitis
    lymphatic c. (LCM)
    lymphocytic c. (LCM)

chorion
    abnormal c.
    c. frondosum
    c. laeve
    mature abnormal c.
chorionic
    c. carcinoma
    c. cavity
    c. epithelioma
    c. gonadotropin (CG, CGT)
    c. gonadotropin assay
    c. gonadotropin test
    c. gonadotropin unit
    c. growth hormone prolactin (CGP)
    c. somatomammotropin (CS)
    c. villi
    c. villus sampling (CVS)
chorionic gonadotropin (CG, CGT)
    c. g.-alpha subunit
    c. g.-beta subunit
    hCG-α subunit
    hCG-β subunit
Chorioptes
chorista
choristoblastoma
choristoma
    neuromuscular c.
choroideremia
choroiditis
choroid plexus papilloma
Chotzen syndrome
chr
    chronic
ChrA
    chromogranin A
    ChrA immunoperoxidase stain
Chr^a antigen
Christeller reaction
Christensen-Krabbe disease
Christensen urea agar
Christian
    C. disease
    C. syndrome
Christian-Hand-Schuller disease
Christian-Weber disease
Christie-Atkins-Munch-Petersen (CAMP)
    C.-A.-M.-P. factor
Christison formula
Christman disease
Christmas
    C. disease
    C. factor
Christopherson nuclear grading system
Christ-Siemens syndrome
Christ-Siemens-Touraine syndrome
chromaffin
    c. body
    c. cell

Gomori method for c.
c. hormone
c. paraganglioma
c. reaction
c. reaction test
c. tumor
chromaffinoma
medullary c.
chromaffinopathy
chromaphil
chromargentaffin
chromate
c. method
c. stain for lead
chromated
c. Cr 51 serum albumin
chromatica
trichomycosis c.
chromatic aberration
chromatid
c. gap
c. interference
nonsister c.
sister c.
chromatin
c. body
c. dust
heteropyknotic c.
Klinger-Ludwig acid-thionin c. for
 sex c.
marginated c.
c. network
nucleolar-associated c.
oxyphil c.
c. particle
c. reservoir
sex c.
X c.
Y c.
chromatinic body
chromatin-negative
chromatinolysis
chromatin-positive
chromation
chromatism
chromatofocusing
chromatogram
chromatograph
gas c.
chromatography
adsorption c.
affinity c.

anion-exchange c.
ascending c.
gas c. (GC)
gas-liquid c. (GLC)
gas-solid c. (GSC)
gel-filtration c.
gel-permeation c.
high-performance liquid c.
high-pressure liquid c. (HPLC)
instant thin-layer c. (ITLC)
ion-exchange c.
liquid-liquid c.
molecular exclusion c.
molecular sieve c.
paper c.
SDS-gel filtration c.
size-exclusion c.
thin-layer c. (TLC)
two-dimensional c.
vapor-phase c. (VPC)
chromatoid
chromatokinesis
chromatolysis
central c.
retrograde c.
transsynaptic c.
chromatolytic
chromatometer
chromatopectic
chromatopexis
chromatophil, chromatophile
chromatophilia
chromatophilic
c. granule
chromatophilous
chromatophobia
chromatophore
chromatophorotropic
c. hormone
chromatotaxis
chromatotropism
chromaturia
chrome
c. alum
c. alum carmine
c. alum hematoxylin-phloxine
 method
c. alum hematoxylin-phloxine stain
c. red
c. violet
c. violet CG
c. yellow

NOTES

127

chromic
    c. acid
    c. acid fixative
chromidial net
chromium
    c. assay
chromium-51
Chromobacterium
    C. violaceum
chromoblastomycosis
chromocenter
chromocyte
chromogen
    Porter-Silber c. (PSC)
    tetramethylbenzidine c.
chromogenesis
chromogenic
    c. bacterium
    c. cephalosporin test
    c. enzyme substrate test
chromogranin
    c. A (ChrA)
Chromohalobacter marismortui
chromolysis
chromolytic method
chromomere
chromometer
chromomycosis
chromonema, pl. **chromonemata**
chromopectic
chromopexis
chromophage
chromophil, chromophile
    c. adenoma
    c. granule
chromophilia
chromophilic
chromophilous
chromophobe
    c. adenoma
    c. cell
    c. granule
chromophobia
chromophobic
chromophore
chromophoric
chromophorous
chromoplastid
chromoprotein
chromosomal
    c. aberration
    c. band
    c. breakage syndrome
    c. deletion
    c. derangement
    c. inversion
    c. linkage
    c. malformation syndrome

    c. mutagen
    nonhistone c. (NHC)
    c. RNA (cRNA)
chromosome
    c. aberration
    accessory c.
    c. alteration
    c. analysis
    Balbiani c.
    c. band
    c. banding
    c. complement
    derivative c. (der)
    double minute c.
    gametic c.
    heteromorphic c.
    homologous c.
    c. map
    marker c.
    metaphase c.
    c. nomenclature
    Philadelphia c., Ph chromosome
      (Ph, Ph$_1$)
    polytene c.
    ring c.
    sex c.
    somatic c.
    c. translocation
    c. trisomy
    X c.
    Y c.
chromotoxic
chromotrope
    c. 2R
chromotropic acid
chronic (chr)
    c. abscess
    c. absorptive arthritis
    c. acholuric jaundice
    c. active hepatitis (CAH)
    c. active inflammation
    c. active liver disease
    c. adhesive pachymeningitis
    c. airway obstruction (CAO)
    c. allograft rejection
    c. anaphylaxis
    c. anemia
    c. anterior poliomyelitis
    c. appendicitis
    c. atrophic gastritis (CAG)
    c. atrophic polychondritis
    c. atrophic thyroiditis
    c. atrophic vulvitis
    c. brain syndrome (CBS)
    c. bronchitis (CB)
    c. bronchitis with asthma (CBA)
    c. bullous dermatosis of childhood
    c. calculous cholecystitis (CCC)

c. cell leukemia
c. cholecystitis
c. cicatrizing enteritis
c. constrictive pericarditis
c. cystic mastitis
c. discoid lupus erythematosus
c. eczema
c. false-positive (CFP)
c. familial icterus
c. familial jaundice
c. fibrosing pancreatitis
c. glomerulonephritis (CG, CGN)
c. granulocytic leukemia (CGL)
c. granulomatous disease (CGD)
c. hypertrophic gastritis
c. hypertrophic vulvitis
c. idiopathic jaundice
c. idiopathic megacolon
c. interstitial hepatitis
c. interstitial nephritis (CIN)
c. interstitial salpingitis
c. lingual papillitis
c. liver disease (CLD)
c. lobular hepatitis (CLH)
c. lung disease (CLD)
c. lymphatic leukemia (CLL)
c. lymphocytic leukemia (CLL)
c. lymphosarcoma cell
c. lymphosarcoma leukemia (CLSL)
c. membranous glomerulonephritis (CMGN)
c. monoblastic leukemia (CMoL)
c. monocytic leukemia (CMoL)
c. myelocytic leukemia (CML)
c. myelogenous leukemia (CML)
c. myelomonocytic leukemia (MLC)
c. nephritis
c. nonleukemic myelosis
c. obstructive lung disease (COLD)
c. obstructive pulmonary disease (COPD)
c. pancreatitis
c. passive congestion (CPC)
c. pneumonitis of infancy (CPI)
c. proliferative arthritis
c. pulmonary emphysema (CPE)
c. pyelonephritis (CPN)
c. renal disease (CRD)
c. renal failure (CRF)
c. respiratory failure
c. rheumatism
c. subdural hematoma (CSH)

c. thyroiditis
c. ulcer
c. ulcerative colitis (CUC)
c. ulcerative proctitis
c. villous arthritis
c. viral hepatitis
chronological age (CA)
chrono-oncology
chronotropic
chronotropism
chrotoplast
CHR reaction
chrysiasis
chrysocyanosis
chrysoidin
Chrysomyia
Chrysops
Chrysosporium parvum
chrysotile
CHS
  Chédiak-Higashi syndrome
Churg-Strauss
  C.-S. angiitis
  C.-S. syndrome
chutta
chylangioma
chylaqueous
chyle
  c. corpuscle
  c. cyst
  c. peritonitis
chylemia
chyliform
  c. ascites
chylocele
  parasitic c.
chyloderma
chylomediastinum
chylomicron, pl. **chylomicra, chylomicrons**
  lipoprotein c.
chylomicronemia
chylopericarditis
chylopericardium
chyloperitoneum
chylopleura
chylopneumothorax
chylorrhea
chylothorax
chylous
  c. arthritis
  c. ascites

NOTES

chylous *(continued)*
    c. effusion
    c. hydrothorax
    c. urine
chyluria
chyme
chymosin
chymotrypsin stain
CI
    cerebral infarction
    chemoimmunotherapy
    chemotherapeutic index
    color index
    Colour Index
    coronary insufficiency
    crystalline insulin
        CI number
Ci
    curie
Ciaccio
    C. fluid
    C. method
    C. stain
Ciaccio-positive lipid
Ciarrocchi disease
cicatricial
    c. horn
    c. pemphigoid
cicatrix, pl. **cicatrices**
    brain c.
    meningocerebral c.
cicatrizant
cicatrization
cicatrizing enterocolitis
Cicuta
cicutoxin
CID
    cytomegalic inclusion disease
CIDS
    cellular immunity deficiency syndrome
CIE
    countercurrent immunoelectrophoresis
CIEP
    counterimmunoelectrophoresis
CIF
    clone-inhibiting factor
cigarette-paper scar
ciguatera
ciguatoxin
Ci-hr
    curie-hour
ciliary dysentery
Ciliata
ciliate dysentery
ciliates
ciliocytophthoria (CCP)
Ciliophora
ciliorum

cilium
Cillobacterium
Cimex lectularius
cimicosis
CIN
    cervical intraepithelial neoplasia
    chronic interstitial nephritis
C/in/
    insulin clearance
cinemicrography
circadian
    c. quotient (CQ)
    c. rhythm
circinata
circinate retinopathy
circle of confusion
circling disease
circuit
    c. breaker
    delay c.
    open c.
    OR c.
    parallel c.
    printed c.
    RC c.
    series c.
    short c.
circuitry
circular dichroism
circulating
    c. anticoagulant
    c. antithromboplastin disorder
    c. atypical lymphocyte
    c. blood volume (CBV)
    c. granulocyte pool (CGP)
    c. reticuloendothelial cell
circulation
    c. rate
    c. time (CT)
circulatory
    c. collapse
    c. failure
    c. insufficiency
    c. overload
circumferential implantation
circummarginata
    placenta c.
circumnevic vitiligo
circumscribed
    c. atrophy
    c. craniomalacia
    c. edema
    c. inflammation
    c. peritonitis
    c. pyocephalus
circumscripta
    osteoporosis c.
circumvallate placenta

cirrhogenic
cirrhogenous
cirrhosis
    alcoholic c.
    biliary c.
    Budd c.
    capsular c. of liver
    cardiac c.
    cholangiolitic c.
    congestive c.
    cryptogenic c.
    diffuse septal c.
    fatty c.
    Glisson c.
    Hanot c.
    Indian childhood c. (ICC)
    juvenile c.
    Laënnec c.
    necrotic c.
    nutritional c.
    obstructive c.
    c. pigment
    pigmentary c.
    pipestem c.
    portal c.
    posthepatic c.
    posthepatitic c.
    postnecrotic c.
    primary biliary c. (PBC)
    stasis c.
    toxic c.
cirrhotic
    c. glomerulosclerosis
cirrose
cirrus, pl. **cirri**
cirsocele
cirsoid
    c. aneurysm
    c. varix
cirsomphalos
CIS
    carcinoma in situ
    central inhibitory state
cis
    c. activation
    c. configuration
cis-**acting locus**
cisterna
    perinuclear c.
    terminal c.
cis/**trans test**
cistron

Citelli syndrome
Citellus
citrate
    c. agar
    c. agar gel electrophoresis
    c. condensing enzyme
    c. intoxication
    lead c.
    c. test
citrated blood
citrate-phosphate-dextrose
citrate-phosphate-dextrose-adenine
citric
    c. acid
    c. acid assay
    c. acid cycle
Citrobacter
    C. diversus
    C. freundii
citrovorum factor (CF)
citrulline
citrullinemia
citrullinuria
Civatte
    C. body
    C. disease
    poikiloderma of Civatte
CJD
    Creutzfeldt-Jakob disease
CK
    creatine kinase
c-Ki-*ras* gene
cL, cl
    centiliter
CLA
    Certified Laboratory Assistant
    cyclic lysine anhydride
Cladorchis watsoni
cladosporiosis
    cerebral c.
Cladosporium
    C. bantianum
    C. carrionii
    C. mansonii
    C. trichoides
    C. werneckii
Cladothrix
clamp connection
Clara
    C. cell
    C. hematoxylin
clarificant

C

NOTES

clarify
Clark
    C. level
    C. malignant melanoma staging
    C. oxygen electrode
    C. rule
    C. test
Clarke fluid
Clarke-Hadfield syndrome
CLAS
    congenital localized absence of skin
clasmatocyte
clasmatocytosis
clasmatosis
class
    c. I, II, III antigens
    immunoglobulin c.
    c. switch
classical
    c. complement pathway
    c. hemophilia
classification
    American Urological System cancer
      staging c.
    Ann Arbor staging c.
    Ann Arbor tumor c.
    Arneth c.
    Astler-Coller modification of
      Dukes c.
    Bergey c.
    Bessman anemia c.
    Borrmann c.
    Broders c.
    Caldwell-Moloy c.
    Denver c.
    Dukes c.
    Eggel tumor c.
    Enzinger tumor c.
    FAB leukemia c.
    Fredrickson dyslipoproteinemia c.
    Gell and Coombs c.
    Horie tumor c.
    Jansky human blood group c.
    Jensen c.
    Kauffman-White c.
    Keith-Wagener c.
    Keith-Wagener-Barker c.
    Kiel c.
    Lancefield c.
    Lennert c.
    Levine-Rosai tumor c.
    Lukes-Butler non-Hodgkin
      lymphoma c.
    Lukes-Collins c.
    McNeer c.
    Moss c.
    Paris c.
    Portmann c.

    Rappaport c.
    Runyon c.
    Rye c.
    Seattle c.
    Skinner c.
clathrate
Clathrochloris
Clathrocystis
Clauberg
    C. test
    C. unit
Claude
    C. Bernard-Horner syndrome
    C. syndrome
claudication
    intermittent c. (IC)
    venous c.
clause
    Delaney c.
clausura
clavate
clavi (*pl. of* clavus)
Claviceps purpurea
claviculus
clavus, pl. **clavi**
claw
    griffin c.
clawfoot
clawhand
CLBBB
    complete left bundle-branch block
CLD
    chronic liver disease
    chronic lung disease
clean-catch
    c.-c. collection method
    c.-c. urine culture
cleaning solution
clear
    c. cell
    c. cell acanthoma
    c. cell adenocarcinoma
    c. cell adenoma
    c. cell carcinoma (CCC)
    c. cell carcinoma of kidney
    c. cell hidradenoma
    c. cell meningioma
    c. cell sarcoma
    c. cell "sugar" tumor
    c. plaque mutation
clearance
    albumin c. (C/alb/)
    p-aminohippurate c. (C/pah/)
    amylase c. (C/am/)
    blood urea c.
    creatinine c. (CC, C/cr/)
    endogenous creatinine c.
    exogenous creatinine c.

free water c.
immune c.
insulin c. (C/in/)
interocclusal c.
inulin c.
iron plasma c.
maximum urea c.
osmolal c.
para-aminohippurate c.
plasma c.
standard urea c.
thyroidal c.
total body c. (Q_B)
urea c. (C/u/, UC)

clearing
c. factor
c. factor lipase
c. medium

Cleary
method of C.

cleavage
c. cell
heterolytic c.
homolytic c.
c. of ovum
c. product
progressive c.

cleaved cell
cleft
c. cheek
c. face
Larrey c.
c. leaflet, mitral valve
c. leaflet, tricuspid valve
c. lip
Maurer c.
c. nose
c. palate
c. spine
c. tongue

cleidocranial, clidocranial
c. dysostosis
c. dysplasia

cleistothecium
Cleland reagent
cleptoparasite
CLH
chronic lobular hepatitis
cutaneous lymphoid hyperplasia

clidocranial (*var. of* cleidocranial)
climacteric
delayed c.

climatic bubo
clindamycin
cline
clinical
c. bacteriologic specimen
c. chemistry
c. chemistry automation
c. chemistry quality control
c. cytogenetics
c. diagnosis
c. diagnostic bacteriology
c. genetics
c. laboratory
C. Laboratory Management Association (CLMA)
c. laboratory maximum area
c. medicine
c. microbiology quality control
c. pathology
c. sensitivity
c. spectrometry
c. spectroscopy
c. spectrum
c. toxicology
c. trials

Clinical Laboratory Scientist (CLS)
clinicopathologic
c. analysis
c. conference (CPC)
c. study

clinilab
Clinistix
Clinitest stool test
clinoscope
exogenous creatinine c.

clip
alligator c.

Clitocybe
clitoridis
smegma c.

clivus
CLL
chronic lymphatic leukemia
chronic lymphocytic leukemia

CLMA
Clinical Laboratory Management Association

cloacogenic
c. carcinoma
c. polyp

C

NOTES

133

clock
    biological c.
    real-time c.
clomiphene test
Clonad monoclonal antibody
clonal
    c. deletion theory
    c. expansion
    c. selection theory
clonazepam
clone
    cDNA c.
    genomic DNA c. (chromosomal)
clone-inhibiting factor (CIF)
clonic
clonidine suppression test
cloning
    cellular c.
    gene c.
    c. inhibitory factor
    molecular c.
    c. vector
clonogenic
    c. assay
clonorchiasis
clonorchiosis
Clonorchis sinensis
clonus
Cloquet canal remnant
closed
    c. dislocation
    c. fracture
closed-loop obstruction
clostridial
    c. myonecrosis
    c. myositis
clostridiopeptidase A
Clostridium
    C. bifermentans
    C. botulinum
    C. butyricum
    C. clostridiiforme
    C. difficile
    C. difficile toxin
    C. difficile toxin assay
    C. histolyticum
    C. histolyticum collagenase
    C. histolyticum collagenase
    C. innocuum
    C. novyi
    C. perfringens
    C. ramosum
    C. septicum
    C. sordelli
    C. sphenoides
    C. tetani
    C. welchii

closure
    delayed primary c. (DPC)
clot
    antemortem c.
    blood c.
    chicken fat c.
    currant jelly c.
    c. lysis
    c. lysis time (CLT)
    postmortem c.
    c. reaction
    c. retraction
    c. retraction time
CLOtest test
clottage
clotting
    c. factor
    c. time (CT)
Cloudman melanoma
cloudy
    c. swelling
    c. swelling degeneration
    c. urine
Clough-Richter syndrome
Clouston syndrome
clove oil
cloverleaf skull
cloxacillin sodium
CLS
    Clinical Laboratory Scientist
CLSL
    chronic lymphosarcoma leukemia
CLSM
    confocal laser scan microscopy
CLT
    clot lysis time
clubbed
    c. digit
    c. finger
    c. toe
clubbing
    hereditary c.
clubfoot
clubhand
clump
clumping
cluster of differentiation
    c. o. d. 2, 3, 4, 8
clusters
    sinusoidal foam cell c.
Clutton joint
cm
    centimeter
CMB
    carbolic methylene blue
CMC
    critical micelle concentration

CM-cellulose
carboxymethyl cellulose
CMF
chondromyxoid fibroma
CMGN
chronic membranous glomerulonephritis
CMI
carbohydrate metabolism index
cell-mediated immunity
CMID
cytomegalic inclusion disease
c/min
cycles per minute
CML
chronic myelocytic leukemia
chronic myelogenous leukemia
CMM
cutaneous malignant melanoma
cmm
cubic millimeter
CMN
cystic medial necrosis
CMN-AA
cystic medial necrosis of ascending aorta
CMO
calculated mean organism
cMo
centimorgan
CMoL
chronic monoblastic leukemia
chronic monocytic leukemia
CMOS logic
CMP
cardiomyopathy
CMP-*N*-acetyl-D-neuraminate
CMR
cerebral metabolic rate
crude mortality ratio
CMRG
cerebral metabolic rate of glucose
CMRO
cerebral metabolic rate of oxygen
CMRR
common mode rejection ratio
CMV
cytomegalovirus
CMV culture
CMV isolation
Cnephia
CNHD
congenital nonspherocytic hemolytic
disease

Cnidospora
Cnidosporidia
CO
corneal opacity
CO_2
carbon dioxide
CO_2 output
CO_2 production
CoA
coenzyme A
coacervate
coacervation
coag
coagulation
Coag-a-mate prothrombin device
coagglutinin
coagula (*pl. of* coagulum)
coagulable
coagulant
coagulase
c. test
coagulate
coagulated albumin
coagulating enzyme
coagulation (coag)
diffuse intravascular c. (DIC)
disseminated intravascular c. (DIC)
exogenous anticoagulant c.
c. factor
c. factor assay
c. factor inhibitor
c. factors I, II, III, IV, V, VII,
VIII, IX, X, XI, XII, XIII
c. factor transfusion
fibrinolysin c.
c. necrosis
c. pathway
plasmin c.
c. time (CT)
c. time test
coagulative
c. necrosis
coagulin
coagulogram
coagulopathy
consumption c.
intravascular consumption c.
(IVCC)
coagulum, pl. coagula
coal
c. tar
c. workers' pneumoconiosis (CWP)

NOTES

135

coalescence
coarctate
coarctation
    c. of aorta
coarsening
coat
    buffy c.
    cell c.
    C. disease
    fuzzy c.
coating fixative
cobalamin
cobalt assay
cobaltinitrite method
cobaltous chloride
Cobas
    C. Fara H centrifugal analyzer
    C. Helios differential analyzer
cobbler's chest
Coblentz test method
cobra
    c. hemotoxin
    c. venom
    c. venom cofactor
    c. venom factor
COBS
    cesarean-obtained barrier-sustained
cocaethylene
cocaine
    c. hydrochloride
    c. metabolite assay
    tetracaine, epinephrine, and c.
    (TAC)
cocarboxylase
cocarcinogen
cocarcinogenesis
cocarde reaction
coccal
cocci (*pl. of* coccus)
Coccidia
coccidia (*pl. of* coccidium)
coccidial
Coccidiasina
coccidioidal
    c. granuloma
Coccidioides
    C. immitis
coccidioidin test
coccidioidoma
coccidioidomycosis
    c. antibodies
    asymptomatic c.
    disseminate c.
    latent c.
    primary c.
    secondary c.
coccidiosis

Coccidium
    C. hominis
coccidium, pl. coccidia
coccinella
coccinellin
coccobacillus
coccobacteria
coccoid
coccus, pl. cocci
    Gram-negative cocci
    Gram-positive cocci
coccygeal fistula
coccygeum
    glomus c.
Cochin China diarrhea
cochineal
cochlear hydrops
Cochliomyia
    C. hominivorax
Cockayne
    C. disease
    C. syndrome
cockroach
cockscomb
    c. polyp
    c. ulcer
coctoprecipitin
cocultivation
cocurrent
COD
    cause of death
code
    degenerate c.
    genetic c.
    Hollerith c.
    mnemonic c.
    object c.
    OP c.
    operation c.
    resistor color c.
    triplet c.
codeine assay
CODE-ON Immunoslide Stainer
coding triplet
Codman tumor
codocyte
codominance
codominant inheritance
codon
    initiation c.
    start c.
    stop c.
    termination c.
coefficient
    absorption c.
    binomial c.
    Bunsen c.
    conversion c.

correlation c.
creatinine c.
decay c.
diffusion c.
dilution c.
distribution c.
extinction c.
extraction c.
hygienic laboratory c.
inbreeding c.
c. of inbreeding
isotonic c.
lethal c.
Long c.
mass attenuation c.
osmotic c.
oxygen utilization c.
partition c.
phenol c.
rank correlation c.
regression c. (R)
Rideal-Walker c.
sedimentation c.
c. of selection
solubility c.
Spearman rank correlation c.
Svedberg unit of sedimentation c. (S)
temperature c. (Q_{10})
urohemolytic c.
urotoxic c.
c. of variation (CV)
velocity c.
volume c.
Coelenterata
coelenterate
coelioscopy
coeloblastula
coelom
coenocyte
coenocytic
coenurosis
Coenurus
coenzyme
c. A (CoA)
D-3-hydroxyacyl c. A
L-hydroxyacyl c. A
malonyl c. A
c. Q (CoQ)
coenzymometer
coeur en sabot
Coe virus

coexpression
COF
cemento-ossifying fibroma
cofactor
cobra venom c.
heparin c.
platelet c.
platelet c. I, II, V
ristocetin c.
c. of thromboplastin
Coffin-Lowry syndrome
Coffin-Siris syndrome
Cogan syndrome
COGTT
cortisone-primcd oral glucose tolerance test
COHB
carboxyhemoglobin
coherent smallpox
cohesion
cohesive termini
Cohnheim theory
cohort
c. labeling
c. study
coil
plectonemic c.
primary c.
random c.
secondary c.
coincidence
c. correction
c. error
c. sum peak
coin lesion
coinlike
Colcemid
Colcher-Sussman method
colchicine
COLD
chronic obstructive lung disease
cold
c. abscess
c. agglutination
c. agglutinin
c. agglutinin disease
c. agglutinin screen
c. agglutinin syndrome
c. agglutinin test
c. agglutinin titer
c. allergy
c. antibody

NOTES

C

137

cold *(continued)*
    c. autoabsorption
    c. autoagglutinin
    c. autoantibody
    c. gangrene
    c. hemagglutinin
    c. hemagglutinin disease
    c. hemoglobinuria
    c. hemolysin
    c. hemolysin test
    c. injury
    c. intolerance
    c. lesion
    c. microtome
    c. nodule
    c. room
    rose c.
    c. sore
    c. stage
    c. ulcer
    c. urticaria
    c. virus
cold-knife conization
cold-reacting antibody
cold-reactive antibody
cold-sensitive mutation
coldsore
colectasia
Cole hematoxylin
coleitis
Coleman-Schiff reagent
Coleoptera
coleoptosis
colestipol hydrochloride
Coley toxin
coli
    Holophyra c.
    melanosis c.
    pseudomelanosis c.
coli-aerogenes group
colibacillary
colibacillemia
colibacilluria
colibacillus
colic
    biliary c.
    endemic c.
    intestinal c.
    c. intussusception
    menstrual c.
    pancreatic c.
    renal c.
    uterine c.
    verminous c.
colicin
colicinogen
colicinogeny
coliform bacillus

colinearity
colipase
    pancreatic c.
coliphage
colistimethate sodium
colistin sulfate
colitis
    acute ulcerative c.
    amebic c.
    antibiotic-associated c. (AAC)
    balantidial c.
    chronic ulcerative c. (CUC)
    collagenous c.
    c. cystica profunda
    c. cystica superficialis
    granulomatous c.
    c. gravis
    hemorrhagic c.
    ischemic c.
    mucous c.
    pseudomembranous c. (PMC)
    radiation c.
    regional c.
    spastic c.
    ulcerative c. (UC)
    uremic c.
colitose
colitoxicosis
colitoxin
coliuria
collagen
    c. bundle
    c. degeneration
    c. deposition
    c. diseases
    c. staining method
collagenase
    Clostridium histolyticum c.
collagenoblast
collagenocyte
collagenosis
collagenous
    c. colitis
    c. fiber
collagen-vascular diseases
collapse
    circulatory c.
    massive c.
    structure c.
collar-button abscess
collectins
collection
    arterial blood c.
    urine specimen c.
collector
College of American Pathologists (CAP)
Collet-Sicard syndrome
Collet syndrome

colliculitis
2,4,6-collidine
collier's lung
colligative
collimate
collimator
colliquation
    ballooning c.
    reticulating c.
colliquative
    c. albuminuria
    c. degeneration
    c. necrosis
collision tumor
collodion
    c. baby
    c. filter
colloid
    c. adenocarcinoma
    c. adenoma
    c. body
    bovine c.
    c. cancer
    c. carcinoma
    c. corpuscle
    c. cyst
    c. degeneration
    c. goiter
    c. milium
    c. osmotic hemolysis
    c. shock
colloidal
    c. dispersion
    c. electrolyte
    c. gold (CG)
    c. gold reaction
    c. gold test
    c. iron stain
    c. osmotic pressure (COP)
    c. silicon dioxide
colloidoclasia
colloid-osmotic lysis
Collyriclum
coloboma, pl. **colobomas, colobomata**
colocholecystostomy
colocolostomy
colocutaneous fistula
coloileal fistula
colon
    c. bacillus
    giant c.
    irritable c. (IC)

    lead-pipe c.
    c. tumor
colonic
    c. fistula
    c. smear
    c. vomitus
colonization
    c. infection
colony
    bitten c.
    butyrous c.
    D c.
    daughter c.
    dwarf c.
    effuse c.
    H c.
    M c.
    mucoid c.
    O c.
    R c.
    raised c.
    rough c.
    S c.
    satellite c.
    smooth c.
colony-forming
    c.-f. unit
    c.-f. unit-culture (CFU-C)
    c.-f. unit-erythroid (CFU-E)
    c.-f. units/mL (CFU/mL)
    c.-f. unit-spleen (CFU-S)
colony-stimulating
    c.-s. activity (CSA)
    c.-s. factor (CSF)
coloproctitis
coloptosia
coloptosis
color
    complementary c.'s
    C. Index
    c. index (CI)
    c. index number
    primary c.'s
    spectral c.
Colorado
    C. tick fever
    C. tick fever virus
color-contrast microscope
colorectal polyp
colorectitis
colorimeter
colorimetric

NOTES

colorimetry
Coloscreen Self test
colosigmoidostomy
colostrum corpuscle
Colour Index (CI)
colovaginal fistula
colovesical fistula
colpatresia
colpectasia
colpitis
colpocystitis
colpocytology
colpohyperplasia
    c. cystica
    c. emphysematosa
Columbia
    C. blood agar
    C. medium
    C. S. K. virus
columbium
columella
columnar
    c. cell
    c. epithelium
coma
    alcoholic c.
    apoplectic c.
    c. cast
    c. dé passé
    diabetic c.
    Harvard criteria of irreversible c.
    hepatic c.
    irreversible c.
    metabolic c.
    uremic c.
comatose
comb-growth test
combination calculus
combined
    c. androgen blockade
    c. immunodeficiency
    c. immunodeficiency disease
    c. immunodeficiency syndrome
    c. pituitary function test
    c. sclerosis
    c. systems disease
    c. ventricular hypertrophy (CVH)
combining site
combustible
    c. gas
    c. gas detector
    c. liquid
    c. vapor
combustion
comedo, pl. comedones
    c. nevus
comedocarcinoma
comedomastitis

comedonecrosis
comedones (pl. of comedo)
comet cell
comma bacillus
command
commensal
commensalism
comment
comminuted
    c. fracture
common
    c. antigen (CA)
    c. cold virus
    c. logarithm
    c. mode rejection ratio (CMRR)
    c. mode signal
    c. opsonin
    c. reference
    c. storage
    c. variable hypogammaglobulinemia (CVH)
    c. variable immunodeficiency
    c. variable immunodeficiency syndrome
    c. wart
commotio
    c. cerebri
communicable
    c. disease
communicating
    c. hydrocephalus
community
commutator
compacta
    pars c.
compact bone
comparative pathology
comparison
    c. eyepiece
    c. microscope
    c. operation
compartmental
    c. analysis
    c. syndrome
compatibility
    ABO c.
    c. test
compatibility test
compatible
compensated
    c. acidosis
    c. alkalosis
    c. eyepiece
compensation
    broken c.
    dosage c.
    temperature c. (TC)

compensatory
c. atrophy
c. emphysema
c. hypertrophy
c. hypertrophy of the heart
c. polycythemia
c. regeneration
competence
embryonic c.
immunologic c.
immunological c.
competition
antigenic c.
c. hybridization
competitive
c. antagonist
c. inhibition
c. protein-binding (CPB)
c. protein-binding assay
competitor DNA
compiler
optimizing c.
compile time
complement
c. activation
c. binding assay
c. chemotactic factor
chromosome c.
c. component
c. deficiency state
c. direct Coombs test
dominant c.
endocellular c.
erythrocyte, antibody, c. (EAC)
c. fixation (CF)
c. inactivation
c. lysis sensitivity test
c. system
c. total
two's c.
c. unit
whole c. (WC')
complemental inheritance
complementarity
c. determining region
dominant c.
complementary
c. base
c. colors
c. DNA (cDNA)
c. gene
c. hypertrophy

c. metal oxide semiconductor logic
c. strand
c. symmetry amplifier
complementation
complement-fixation
c.-f. reaction
Reiter protein c.-f. (RPCF)
c.-f. test (CFT)
Treponema pallidum c.-f. (TPCF)
complement-fixing (CF)
c. antibody (CFA)
complement-mediated cytotoxicity
complementophil
complete
c. abortion
c. anterior dislocation
c. antibody
c. antigen
c. blood count (CBC)
c. carcinogen
c. fistula
c. heart block (CHB)
c. inferior dislocation
c. left bundle-branch block (CLBBB)
c. obstruction
c. penetrance
c. posterior dislocation
c. reaction of degeneration (CRD)
c. right bundle-branch block (CRBBB)
c. superior dislocation
c. transduction
complex
activated c.
c. adrenal endocrine disorder
AIDS-related c. (ARC)
antigen-antibody c.
antigenic c.
c. atypical hyperplasia/metaplasia (CAHM)
avian leukosis-sarcoma c.
avidin-biotin c.
avidin-biotin-peroxidase c. (ABC)
Carney c.
charge-transfer c.
feline leukemia-sarcoma virus c.
Ghon c.
Golgi c.
c. gonadal endocrine disorder
H-2 c.
histocompatibility c.

NOTES

141

complex *(continued)*
    HLA c.
    immune c.
    junctional c.
    major histocompatibility c. (MHC)
    membrane attack c.
    Meyenburg c.
    minor histocompatibility c.
    c. number
    c. odontoma
    PAP c.
    peroxidase-antiperoxidase c.
    c. pituitary endocrine disorder
    primary c.
    prothrombin c.
    ribonucleoprotein c.
    ribosome-lamella c.
    RNP c.
    sicca c.
    steroid-receptor c.
    synaptonemal c.
    Tacaribe c. of viruses
    c. thyroid endocrine disorder
    triple symptom c.
    VATER c.
    vitamin B c.
    von Meyenburg c.
complexity
    DNA c.
compliance
complication
component
    c. A of prothrombin
    blood c.
    c. of complement
    complement c.
    late positive c. (LPC)
    M c.
    micropapillary c. (MPC)
    plasma thromboplastin c. (PTC)
    secretory c.
    thromboplastic plasma c. (TPC)
composite tumor
composition resistor
compound
    acetone c.
    c. aneurysm
    aromatic c.
    carbamino c.
    carbon inorganic c.
    c. comminuted fracture (CCF)
    condensation c.
    c. cyst
    c. dislocation
    c. fracture
    c. granular corpuscle
    heterocyclic c.
    c. leukemia

    meso c.
    c. microscope
    c. multiple fractures
    c. nevus
    c. odontoma
    organometallic c.
    organophosphate c.
    polar c.
    c. presentation
    c. tumor
    c. X
compressed
    c. fracture
    c. gas storage
    c. spectral assay (CSA)
compression
    c. of brain
    cerebral c.
    cord c. (CC)
    c. injury
compromised
Con A, conA, con A
    concanavalin A
conc
    concentrated
    concentration
concanavalin A (Con A, con A, conA)
concatenate
concatenation
Concato disease
concentrate
    granulocyte c.
    intrinsic factor c. (IFC)
    marine protein c. (MPC)
    platelet c.
concentrated (conc)
concentration (conc)
    approximate lethal c. (ALC)
    bactericidal c. (BC)
    blood alcohol c. (BAC)
    carbon dioxide c.
    critical micelle c. (CMC)
    hazardous c.
    hydrogen ion c. (pH)
    hydroxyl c. (pOH)
    ionic c.
    lethal c. (LC)
    limiting isorrheic c. (LIC)
    M c.
    mass c.
    maximum permissible c. (MPC)
    maximum urinary c. (MUC)
    mean cell hemoglobin c. (MCHC)
    mean corpuscular hemoglobin c.
      (MCC, MCHC)
    minimal bactericidal c. (MBC)
    minimal inhibitory c. (MIC)
    minimal isorrheic c. (MIC)

minimal lethal c.
minimum bactericidal c.
minimum complete-killing c. (MCC)
minimum detectable c. (MDC)
minimum inhibitory c. (MIC)
minimum lethal c. (MLC)
minimum mycoplasmacidal c. (MPC)
molar c.
c. procedure
radioactive c.
renal vein renin c. (RVRC)
substance c.
c. test
time of maximum c. (T_{max})
total L-chain c. (TLC)

concentric
c. fibroma
c. hypertrophy

conception
retained products of c.

conchoidal body
concomitant immunity
concordance
concrement
concrescence
concretio
c. cordis
c. pericardii

concretion
calcific c.

concussion
brain c.
c. myelitis
spinal cord c.

condensans
osteitis c.

condensation
c. compound
c. fibrosis
c. polymer

condenser
Abbé c.
dark-field c.

condensing
c. osteitis
c. vacuole

condition
steady-state c.
sufficient c.

conditional
c. jump
c. lethal mutation
c. probability

conditional-lethal mutant
conditionally lethal mutant
conductance
conduction
c. electron
saltatory c.
volume c.

conductivity
c. cell volume (CCV)
thermal c. (TC)
water c.

conductometry
conductor
conduit
condyloma, pl. **condylomata**
c. acuminatum
Buschke-Löwenstein giant c.
flat c.
genital c.
giant c.
giant c. of Buschke-Löwenstein
c. latum
pointed c.

condylomatous
cone biopsy
cone-nose bug
conference
clinicopathologic c. (CPC)

confidence
c. interval
c. level

configuration
cis c.
germline c.
villiform c.

confluent
c. bronchopneumonia
c. inflammation
c. pneumonia
c. and reticulate papillomatosis
c. smallpox

confocal laser scan microscopy (CLSM)
conformation
conformer
confusion
circle of c.

congelation urticaria
congener

C

NOTES

congenita
  amyoplasia c.
  amyotonia c.
  pachyonychia c.
  paramyotonia c.
congenital
  c. absence
  c. absence of vagina (CAV)
  c. achromia
  c. adrenal hyperplasia (CAH)
  c. adrenal virilism (CAV)
  c. afibrinogenemia
  c. agammaglobulinemia
  c. aganglionosis
  c. anomaly
  c. aplasia of thymus
  c. aplastic anemia
  c. aregenerative anemia
  c. atransferrinemia
  c. atresia
  c. contracture
  c. cyst
  c. deformity
  c. dislocation
  c. dislocation of hip (CDH)
  c. duplication
  c. dyserythropoietic anemia (types
    I–III) (CDA)
  c. dysphagocytosis
  c. dysplastic angiectasia
  c. dysplastic angiomatosis
  c. dysplastic angiopathy
  c. ectodermal defect
  c. ectodermal dysplasia
  c. elephantiasis
  c. erythropoietic porphyria (CEP)
  c. familial icterus
  c. familial non-hemolytic jaundice
  c. generalized fibromatosis
  c. glaucoma
  c. goiter
  c. hemidysplasia with ichthyosiform
    erythroderma and limb defects
    (CHILD)
  c. hemolytic anemia
  c. hemolytic icterus
  c. hemolytic jaundice
  c. hypophosphatasia
  c. hypoplastic anemia (CHA)
  c. lobar emphysema
  c. localized absence of skin
    (CLAS)
  c. lymphedema
  c. malformation
  c. megacolon
  c. methemoglobinemia
  c. myopathy
  c. nevus

  c. nonregenerative anemia
  c. nonspherocytic hemolytic anemia
  c. nonspherocytic hemolytic disease
    (CNHD)
  c. pancytopenia
  c. porphyria
  c. pterygium
  c. pyloric stenosis
  c. rest
  c. rubella syndrome
  c. ruptured aneurysm
  c. sebaceous hyperplasia
  c. sutural alopecia
  c. thymic aplasia
  c. thymic dysplasia (CTD)
  c. torticollis
  c. total lipodystrophy
  c. toxoplasmosis
  c. valve
congestion
  brain c.
  chronic passive c. (CPC)
  hypostatic c.
  passive c.
  pulmonary c.
  pulmonary venous c. (PVC)
  venous c.
congestive
  c. cardiac failure (CCF)
  c. cirrhosis
  c. edema
  c. heart disease (CHD)
  c. heart failure (CHF)
  c. splenomegaly
conglobata
  acne c.
**conglutinating complement absorption
  test (CCAT)**
conglutination
conglutinin
conglutinogen-activating factor
Congo
  C. Corinth
  C. floor maggot
  C. red
  C. red paper
  C. red stain
  C. red test
  rubrum C.
congophilic
  c. angiopathy
conidia
conidial
Conidiobolus
  C. incongruus
conidiogenous
conidiophore
  Phialophore-type c.

conidiospore
conidium
coniine
coniofibrosis
coniolymphstasis
coniosis
Coniosporium
Conium
conization
    cold-knife c.
conjoined twins
conjugal cancer
conjugant
conjugate
    c. acid
    c. acid-base pairs
    c. base
    c. division
    c. focus
    c. redox pair
conjugated
    c. antigen
    c. bilirubin
    c. estriol
    c. hapten
    c. hyperbilirubinemia, type III
    c. protein
conjugation
    c. bridge
conjugative plasmid
conjunctiva, pl. **conjunctivae**
    bulbar c.
conjunctival
    c. fungus culture
conjunctivitis
    acute contagious c.
    acute epidemic c.
    acute follicular c.
    adult gonococcal c.
    allergic c.
    angular c.
    blennorrheal c.
    catarrhal c.
    follicular c.
    gonococcal c.
    granular c.
    inclusion c.
    infantile purulent c.
    meningococcus c.
    Moraxella c.
    c. neonatorum
    phlyctenular c.

    spring catarrhal c.
    swimming pool c.
    toxicogenic c.
    trachoma-inclusion c. (TRIC)
    tularemic c.
    vernal c.
    welder's c.
conjunctivoma
connection
    anomalous venous c.
    clamp c.
    partial anomalous pulmonary
    venous c. (PAPVC)
connective
    c. tissue
    c. tissue nevus
    c. tumor
connective-tissue diseases
Conn syndrome
conoid
Conor and Bruch disease
Conradi disease
consanguineous
    c. donor (CD)
    c. mating
consanguinity
consecutive
    c. aneurysm
    c. angiitis
consistent estimate
console
consolidation
conspecific
constant (k)
    absorption c.
    acid ionization c.
    affinity c.
    Ambard c.
    association c.
    base ionization c.
    binding c.
    Boltzmann c.
    decay c.
    dielectric c.
    diffusion c.
    disintegration c.
    dissociation c.
    equilibrium c.
    Faraday c.
    gas c.
    ionization c.
    Planck c.

C

NOTES

145

constant *(continued)*
    radioactive c.
    rate c.
    c. region (C region)
constituent
    endocrine granule c. (EGC)
constitution
constitutional
    c. cause
    c. disease
    c. dwarf
    c. hepatic dysfunction
    c. hyperbilirubinemia
    c. reaction
    c. thrombopathy
    c. ulcer
constitutive
    c. enzyme
    c. expression
    c. heterochromatin
    c. heterochromatin method
    c. mutation
constriction
    primary c.
    secondary c.
constrictive
    c. endocarditis
    c. pericarditis
construct
constructable
construction
constructive
    c. interference
    c. proof
consumption
    c. coagulopathy
    oxygen c.
contact (c)
    c. activation product
    c. allergy
    c. autoradiography
    c. catalysis
    c. dermatitis
    hospital-acquired penetration c.
    c. hypersensitivity
    c. inhibition
    c. sensitivity
contactant
contact-type dermatitis
contagion
    immediate c.
    mediate c.
contagious
    c. disease
    c. ecthyma
    c. ecthyma (pustular dermatitis) virus of sheep

    c. pustular dermatitis
    c. pustular stomatitis virus
contagiousness
contagium
    c. animatum
    c. vivum
contain
    to c. (TC)
container size limitations
containment
contaminant
contaminate
contamination
content
    carbon dioxide c.
    dye c.
    gastrointestinal c.'s
    heat c.
contiguum
    per c.
continence
continent
contingency table
contingent negative variation
continua
    acrodermatitis c.
    epilepsia partialis c. (EPC)
continued fever
continuous
    c. distending pressure (CDP)
    c. endothelium
    c. flow culture
    c. function
    c. phase
    c. spectrum
continuum
    per c.
contour
contract
contracted kidney
contractile
    c. ring
    c. vacuole
contraction
    c. band
    isovolumic c. (IC)
contracture
    congenital c.
    Dupuytren c.
    ischemic c.
    organic c.
    Volkmann c.
contrafissura
contraindication
contralateral
    c. axillary metastasis (CAM)
    c. infiltrating duct carcinoma

contrast
  bright c.
  c. media reaction
  c. medium
  c. stain
contrasuppressor cell
contrecoup
control
  c. animal
  ChemTRAK liquid chemistry c.
  clinical chemistry quality c.
  clinical microbiology quality c.
  c. experiment
  c. group
  ignition source c.
  c. material
  process c.
  quality c. (QC)
  spill c.
controlled
  c. access laboratory
  c. substance
contused wound
contusion
  brain c.
  scalp c.
  wind c.
convalescent
  c. carrier
  c. serum
convection
conventional animal
convergence
conversational mode
conversion
  c. coefficient
  c. electron
  internal c.
  Mantoux c.
  c. ratio
convertase
converter
  analog-to-digital c.
  D/A c.
  digital-to-analog c. (DAC)
  voltage-to-frequency c.
convertin
converting enzyme
convexobasia
Conway cell
cooled-knife method

Cooley
  C. anemia
  C. disease
Coomassie brilliant blue R-250
Coombs
  C. serum
  C. test (CT)
Cooper disease
Cooperia
coordinate
  cartesian c.'s
  c. covalent bond
  polar c.'s
  spherical polar c.'s
  X-Y-Z beam scanning method c.
COP
  colloidal osmotic pressure
COPD
  chronic obstructive pulmonary disease
Cope method of bronchography
copepod
Copepoda
Coplin jar
copolymer
copper
  c. assay
  c. deposit demonstration
  c. reduction test
  c. storage protein
  c. sulfate
  c. sulfate method
copper-binding protein test
coprecipitation
coprecipitin
copremesis
Coprinus
coproantibody
coprohematology
coprolith
coprology
coproma
Copromastix
  C. prowazeki
Copromonas
  C. subtilis
coprophagous
coprophagy
coprophil
coprophilia
coproporphyria
  free erythrocyte c. (FECP)
coproporphyrin (CP)

NOTES

coproporphyrin *(continued)*
    c. assay
    free erythrocyte c. (FEC)
    c. test
    urinary c. (UCP)
coproporphyrinogen oxidase
coproporphyrinuria
coprostanol
coprostasis
coprosterol
coprozoa
coprozoic
    c. ameba
copulation
CoQ
    coenzyme Q
cor, gen. **cordis**
    c. adiposum
    c. biloculare
    c. bovinum
    concretio cordis
    c. mobile
    c. pendulum
    c. pseudotriloculare biatriatum
    c. pulmonale
    c. triatriatum
    c. triloculare biatriatum
    c. triloculare biventriculare
coracidium
coral calculus
corallin
    yellow c.
Corbin technique
Corbus disease
cord
    c. blood
    c. blood screen
    c. compression (CC)
    c. factor
    marginal insertion of umbilical c.
    prolapsed umbilical c.
    ruptured umbilical c.
    sex c.'s
cordis (*gen. of* cor)
Cordylobia
    C. anthropophaga
cordylobiasis
core
    air c.
    c. antigen
    hyaline c.
    magnetic c.
    c. memory
    c. pneumonia
corectasis
coremium
corepressor
Cori disease

Corinth
    Congo C.
coriphosphine O
corneal
    c. opacity (CO)
    c. ulcer
    c. vascularization
Cornelia de Lange syndrome
corneous
Corner-Allen
    C.-A. test
    C.-A. unit
corn ergot
cornification
cornified
cornmeal agar
cornoid lamella
cornu, gen. **cornus**, pl. **cornua**
    c. cutaneum
corona, pl. **coronae**
    c. veneris
coronal section
coronary
    c. artery bypass graft (CABG)
    c. artery disease (CAD)
    c. atherosclerotic heart disease (CAHD)
    c. blood flow (CBF)
    c. embolism
    c. heart disease (CHD)
    c. insufficiency (CI)
    c. ostial stenosis
    c. prognostic index (CPI)
    c. thrombosis (CT)
Coronaviridae
Coronavirus
coronavirus
coroner
corpora (*pl. of* corpus)
    c. amylacea
    c. arenacea
    c. lutea cysts
corporea lutea twin
corporis
corps ronds
corpulence
corpulency
corpus, pl. **corpora**
    c. albicans
    c. amylaceum, pl. corpora amylacea
    corpora arenacea
    c. hemorrhagicum
    c. hemorrhagicum cyst
    c. luteum
    c. luteum hematoma
    c. luteum hormone
    c. luteum hormone unit
    c. luteum of pregnancy

corpuscle
    amniotic c.
    amylaceous c.
    amyloid c.
    Bizzozero c.
    blood c.
    chyle c.
    colloid c.
    colostrum c.
    compound granular c.
    Donné c.
    dust c.
    Eichhorst c.
    exudation c.
    ghost c.
    Gluge c.
    Hassall c.
    inflammatory c.
    lymph c., lymphoid c.
    lymphatic c.
    Merkel c.
    Mexican hat c.
    molluscum c.
    Negri c.
    Norris c.
    pessary c.
    phantom c.
    plastic c.
    pus c.
    red c.
    reticulated c.
    salivary c.
    shadow c.
    third c.
    Traube c.
    white c.
    Zimmermann c.
corpuscular lymph
corralin yellow
corrected
    c. blood volume (CBV)
    c. dextrocardia
    c. retention time
    c. reticulocyte count
    c. sedimentation rate (CSR)
    c. transposition (CT)
correction
    Allen c.
    coincidence c.
correlation coefficient
corresponding ray
Corrigan disease

corrin ring
corrosion
    c. cast
    c. preparation
corrosive esophagitis
corrosivity
cortex
    adrenal c.
cortical
    c. achromia
    c. bone
    c. defect
    c. dysplasia
    c. hormone
    c. necrosis
    c. osteitis
    c. stromal hyperplasia (CSH)
corticale
    Cryptostroma c.
corticalization
corticoid
    anti-inflammatory c. (AC)
    17-OH-c.'s test
corticosteroid-binding
    c.-b. globulin (CBG)
    c.-b. protein
corticosteroid myopathy
corticosterone
corticotrope
corticotropin
corticotropin-releasing factor (CRF)
Corticoviridae
cortisol
    c. assay
    c. production rate (CPR)
    c. secretion rate (CSR)
    urinary free c.
cortisol-binding globulin (CBG)
cortisone
cortisone-glucose tolerance test (CGTT)
cortisone-primed oral glucose tolerance test (COGTT)
cortol
cortolone
Cortrosyn
Corvisart disease
corymbiform
Corynebacteriaceae
corynebacteriophage
    β-c.
    beta c.

NOTES

Corynebacterium
>   *C. acnes*
>   *C. diphtheriae*
>   *C. diphtheriae* throat culture
>   *C. enzymicum*
>   *C. equi*
>   *C. genitalium*
>   *C. hoagii*
>   *C. hofmannii*
>   *C. infantisepticum*
>   *C. minutissimum*
>   *C. mycetoides*
>   *C. necrophorum*
>   *C. parvulum*
>   *C. pseudodiphtheriticum*
>   *C. pseudotuberculosis*
>   *C. renale*
>   *C. tenuis*
>   *C. ulcerans*
>   *C. vaginale*
>   *C. xerosis*

coryneform group
coryza
>   allergic c.

Coryzavirus
coryzavirus
cosine
cosmid
cosmopolitan
costa
costal pleurisy
costaricensis
>   *Morerastrongylus c.*

Costen syndrome
cosynthase
>   uroporphyrinogen III c.

cosyntropin
>   c. test

Cotard syndrome
Cotasil silicone slide coating material
cothromboplastin
cotinine
Cotlove titrator
cotransport
cotton dust asthma
cotton-fiber embolism
cotton-wool appearance
Cotugno disease
Cotunnius disease
cot value
Cotylogonimus
cough
>   c. plate
>   whooping c.

coulomb (Q)
Coulomb law
coulometer
coulometric titration

coulometry
Coulter
>   C. counter
>   C. STKS hematology analyzer

coumachlor
Coumadin
coumarin
Coumatrak prothrombin time device
Councilman
>   C. hyaline body
>   C. lesion

Councilmania
counseling
>   genetic c.

count
>   absolute eosinophil c.
>   Addis c.
>   agar plate c.
>   Arneth c.
>   background c.
>   blood c.
>   blood cell c.
>   bone marrow differential c.
>   CD4/CD8 c.
>   cell c.
>   complete blood c. (CBC)
>   complete blood c. (CBC)
>   corrected reticulocyte c.
>   differential c.
>   differential leukocyte c. (DLC)
>   differential white blood c.
>   egg c.
>   eosinophil c.
>   fecal leukocyte c.
>   filament-nonfilament c.
>   c. information density
>   c.'s per minute (cpm)
>   platelet c. (PC)
>   proportional c.
>   c. rate
>   c. rate meter
>   red blood c. (rbc, RBC)
>   red blood cell c.
>   Response GM granulocyte c.
>   reticulocyte c.
>   Schilling blood c.
>   Schilling blood c.
>   scintillation c.
>   spinal fluid leukocyte c.
>   too numerous to c. (TNTC)
>   total cell c.
>   total ridge c. (TRC)
>   viable cell c.
>   white blood cell c.
>   white cell c. (WCC)

counter
>   automated differential leukocyte c.
>   cell c.

Coulter c.
decade c.
electronic cell c.
frequency c.
gamma-well c.
Geiger-Müller c.
ion c.
liquid scintillation c.
proportional c.
radiation c.
ring c.
ripple c.
scintillation c.
shift c.
synchronous c.
Sysmex R-1000 reticulocyte c.
counterclockwise (CCW)
countercurrent
c. extraction
c. immunoelectrophoresis (CIE)
c. mechanism
counterimmunoelectrophoresis (CIEP)
counterstain
counting
automated reticulocyte c.
c. cadence
c. chamber
photon c.
c. plate
couple
redox c.
coupler
acoustic c.
coupling
c. capacitor
c. defect
Courvoisier law
Courvoisier-Terrier syndrome
covalent bond
Covalink MicroElisa culture plate
covariance
covariate
coverglass
cover glass
coverslip
Coverslipper
Jung CV 5000 Robotic C.
Cowden disease
Cowdria ruminantium
Cowdry
C. type A inclusion body
C. type B inclusion body

cow kidney
Cowper cyst
cowperitis
cowpox
c. virus
coxa, pl. **coxae**
c. magna
c. plana
Coxiella
C. burnetii
coxitis
Coxsackievirus
C. A, B virus titer (C virus)
C. A, type 1
C. B, type 1
C. encephalitis
Cox vaccine
CP
cerebral palsy
chemically pure
coproporphyrin
cystosarcoma phyllodes
C/P
cholesterol-phospholipid ratio
cP
centipoise
C/pah/
p-aminohippurate clearance
CPB
cardiopulmonary bypass
competitive protein-binding
CPB assay
CPC
chronic passive congestion
clinicopathologic conference
CPD
cephalopelvic disproportion
CPD-adenine
CPE
chronic pulmonary emphysema
cytopathic effect
C-peptide
C-p. test
CPI
chronic pneumonitis of infancy
coronary prognostic index
cpm
counts per minute
CPN
chronic pyelonephritis
CPPD
calcium pyrophosphate deposition disease

NOTES

151

CPR
    cerebral cortex perfusion rate
    cortisol production rate
C_3 proactivator
cps
    cycles per second
CQ
    circadian quotient
C_1q immune complex detection
CR
    crown rump
crab
    c. hand
    c. louse
    c. yaws
Crabtree effect
cracked heel
cradle cap
Craigia
Craigie tube method
Crandall syndrome
craniad
cranial
    c. arteritis
    c. insufflation
    c. monocephalus duplication
craniocarpotarsal
    c. dysplasia
    c. dystrophy
craniocele
craniocleidodysostosis
craniodiaphysial dysplasia
craniofacial dysostosis
craniomalacia
    circumscribed c.
craniomeningocele
craniometaphysial dysplasia
craniopagus
craniopathy
    metabolic c.
craniopharyngioma
    ameloblastomatous c.
    cystic papillomatous c.
craniorachischisis
cranioschisis
craniosclerosis
craniostenosis
craniosynostosis
craniotabes
craniotrypesis
cranium
    c. bifidum
crassamentum
crater
crateriform
craw-craw
CRBBB
    complete right bundle-branch block

CRD
    chronic renal disease
    complete reaction of degeneration
C-reactive
    C.-r. protein (CRP)
    C.-r. protein assay
    C.-r. protein test
cream
    leukocyte c.
crease
    palmar c.
    simian c.
creatine
    c. kinase (CK)
    c. kinase assay
    c. kinase isoenzyme
    c. kinase isoenzyme electrophoresis
    c. kinase test
    c. phosphate
    c. phosphokinase
creatinemia
creatinine
    amniotic fluid c.
    c. assay
    c. clearance (CC, C/cr/)
    c. clearance test
    c. coefficient
creatinuria
Credé method
creeping
    c. disease
    c. eruption
    c. substitution of bone
    c. ulcer
crenate
crenated cell
crenation
crenocyte
crenocytosis
Crenosoma vulpis
crenulate
creola body
crepitans
    tenosynovitis c.
crescent
    c. cell
    c. cell anemia
    glomerular c.
    c. sign
crescentic glomerulopathy
cresol
    c. assay
    c. red
CREST
    calcinosis, Raynaud phenomenon, esophageal motility disorders, sclerodactyly, and telangiectasia
    CREST syndrome

cresta
cresyl
    c. blue
    c. blue brilliant
    c. blue brilliant stain
    c. echt
    c. fast violet
    c. violet (CV)
    c. violet acetate
    c. violet stain
cretinism
Creutzfeldt-Jakob
    C.-J. disease (CJD)
    C.-J. syndrome
CRF
    chronic renal failure
    corticotropin-releasing factor
crib death
cribriform carcinoma
cribrosa
    area c.
cri du chat syndrome
Crigler-Najjar
    C.-N. disease
    C.-N. syndrome
Crimean-Congo
    C.-C. hemorrhagic fever
    C.-C. hemorrhagic fever virus
Crimean hemorrhagic fever virus
criminal abortion
crinophagy
Crippa lead tetraacetate method
crisis, pl. crises
    addisonian c.
    adrenal c.
    anaphylactoid c.
    aplastic c.
    blast c.
    blood c.
    celiac c.
    myclocytic c.
    salt-losing c.
    sickle cell c.
    thyroid c., pl. crises
criteria, sing. criterion
    Azzopardi c.
    Child hepatic risk c.
    Katzenstein and Peiper c.
    Krauss and Neubecker
      morphologic c.
    Masaoka staging c.

    Muller-Hermelink c.
    van Diest c.
Crithidia
    C. immunofluorescence testing
critical
    c. angle
    c. flicker fusion (CFF)
    c. flicker fusion test
    c. illumination
    c. mass
    c. micelle concentration (CMC)
    c. path analysis
    c. region
    c. temperature
CRM
    cross-reacting material
cRNA
    chromosomal RNA
crocein
    brilliant c.
crocidolite
Crocq disease
Crohn disease
Cronkhite-Canada syndrome
Crooke
    C. granule
    C. hyaline change
    C. hyaline degeneration
cross
    c. activation
    c. agglutination
    c. hybridization
    c. infection
    c. product
    c. reaction
    three-point c.
    c. wall
cross-assembler
cross-compiler
crossed
    c. grid
    c. immunoelectrophoresis
cross-linking
crossmatch (XM)
cross-matching, crossmatching
crossover frequency
cross-reacting
    c.-r. agglutinin
    c.-r. antibody
    c.-r. antigen
    c.-r. material (CRM)
cross-reactivity

NOTES

C

cross-sectional survey
crotalin
Crotalus
    C. antitoxin
croton oil
crot value
croup
croup-associated virus
croupous
    c. bronchitis
    c. inflammation
    c. lymph
    c. membrane
    c. pharyngitis
Crouzon
    C. craniofacial dysostosis
    C. disease
    C. syndrome
crowded cell index
crowding effect
Crow-Fukase syndrome
crown
    C. needle
    c. rump (CR)
crown-heel (CH)
CRP
    C-reactive protein
^{51}Cr red cell survival
CRS
    Chinese restaurant syndrome
CRST
    calcinosis cutis, Raynaud phenomenon,
    sclerodactyly, and telangiectasia
    CRST syndrome
CRT
    cathode ray tube
    CRT terminal
cruciate
crucible
crude
    c. mortality ratio (CMR)
    c. rate
    c. urine
cruor
cruris
crush
    c. injury
    c. kidney
    c. syndrome
crusta, pl. crustae
    c. inflammatoria
    c. phlogistica
Crustacea
crusted ringworm
Cruveilhier-Baumgarten
    C.-B. disease
    C.-B. syndrome
Cruveilhier disease

Cruz-Chagas disease
cruzi
    Schizotrypanum c.
cryalgesia
crymophilic
crymophylactic
cryoablation
cryobank
cryobiology
cryocrit
cryofibrinogen
cryofibrinogenemia
cryogammaglobulin
Cryo-Gel embedding medium
cryogenic
cryoglobulin
cryoglobulinemia
    crystal c.
cryohydrocytosis
Cryokwik
cryolysis
cryopathic hemolytic syndrome
cryophile
cryophilic
cryophylactic
cryoprecipitate
cryoprecipitated antihemophilic factor
cryoprecipitation
cryopreservation
cryopreservative
    Microbank c.
cryoprobe
cryoprotectant
cryoprotein
CRYO rubber mold
cryoscope
cryoscopy
cryostat
    C. Frozen Sectioning Aid
cryotolerant
CRYO-VAC-A cryostat vacuum system
crypt
    c. abscess
    adenomatous c.
    c. distortion
    c. epithelium
    c.'s fof Lieberkühn
cryptic enzyme
cryptitis
Cryptococcaceae
cryptococcal
    c. antigen
    c. antigen titer
    c. meningitis
    c. polysaccharide
cryptococcemia
cryptococci
cryptococcoma

cryptococcosis
Cryptococcus
    C. antibody titer
    C. neoformans
Cryptocystis trichodectis
Cryptogamia
cryptogenic
    c. cirrhosis
    c. infection
    c. pyemia
    c. septicemia
cryptolith
cryptomenorrhea
cryptophthalmos
cryptophthalmus syndrome
cryptorchidism
cryptorchid testis
cryptorchism
cryptosporidia
cryptosporidiosis
Cryptosporidium
    C. diagnostic procedure
Cryptostroma corticale
cryptostromosis
cryptoxanthin
cryptozoite
crystal
    asthma c.
    birefringent c.
    blood c.
    Böttcher c.
    c. cell
    Charcot-Leyden c.
    Charcot-Neumann c.
    Charcot-Robin c.
    chiral c.
    c. cryoglobulinemia
    c. deposition disease
    Florence c.
    hematoidin c.
    knife-rest c.
    leukocytic c.
    Leyden c.
    liquid c.
    c. of Lubarsch
    Lubarsch c.
    Reinke c.
    scintillation c.
    sperm c.
    spermin c.
    thorn apple c.
    twin c.

    tyrosine c.
    urate c.
    uric acid c.
    c. urinary cast
    c.'s in urine sediment
    urine sediment c.
    c. violet
    c. violet vaccine
    Virchow c.
    whetstone c.
crystal-induced chemotactic factor
crystalline
    c. amylose
    c. birefringence
    c. egg albumin (CEA)
    c. insulin (CI)
    c. macromolecule alteration
crystallization
crystallography
    x-ray c.
crystalloid
    Charcot-Böttcher c.
crystalluria
CS
    chorionic somatomammotropin
C&S
    culture and sensitivity
        C&S test
CSA
    colony-stimulating activity
    compressed spectral assay
CSF
    cerebrospinal fluid
    colony-stimulating factor
        CSF glutamine test
CSH
    capsular synovial-like hyperplasia
    chronic subdural hematoma
    cortical stromal hyperplasia
Csillag disease
CSM
    cerebrospinal meningitis
CSR
    corrected sedimentation rate
    cortisol secretion rate
cSt
    centistoke
CT
    cerebral thrombosis
    circulation time
    clotting time
    coagulation time

NOTES

C

CT *(continued)*
 Coombs test
 coronary thrombosis
 corrected transposition
 cytotechnologist
  CT number
CTCL
 cutaneous T-cell lymphoma
CTD
 carpal tunnel decompression
 congenital thymic dysplasia
Ctenocephalides
  C. canis
C-terminal
ctetosome
CT-guided stereotactic biopsy
CTL
 cytologic T lymphocyte
CTP
 cytidine triphosphate
 cytosine triphosphate
C/u/
 urea clearance
cu
 cubic
Cuban itch
cubic (cu)
  c. centimeter (cu cm)
  c. millimeter (cmm)
CUC
 chronic ulcerative colitis
cu cm
 cubic centimeter
cuff
  perivascular c.
cuffing
  lymphocytic c.
culbertsoni
  Acanthamoeba c.
cul-de-sac smear
Culex
Culicidae
culicis
  Agamomermis c.
Culicoides
culicosis
Culiseta melanura
Cullen sign
Cult-Dip Plus bacteriologic culture
cultivation
culture
  abscess aerobic c.
  Actinomyces c.
  adenovirus c.
  aerobic and anaerobic blood c.
  anaerobic bacteria c.
  animal cell c.
  arterial line c.

  attenuated c.
  bacterial c.
  blood c.
  bronchial aspirate anaerobic c.
  burn c.
  cell wall defective bacteria c.
  cerebrospinal fluid c.
  cervical c.
  Chlamydia c.
  chorioallantoic c.
  clean-catch urine c.
  CMV c.
  colony-forming unit-c. (CFU-C)
  conjunctival fungus c.
  continuous flow c.
  Corynebacterium diphtheriae
   throat c.
  Cult-Dip Plus bacteriologic c.
  cytomegalovirus c.
  direct c.
  ear c.
  EBV c.
  elective c.
  endometrium anaerobic c.
  enrichment c.
  enterovirus c.
  Epstein-Barr virus c.
  flask c.
  fungus c.
  genital c.
  gonorrhea c. (GC)
  gravity-settling c. (GSC)
  group A beta hemolytic
   streptococci throat c.
  group A β-hemolytic streptococci
   throat c.
  hanging-block c.
  hanging-drop c.
  Helicobacter pylori urease test
   and c.
  herpes simplex virus c.
  HIV c.
  HSV c.
  human immunodeficiency virus c.
  influenza virus c.
  Legionella pneumophila c.
  Leptospira c.
  c. medium
  mixed c.
  mixed leukocyte c. (MLC)
  mixed lymphocyte c. (MLC)
  mumps virus c.
  mycobacteria c.
  nasopharyngeal c.
  needle c.
  Neisseria gonorrhoeae c.
  Nocardia c.
  organ c.

parainfluenza virus c.
plate c.
primary c.
pure c.
radioisotopic c.
respiratory syncytial virus c.
RSV c.
rubella virus c.
secondary c.
semiquantitative viral c.
c. and sensitivity (C&S)
shake c.
skin fungus c.
skin mycobacteria c.
slant c.
slope c.
spinal fluid c.
sputum fungus c.
sputum mycobacteria c.
stab c.
Staphylococcus aureus
  nasopharyngeal c.
sterility c.
stock c.
stool fungus c.
stool mycobacteria c.
streak c.
synchronized c.
throat c.
thrust c.
tissue c. (TC)
tube c.
type c.
Ureaplasma urealyticum genital c.
urine fungus c.
urine mycobacteria c.
varicella-zoster virus c.
viral c.
VZV c.
wound c.
culturing
bacterial c.
cumulated activity ratio
cumulative
c. action
c. distribution
cumulus oophorous
cuneate
cuneiform
cuniculus
Cunninghamella elegans

cup
cytospin c.
cupremia
cupric ion-inhibited acid phosphatase
cupriuresis
cuprous
curative dose (CD)
curdy pus
curet, curette
curettage
endometrial c.
curie (C, c, Ci)
curie-hour (Ci-hr)
curium
Curling ulcer
currant jelly clot
currens
larva c.
current
alternating c.
dark c.
diffusion c.
direct c.
eddy c.
c. gain
c. regulator
saturation c.
three-phase c.
Curschmann
C. disease
C. spiral
cursor
Curtis-Fitz-Hugh syndrome
Curtius syndrome
curve
calibration c.
carbon dioxide dissociation c.
carbon dioxide response c.
characteristic c.
dye-dilution c.
epidemic c.
c. fitting
indicator-dilution c.
logarithmic c.
multiple event c.
oxygen-hemoglobin dissociation c.
precipitin c.
pressure-volume c.
Price-Jones c.
regression c.
standard c.
whole-body titration c.

NOTES

C

Curvularia
    C. geniculate
Cushing
    C. basophilism
    C. disease
    C. syndrome
    C. ulcer
cushingoid
    c. facies
customary temperature scale
cutaneomandibular polyoncosis
cutaneomeningospinal angiomatosis
cutaneomucouveal syndrome
cutaneous
    c. anthrax
    c. emphysema
    c. focal mucinosis
    c. fungus
    c. hemorrhoid
    c. horn
    c. leishmaniasis
    c. leprosy
    c. lymphoid hyperplasia (CLH)
    c. lymphoma
    c. malformation
    c. malignant melanoma (CMM)
    c. meningioma
    c. myiasis
    c. reaction
    c. systemic angiitis
    c. T-cell lymphoma (CTCL)
    c. tuberculin test
    c. tuberculosis
    c. vasculitis
cutdown
Cuterebra
cuticle
cutireaction
    c. test
cutis
    c. anserina
    atrophia maculosa varioliformis c.
    c. elastica
    c. hyperelastica
    c. laxa
    c. verticis gyrata
cutoff frequency
cutter
    agar c.
cutting
    section c.
cuvet
    c. oximeter
CV
    cell volume
    coefficient of variation
    cresyl violet

CVA
    cardiovascular accident
    cerebrovascular accident
CVD
    cardiovascular disease
CVH
    combined ventricular hypertrophy
    common variable
      hypogammaglobulinemia
CVOD
    cerebrovascular obstructive disease
CVP
    cell volume profile
CVR
    cardiovascular-renal
    cerebrovascular resistance
CVRD
    cardiovascular renal disease
CVS
    chorionic villus sampling
CWDF
    cell wall-deficient bacterial forms
CWP
    coal workers' pneumoconiosis
cyanemia
cyanhemoglobin
cyanide
    c. anion
    c. assay
    ethyl c.
    hydrogen c.
    mercuric c.
    c. poisoning
    potassium c.
cyanide-ascorbate test
cyanide-nitroprusside test
cyanidol
cyanmethemoglobin
cyanoacrylate
Cyanobacteria
cyanochroic
cyanochrous
cyanocobalamin
    c. Co 57
cyanogen
cyanophil, cyanophile
cyanophilous
cyanophoric glycoside
cyanosed
cyanosis
    enterogenous c.
    false c.
    hereditary methemoglobinemic c.
    toxic c.
cyanotic
    c. atrophy
    c. atrophy of liver
    c. induration

cyanuria
Cyathostoma
Cyathostomum
cybrid
cyclamate
cyclase
    adenyl c.
    adenylate c.
cycle
    cell c.
    citric acid c.
    eukaryotic cell c.
    Krebs c.
    Krebs-Henseleit c.
    menstrual c.
    mitotic c.
    operating c.
    c.'s per minute (c/min)
    c.'s per second (cps)
    pregnancy c.
    RANTES c.
    replication c.
    TCA c.
    tricarboxylic acid c.
    urea c.
Cycler
    Perkin-Elmer/Cetus DNA
      Thermal C.
cyclic
    c. adenosine monophosphate
    c. albuminuria
    c. AMP
    c. AMP test
    c. GMP
    c. guanosine monophosphate
    c. hydrocarbon
    c. lysine anhydride (CLA)
    c. neutropenia
    c. nucleotide
    c. tissue alteration
cyclin
    c. D1 gene
    c. D1 oncogene
cyclitis
cyclitol
cyclization
cycloalkane
cycloalkene
cyclodiene hydrocarbon pesticide
cyclodimerization
cyclogeny
cyclohexane

cycloheximide
cyclohexylamine
cyclonite
cyclopentane
cyclopentanoperhydrophenanthrene
cyclophosphamide
    c., doxorubicin hydrochloride,
      vincristine (Oncovin), prednisone
      (CHOP)
    c., THP-doxorubicin, vincristine,
      prednisone (THPCOP)
Cyclophyllidea
cyclopia
Cyclops
cycloserine
cyclosis
Cyclospora
cyclosporiasis
cyclosporine
cyclotron
cyclozoonosis
cylinder
    Bence Jones c.
    graduated c.
    Külz c.
cylindrical
    c. bronchiectasis
    c. embryo
cylindroadenoma
cylindroid
    c. aneurysm
cylindroma
    dermal eccrine c.
cylindromatous carcinoma
cylindrosarcoma
cylindruria
cynanche
    c. maligna
    c. tonsillaris
cyproheptadine hydrochloride
Cyriax syndrome
cyrtometer
Cys
    cysteine
cyst
    adventitious c.
    allantoic c.
    alveolar hydatid c.
    aneurysmal bone c.
    apoplectic c.
    arachnoid c.
    Baker c.

C

NOTES

cyst *(continued)*
 Bartholin c.
 blood c.
 blue dome c.
 bone c.
 branchial cleft c.
 bronchial c.
 bronchogenic c.
 bursal c.
 cerebellar c.
 chocolate c.
 choledochal c.
 chyle c.
 colloid c.
 compound c.
 congenital c.
 corpora lutea c.'s
 corpus hemorrhagicum c.
 Cowper c.
 daughter c.
 dental follicular c.
 dentigerous c.
 dermoid c.
 dermoid c. of ovary
 developmental jaw c.
 distention c.
 duplication c.
 echinococcus c.
 embryonal duct c.
 endometrial c.
 endothelial c.
 enterogenous c.
 ependymal c.
 epidermal inclusion c.
 epidermoid inclusion c.
 epididymal c.
 epithelial inclusion c.
 extravasation c.
 exudation c.
 false c.
 fissural c.
 c. fluid cytology
 follicle c.
 follicular c.
 ganglion c.
 Gartner c.
 gas c.
 germinal epithelial inclusion c.
 globulomaxillary c.
 glomerular c.
 granddaughter c.
 hemorrhagic c.
 hepatic c.
 hydatid c.
 implantation c.
 inclusion c.
 inflammatory c.
 involution c.

iodine c.
junctional c.
keratinous c.
Kobelt c.
lacteal c.
leptomeningeal c.
luteal c.
luteinized follicular c.
meibomian c.
mesonephric c.
mesothelial c.
milium c.
milk c.
Morgagni c.
mother c.
mucinous c.
mucous c.
multilocular hydatid c.
multiloculate hydatid c.
myxoid c.
nabothian c.
necrotic c.
neural c.
odontogenic c.
oil c.
oophoritic c.
osseous hydatid c.
ovarian c.
paraphysial c.
parasitic c.
parathyroid c.
parent c.
paroophoritic c.
parvilocular c.
pericardial c.
periodontal c.
phaeomycotic c.
pilar c.
piliferous c.
pilonidal c.
pineal c.
posttraumatic leptomeningeal c.
proliferating tricholemmal c.
proliferation c.
proliferative c.
proliferous c.
pseudomucinous c.
radicular c.
ranular c.
Rathke cleft c.
renal c.
retention c.
rete c. of ovary
sanguineous c.
sebaceous c.
secretory c.
seminal vesical c.
sequestration c.

serous c.
simple bone c.
solitary bone c.
sterile c.
sublingual c.
suprasellar c.
synovial c.
Tarlov c.
tarry c.
tarsal c.
tension c.
teratomatous c.
theca-lutein c.
thyroglossal duct c.
thyrolingual c.
traumatic bone c.
trichilemmal c.
tubular c.
umbilical c.
unicameral bone c.
unilocular hydatid c.
urachal c.
urinary c.
utricular c.
vitellointestinal c.
wolffian c.
cystacanth
cystadenocarcinoma
mucinous c.
papillary serous c.
pseudomucinous c.
serous c.
cystadenofibroma
cystadenoma
hepatobiliary c.
c. lymphomatosum
mucinous c.
oncocytic papillary c.
papillary c.
papillary c. lymphomatosum
pseudomucinous c.
serous c.
cystathionase
cystathionine
cystathionine-γ-lyase
cystathionine-β-synthase
cystathioninuria
cystauchenitis
cysteamine
cystectasia
cystectasy

cysteic acid method
cysteine (Cys)
cysteinyl
cystic
c. acute inflammation
c. adenomatoid malformation
c. atrophy
c. bronchiectasis
c. carcinoma
c. chronic cervicitis
c. chronic inflammation
c. corpus hemorrhagicum
c. corpus luteum
c. degeneration
c. dermoid teratoma
c. diathesis
c. disease
c. disease of the breast
c. disease of lung
c. disease of renal medulla
c. endometrial hyperplasia
c. fibrosis (CF)
c. fibrosis of pancreas (CFP)
c. fibrosis test
c. goiter
c. granulomatous inflammation
c. hygroma
c. hyperplasia
c. hyperplasia of the breast
c. hyperplasia of endometrium
c. kidney
c. lymphangiectasis
c. mastitis
c. mastopathy
c. medial necrosis (CMN)
c. medial necrosis of ascending aorta (CMN-AA)
c. medionecrosis
c. mole
c. myxoma
c. ovarian follicle
c. papillomatous craniopharyngioma
c. polyp
cystica
osteitis fibrosa c.
pneumatosis intestinalis c.
pyelitis c.
spina bifida c.
ureteritis c.
cysticerci (*pl. of* cysticercus)
cysticercoid

NOTES

cysticercosis
    c. titer
Cysticercus
    C. bovis
    C. cellulosae
    C. fasciolaris
    C. ovis
    C. tenuicollis
cysticercus, pl. **cysticerci**
cystides (*pl. of* cystis)
cystiform
cystigerous
cystine
    c. calculus
    c. storage disease
    c. trypticase agar
cystinemia
cystinosis
cystinotic leukocyte
cystinuria
    familial c.
    c. test
cystiphorous
cystis, pl. **cystides**
cystitis
    acute hemorrhagic c.
    c. colli
    c. cystica
    follicular c.
    c. follicularis
    c. glandularis
    hemorrhagic c.
    Hunner c.
    interstitial c.
    c. pneumatoides
    ulcerative c.
cystoadenoma
cystocarcinoma
cystocele
cystocolostomy
cystodiverticulum
cystoenterostomy
cystoepithelioma
cystofibroma
cystogastrostomy
cystogenic aneurysm
cystoid
    c. macular degeneration
cystojejunostomy
cystolith
cystolithiasis
cystolithic
cystoma
    serous c.
cystomorphous
cystomyoma
cystomyxoadenoma
cystomyxoma

cystopherous
cystoptosia
cystoptosis
cystopyelitis
cystopyelonephritis
cystosarcoma
    c. phyllodes (CP)
cystoureteritis
cystourethritis
cystourethrocele
cystous
Cystoviridae
cystyl
cytapheresis
cytase
Cytauxzoon
cytauxzoonosis
cythemolytic icterus
cytidine
    c. diphosphate
    c. monophosphate
    c. triphosphate (CTP)
cytidine-5'-phosphate
cytidylic acid
cytidylyl
cytoanalyzer
cytobiology
cytoblast
cytoblastema
cytocentrifugation
cytocentrifuge
cytochalasin
cytochemical
cytochemistry
cytochrome
    c. b_5 reductase
    c. b_5 reductase assay
    c. oxidase test
cytocidal
cytocide
cytoclasis
cytoclastic
cytocyst
cytode
cytodegenerative
    c. necrosis
cytodiagnosis
    exfoliative c.
cytodifferentiation
cytofluorography
cytogene
cytogenetic map
cytogenetics
    clinical c.
    population c.
cytoglucopenia
cytoid
    c. body

cytokeratin
- c. 7
- c. 20
- c. 19 antigen

cytokine
- c. network

cytokinesis
cytolipin H
cytologic
- c. abnormality
- c. alteration
- c. degeneration
- c. diagnosis
- c. engulfment
- c. examination
- c. filter preparation
- c. screening
- c. smear
- c. specimen
- c. T lymphocyte (CTL)

cytology
- >cerebrospinal fluid c.
- analytic c.
- aspiration c.
- aspiration-biopsy c.
- bronchial washings c.
- brushings c.
- cervical/vaginal c.
- effusion c.
- exfoliative c.
- image c.
- ThinPrep c.

cytolysate
- blood c.

cytolysin
cytolysis
- immune c.

cytolysosome
CytoLyt fixative
cytolytic
- T (cell) c. (Tc)

cytoma
cytomegalic
- c. cell
- c. inclusion disease (CID, CMID)
- c. inclusion disease cytology
- c. inclusion disease virus

cytomegalovirus (CMV)
- c. antibody
- c. culture
- c. disease
- c. isolation

cytomegaly
cytomere
cytometaplasia
cytometer
- Bayer/Technicon H1 automated flow c.
- Epics C flow c.
- Epics Profile flow c.
- flow c.

cytometric image analysis
cytometry
- DNA flow c.
- flow c. (FCM)
- image c.

cytopathic
- c. effect (CPE)

cytopathogenesis
cytopathogenic
- c. virus

cytopathologic, cytopathological
cytopathologist
cytopathology
cytopathy
cytopenia
cytophagic histiocytic panniculitis
cytophagous
cytophagy
cytophanere
cytopharynx
cytophil group
cytophilic
- c. antibody

cytophotometer
cytophotometry
- DNA c.
- flow c.

cytophylactic
cytophylaxis
cytopipette
cytoplasm
- amphophilic c.
- ground-glass c.

cytoplasmic
- c. CD3
- c. crystalline aggregate
- c. fiber alteration
- c. fibril alteration
- c. filament alteration
- c. glycogen
- c. inclusion
- c. inclusion body
- c. inheritance

C

NOTES

cytoplasmic *(continued)*
    c. lipid aggregate
    c. lipid droplet alteration
    c. macromolecule aggregate
    c. matrix alteration
    c. membrane
    c. vacuole
    c. vacuolization
cytoplast
cytopreparation
cytopyge
cytoreductive therapy
Cyto-Rich cervical cytology monolayer system
cytorrhyctes
cytoryctes
cytoscopy
cytosine
    c. arabinoside (CA)
    guanine c. (GC)
    c. triphosphate (CTP)
cytosis
cytoskeletal filament
cytoskeleton
cytosmear
cytosol
cytosome
    lipid c. (LC)
cytospin
    c. analysis
    c. cup
    c. slide centrifuge Gram-stained smear
cytostasis
cytostatic
cytostome
cytotactic

cytotaxia
cytotaxis
    negative c.
    positive c.
cytotechnologist (CT)
cytothesis
cytotoxic
    c. necrosis
    c. reaction
    T (cell) c. (Tc)
    c. T cell
cytotoxicity
    antibody-dependent cell-mediated c. (ADCC)
    complement-mediated c.
    lymphocyte-mediated c.
cytotoxin
cytotrophic serum
cytotrophoblast
cytotropic
    c. antibody
    c. antibody test
cytotropism
Cytoxan
cytozoic
cytozoon
cytozyme
cyturia
Cytyc
    C. CytoLyt preservative solution
    C. Preservcyt preservative solution
Czapek-Dox
    C.-D. agar
    C.-D. medium
Czapek solution agar
Czerny disease

Δ (*var. of* Delta)
δ (*var. of* delta)
    δ agent
    δ antigen
    δ cell islet
    δ check
    δ hepatitis
    δ ray
    δ staphylolysin
    δ virus

D
    D antigen
    D colony
    D line
    D value

D_{CO}
    diffusing capacity for carbon monoxide

d
    decigram

D-
    sterically related to D-glyceraldehyde

d-
    dextrorotatory

2,4-D
D10 antigen
D-3-hydroxyacyl coenzyme A
DA
    degenerative arthritis
    direct agglutination
    disaggregated
        DA pregnancy test
Daae disease
Daae-Finsen disease
DAB
    diaminobenzidine
        DAB reaction
Dabska tumor
DAC
    diazacholesterol
    digital-to-analog converter
D/A converter
DaCosta
    D. disease
    D. syndrome
dacroyte
dacryadenitis
dacryoadenitis
dacryoblennorrhea
dacryocyst
dacryocystitis
dacryocyte
dacryolith
    Desmarres d.
    Nocardia d.
dacryoma

dacryosolenitis
dactinomycin
Dactylaria
dactylitis
dactylolysis spontanea
Dade Hepzyme heparinase
Da Fano stain
DAGT
    direct antiglobulin test
DAH
    disordered action of heart
dahlia
daisy
Dakin solution
DAKO
    D. Envision System Peroxidase
    D. target retrieval solution
dalapon
Dale-Laidlaw clotting time method
Dalen-Fuchs nodule
Dale reaction
Dalrymple disease
dalton
Dalton law
dam
damage
    irradiation d.
    minimal brain d. (MBD)
    myocardial d. (MD)
    radiation d.
Damalinia
D-amino acid oxidase
dAMP
    deoxyadenosine monophosphate
damping
Dam unit
Danbolt-Closs syndrome
dandy fever
Dandy-Walker syndrome
Dane
    D. and Herman keratin stain
    D. method
    D. particle
Danielssen-Boeck disease
Danielssen disease
Danlos syndrome
DANS
    1-dimethylaminoaphthalene-5 sulfonic
        acid
dansyl chloride
Danubian endemic familial nephropathy
Danysz phenomenon
DAP
    direct agglutination pregnancy

D

DAPI
4′6-diamidino-2-phenylindole-2 HCl
DAPI stain
DAPT
direct agglutination pregnancy test
D-arabitol dehydrogenase
Darier disease
dark
d. current
d. reaction
d. reactivation
dark-field
d.-f. condenser
d.-f. examination
fluorescent antibody d.-f. (FADF)
d.-f. microscope
dark-ground microscope
Darling disease
Darlington amplifier
Darrow
D. red
D. red stain
d'Arsonval meter
Dasyprocta
DAT
differential agglutination titer
diphtheria antitoxin
direct agglutination test
data
analog d.
categorical d.
metric d.
ranked d.
date fever
Datril
daughter
d. colony
d. cyst
daunomycin
daunorubicin
d., cytarabine, 6-mercaptopurine,
prednisone (DCMP)
Davainea
Davaineidae
Davenport graph
David disease
Davidsohn differential absorption test
Davies disease
davtiani
Teladorsagia d.
Dawson encephalitis
Day test
DB
dextran blue
DBC
dye-binding capacity
DBCL
dilute blood clot lysis (method)

DBI
development-at-birth index
DCA
deoxycholate-citrate agar
DCF
direct centrifugal flotation
DCIS
ductal carcinoma in situ
DCMP
daunorubicin, cytarabine, 6-
mercaptopurine, prednisone
DCT
direct Coombs test
DDD
dense-deposit disease
dihydroxydinaphthyl disulfide
D-dimer
D-d. assay
D-d. test
DDS
dystrophy-dystocia syndrome
DDT assay
DDVP
dimethyldichlorovinyl phosphate
de
D. Castro fluid
d. Clerambault syndrome
d. Galantha method for urates
d. Lange syndrome
D. Morgan spot
d. Quervain disease
d. Quervain thyroiditis
D. Ritis ratio
D. Sanctis-Cacchione syndrome
D. Toni-Fanconi syndrome
DEA
dehydroepiandrosterone
deactivation
deacylase
acylsphingosine d.
deacylate
dead
d. of disease (DOD)
d. fetus in utero (DFU)
d. finger
d. on arrival (DOA)
d. time
dead-end host
deadly agaric
DEAE-cellulose
diethylaminoethyl cellulose
dealbation
dealcoholization
deallergization
deallergize
deaminase
adenosine d. (ADA)
guanine d.

histidine α-d.
histidine alpha d.
porphobilinogen d.
deaquation
dearterialization
death
brain d.
cause of d. (COD)
cell d.
cerebral d.
crib d.
early neonatal d.
fetal d.
d. fever
functional d.
indirect maternal d.
infant d.
intrauterine d. (IUD)
late neonatal d.
local d.
maternal d.
natural d.
neonatal d. (ND, NND)
nonrenal d. (NRD)
perinatal d.
somatic d.
sudden cardiac d. (SCD)
sudden coronary d. (SCD)
sudden unexpected d. (SUD)
sudden unexpected, unexplained d.
  (SUUD)
sudden unexplained d. (SUD)
sudden unexplained infant d.
  (SUID)
d. trance
DeBakey aortic assay
Debaryomyces
D. hansenii
D. hominis
D. neoformans
debrancher deficiency limit dextrinosis
debranching enzyme
Debré phenomenon
Debré-Semelaigne syndrome
débridement, debridement
debris
debubbling
debug
debye
decacurie
decade counter
decagram

decalcification
decalcify
decalcifying
decaliter
decameter
decanoic acid
decant
decantation
decarboxylase
branched-chain alpha ketoacid d.
branched-chain α-ketoacid d.
d. broth
glutamate d.
glutamic acid d. (GAD)
histidine d. (HDC)
methylmalonyl-CoA d.
ornithine d.
orotidine-5'-phosphate d.
orotidylate d.
oxaloacetate d.
uroporphyrinogen d.
decarboxylation
amine precursor uptake and d.
  (APUD)
decay (DK)
α-d.
alpha d.
d. antibody-accelerating factor
β-d.
beta d.
branching d.
d. coefficient
d. constant
exponential d.
d. mode
positron beta d.
d. product
radioactive d.
d. rate
d. scheme
deceration
decerebrate
d. rigidity
decibel
decidua
ectopic d.
decidual
d. alteration
d. cast
d. cell
d. change
d. endometritis

D

NOTES

decidual *(continued)*
    d. membrane
    d. metaplasia
    d. reaction
deciduitis
deciduoid
deciduoma
    Loeb d.
deciduous skin
decigram (d)
decile
deciliter (dL, dl)
    milligrams per d. (mg%)
decimal reduction time
decimeter (dm)
decinem (dn)
decision table
decoagulant
decode
decoder
decolorize
decompensation
    cardiac d.
    d. injury
    d. sickness
decomposition potential
decompression
    carpal tunnel d. (CTD)
    d. injury
    d. sickness
decontamination
decortication
decoy cell
decrement
decubation
decubitus
    d. calculus
    d. ulcer
decussate
decussation
dedifferentiated liposarcoma
dedifferentiation
de-efferentation
deep agar
deer fly, deerfly
Deetjen body
def
    deficiency
defect
    acquired d.
    aldosterone secretion d. (ASD)
    aortic septal d.
    atrial septal d. (ASD)
    congenital ectodermal d.
    cortical d.
    coupling d.
    ectodermal d.
    endocardial cushion d.

    fibrous cortical d.
    filling d.
    Gerbode d.
    hydrogen-detected ventricular
      septal d. (HVSD) ·
    interatrial septal d. (IASD)
    interventricular septal d. (IVSD)
    intraventricular conduction d.
      (IVCD)
    iodide transport d.
    iodotyrosine deiodinase d.
    labyrinthine d. (LD)
    neural tube d.
    no significant d. (NSD)
    organification d.
    plasma d. (PD)
    platelet d. (PLD)
    septal d. (SD)
    serum d. (SD)
    surgical d.
    ventricular septal d. (VSD)
    zero d.'s (Z/D)
defective
    d. bacteriophage
    d. interfering particle
    d. phage
    d. probacteriophage
    d. prophage
    d. virus
defense
    host d.'s
    d. mechanism
defensins
deferentitis
deferoxamine
    d. mesylate
    d. mesylate infusion test
defervescent stage
defibrinated blood
defibrination
    d. syndrome
deficiency (def)
    adenosine deaminase d.
    ADH d.
    alpha-1 antitrypsin d.
    d. anemia
    antidiuretic hormone deficiency
    antitrypsin d.
    α_1-antitrypsin d.
    argininosuccinate synthetase d.
    beta-*d*-glucuronidase d.
    brancher d.
    carbamoyl phosphate synthetase
      I d.
    20,22-desmolase d.
    dihydropteridine reductase d.
    disaccharidase d.
    d. disease

duplication d.
d. factor (DF)
d. factors I, II, V, VII, VIII, IX, X, XI
galactokinase d.
glucose-6-phosphate dehydrogenase d.
glucosephosphate isomerase d.
β-d-glucuronidase d.
glutathione reductase d.
glutathione synthetase d.
growth hormone d. (GHD)
hereditary plasmathromboplastin component d.
immune d.
immunity d.
immunological d.
lactase d.
LCAT d.
lecithin-cholesterol acyltransferase d.
leukocyte adhesion d. (LAD)
lipoprotein lipase d.
myeloperoxidase d.
ornithine carbamoyltransferase d.
ornithine transcarbamylase d.
phosphofructokinase d.
phosphohexose isomerase d.
phosphorylase d.
placental steroid sulfatase d.
plasma thromboplastin antecedent d.
prothrombin d.
pseudocholinesterase d.
PTA d.
PTC d.
pyruvate kinase d.
secondary antibody d.
serum prothrombin conversion accelerator d.
SPCA d.
specific coagulation factor d.
stable factor d.
sulfite oxidase d.
thiamine d.
thromboplastin antecedent d.
triosephosphate isomerase d.
tuftsin d.
vitamin d.
deficit
base d. (BD)
defined
serologically d. (SD)
d. substrate (DS)

definition
recursive d.
definitive
d. callus
d. erythroblast
d. host
d. method
d. organism identification
deflection signal
deflorescence
defoliant
deformability
deformans
osteitis d.
osteochondrodystrophia d.
deformation
deforming
deformity
acquired d.
Arnold-Chiari d.
congenital d.
J-sella d.
Klippel-Feil d.
lobster claw d.
pigeon breast d.
swan-neck d.
valgus d.
varus d.
deg
degeneration
degree
degeneracy
degenerate
d. code
degenerated
d. intervertebral disk
d. intervertebral fibrocartilage
d. meniscus
degenerating myelin demonstration
degeneratio
degeneration (deg)
adipose d.
albuminoid d.
albuminous d.
Alzheimer fibrillary d.
amyloid d.
angiolithic d.
ascending d.
atheromatous d.
axonal d.
ballooning d.
basophilic granular d.

D

NOTES

degeneration *(continued)*
    calcareous d.
    capsular lipochondral d.
    carneous d.
    caseous d.
    cellular d.
    cloudy swelling d.
    collagen d.
    colliquative d.
    colloid d.
    complete reaction of d. (CRD)
    Crooke hyaline d.
    cystic d.
    cystoid macular d.
    cytologic d.
    descending d.
    elastoid d.
    elastotic d.
    fatty d.
    feathery d.
    fibrinoid d.
    fibrinous d.
    fibrous d.
    floccular d.
    foamy d.
    granular d.
    granulovacuolar d.
    gray d.
    hepatolenticular d.
    hyaline d.
    hydatid d.
    hydropic d.
    lenticular progressive d.
    lipid d.
    lipochondral d. (LCD)
    lipoid d.
    liquefaction d.
    liquefactive d.
    medial d.
    Mönckeberg d.
    mucinoid d.
    mucinous d.
    mucoid medial d.
    myelin d.
    myelinic d.
    myxoid d.
    myxomatous d.
    neurofibrillary d.
    parenchymatous d.
    partial reaction of d. (PRD)
    pigmentary d.
    pseudomucinous d.
    pseudotubular d.
    reaction of d. (DeR, DR)
    reaction of (to) d. (RD)
    red d.
    reticular d.
    retrograde d.

    secondary d.
    senile d.
    spongy d. of infancy
    striatonigral d.
    subacute combined d. (SACD)
    subacute combined d. of the spinal cord
    transsynaptic d.
    Türck d.
    vacuolar d.
    wallerian d. (WD)
    waxy d.
    Zenker d.
degenerative
    d. arthritis (DA)
    d. change
    d. index
    d. inflammation
    d. joint disease (DJD)
deglycerolization
Degos
    D. disease
    D. syndrome
degradation
degranulation
degree (deg)
    d.'s of freedom (df)
    second d.
dehiscence
dehydrase
    aminolevulinic acid d. (ALAD)
dehydratase
    carbonate d.
dehydrate
dehydrated alcohol
dehydration
dehydroascorbic acid
dehydrobilirubin
dehydroepiandrosterone (DEA, DHA, DHEA)
dehydroepiandrosterone sulfate (DHEAS, DS)
dehydrogenase
    acyl-CoA d.
    alcohol d. (ADH)
    aldehyde d.
    branched-chain alpha ketoacid d.
    branched-chain α-ketoacid d.
    D-arabitol d.
    glucose-6-phosphate d. (G-6-PD)
    glutamate d.
    glyceraldehyde phosphate d. (GAPD, GAPDH)
    heat-stable lactic d. (HLDH)
    hexosephosphate d.
    3-hydroxybutyrate d.
    iditol d.
    isocitrate d.

isocitric d.
isovaleryl-CoA d.
lactate d. (LD, LDH)
lactic d. (LD)
ʟ-arabinose d.
ʟ-arabitol d.
lysine d.
malate d.
malic d. (MD)
oxoglutarate d.
2-oxoisovalerate d.
phosphogluconate d.
polyol d.
proline d.
1-pyrroline-5-carboxylate d.
saccharopine d.
sarcosine d.
serum hydroxybutyrate d. (SHBD)
serum isocitric d. (SICD)
sorbitol d.
tetrahydrofolate d.
triosephosphate d.
xylitol d.
ʟ-xylulose d.
dehydrogenate
dehydrogenation
dehydroisoandrosterone (DHIA)
deiminase
arginine d.
deionization
Dejerine
D. disease
D. syndrome
Dejerine-Klumpke syndrome
Dejerine-Roussy syndrome
Dejerine-Sottas
D.-S. disease
D.-S. syndrome
dekanem (Dn)
Del
D. Castillo syndrome
D. Rio Hortega stain
Delafield
D. fixative solution
D. hematoxylin
D. hematoxylin stain
Delaney clause
delay
d. circuit
d. line
delayed
d. adrenarche

d. allergy
d. climacteric
d. hemolytic transfusion reaction
d. hypersensitivity
d. hypersensitivity reaction
d. menopause
d. primary closure (DPC)
d. puberty
delayed-type hypersensitivity (DTH)
deletion
antigenic d.
chromosomal d.
intercalary d.
interstitial d.
d. mutation
terminal d.
d. theory
deliquescence
deliquescent
delirium tremens (DT)
delitescence
deliver
to d. (TD)
delivery
spontaneous d. (SD)
delle
delphian node
Delta, Δ
delta, δ
d. agent
d. aminolevulinic acid
d. antigen
d. base
d. cell
d. cell islet
d. check
d. hepatitis
d. ray
d. staphylolysin
demarcation
line of d.
Dematiaceae
dematiaceous
d. fungi
Dematium
demeclocycline
dementia
transmissible d.
demethylchlortetracycline
demeton
methyl d.

D

NOTES

demilune
    d. body
demineralization
Demodex
    D. folliculorum
demonstration
    calcium deposit d.
    copper deposit d.
    degenerating myelin d.
    iron-positive pigment d.
demyelinate
demyelinated myelitis
demyelinating
    d. diseases
    d. encephalopathy
demyelination
    axonal d.
denaturation
    protein d.
denaturing
    d. gels
    d. gradient gel electrophoresis
    (DGGE)
dendritic
    d. calculus
    d. cell
    d. cell tumor
dendrocyte
    dermal d.
dengue
    hemorrhagic d.
    d. hemorrhagic fever
    d. shock syndrome
    d. virus
    d. virus, types 1, 2, 3, 4
denitrifying bacterium
Dennie-Marfan syndrome
Dennis technique
dense body
dense-core neurosecretory granule
dense-deposit disease (DDD)
densimeter
densitometer
densitometry
density
    buoyant d.
    character d.
    count information d.
    fiber d.
    d. function
    d. gradient centrifugation
    luminous flux d.
    optical d. (OD)
    scan information d.
    subplasmalemmal d.
    total body d. (TBD)
density-dependent repair

dental
    d. calculus
    d. caries
    d. fluorosis
    d. follicular cyst
    d. granuloma
    d. lymph
    d. pathology
    d. plaque
dentate nucleus
dentatus
    Stephanurus d.
denticulated
dentigerous
    d. cyst
    d. mixed tumor
dentin
    d. crystal alteration
    d. dysplasia
dentinal fluid
dentinogenesis imperfecta
dentinoma
    fibroameloblastic d.
Denver classification
Denys-Leclef phenomenon
deossification
deoxyadenosine monophosphate (dAMP)
deoxyadenosine-'5-phosphate
deoxyadenylic acid
6-deoxy-beta-L-mannose
deoxycholate
deoxycholate-citrate agar (DCA)
deoxycholic acid
deoxycorticoids (DOCS)
deoxycorticosterone (DOC)
    d. acetate (DOCA)
    11-d. test
deoxycortisol
    11-d. test
deoxycytidine monophosphate
deoxycytidine-5'-phosphate
deoxycytidylic acid
6-deoxy-L-galactose
deoxygenated hemoglobin
deoxyguanosine
    d. monophosphate (dGMP)
    d. phosphate
deoxyguanosine-5'-phosphate
2-deoxyguanosine-5'-triphosphate (dGTP)
deoxyguanylic acid
deoxyhemoglobin
6-deoxy-β-L-mannose
deoxynucleotidyl transferase
deoxyribonuclease (DNase, DNAse)
    d. agar
    d. digestion
    d. I

d. II
d. test
deoxyribonucleic
    d. acid (DNA)
    d. acid stain
    d. acid staining
deoxyribonucleic acid (DNA)
    competitor DNA
deoxyribonucleoprotein (DNP)
deoxyribonucleoside
deoxyribonucleotide
deoxyribose
deoxysugar
deoxythymidine triphosphate (dTTP)
deoxyuridine
    d. monophosphate (dUMP)
    d. phosphate
    d. suppression test
deoxyuridine-5′-phosphate
deoxyuridylic acid
deoxyvirus
deparaffinization
Department of Public Health (DPH)
dependence
    anchorage d.
    drug d.
dependent
    d. edema
    d. variable
Dependovirus
depigmentation
deplasmolysis
depletion
    d. layer
    lipid d.
    ovarian ascorbic acid d. (OAAD)
    plasma d.
depolarization
deposit
    brickdust d.
    posterior corneal d. (PCD)
deposition
    bilharzial pigment d.
    calcium d.
    cholesterol d.
    collagen d.
    fatty d.
    ferrocalcinotic d.
    foreign material d.
    hemosiderin d.
    Kupffer cell iron d.
    malarial pigment d.

    particulate crystalline material d.
    xanthomatous d.
depot
    fat d.
    d. reaction
depramine assay
depressant
depressed
    d. adenoma
    d. fracture
depression
    bone marrow d.
    myeloid d.
deprivation
    d. disease
deproteinization
depth
    d. dose
    d. of field
    d. of focus
    relative sagittal d. (RSD)
depulization
DeR
    reaction of degeneration
der
    derivative chromosome
deradelphus
derangement
    chromosomal d.
Dercum disease
derepressed gene
derepression
    transient d.
derivation
derivative
    d. chromosome (der)
    purified protein d. (PPD)
derivative-standard
    purified protein d. (PPD-S)
derived
    d. albumin
    d. protein
Dermacentor
    D. andersoni
    D. occidentalis
    D. reticulatus
    D. variabilis
Dermacentroxenus
    D. akari
    D. australis
    D. conori
    D. orientalis

D

NOTES

Dermacentroxenus (continued)
    D. rickettsi
    D. sibericus
dermal
    d. bone
    d. dendritic cell
    d. dendrocyte
    d. duct tumor
    d. eccrine cylindroma
    d. epidermal nevus
    d. nevus
    d. papilla
    d. sinus
    d. tuberculosis
dermal-epidermal nevus
Dermanyssus gallinae
dermatan sulfate
dermatitidis
    Ajellomyces d.
    Blastomyces d.
dermatitis, pl. **dermatitides**
    actinic d.
    allergic d.
    atopic d.
    d. atrophicans
    d. atrophicans diffusa
    d. atrophicans maculosa
    d. chronica atrophicans idiopathica
    contact d.
    contact-type d.
    contagious pustular d.
    eczematoid d.
    d. escharotica
    d. exfoliativa
    d. exfoliativa infantum
    d. exfoliativa neonatorum
    exfoliative d.
    factitious d.
    d. gangrenosa infantum
    d. herpetiformis
    infectious eczematoid d.
    lichenoid d.
    d. medicamentosa
    nummular d.
    photocontact d.
    phototoxic contact d.
    pigmented purpuric lichenoid d.
    psoriasiform d.
    radiation d.
    d. repens
    Schamberg d.
    seborrheic d.
    stasis d.
    subcorneal pustular d.
    toxic d.
    d. venenata
    d. verrucosa

dermatoarthritis
    lipoid d.
Dermatobia
    D. hominis
dermatobiasis
dermatocele
dermatocellulitis
dermatochalasis
dermatocyst
dermatofibroma
dermatofibrosarcoma protuberans (DFSP)
    pigmented d. p.
dermatofibrosis lenticularis disseminata
dermatogen
dermatographism
dermatolysis
dermatoma
dermatomegaly
dermatomycosis
    d. pedis
dermatomyoma
dermatomyositis
dermatopathia
    d. pigmentosa reticularis
dermatopathic
    d. lymphadenitis
    d. lymphadenopathy
dermatopathology
Dermatophagoides pteronyssinus
Dermatophilaceae
dermatophilosis
Dermatophilus
    D. congolensis
    D. penetrans
dermatophylaxis
dermatophyte
    d. test medium (DTM)
dermatophytid
dermatophytosis
dermatorrhagia
dermatorrhexis
dermatosclerosis
dermatosis, pl. **dermatoses**
    benign chronic bullous d. of childhood
    Bowen precancerous d.
    chronic bullous d. of childhood
    dermolytic bullous d.
    d. papulosa nigra
    pigmentary d.
    progressive pigmentary d.
    radiation d.
    subcorneal pustular d.
    ulcerative d.
dermatozoiasis
dermatozoon
dermatozoonosis

dermatrophia
dermatrophy
dermis
dermographia
dermoid
    d. cyst
    d. cyst of ovary
    implantation d.
    inclusion d.
    sequestration d.
    d. tumor
dermolysis
dermolytic bullous dermatosis
dermonecrotic
dermopathy
    diabetic d.
dermophlebitis
dermostenosis
dermostosis
dermosyphilopathy
dermotoxin
dermotuberculin reaction
derodidymus
DES
    diethylstilbestrol
desalt
desaturation
descending
    d. degeneration
descensus
    d. ventriculi
descent
desensitization
    drug d.
    heterologous d.
    homologous d.
desensitize
desert fever
desetope
desferrioxamine
deshydremia
desiccant
desiccate
desiccation
desiccative
desiccator
designated blood donation
desipramine assay
Desmarres dacryolith
desmectasia
desmectasis

desmin
    d. antibody
desmitis
Desmodus
desmogenous
desmoglein
desmoid
    extra-abdominal d.
    d. tumor
desmolase
    17,20-d.
    20,22-d.
    20,22-d. deficiency
desmon
desmoplasia
desmoplastic
    d. cerebral astrocytoma
    d. fibroma
    d. infantile ganglioglioma
    d. medulloblastoma
    d. melanoma
    d. small round-cell tumor (DSRCT)
    d. stroma
    d. trichoblastoma
    d. trichoepithelioma
desmosine
desmosome
desmosterol
desolvation
desoxycholate
    bromocresol purple d. (BCP-D)
11-desoxycorticosterone
despeciate
despeciated antitoxin
despeciation
despumation
desquamate
desquamation
desquamativa
    otitis d.
desquamative
    d. inflammatory vaginitis
    d. interstitial pneumonia (DIP)
    d. interstitial pneumonitis (DIP)
    d. interstitial poisoning
destructive
    d. distillation
    d. interference
destruens
    chorioadenoma d.
    Hyphomyces d.
desynapsis

D

NOTES

desynchronization
detached cranial section
detachment
    retinal d.
detection
    antibody d.
    cardiac shunt d.
    C_1q immune complex d.
detector
    alpha-particle d.
    cadmium telluride d.
    combustible gas d.
    EC d.
    electron capture d.
    error d.
    flame ionization d. (FID)
    lithium-drifted d.
    paralyzable d.
    α-particle d.
    surface-barrier d.
    TC d.
    thermal conductivity d.
    thermoluminescent d.
    d. transfer function (DTF)
detergent
    anionic d.
    nonionic d.
determinant
    allotypic d.
    antigenic d.
    genetic d.
    d. group
    idiotypic antigenic d.
    immunogenic d.
    isoallotypic d.
    R d.
    resistance d. (RD)
    rough d.
determination
    activity d.
    lactate dehydrogenase isoenzymes d.
    lecithin-sphingomyelin ratio d.
    sex d.
    Shimadzu hemoglobin d.
deterministic
detersive
detoxicate
detoxication
detoxification
    metabolic d.
detoxify
detritic synovitis
detrition
detritus
detumescence
deuteranomaly
deuteranopia

deuterium
deuterohemophilia
deuteromycetes
Deuteromycota
deuteron
deuterosome
deuterotocia
deuterotoky
deutomerite
Deutschländer disease
DEV
    duck embryo vaccine
development
developmental
    d. arrest
    d. jaw cyst
    d. mixoploid
    d. synchronism
development-at-birth index (DBI)
Devergie disease
deviant
deviate
    standardized d.
deviation
    average d. (AD)
    immune d.
    d. to the left
    mean d.
    mean square d.
    no significant d. (NSD)
    relative standard d. (RSD)
    d. to the right
    right axis d. (RAD)
    standard d. (SD)
    sum of square d.'s (SSD)
Devic disease
device
    Boyden chamber assay d.
    Coag-a-mate prothrombin d.
    Coumatrak prothrombin time d.
    I/O d.
    OraSure HIV-1 Oral Specimen Collection D.
    Riechert-Mundiger stereotactic d.
    semiconductor d.
devil's grip
devolution
Dewar flask
dexamethasone (DXM)
    d. suppression test (DST)
dexiocardia
dextran
    d. blue (DB)
    low molecular weight d. (LMD, LMDX)
dextrin
    limit d.

dextrinosis
 debrancher deficiency limit d.
 limit d.
dextrinuria
dextrocardia
 corrected d.
 false d.
 isolated d.
 secondary d.
 type 1, 2, 3, 4 d.
 d. with situs inversus
dextrogastria
dextroposition
 d. of the heart
dextrorotatory (*d*-)
dextrose
 d. solution mixture (DSM)
 d. test
dextrose-nitrogen ratio (DN)
dextrose-saline (DS)
dextrose in water (percent) (D/W)
dextrosuria
dextrothyroxine sodium
dextroversion
 d. of the heart
DF
 deficiency factor
 disseminated foci
df
 degrees of freedom
DFA
 direct fluorescent antibody
 direct fluorescent assay
DFA-TP
 direct fluorescent antibody-*Treponema*
 pallidum test
 DFA-TP test
DFB
 diffuse panbronchiolitis
DFSP
 dermatofibrosarcoma protuberans
DFU
 dead fetus in utero
 dideoxyfluorouridine
DGGE
 denaturing gradient gel electrophoresis
 DGGE technique
D-glucaric acid
β-*d*-glucuronidase deficiency
dGMP
 deoxyguanosine monophosphate

dGTP
 2-deoxyguanosine-5'-triphosphate
DHA
 dehydroepiandrosterone
Dharmendra antigen
DHE
 dihydroergotamine
DHEA
 dehydroepiandrosterone
 DHEA test
DHEAS
 dehydroepiandrosterone sulfate
d'Herelle phenomenon
DHFR
 dihydrofolate reductase
DHIA
 dehydroisoandrosterone
DHL
 diffuse histocytic lymphoma
DHMA
 dihydroxymandelic acid
dhobie itch
DHT
 dihydrotachysterol
 dihydrotestosterone
 DHT test
DI
 diabetes insipidus
Di
 D. antigen
 D. Guglielmo disease
 D. Guglielmo syndrome
diabetes
 adult-onset d.
 alimentary d.
 bronze d.
 calcinuric d.
 d. innocens
 d. insipidus (DI)
 insulin-dependent d. mellitus
 (IDDM)
 juvenile-onset d.
 lipoatrophic d.
 maturity-onset d.
 d. mellitus (DM)
 Mosler d.
 noninsulin-dependent d. mellitus
 (NIDDM)
 phloridzin d.
 renal d.
diabetic
 d. acidosis

D

NOTES

177

diabetic *(continued)*
    d. amyotrophy
    d. angiopathy
    d. coma
    d. dermopathy
    d. gangrene
    d. glomerulosclerosis
    hyperosmolar d. coma
    d. ketoacidosis
    d. lipemia
    d. microangiopathy
    d. myelopathy
    d. nephropathy
    d. neuropathy
    d. retinopathy (DR)
    d. ulcer
    d. urine
diabeticorum
    bullosis d.
diabetogenic hormone
diacetemia
diacetic acid
diacetonuria
diaceturia
diaclasia
diaclasis
diacylglycerol
diag
    diagnosis
Diagnex
    D. Blue
    D. Blue test
diagnosis (diag)
    clinical d.
    cytologic d.
    differential d.
    laboratory d.
    pathologic d.
    physical d.
    prenatal d.
    provocative d.
    serum d.
diagnostic
    d. diphtheria toxin
    d. sensitivity
    d. specificity
diagram
    acid-base d.
    block d.
    scatter d.
    Venn d.
diakinesis
dial
    d. unit
    vernier d.
Dialister
dialysance
dialysate

dialysis
    equilibrium d.
    extracorporeal d.
    peritoneal d.
dialyzer
diamagnetic
diameter
    Mantoux d. (MD)
    mean cell d. (MCD)
    mean corpuscular d. (MCD)
    outside d. (OD)
diamide
4′6-diamidino-2-phenylindole-2 HCl (DAPI)
diamine
diaminobenzidine (DAB)
    d. reaction
    d. stain
    3-3′-d. tetrahydrochloride
Diamond-Blackfan
    D.-B. anemia
    D.-B. syndrome
diamond fuchsin
Diamyl
diapedesis
Diaphane
    D. solution
diaphanometer
diaphanoscope
diaphragm
    eventration of d.
diaphragmatic
    d. hernia
    d. peritonitis
    d. pleurisy
diaphysial, diaphyseal
    d. aclasis
    d. dysplasia
    d. juxtaepiphysial exostosis
diaphysitis
Diaptomus
diarrhea
    bovine virus d.
    Brainerd d.
    Cochin China d.
    tropical d.
diarrheagenic *E. coli*
diastase digestion
diastasic action
diastasis
diastasuria
diastatic
diastematocrania
diastematomyelia
diastereoisomer
diastereoisomerism
diastereomer

diastolic hypertension
diathesis, pl. diatheses
    cystic d.
    hemorrhagic d.
diathetic
diatom
diatomaceous earth
diauxic
diauxie
diazacholesterol (DAC)
diazepam
    d. assay
    d. breath test
diazinon
diazo
    d. reaction
    d. reagent
    d. stain for argentaffin granules
    d. staining method
diazomethane generator
diazonium salt
diazotize
dibasic
    d. acid
    d. potassium phosphate
dibenz[*a,h*]anthracene
dibenzopyridine
diborane
dibothriocephaliasis
Dibothriocephalus
dibrachius
    monocephalus tetrapus d.
    monocephalus tripus d.
1,2-dibromethane
dibromide
    ethylene d.
dibucaine number (DN)
DIC
    diffuse intravascular coagulation
    disseminated intravascular coagulation
dicarbamylamine
dicarboxylic acid
dicentric
dicephalus
    d. dipus dibrachius
    d. dipus tetrabrachius
    d. dipus tribrachius
    d. dipygus
    d. tripus tribrachius
dicheirus
dichlobenil

dichloride
    ethylene d.
    ethylidene d.
p-dichlorobenzene
dichlorodiethyl sulfide
dichlorodiphenyl-trichloroethane
1,1-dichloroethane
1,2-dichloroethane
sym-dichloroethylene
2,6-dichloroindophenol
dichloromethane
2,6-dichlorophenol-indophenol
(2,4-dichlorophenoxy)acetic acid
dichloropropene-dichloropropene mixture
dichlorvos
    dimethyldichlorovinyl phosphate
dichorionic
    d. diamniotic placenta
    d. placenta twins
dichotomous variable
dichotomy
dichroic filter system
dichroism
    circular d.
dichromate
    potassium d.
dichromophil, dichromophile
Dick
    D. method
    D. test
    D. test toxin
dicloxacillin
dicofol
dicrocoeliosis
Dicrocoelium
    D. dendriticum
Dictyocaulus
    D. viviparus
dictyotene
dicumarol
Didelphis
dideoxyfluorouridine (DFU)
didymitis
Diego antigen
diel
dieldrin
dielectric
    d. constant
    d. strength
diener
Dientamoeba fragilis
dieretic

D

NOTES

diet
    elimination d.
dietary protein
Dieterle
    D. method
    D. stain
dietetic albuminuria
diethylamide
    lysergic acid d. (LSD)
diethylamine
diethylaminoethyl cellulose (DEAE-cellulose)
diethyldithiocarbamate
diethylenetriaminepentaacetic acid
diethylstilbestrol (DES)
diethyl sulfate
Difco ESP testing system
difference
    alveolar-arterial carbon dioxide d.
    alveolar-arterial oxygen d.
    d. amplifier
    arteriovenous carbon dioxide d.
    arteriovenous oxygen d.
    cation-anion d.
    electric potential d.
    d. limen (DL)
    mean of consecutive d.'s (MCD)
    no significant d. (NSD)
differential
    d. agglutination titer (DAT)
    d. count
    d. diagnosis
    d. leukocyte count (DLC)
    d. leukocyte count automation
    d. renal function test
    d. stain
    d. thermometer
    d. ureteral catheterization test
    d. white blood count
differentiation
    amphicrine d.
    biphenotypic d.
    cell d.
    endothelial d.
    epithelial d.
    meissnerian d.
    mesenchymal d.
    myofibroblastic d.
    neuroendocrine d.
    rhabdomyoblastic d.
    sex d.
differentiator
Diff-Quik smear
diffraction grating
diffusate
diffuse
    d. abscess
    d. acute inflammation

d. acute peritonitis
d. amyloidosis
d. aneurysm
d. angiokeratoma
d. arterial ectasia
d. bronchopneumonia
d. chronic inflammation
d. emphysema
d. enlargement
d. esophageal spasm
d. ganglion
d. glomerulonephritis
d. goiter
d. histocytic lymphoma (DHL)
d. hyperplasia
d. hypertrophy
d. illumination
d. infantile familial sclerosis
d. infiltrative lung disease (DILD)
d. inflammation
d. interstitial fibrosis
d. interstitial pneumonia
d. interstitial pulmonary disease
d. intravascular coagulation (DIC)
d. lymphatic tissue
d. meningiomatosis
d. mesangial proliferation
d. necrosis
d. neuroendocrine system
d. nontoxic goiter
d. panbronchiolitis (DFB)
d. peritonitis
d. phlegmon
d. poorly differentiated lymphoma (DPDL)
d. pulmonary disease (DPD)
d. pyelonephritis
d. reflection
d. septal cirrhosis
d. small cleaved cell lymphoma
d. ulceration
d. waxy spleen
diffusible
diffusing
    d. capacity for carbon monoxide (D_{CO})
    d. capacity of lung
diffusion
    d. coefficient
    d. constant
    d. current
    facilitated d.
    gel d.
    d. method
    d. potential
    d. shell
diffusivity
Digenea

digenesis
digenetic
DiGeorge syndrome
digestion
    deoxyribonuclease d.
    diastase d.
    glycogen d.
    hyaluronidase d.
    neuraminidase d.
    sialidase d.
    d. vacuole
digestive
    d. albuminuria
    d. disorder
    d. glycosuria
    d. leukocytosis
digit
    check d.
    clubbed d.
    significant d.'s
Digitalis
digitalis
    d. glycoside
    d. unit
digital-to-analog converter (DAC)
digital voltmeter
digitate wart
digiti (*pl. of* digitus)
digitize
digitizer
digitonin
    d. method
    d. reaction
digitoxin
digitus, pl. **digiti**
    digiti hippocratici
diglyceride
digoxigenin-labeled riboprobe
digoxin
Digramma
    D. brauni
dihydric alcohol
dihydrobiopterin
dihydroergotamine (DHE)
dihydrofolate reductase (DHFR)
dihydrofolic acid
dihydrofolliculin
dihydropteridine
    d. reductase
    d. reductase deficiency
dihydropyrimidinase
dihydropyrimidine

dihydropyrimidinuria
dihydrosphingosine
dihydrotachysterol (DHT)
dihydrotestosterone (DHT)
dihydroubiquinone
dihydrouridine
dihydroxyacetone phosphate
dihydroxycholecalciferol
    1,25-d. assay
dihydroxydinaphthyl disulfide (DDD)
dihydroxymandelic
    d. acid (DHMA, DOMA)
    3,4-d. acid
2,5-dihydroxyphenylacetic acid
dihydroxyphenylalanine (DOPA)
diiodothyronine
diiodotyrosine (DIT)
2,4-diisocyanate
    toluene 2,4-diisocyanate
diisopropyl phosphofluoridate
dikaryon
diktyoma
dil
Dilantin
dilatation
    aneurysmal d.
    balloon d.
    poststenotic d.
    d. thrombosis
dilate
dilation
    cardiac d.
DILD
    diffuse infiltrative lung disease
diluent
dilute blood clot lysis (method) (DBCL)
diluted whole blood clot lysis
dilution
    d. anemia
    d. coefficient
    doubling d.
    log d.
    maximum inhibiting d. (MID)
    nitrogen d.
    routine test d. (RTD)
    serial d.
    d. test
dilution-filtration technique
DIM
    divalent ion metabolism
Dimastigamoeba
dimefox

D

NOTES

dimension
dimer
    thymine d.
dimercaprol
dimercaptopropanol
dimerization
dimethoate
dimethyl
    d. ether
    d. ketone
    d. sulfate
    d. sulfoxide
N,N-dimethylacetamide
dimethylallyl diphosphate
dimethylaminoaphthalene
    1-d.-5 sulfonic acid (DANS)
dimethylaminoazobenzene
7,12-dimethylbenz[a]anthracene
dimethylbenzene
dimethyldichlorovinyl phosphate (DDVP, dichlorvos)
N,N-dimethylformamide
dimethylguanosine
dimethyl ketone
dimethylnitrosamine
5,5-dimethyl-2,4-oxazolidinedione
diminazene aceturate
dimorphic
    d. anemia
    d. pathogenic fungi
dimorphism
dimorphous
    d. leprosy
dimple sign
dinitrate
    ethylene glycol d.
dinitrobenzene
dinitrochlorobenzene (DNCB)
dinitrogen tetroxide
dinitro-orthocresol (DNOC)
dinitrophenol
dinitrophenylhydrazine test
Dinobdella
    D. ferox
dinoflagellate
    d. toxin
dinormocytosis
dinucleotide
    flavin adenine d. (FAD)
    nicotinamide adenine d. (NAD)
    reduced nicotinamide-adenine d.
Dioctophyma
    D. renale
dioctophymiasis
gem-diol
diopter
1,4-dioxane
    dioxane 1,4-dioxane

dioxane 1,4-dioxane
dioxathion
dioxide
    carbamino-carbon d.
    carbon d. (CO_2)
    colloidal silicon d.
    silicon d.
    solid carbon d.
dioxin
dioxygenase
    p-hydroxyphenylpyruvate d.
    proline,2-oxoglutarate d.
1,2-dioxygenase
    homogentisate 1,2-dioxygenase
DIP
    desquamative interstitial pneumonia
    desquamative interstitial pneumonitis
dipalmitoylphosphatidylcholine
DI particle
dip-coating autoradiography
dipeptidase
    aminoacyl-histidine d.
Dipetalonema
    D. perstans
    D. streptocerca
dipetalonemiasis
diphacinone
diphasic
    d. meningoencephalitis virus
    d. milk fever
    d. milk fever virus
    d. wave
diphenadione
diphenhydramine (DPH)
    d. hydrochloride
diphenyl
diphenylhexatriene (DPH)
diphenylhydantoin (DPH)
    d. gingivitis
diphenylmethane dye
diphosphate
    adenosine d.
    adenosine 5'-d. (ADP)
    cytidine d.
    dimethylallyl d.
    fructose d.
    geranyl geranyl d.
    guanosine d.
    hexose d.
    inosine d.
    Δ^3-isopentenyl d.
    Δ^2-isopentenyl d.
    thymidine d. (dTDP)
    uridine d. (UDP)
diphosphatidylglycerol
diphosphoglycerate
    2,3-d. mutase
    d. phosphatase

diphosphoinositide
diphosphonate
diphosphopyridine nucleotide (DPN, DPNH)
diphosphosulfate
    phosphoadenosine d.
diphtheria
    d. antitoxin (DAT)
    d. antitoxin unit
    avian d.
    d. bacillus
    false d.
    fowl d.
    d., pertussis, and tetanus (vaccine) (DPT)
    d., tetanus, and pertussis (vaccine) (DTP)
    d. toxin
    d. toxin immunization reaction
    d. toxin normal (DTN)
    d. toxoid, tetanus toxoid, and pertussis vaccine
diphtheritic
    d. enteritis
    d. membrane
    d. ulcer
diphtheritica
    otitis d.
diphtheroid
    aerobic d.
    anaerobic d.
    d. bacilli
diphtherotoxin
diphyllobothriasis
Diphyllobothrium
    D. anemia
    D. latum
dipicolinic acid
diploalbuminuria
diplobacillus
diplobacterium
diploblastic
diplochromosome
diplococcemia
diplococci (*pl. of* diplococcus)
diplococcin
Diplococcus
    D. constellatus
    D. magnus
    D. morbillorum
    D. mucosus
    D. paleopneumoniae

    D. plagarumbelli
    D. pneumoniae
diplococcus, pl. **diplococci**
    Gram-negative intracellular diplococci (GNID)
    d. of Morax-Axenfeld
    d. of Neisser
    Weichselbaum d.
Diplogaster
Diplogonoporus
    D. brauni
    D. grandis
diploid
    d. merogony
    d. number
diploidy
Diplomate of the National Board of Medical Examiners
diplomelituria
diplomyelia
diplonema
diplont
diplopod
diplopoda
diplosome
Diplosporium
diplotene
dipolar
    d. ion
    d. structure
dipole moment
dipstick
Diptera
dipteran
dipterous
Dipus sagitta
dipygus
    d. parasiticus
dipylidiasis
Dipylidium caninum
diquat assay
direct
    d. agglutination (DA)
    d. agglutination pregnancy (DAP)
    d. agglutination pregnancy test (DAPT)
    d. agglutination test (DAT)
    d. antiglobulin test (DAGT)
    d. bilirubin
    d. bilirubin test
    d. centrifugal flotation (DCF)
    d. Coombs test (DCT)

D

NOTES

direct *(continued)*
    d. culture
    d. current
    d. detection
    d. fluorescent antibody (DFA)
    d. fluorescent antibody stain
    d. fluorescent antibody test
    d. fluorescent antibody test -
        Treponema pallidum (DFA-TP test)
    d. fluorescent antibody-*Treponema*
        pallidum test (DFA-TP)
    d. fluorescent assay (DFA)
    d. hernia
    d. maternal death
    d. reacting bilirubin
    d. transport
    d. vision spectroscope
direct-coupled amplifier
directional selection
directory
direct-reading potentiometer
Dirofilaria
    D. conjunctivae
    D. immitis
    D. repens
    D. tenuis
dirofilariasis
disaccharidase deficiency
disaccharide
    d. tolerance test
disaggregated (DA)
disappearance
    plasma iron d. (PID)
disappearing bone disease
disarray
    lobular d.
disc (*var. of* disk)
discharge
    double d.
    epileptiform d. (ED)
    exit d.
    d. frequency
    urethral d. (UD)
discitis
disclosing solution
discocyte
discoid lupus erythematosus (DLE)
discontinu
    tracé d.
discontinuous
    d. endothelium
    d. sterilization
discordance
discordant lymphoma
discrete
    d. smallpox
    d. subaortic stenosis

discriminant
    d. analysis
    d. function
discriminator
discussive
discutient
disease
    ABO hemolytic d. of the newborn
    abortive viral d.
    accumulation d.
    Acosta d.
    acute cardiovascular d. (ACVD)
    acute infectious d. (AID)
    acute respiratory d. (ARD)
    Adams-Stokes d. (AS)
    Addison d.
    Addison-Biermer d.
    adrenal d.
    adult celiac d.
    adult polycystic d.
    akamushi d.
    Akureyri d.
    Albarrán d.
    Albers-Schönberg d.
    Albert d.
    Albright d.
    Aleutian d. (AD)
    Aleutian mink d.
    Alexander d.
    Aliber d.
    Almeida d.
    Alpers d.
    alpha-chain d.
    alpha heavy-chain d.
    altitude d.
    Alzheimer d.
    Anders d.
    Andes d.
    antibody deficiency d.
    anti-GBM d.
    aortoiliac occlusive d.
    Apert d.
    Apert-Crouzon d.
    Aran-Duchenne d.
    arboviral virus d.
    arc-welder's d.
    Armanni-Ebstein d.
    Armstrong d.
    arterial occlusive d. (AOD)
    arteriosclerotic cardiovascular d.
      (ASCVD)
    arteriosclerotic heart d. (AHD)
    arthropod-borne viral d.
    atherosclerotic cardiovascular d.
      (ASCVD)
    atherosclerotic heart d. (AHD)
    atopic d.
    Aujeszky d.

Australian X d.
autoimmune d.
Ayerza d.
Baelz d.
Balfour d.
Ballet d.
Ballingall d.
Baló d.
Bamberger d.
Bamberger-Marie d.
Bamle d.
Bang d.
Bannister d.
Banti d.
Barclay-Baron d.
Barcoo d.
Barlow d.
Barraquer d.
Basedow d.
Batten d.
bauxite workers' d.
Bayle d.
Bazin d.
Beard d.
Beau d.
Beauvais d.
Bechterew d.
Beck d.
Becker d.
Begbie d.
Béguez César d.
Behçet d.
Behr d.
Beigel d.
Bekhterev d.
Bell d.
Bennett d.
Benson d.
Berger d.
Bergeron d.
Berlin d.
Bernhardt d.
Besnier-Boeck d.
Besnier-Boeck-Schaumann d.
Best d.
Biedl d.
Bielschowsky d.
Bielschowsky-Jansky d.
Biermer d.
Bilderbeck d.
biliary tract d.
Billroth d.

Binswanger d.
Bird d.
bird-breeder's d.
black lung d.
Bloch-Sulzberger d.
Blocq d.
Bloodgood d.
Blount d.
Blount-Barber d.
bluecomb d. of chickens
bluecomb d. of turkeys
Blumenthal d.
Boeck d.
Bogaert d.
Borna d.
Bornholm d.
Bostock d.
Bouchard d.
Bouillaud d.
Bourneville d.
Bourneville-Pringle d.
Bouveret d.
Bowen d.
Bradley d.
Brailsford-Morquio d.
branching glycogen storage d.
Breda d.
Breisky d.
Bretonneau d.
Bright d.
Brill d.
Brill-Symmers d.
Brill-Zinsser d.
Brinton d.
Brion-Kayser d.
Brissaud d.
broad-beta d.
Brocq d.
Brodie d.
bronzed d.
Brooke d.
Brown-Symmers d.
Bruck d.
Bruton d.
Budd d.
Buerger d.
Buhl d.
bullous d.
Bury d.
Buschke d.
Busquet d.
Buss d.

D

NOTES

185

disease *(continued)*

Busse-Buschke d.
Byler d.
Caffey d.
caisson d.
calcium pyrophosphate deposition d. (CPPD)
caloric d.
Calvé-Perthes d.
Calvé-Perthes-Legg d.
Camurati-Engelmann d.
Canavan d.
Capdepont d.
carcinoid heart d.
cardiac d. (CD)
cardiovascular d. (CD, CVD)
cardiovascular renal d. (CVRD)
Caroli d.
Carrión d.
Castellani d.
Castleman d.
cat-scratch d.
Cavare d.
Cazenave d.
celiac d.
Centers for D. Control (CDC)
central core d.
central Recklinghausen d. type II
cerebrovascular obstructive d. (CVOD)
ceroid storage d.
Chabert d.
Chagas d.
Chagas-Cruz d.
γ-chain d.
μ-chain d.
Championnière d.
Charcot d.
Charcot-Marie-Tooth d.
Charlouis d.
Cheadle d.
Chédiak-Higashi d.
cheese washer's d.
Cherchevski d.
Cherchewski d.
Chester d.
Chiari d.
chlamydial d.
cholesterol ester storage d.
Christensen-Krabbe d.
Christian d.
Christian-Hand-Schuller d.
Christian-Weber d.
Christman d.
Christmas d.
chronic active liver d.
chronic granulomatous d. (CGD)
chronic liver d. (CLD)

chronic lung d. (CLD)
chronic obstructive lung d. (COLD)
chronic obstructive pulmonary d. (COPD)
chronic renal d. (CRD)
Ciarrocchi d.
circling d.
Civatte d.
Coat d.
Cockayne d.
cold agglutinin d.
cold hemagglutinin d.
collagen d.'s
collagen-vascular d.'s
combined immunodeficiency d.
combined systems d.
communicable d.
Concato d.
congenital nonspherocytic hemolytic d. (CNHD)
congestive heart d. (CHD)
connective-tissue d.'s
Conor and Bruch d.
Conradi d.
constitutional d.
contagious d.
Cooley d.
Cooper d.
Corbus d.
Cori d.
coronary artery d. (CAD)
coronary atherosclerotic heart d. (CAHD)
coronary heart d. (CHD)
Corrigan d.
Corvisart d.
Cotugno d.
Cotunnius d.
Cowden d.
creeping d.
Creutzfeldt-Jakob d. (CJD)
Crigler-Najjar d.
Crocq d.
Crohn d.
Crouzon d.
Cruveilhier d.
Cruveilhier-Baumgarten d.
Cruz-Chagas d.
crystal deposition d.
Csillag d.
Curschmann d.
Cushing d.
cystic d.
cystic d. of the breast
cystic d. of renal medulla
cystine storage d.
cytomegalic inclusion d. (CID, CMID)

cytomegalovirus d.
Czerny d.
Daae d.
Daae-Finsen d.
DaCosta d.
Dalrymple d.
Danielssen d.
Danielssen-Boeck d.
Darier d.
Darling d.
David d.
Davies d.
dead of d. (DOD)
deerfly d.
deficiency d.
degenerative joint d. (DJD)
Degos d.
Dejerine d.
Dejerine-Sottas d.
demyelinating d.'s
dense-deposit d. (DDD)
deprivation d.
de Quervain d.
Dercum d.
Deutschländer d.
Devergie d.
Devic d.
diffuse infiltrative lung d. (DILD)
diffuse interstitial pulmonary d.
diffuse pulmonary d. (DPD)
Di Guglielmo d.
disappearing bone d.
diverticular d.
dog d.
Döhlc d.
dominantly inherited Lévi d.
Dubini d.
Dubois d.
Duchcnne d.
Duchenne-Aran d.
Duchenne-Griesinger d.
Duhring d.
Dukes d.
Duncan d.
Dupuytren d. of the foot
Durand d.
Durand-Nicolas-Favre d.
Durante d.
Duroziez d.
Dutton d.
Eales d.
Ebola virus d.

Ebstein d.
echinococcus d.
Economo d.
Edsall d.
endemic d.
endocrine d.
Engelmann d.
Engel-von Recklinghausen d.
English d.
Engman d.
eosinophilic endomyocardial d.
epidemic d.
epithelial cell d.
epizootic hemorrhagic d. of deer
Epstein d.
Erb d.
Erb-Charcot d.
Erb-Goldflam d.
Erdheim d.
Eulenburg d.
exanthcmatous d.
extramammary Paget d.
extrapyramidal d.
Fabry d.
Fahr d.
Farber d.
fatal granulomatous d. (FGD)
fat-deficiency d.
Fauchard d.
Favre-Racouchot d.
Fede d.
Feer d.
femoropopliteal occlusive d.
Fenwick d.
fibrocystic d. of the breast
fibrocystic d. of the breast
Fiedler d.
fifth d.
Filatov d.
fish-slime d.
Flajani d.
Flatau-Schilder d.
Flegel d.
flint d.
floating beta d.
focal d.
Folling d.
foot-and-mouth d. (FMD)
Forbes d.
Fordycc d.
Forestier d.
Förster d.

D

NOTES

disease *(continued)*
    Fothergill d.
    Fournier d.
    fourth venereal d.
    Fox-Fordyce d.
    Francis d.
    Frankl-Hochwart d.
    Franklin d.
    Frei d.
    Freiberg d.
    Friedländer d.
    Friedmann d.
    Friedreich d.
    Friend d.
    Frommel d.
    functional d.
    Furstner d.
    Gairdner d.
    Gaisböck d.
    gamma chain d.
    gamma heavy-chain d.
    Gamna d.
    Gandy-Nanta d.
    gannister d.
    Garré d.
    gasping d.
    gastroesophageal reflux d. (GERD)
    gastrointestinal d.
    Gaucher d.
    gay-related immunodeficiency d.
    Gee d.
    Gee-Herter d.
    Gee-Herter-Heubner d.
    Gee-Thaysen d.
    Gensoul d.
    Gerhardt d.
    Gerlier d.
    gestational trophoblastic d. (GTD)
    giant platelet d.
    Gibney d.
    Gierke d.
    Gilbert d.
    Gilchrist d.
    Glanzmann d.
    Glénard d.
    Glisson d.
    glomerular basement membrane disease
    glomerulocystic d.
    glycogen storage d.
    Goldflam d.
    Goldflam-Erb d.
    Goldscheider d.
    Goldstein d.
    Gorham d.
    Gougerot-Blum d.
    Gougerot-Ruiter d.
    Gougerot-Sjögren d.

    Graefe d.
    graft-versus-host d. (GVHD)
    granulomatous d.
    Graves d.
    Greenfield d.
    Greenhow d.
    Griesinger d.
    Gross d.
    Grover d.
    Guinon d.
    Gull d.
    Günther d.
    GVH d.
    Habermann d.
    Haff d.
    Haglund d.
    Hagner d.
    Hailey-Hailey d.
    Hall d.
    Hallervorden-Spatz d.
    Hallopeau d.
    Hamman d.
    Hammond d.
    Hand d.
    hand-foot-and-mouth d.
    Hand-Schüller-Christian d.
    Hanot d.
    Hansen d.
    d. of Hapsburgs
    hard pad d.
    Harley d.
    Hartnup d.
    Hashimoto d.
    heavy-chain d.
    α-heavy-chain d.
    γ-heavy-chain d.
    μ-heavy-chain d.
    Heberden d.
    Hebra d.
    Heerfordt d.
    Heine-Medin d.
    Heller-Döhle d.
    helminthic d.
    hemoglobin C d.
    hemoglobin E-thalassemia d.
    hemoglobin H d.
    hemolytic d. of newborn (HDN)
    hemorrhagic d. of deer
    hemorrhagic d. of the newborn
    Henderson-Jones d.
    hepatic veno-occlusive d.
    hepatolenticular d.
    hepatorenal glycogen storage d.
    hereditary d.
    heredodegenerative d.
    herpetic viral d.
    herring-worm d.
    Hers d.

Herter d.
Herter-Heubner d.
Heubner d.
hidebound d.
Hildenbrand d.
Hippel d.
Hippel-Lindau d.
Hirschfeld d.
Hirschsprung d. (HD)
His d.
His-Werner d.
Hjärre d.
hock d.
Hodara d.
Hodgkin d. (HD)
Hodgson d.
Hoffa d.
holoendemic d.
hoof-and-mouth d.
hookworm d.
Hoppe-Goldflam d.
Horton d.
Huchard d.
Hunt d.
Huntington d.
Hurler d.
Hutchinson-Boeck d.
Hutchinson-Gilford d.
Hutinel d.
hyaline membrane d. of the
  newborn
hydatid d. (HD)
Hyde d.
hydrocephaloid d.
hyperendemic d.
hypertensive arteriosclerotic heart d.
  (HASHD)
hypertensive cardiovascular d.
  (HCVD)
hypertensive pulmonary vascular d.
  (HPVD)
hypertensive vascular d. (HVD)
hypopigmentation-
  immunodeficiency d.
I-cell d.
idiopathic Bamberger-Marie d.
immune complex d.
immunodeficiency d.
immunoproliferative small
  intestinal d. (IPSID)
inborn lysosomal d.
inclusion body d.

inclusion cell d.
incompatible hemolytic blood
  transfusion d. (IHBTD)
infantile celiac d.
infectious d.
inflammatory bowel d.
inflammatory pelvic d. (IPD)
inherited d.
intercurrent d.
interstitial lung d.
iron storage d.
Isambert d.
ischemic bowel d.
ischemic heart d. (IHD)
ischemic leg d. (ILD)
ischemic limb d. (ILD)
island d.
Itai-Itai d.
Jaffe-Lichtenstein d.
Jakob d.
Jakob-Creutzfeldt d.
Jaksch d.
Janet d.
Jansen d.
Jansky-Bielschowsky d.
Jensen d.
Johne d.
Johnson-Steven d.
Jourdain d.
jumping d.
Jüngling d.
Kahlbaum d.
Kahler d.
Kalischer d.
Kashin-Bek d.
Kawasaki d.
Kayser d.
kedani d.
Keshan d.
Kienböck d.
Kikuchi d.
Kikuchi-Fujimoto d.
Kimmelstiel-Wilson d.
Kimura d.
kinky hair d.
Kinnier Wilson d.
Kirkland d.
kissing d.
Klebs d.
Klemperer d.
Klippel d.
knight d.

D

NOTES

disease *(continued)*

Köhler d.
Köhlmeier-Degos d.
Koshevnikoff d.
Krabbe d.
Krishaber d.
Kufs d.
Kugelberg-Welander d.
Kuhnt-Junius d.
Kümmell d.
Kümmell-Verneuil d.
Kussmaul d.
Kussmaul-Maier d.
Kyasanur Forest d.
Kyrle d.
Laënnec d.
Lafora d.
Lancereaux-Mathieu d.
Landouzy d.
Landry d.
Lane d.
Langdon Down d.
Larrey-Weil d.
Larsen d.
Larsen-Johansson d.
Lasègue d.
Lauber d.
L-chain d.
Leber d.
Legal d.
Legg d.
Legg-Calvé-Perthes d.
Legg-Perthes d.
Legionnaire's d. (LD)
Leigh d.
Leiner d.
Leloir d.
Lenègre d.
Leri-Weill d.
Leroy d.
Letterer-Siwe d.
Lev d.
Lewandowski-Lutz d.
Leyden d.
Libman-Sacks d.
Lichtheim d.
light-chain d.
Lignac d.
Lindau d.
Lindau-von Hippel d.
linear IgA bullous d. in children
lipid storage d.
Lipschütz d.
Little d.
Lobo d.
Lobstein d.
Löffler d.
Lorain d.

Lou Gehrig d.
Lowe d.
Lucas-Championnière d.
Luft d.
lumpy skin d.
lunger d.
Lutz-Splendore-Almeida d.
Lyell d.
Lyme d.
lymphocyte predominance
  Hodgkin d. (LPHD)
lymphoproliferative d. (LPD)
lymphoreticular d.
lysosomal storage d.
MacKenzie d.
Madelung d.
Magitot d.
Maher d.
Majocchi d.
Malassez d.
Malherbe d.
Malibu d.
mammary Paget d.
Manson d.
maple bark strippers' d.
maple syrup urine d. (MSUD)
marble bone d.
Marburg virus d.
March d.
Marchiafava-Bignami d.
Marek d. (MD)
Marek herpesvirus d. (MDHV)
Marfan d.
Marie d.
Marie-Bamberger d.
Marie-Strümpell d.
Marie-Tooth d.
Marion d.
Marsh d.
Martin d.
mast cell d.
Mathieu d.
Maunier-Kuhn d.
Maxcy d.
McArdle d.
McArdle-Schmid-Pearson d.
McLean-Maxwell d.
Medin d.
Mediterranean-hemoglobin E d.
medullary cystic d. (MCD)
Meige d.
Meleda d.
Ménétrier d. (MD)
Ménière d.
Merzbacher-Pelizaeus d.
metabolic bone d.
Meyenburg d.
Meyer d.

Mibelli d.
microcystic d. of renal medulla
microdrepanocytic d.
micrometastatic d.
microvillous inclusion d.
Mikulicz d.
Mills d.
Milroy d.
Milton d.
Minamata d.
minimal-change d.
Minor d.
Mitchell d.
mixed connective-tissue d. (MCTD)
Miyasato d.
Möbius d.
Moeller-Barlow d.
molecular d.
Molten d.
Mondor d.
Monge d.
Morel-Kraepelin d.
Morgagni d.
Morquio d.
Morquio-Ullrich d.
Morton d.
Morvan d.
Moschcowitz d.
motor neuron d.
Mucha d.
Mucha-Habermann d.
mu chain d.
mucopolysaccharide storage d.
mucosal d.
multicore d.
Munchmeyer d.
Myá d.
myeloproliferative d.
myocardial d. (MD)
Nairobi sheep d.
Neftel d.
Neumann d.
neutral lipid storage d.
newborn hemolytic d.
newborn hemorrhagic d.
Newcastle d. (ND)
Newcastle virus d. (NVD)
Nicolas-Favre d.
Nidoko d.
Nieden d.
Niemann d.
Niemann-Pick d. (NPD)

nil d.
nodular sclerosing Hodgkin d.
 (NSHD)
no evidence of d. (NED)
Nonne-Milroy d.
Nordau d.
Norwalk d.
no significant d. (NSD)
Novy rat d.
oasthouse urine d.
obstructive airway d. (OAD)
occupational lung d.
Oguchi d.
Ohara d.
Ollier d.
Olmer d.
Opitz d.
Oppenheim d.
Oppenheim-Urbach d.
organic d.
Oriental lung fluke d.
Ormond d.
Osgood-Schlatter d.
Osler d.
Osler-Vaquez d.
Osler-Weber-Rendu d.
Otto d.
Owren d.
Paas d.
Paget d.
Paget d. of bone
Paget d. of breast
Panner d.
paper mill worker's d.
Parkinson d. (PD)
Parrot d.
Parry d.
Parson d.
Patella d.
Pauzat d.
Pavy d.
Payr d.
pearl-worker's d.
Pel-Ebstein d.
Pelizaeus-Merzbacher d.
Pellegrini d.
Pellegrini-Stieda d.
pelvic inflammatory d. (PID)
periodic d.
periodontal d.
peripheral arterial occlusive d.
 (PAOD)

D

NOTES

disease *(continued)*
peripheral arteriosclerotic
  occlusive d. (PAOD)
peripheral vascular d. (PVD)
Perrin-Ferraton d.
Perthes d.
Pette-Döring d.
Peyronie d.
Pfeiffer d.
Phocas d.
Pick d.
pickwickian d.
pigeon breeder d.
Pinkus d.
Plummer d.
polycystic d. (PCD)
polycystic d. of kidneys
polycystic liver d.
polycystic ovary d.
polycystic renal d.
polyendocrine autoimmune d.
Pompe d.
Poncet d.
Posada d.
Posada-Wernicke d.
posttransplant lymphoproliferative d.
  (PTLD)
Pott d.
Potter d.
Poulet d.
poultry handler's d.
Preiser d.
primary myocardial d. (PMD)
Pringle d.
Profichet d.
proliferative breast d. (PBD)
pulmonary d. (PD)
pulmonary thromboembolic d.
  (PTED)
pulseless d.
Purtscher d.
Pyle d.
pyramidal d.
quiet hip d.
Quincke d.
Quinquaud d.
Ranikhet d.
rat-bite d.
Rayer d.
Raynaud d. (RD)
Recklinghausen d.
Recklinghausen d. of bone
Recklinghausen d. type I
Reclus d.
redwater d.
Reed-Hodgkin d.
Refsum d.
Reichmann d.

Reiter d.
renal cystic d.
Rendu-Weber-Osler d.
respiratory viral d.
rheumatic d.
rheumatic heart d. (RHD)
rheumatoid heart d.
Ribas-Torres d.
Riedel d.
Riga-Fede d.
Rigg d.
Ritter d.
Robinson d.
Roble d.
Roger d.
Rokitansky d.
Romberg d.
Rosai-Dorfman d.
Rosenbach d.
Rossbach d.
Roth d.
Roth-Bernhardt d.
Rougnon-Heberden d.
Roussy-Lévy d.
Rubarth d.
Rummo d.
runt d.
Rust d.
Ruysch d.
Sachs d.
salivary gland virus d.
Sanders d.
Sandhoff d.
Saunders d.
Savill d.
Schamberg d.
Schanz d.
Schaumann d.
Schenck d.
Scheuermann d.
Schilder d.
Schimmelbusch d.
Schlatter d.
Schlatter-Osgood d.
Schmorl d.
Scholz d.
Schönlein d.
Schönlein-Henoch d.
Schottmüller d.
Schroeder d.
Schüller d.
Schüller-Christian d.
Schultz d.
Schweninger-Buzzi d.
sea-blue histiocyte d.
secondary d.
Seitelberger d.
self-limited d.

Selter d.
Senear-Usher d.
senile hip d.
septic d.
serum d.
severe combined
  immunodeficiency d.
sexually transmitted d. (STD)
Shaver d.
Shichito d.
shimamushi d.
sickle cell hemoglobin C d.
sickle cell hemoglobin D d.
sickle cell-thalassemia d.
Simmonds d.
Simons d.
Siwe-Letterer d.
sixth venereal d.
Sjögren d.
Skevas-Zerfus d.
skinbound d.
slow virus d.
Sly d.
Smith d.
Smith-Strang d.
Sneddon-Wilkinson d.
specific d.
Spencer d.
sphingolipid storage d.
Spielmeyer-Stock d.
Spielmeyer-Vogt d.
Stanton d.
Stargardt d.
Steinert d.
Sternberg d.
Sticker d.
Stieda d.
Still d.
Stokes-Adams d.
storage pool d.
Strümpell d.
Strümpell-Leichtenstern d.
Strümpell-Lorrain d.
Strümpell-Marie d.
Strümpell-Westphal d.
Sudeck d.
Sutton d.
Swediaur d.
Sweet d.
Swift d.
Swift-Feer d.
swine vesicular d.

Sydenham d.
Sylvest d.
Symmers d.
systemic autoimmune d.
systemic febrile d.
Takahara d.
Takayasu d.
Talfan d.
Talma d.
Tangier d.
Tarui d.
Taussig-Bing d.
Tay d.
Taylor d.
Tay-Sachs d. (TSD)
Teschen d.
thalassemia-sickle cell d.
Thaysen d.
Theiler d.
Thiemann d.
third d.
Thomsen d.
Thomson d.
thromboembolic d. (TED)
Thygeson d.
thyrocardiac d.
thyrotoxic heart d.
Tillaux d.
Tommaselli d.
Tooth d.
Tornwaldt d.
Tourette d.
transfusion-associated graft-vs
  host d.
transport d.
Trevor d.
trophoblastic d.
tropical d.
tsutsugamushi d.
tuberculosis-respiratory d. (TB-RD)
Tyzzer d.
Underwood d.
Unna d.
unstable hemoglobin d.
Unverricht d.
upper respiratory d. (URD)
Urbach-Oppenheim d.
Urbach-Wiethe d.
urinary tract d.
vagabond's d.
van Bogaert d.
van Buren d.

D

NOTES

disease *(continued)*

    Vaquez d.
    Vaquez-Osler d.
    venereal d. (VD)
    veno-occlusive d. of the liver
    Verneuil d.
    Verse d.
    Vidal d.
    Vincent d.
    vinyl chloride d.
    viral hematodepressive d. (VHD)
    Virchow d.
    virus X d.
    Vogt-Spielmeyer d.
    Volkmann d.
    Voltolini d.
    von Bechterew d.
    von Economo d.
    von Gierke d.
    von Hippel d.
    von Hippel-Lindau d.
    von Jaksch d.
    von Meyenburg d.
    von Recklinghausen d.
    von Willebrand d. (VW)
    Voorhoeve d.
    Vrolik d.
    Wagner d.
    Waldenström d.
    Wardrop d.
    Wartenberg d.
    Wassilieff d.
    wasting d.
    Weber-Christian d.
    Weber-Rendu-Osler d.
    Wegner d.
    Weil d.
    Weir Mitchell d.
    Wenckebach d.
    Werdnig-Hoffmann d.
    Werlhof d.
    Werner-His d.
    Werner-Schultz d.
    Wesselsbron d.
    Westphal d.
    Westphal-Strümpell d.
    Whipple d.
    White d.
    white muscle d.
    white spot d.
    Whitmore d.
    Whytt d.
    Wilkie d.
    Willis d.
    Wilson d.
    Winckel d.
    Windscheid d.
    Winiwarter-Buerger d.
    Winkler d.
    Winton d.
    Witkop d.
    Wohlfart-Kugelberg-Welander d.
    Wolman d.
    woolsorter's d.
    Woringer-Kolopp d.
    X-linked lymphoproliferative d.
    Zahorsky d.
    Ziehen-Oppenheim d.
    Zinsser-Brill d.

diseased kidney (DK)
disfigurative
disgerminoma
dish

    Petri d.
    Stender d.

disinfect
disinfectant
disinfection
disinsection
disintegration constant
disjunction
disjunctive absorption
disk, disc

    blood d.
    d. capacitor
    degenerated intervertebral d.
    d. diffusion test
    d. electrophoresis
    intercalated d.
    d. kidney
    d. sensitivity method

diskitis
diskocyte
dislocation

    anterior complete d.
    closed d.
    complete anterior d.
    complete inferior d.
    complete posterior d.
    complete superior d.
    compound d.
    congenital d.
    fracture d.
    pathologic d.

dismutase

    superoxide d.

disomic population
disomy
disopyramide
disorder

    antifactor I–IX d.
    autosomal dominant d.
    autosomal recessive d.
    blood coagulation d.
    circulating antithromboplastin d.
    complex adrenal endocrine d.

complex gonadal endocrine d.
complex pituitary endocrine d.
complex thyroid endocrine d.
element d.
functional d.
immune complex d.
immunoproliferative d.
intestinal flow d.
ion d.
lipid transport d.
lymphoproliferative d.
lymphoreticular d.
myeloproliferative d.
peristalsis d.
pituitary endocrine d.
plasma iodoprotein d.
posttransplant lymphoproliferative d.
  (PTLPD)
thyroid endocrine d.
ureteral peristalsis d.
urogenital d.

disordered action of heart (DAH)
disorganization
dispermic chimera
dispermy
disperse phase
dispersion
colloidal d.
molecular d.
optical rotary d. (ORD)

dispersive medium
displaceability
displacement
d. analysis
anterior d.

display
seven-segment d.

disposable
disproportion
cephalopelvic d. (CPD)

dissect
dissecting aneurysm
dissection
aortic d.
d. tubercle

disseminata
dermatofibrosis lenticularis d.

disseminate coccidioidomycosis
disseminated
d. acute lupus erythematosus
d. aspergillosis
d. condensing osteopathy

d. foci (DF)
d. inflammation
d. intravascular coagulation (DIC)
d. lipogranulomatosis
d. lupus erythematosus (DLE)
d. sclerosis
d. superficial actinic porokeratosis
  (DSAP)
d. tuberculosis

dissemination
disseminatum
xanthoma d. (XD)

disseminatus
lupus erythematosus d. (LED)

dissociation
albuminocytologic d.
bacterial d.
d. constant
microbic d.

dissolution
dissolve
dissymmetry
distal
d. ileitis
d. latency
d. muscular dystrophy
d. myopathy

distal-type
d.-t. muscular dystrophy
d.-t. progressive muscular dystrophy

distance
focal d.
interelectrode d.
skin to tumor d. (STD)
working d.

distemper
feline d.
d. virus

distention, distension
d. cyst
d. ulcer

distill
distillate
distillation
destructive d.
fractional d.
molecular d.
vacuum d.

distilled oil
Distoma
distome

D

NOTES

distomiasis
    pulmonary d.
Distomum
distortion
    barreling d.
    crypt d.
distribution
    anomalous vascular d.
    binomial d.
    chi-squared d.
    d. coefficient
    cumulative d.
    d. curve
    dose d.
    F d.
    frequency d.
    d. function
    gaussian d.
    d. leukocytosis
    lognormal d.
    nitrogen d.
    Poisson d.
    probability d.
    reference d.
    sample d.
    skewed d.
    symmetric d.
    t d.
disulfide
    d. bond
    carbon d.
    dihydroxydinaphthyl d. (DDD)
disulfiram assay
disulfoton
disuse atrophy
DIT
    diiodotyrosine
    drug-induced thrombocytopenia
dithionite test
dithiothreitol
Dittrich
    D. plug
    D. stenosis
diuresis, pl. **diureses**
diuretic
    cardiac d.
    hemopoiesic d.
    loop d.
    mechanical d.
    osmotic d.
    thiazide d.
diurnal
diuron
divalent ion metabolism (DIM)
divarication
diverticula (*pl. of* diverticulum)
diverticular disease

diverticulitis
    hemorrhagic d.
    obstructive d.
    perforated d.
diverticuloma
diverticulosis
diverticulum, pl. **diverticula**
    cervical d.
    duodenal d.
    epiphrenic d.
    false d.
    hypopharyngeal d.
    Meckel d.
    Pertik d.
    pharyngoesophageal d.
    pulsion d.
    traction d.
    true d.
    urethral d.
    ventricular d.
    vesical d.
    Zenker d.
divided dose
divider
    voltage d.
diving goiter
division
    cell d.
    conjugate d.
    equational d.
    maturation d.
    reduction d.
Dixon test
dizygotic twins
DJD
    degenerative joint disease
DK
    decay
    diseased kidney
DL
    difference limen
    Donath-Landsteiner
dL, dl
    deciliter
D-L Ab
    Donath-Landsteiner antibody
DLC
    differential leukocyte count
DLE
    discoid lupus erythematosus
    disseminated lupus erythematosus
D-L hemolysin
DM
    diabetes mellitus
dm
    decimeter
DMD
    Duchenne muscular dystrophy

DN
dextrose-nitrogen ratio
dibucaine number
Dn
dekanem
dn
decinem
DNA
deoxyribonucleic acid
DNA aneuploidy
complementary DNA (cDNA)
DNA complexity
DNA cytophotometry
DNA fingerprint
DNA fingerprinting
DNA flow cytometry
DNA homology
DNA hybridization
DNA ligase
DNA marker
DNA nucleotidylexotransferase
DNA nucleotidyltransferase
DNA ploidy
DNA polymerase
DNA probe
DNA reassociation
recombinant DNA (rDNA)
DNA renaturation
DNA repair
ribosomal DNA (rDNA)
DNA synthesis
DNA virus
DNAase (*var. of* DNAse)
DNA-DNA hybridization
DNA-RNA hybridization
DNase, DNAse
deoxyribonuclease
DNase agar
DNase test
DNCB
dinitrochlorobenzene
D^u negative
DNOC
dinitro-orthocresol
DNP
deoxyribonucleoprotein
DOA
dead on arrival
DOC
deoxycorticosterone
DOCA
deoxycorticosterone acetate

docimasia
auricular d.
hepatic d.
pulmonary d.
DOCS
deoxycorticoids
DOD
dead of disease
Döderlein bacillus
dog
d. disease
d. distemper virus
d. flea
d. fly
d. hookworm
d. louse
d. nose
d. unit
Döhle
D. disease
D. inclusion
D. inclusion body
Döhle-Heller aortitis
Dold
D. reaction
D. test
dolichocolon
dolichoectatic artery
dolichol phosphate
dolipore
doll's eye movements
dolor
DOMA
dihydroxymandelic acid
domain
domiciliated
dominance
incomplete d.
dominant
d. character
d. complement
d. complementarity
d. gene
d. inheritance
dominantly inherited Lévi disease
Donath-Landsteiner (DL)
D.-L. antibody (D-L Ab)
D.-L. cold autoantibody
D.-L. phenomenon
D.-L. test
Donnan potential

D

NOTES

Donné
>D. body
>D. corpuscle
>D. test

Donohue syndrome

donor
>cadaver d. (CD)
>consanguineous d. (CD)
>F d.
>living d. (LD)
>proton d.
>universal d.

Donovan body

Donovania
>*D. granulomatis*

DOPA
>dihydroxyphenylalanine
>DOPA stain

dopa
>d. reaction

dopamine
>d. hydroxylase
>d. monooxygenase

dopaminergic

dopaquinone

Doppler effect

d'orange
>peau d.

Doriden

dormancy

dormant

Dorner stain

Dorothy Reed cell

dorsalis
>tabes d.

dosage
>d. compensation
>gene d.
>high d. (HD)

dose
>absorbed d.
>d. account
>air d.
>booster d.
>d. calibrator
>curative d. (CD)
>depth d.
>d. distribution
>divided d.
>effective d. (ED)
>epilating d.
>erythema d.
>d. estimate
>exit d.
>fatal d. (FD)
>genetically significant d. (GSD)
>infecting d. (ID)
>infective d. (ID)

integral d.
L d.
L^+ d.
L_0 d.
lethal d. (LD)
Lf d.
loading d.
Lr d.
maximal permissible d. (MPD)
mean d.
mean hemolytic d. (MHD)
mean d. per unit cumulated
>activity

median effective d. (ED_{50})
median fatal d. (FD_{50})
median infectious d. (ID_{50})
median lethal d. (LD_{50})
median tissue culture d. (TCD_{50})
median tissue culture infective d.
>($TCID_{50}$)

medical internal radiation d.
>(MIRD)

minimal erythema d. (MED)
minimal infecting d. (MID)
minimal lethal d.
minimal morbidostatic d. (MMD)
minimal reacting d. (MRD)
minimum hemolytic d. (MHD)
minimum infective d. (MID)
minimum lethal d. (MLD)
normal single d. (NSD)
organ tolerance d. (OTD)
radiation d.
radiation absorbed d. (rad)
d. rate
sensitizing d.
shocking d.
skin d.
skin test d. (STD)
threshold d.
threshold erythema d. (TED)
tissue culture d. (TCD)
tissue culture infectious d.
>($TCID_{50}$)

tissue culture infective d. (TCID)
tissue tolerance d. (TTD)
titrated initial d. (TID)
tumor lethal d. (TLD)

dose-reduction factor (DRF)

dosimeter
>pencil d.
>pocket d.
>thermoluminescent d.
>ultraviolet fluorescent d.

dosimetry

dot
>d. blot test
>Maurer d.'s

Mittendorf d.'s
d. product
d. scan
Schüffner d.'s
Ziemann d.'s
double
d. albuminemia
d. antibody immunoassay
d. antibody method
d. antibody precipitation
d. antibody sandwich assay
d. blind experiment
d. diffusion test
d. discharge
d. ductus arteriosus
d. (gel) diffusion precipitin test in one dimension
d. (gel) diffusion precipitin test in two dimensions
d. helix
d. immunodiffusion
d. immunolabeling
d. intussusception
d. minute chromosome
d. oxalate
d. pneumonia
d. refraction
d. stain
d. tertian malaria
d. trisomy
double-beam photometer
double-blind
double-contrast
d.-c. examination
d.-c. study
double-masked experiment
double-pole
d.-p. double-throw switch
d.-p. single-throw switch
double-precision variable
doubling
d. dilution
d. time
Douglas abscess
dourine
Dowex
Downey cell
Downey-type lymphocyte
down-regulation
downstream
Down syndrome (DS)

doxepin
d. hydrochloride
d. hydrochloride assay
doxorubicin
d. (Adriamycin), cyclophosphamide, etoposide, ifosfamide, vincristine (Oncovin), methotrexate, bleomycin (CAMBO-VIP)
vincristine, cyclophosphamide, prednisone, d. (Adriamycin) (VEPA)
doxycycline
D-PAS stain
DPC
delayed primary closure
DPD
diffuse pulmonary disease
DPDL
diffuse poorly differentiated lymphoma
2,3-DPGM
DPH
Department of Public Health
diphenhydramine
diphenylhexatriene
diphenylhydantoin
DPN
diphosphopyridine nucleotide
DPNH
diphosphopyridine nucleotide
D^u positive
DPT
diphtheria, pertussis, and tetanus (vaccine)
DR
diabetic retinopathy
reaction of degeneration
Drabkin reagent
dracontiasis
dracunculiasis
dracunculosis
Dracunculus
D. medinensis
Dragendorff
D. solution
D. test
dragon
d. worm
d. worm infection
drainage
anomalous venous d.
drain-trap stomach
Drechslera hawaiiensis

D

NOTES

199

drench hose
drepanidium
Drepanidotaenia
    D. lanceolata
drepanocyte
drepanocytemia
drepanocythemia
drepanocytic
drepanocytosis
Drepanospira
Dresbach
    D. anemia
    D. syndrome
Dressler syndrome
DRF
    dose-reduction factor
dried
    d. human serum
    d. yeast
drift
    antigenic d.
    genetic d.
    random genetic d.
drive
    tape d.
drop
    d. heart
    voltage d.
droplet
    electron-dense d.
    d. infection
    d. nuclei
dropsical
dropsy
    abdominal d.
Drosophila
drug
    d. abuse screen
    d. addiction
    d. allergy
    antibiotic antitumor d.
    d. dependence
    d. desensitization
    d. interaction
    d. interference
    ototoxic d.
    radioactive d.
    d. screening assay
    sulfa d.
    d. tolerance
drug-fast
drug-induced
    d.-i. hepatitis
    d.-i. thrombocytopenia (DIT)
drug-resistant
drumstick
    d. finger
    d. spore

drusen
dry
    d. abscess
    d. bronchiectasis
    d. catarrh
    d. gangrene
    d. leprosy
    d. objective
    d. pleurisy
drying agent
DS
    defined substrate
    dehydroepiandrosterone sulfate
    dextrose-saline
    Down syndrome
DSAP
    disseminated superficial actinic
      porokeratosis
DSM
    dextrose solution mixture
DSRCT
    desmoplastic small round-cell tumor
DST
    dexamethasone suppression test
DT
    delirium tremens
    dye test
dTDP
    thymidine diphosphate
DTF
    detector transfer function
DTH
    delayed-type hypersensitivity
DTM
    dermatophyte test medium
DTN
    diphtheria toxin normal
DTP
    diphtheria, tetanus, and pertussis
      (vaccine)
dTTP
    deoxythymidine triphosphate
dual-contrast study
dual-in-line package
dualism
Duane-Hunt relation
Duane syndrome
Dubini disease
Dubin-Johnson syndrome
Dubin-Sprinz syndrome
Dubois
    D. abscess
    D. disease
Duboisia
Dubreuil-Chambardel syndrome
Duchenne
    D. disease

D. muscular dystrophy (DMD)
D. syndrome
Duchenne-Aran disease
Duchenne-Erb syndrome
Duchenne-Griesinger disease
Duchenne-type muscular dystrophy
duck
d. embryo origin vaccine
d. embryo vaccine (DEV)
d. hepatitis virus
d. influenza virus
d. plague
d. plague virus
Ducrey
D. bacillus
D. test
duct
d. carcinoma
d. papilloma
ductal
d. carcinoma
d. carcinoma in situ (DCIS)
d. hyperplasia
ductopenia
ductular piecemeal necrosis
ductule
aberrant d.
ductus deferens tumor
Duffy
D. antibodies, Fy^a, Fy^b
D. antigen
D. blood group system
Duhring disease
Duke
D. bleeding time test
D. method
D. method of bleeding time
Dukes
D. classification
D. disease
D. staging
dullness
relative hepatic d. (RHD)
dumbbell ganglioneuroma
dumdum fever
dummy variable
dUMP
deoxyuridine monophosphate
dumping syndrome
Duncan
D. disease
Dunnet multiple component test

duodenal
d. atresia
d. contents examination
d. diverticulum
d. fistula
d. smear
d. ulcer
duodenitis
duodenocholangitis
duodenocholecystostomy
duodenocystostomy
duodenoenterostomy
duodenostomy
duovirus
DU-PAN-2 stain
Duplay syndrome
duplex
d. ileum
d. kidney
d. placenta
duplication
caudal dipygus d.
congenital d.
cranial monocephalus d.
d. cyst
d. deficiency
facial diprosopus d.
fetal d.
trunk d.
Dupré syndrome
Dupuytren
D. contracture
D. disease of the foot
D. fibromatosis
Durand disease
Durand-Nicolas-Favre disease
Duran-Reynals permeability factor
Durante disease
Dürck node
Duroziez disease
dust
blood d.
d. cell
chromatin d.
d. corpuscle
nuclear d.
Dutcher body
Dutton
D. disease
D. relapsing fever
Duttonella

NOTES

D5W, D5 & W, D₅W
    5 percent dextrose in water
D/W
    dextrose in water (percent)
dwarf
    achondroplastic d.
    d. colony
    constitutional d.
    pituitary d.
    primordial d.
    d. tapeworm
dwarfism
    achondroplastic d.
    acromelic d.
    chondrodystrophic d.
    Fröhlich d.
    lethal d.
    mesomelic d.
    micromelic d.
    phocomelic d.
    pituitary d.
    polydystrophic d.
    senile d.
    Silver-Russell d.
    snub-nose d.
    thanatophoric d.
DXM
    dexamethasone
dyad
dydrogesterone
dye
    acid d.
    acidic d.
    acridine d.
    aminoanthraquinone d.
    aminoketone d.
    amphoteric d.
    aniline d.
    anionić d.
    anthraquinone d.
    azin d.
    azo d.
    azocarmine d.
    azoic d.
    basic d.
    cationic d.
    d. content
    diphenylmethane d.
    endolymphatic d.
    d. exclusion test
    d. excretion test
    fluorescent d.
    hydroxyketone d.
    indamine d.
    indigoid d.
    indophenol d.
    ketonimine d.
    lactone d.

    metachromatic d.
    methine d.
    methylene blue d. (MBD)
    natural d.
    NBT d.
    nitro d.
    nitroblue tetrazolium d.
    nitroso d.
    oxazin d.
    oxazine d.
    patent blue V d.
    phthalocyanine d.
    polymethine d.
    quinoline d.
    rosanilin d.
    salt d.
    stilbene d.
    sulfur d.
    synthetic d.
    d. test (DT)
    thiazin d.
    thiazole d.
    triarylmethane d.
    triphenylmethane d.
    vital d.
    xanthene d.
dye-binding capacity (DBC)
dye-dilution curve
dyed starch method
Dyggve-Melchior-Clausen syndrome
Dyke-Davidoff-Masson syndrome
dyn
    dyne
dynamic
    d. equilibrium
    d. ileus
    d. isomerism
    d. storage allocation
    d. viscosity
dyne (dyn)
dynein
dyphylline
Dyrenium
dysautonomia
    familial d.
dysbarism
dysbetalipoproteinemia
    familial d.
dysbolism
dyscephalia
    d. mandibulo-oculofacialis
dyschondrogenesis
dyschondroplasia
    d. with hemangiomas
dyschondrosteosis
dyscrasia
    blood d.

lymphatic d.
plasma cell d.
dyscrasic
dyscratic
dysembryoma
dysembryoplastic
    d. neuroepithelial tumor
dysemia
dysencephalia splanchnocystica
dysentery
    amebic d.
    d. antitoxin
    bacillary d.
    d. bacilli
    balantidial d.
    bilharzial d.
    catarrhal d.
    ciliary d.
    ciliate d.
    epidemic d.
    flagellate d.
    Flexner d.
    fulminant d.
    giardiasis d.
    malarial d.
    protozoal d.
    scorbutic d.
    Sonne d.
    spirillar d.
    sporadic d.
    viral d.
    winter d. of cattle
dyserythropoiesis
dyserythropoietic congenital anemia
dysfibrinogenemia
dysfunction
    constitutional hepatic d.
    minimal brain d. (MBD)
    papillary muscle d.
    phagocyte d.
dysfunctional
    d. bleeding
dysgammaglobulinemia
dysgenesis
    familial gonadal d.
    gonadal d.
    seminiferous tubule d.
    testicular d.
    XO gonadal d.
    XX gonadal d.
    XY gonadal d.
dysgenetic

dysgerminoma
dysglobulinemia
dysgonic
dyshematopoiesis
dyshematopoietic
dyshemopoiesis
dyshemopoietic
    d. anemia
dyshesion
dyshesive
dyshidrosis
dyshormonogenesis
dyshormonogenic goiter
dyskaryosis
dyskaryotic
dyskeratoma
    warty d.
dyskeratosis
    benign d.
    d. congenita
    hereditary benign intraepithelial d.
    intraepithelial d.
    isolated d. follicularis
    malignant d.
dyskeratotic
dyskinesia
    tracheobronchial d.
dyslipoproteinemia
dysmenorrhea
dysmorphia
    mandibulo-oculofacial d.
dysmorphism
dysmyelopoietic syndrome
dysosteogenesis
dysostosis
    acrofacial d.
    cleidocranial d.
    craniofacial d.
    Crouzon craniofacial d.
    mandibuloacral d.
    mandibulofacial d.
    metaphysial d.
    d. multiplex
    orodigitofacial d.
    otomandibular d.
    peripheral d.
dysoxidative carbonuria
dyspallia
dysphagia
    sideropenic d.
dysphagocytosis
    congenital d.

D

NOTES

dyspigmentation
dysplasia
    acquired d.
    anhidrotic ectodermal d.
    anterofacial d.
    anteroposterior facial d.
    asphyxiating thoracic d.
    atriodigital d.
    bronchopulmonary d. (BPD)
    cerebral d.
    cervical d.
    chondroectodermal d.
    cleidocranial d.
    congenital ectodermal d.
    congenital thymic d. (CTD)
    cortical d.
    craniocarpotarsal d.
    craniodiaphysial d.
    craniometaphysial d.
    dentin d.
    diaphysial d.
    ectodermal hereditary d.
    d. epiphysialis hemimelia
    d. epiphysialis multiplex
    d. epiphysialis punctata
    epithelial d.
    faciodigitogenital d.
    familial fibrous d. of jaws
    fibromuscular d.
    fibrous d. of bone
    fibrous familial d.
    fibrous d. of jaws
    fibrous monostotic d.
    hereditary renal-retinal d.
    hidrotic ectodermal d.
    hypohidrotic ectodermal d.
    lymphopenic thymic d.
    mammary d.
    mandibulofacial d.
    metaphysial d.
    monostotic fibrous d.
    mucoepithelial d.
    multiple epiphysial d.
    neuronal intestinal d.
    OAV d.
    oculoauriculovertebral d.
    oculodentodigital d.
    oculovertebral d.
    ODD d.
    OMM d.
    ophthalmomandibulomelic d.
    polyostotic fibrous d.
    postradiation d. (PRDX)
    precancerous d.
    pseudoachondroplastic
      spondyloepiphysial d.

    septo-optic d.
    spondyloepiphysial d. (SED)
    thymic d.
    T-zone d.
    ventriculoradial d.
    vesical d.
    Zenker d.
dysplastic
    d. nevus
    d. nevus syndrome
dyspoiesis
dysprosium
dysproteinemia
dysproteinemic
dysprothrombinemia
dyssebacia
dysspondylism
dyssynergia
    progressive cerebellar d.
dystonia
dystonic
dystopia
dystopic
dystrophia
    d. brevicollis
    d. unguium
dystrophic
    d. calcification
    d. calcinosis
dystrophin antibody
dystrophy
    adiposogenital d.
    asphyxiating thoracic d. (ATD)
    Becker d.
    craniocarpotarsal d.
    distal muscular d.
    distal-type muscular d.
    Duchenne muscular d. (DMD)
    Duchenne-type muscular d.
    infantile neuroaxonal d. (INAD)
    Landouzy-Dejerine progressive
      muscular d.
    limb-girdle muscular d.
    lipoid d.
    muscular d. (MD)
    myotonic d.
    ocular muscle d. (OMD)
    ophthalmoplegic-type progressive
      muscular d.
    progressive muscular d. (PMD)
    thoracic asphyxiant d. (TAD)
    thoracic-pelvic-phalangeal d.
    vulvar d.
dystrophy-dystocia syndrome (DDS)
dysuria-pyuria syndrome

ε (*var. of* epsilon)
    ε staphylolysin
E
    erythrocyte
    extraction fraction
        E antigen
        E erythrocyte rosette assay
        E rosette
E$_1$
    estrone
E$_2$
    estradiol
E$_3$
    estriol
E$_4$
    estetrol
eos (*var. of* eo)
EA
    early antigen
EAC
    Ehrlich ascites carcinoma
    erythrocyte, antibody, complement
        EAC rosette
        EAC rosette assay
Eadie-Hofstee equation
EAE
    experimental allergic encephalomyelitis
Eagle
        E. basal medium
        E. minimum essential medium
        E. syndrome
EAHF
    eczema, asthma, hay fever
EAHLG
    equine antihuman lymphoblast globulin
EAHLS
    equine antihuman lymphoblast serum
Eales disease
EAN
    experimental allergic neuritis
EAP
    epiallopregnanolone
ear
        cauliflower e.
        e. culture
        e. lobule
        scroll e.
Earle
        E. L fibrosarcoma
        E. solution
early
        e. antigen (EA)
        e. neonatal death
        e. reaction

early-phase response
earth
    diatomaceous e.
eastern
        e. equine encephalitis
        e. equine encephalitis virus titer
        e. equine encephalomyelitis (EEE)
        e. equine encephalomyelitis virus
Eaton
        E. agent
        E. agent pneumonia
Eaton-Lambert syndrome
EB
    epidermolysis bullosa
    estradiol benzoate
        EB virus
EBER1 riboprobe
Eberthella
    E. typhi
Eberth line
EBL
    estimated blood loss
EBNA
    Epstein-Barr nuclear antigen
Ebola
        E. hemorrhagic fever
        E. virus
        E. virus disease
Ebstein
        E. anomaly
        E. disease
        E. malformation
eburnation
EBV
    Epstein-Barr virus
        EBV culture
        EBV virus
EC
    electron capture
    enteric-coated
    enterochromaffin-cell hyperplasia
    Escherichia coli
    extracellular
        EC detector
ECA
    ethacrynic acid
ECBO virus
    enteric cytopathogenic bovine orphan
    virus
ECBV
    effective circulating blood volume
eccentric hypertrophy
eccentrochondroplasia
ecchondroma

E

ecchondrosis
  e. physaliformis
  e. physaliphora
ecchordosis
  e. physalifora
  e. physaliformis
ecchymoma
ecchymosed
ecchymosis, pl. **ecchymoses**
  Tardieu ecchymoses
ecchymotic
eccrine
  e. acrospiroma
  e. poroma
  e. spiradenoma
  e. tumor
ECDO virus
ECF-A
  eosinophil chemotactic factor of
    anaphylaxis
ECFV
  extracellular fluid volume
ecgonine
echidninus
  Laelaps e.
Echidnophaga gallinacea
echinate
Echinochasmus
echinococciasis
echinococcosis
  e. serological test
  unilocular e.
Echinococcus
  E. granulosus
  E. multilocularis
echinococcus
  e. cyst
  e. disease
echinocyte
echinocytosis
Echinorhynchus
echinosis
Echinostoma
  E. ilocanum
  E. lindoensis
  E. malayanum
  E. perfoliatum
  E. revolutum
echinostomiasis
echinulate
echo
  M-mode e.
ECHO virus
  enteric cytopathogenic human orphan
    virus
  E. v. type 1, 12, 28
echovirus

echt
  cresyl e.
ECIS
  endometrial carcinoma in situ
ECL
  electrogenerated chemiluminescence
  emitter-coupled logic
  enterochromaffin-like
  extracapillary lesion
eclampsia
  puerperal e.
  uremic e.
eclipse
  e. period
  e. phase
eclipsed
ECLT
  euglobulin clot lysis time
ECM
  erythema chronicum migrans
  extracellular material
ECMO virus
  enteric cytopathogenic monkey orphan
    virus
ECoG
  electrocorticogram
  electrocorticography
ecoid
E. coli
  Escherichia coli
ecologic niche
ecology
Economo disease
EcoR1 enzyme
ecospecies
ecosystem
ecotaxis
ecotropic virus
ecphyma
ECSO virus
  enteric cytopathogenic swine orphan
    virus
ecstrophe
ECT
  ectomesenchymal chondromyxoid tumor
  euglobulin clot test
ectacolia
ectasia
  e. cordis
  diffuse arterial e.
  hypostatic e.
  mammary duct e.
  papillary e.
  senile e.
  e. ventriculi paradoxa
ectasis
ectatic
  e. aneurysm

ecthyma
    contagious e.
    e. gangrenosum
    e. infectiosum
    e. infectiosum virus
ecthymatiform
ecthymiform
ectoantigen
ectocervical smear
ectocyst
ectodermal
    e. defect
    e. hereditary dysplasia
ectodermatosis
ectodermosis
    e. erosiva pluriorificialis
ectogenous
ectoglobular
ectomerogony
ectomesenchymal chondromyxoid tumor (ECT)
ectomesenchyme
ectoparasite
ectoparasiticide
ectoparasitism
ectoperitonitis
ectophyte
ectopia
    e. cloacae
    e. renis
    e. testis
    e. vesicae
ectopic
    e. ACTH syndrome
    e. anus
    e. decidua
    e. focus (EF)
    e. hormone
    e. pinealoma
    e. pregnancy (EP)
    e. testis
ectoplasm
ectopy
ectosarc
ectostosis
ectothrix
    e. infection
ectotoxin
ectozoic
ectozoon, pl. ectozoa
ectromelia
    e. virus

ectromelus
ectrometacarpia
ectropion
ECV
    extracellular volume
ECW
    extracellular water
eczema
    allergic e.
    baker's e.
    chronic e.
    e. erythematosum
    facial e.
    e. herpeticum
    e. hypertrophicum
    lichenoid e.
    e. marginatum
    nummular e.
    e. verrucosum
    e. vesiculosum
eczema, asthma, hay fever (EAHF)
eczematoid dermatitis
ED
    effective dose
    epileptiform discharge
ED$_{50}$
    median effective dose
E-DCIS
    endocrine ductal carcinoma in situ
Eddowes syndrome
eddy current
eddy-current loss
edema
    angioneurotic e.
    blue e.
    brain e.
    brown e.
    bullous e.
    bullous e. vesicae
    cardiac e.
    cerebral e.
    circumscribed e.
    congestive e.
    dependent e.
    heat e.
    hereditary angioneurotic e. (HANE)
    inflammatory e.
    lymphatic e.
    malignant e.
    e. neonatorum
    noninflammatory e.
    periodic e.

E

NOTES

edema *(continued)*
    peripheral e.
    pitting e.
    pulmonary e. (PE)
    Quincke e.
    solid e.
edematization
edematous
edetate
    calcium disodium e.
edetic acid
Edinger-Westphal nucleus
Edlefsen reagent
Edman reaction
Edmondson tumor grading system
EDRF
    endothelium-derived relaxing factor
edrophonium
    e. chloride
    e. chloride test
EDS
    Ehlers-Danlos syndrome
Edsall disease
EDTA
    ethylenediaminetetraacetic acid
EDTA-associated leukoagglutination
EDTA-dependent
    pseudothrombocytopenia
Edwardsiella
    E. tarda
Edwardsielleae
Edwards-Patau syndrome
Edwards syndrome
EEE
    eastern equine encephalomyelitis
        EEE virus
EF
    ectopic focus
    encephalitogenic factor
EFA
    essential fatty acids
EFC
    endogenous fecal calcium
EFE
    endocardial fibroelastosis
effect
    Arias-Stella e.
    Auger e.
    Bohr e.
    Crabtree e.
    crowding e.
    cytopathic e. (CPE)
    Doppler e.
    Faraday e.
    founder e.
    Haldane e.
    oxygen e.
    Pasteur e.

    photoelectric e.
    photographic e.
    piezoelectric e.
    radiation e.'s
    side e.
    Somogyi e.
    Staub-Traugott e.
    Whitten e.
    Wolff-Chaikoff e.
effective
    e. circulating blood volume
        (ECBV)
    e. dose (ED)
    e. half-life
    e. oxygen transport (EOT)
    e. refractory period (ERP)
    e. renal blood flow (ERBF)
    e. renal plasma flow
    e. temperature (ET)
effectiveness
    relative biological e. (RBE)
effector
    allosteric e.
    e. cell
effemination
efficacy
efficiency
    geometric e.
    photopeak detection e.
efflorescence
effuse colony
effusion
    chylous e.
    e. cytology
    lymphoid-rich e.
    serofibrinous e.
    serosanguineous e.
    serous e.
EFV
    extracellular fluid volume
EGC
    endocrine granule constituent
EGE
    eosinophilic gastroenteritis
EGFR
    epidermal growth factor receptor
egg count
Eggel tumor classification
egg-white lysozyme (EWL)
egg-yolk agar
EGL
    eosinophilic granuloma of lung
eglandulous
EGOT
    erythrocyte glutamic oxaloacetic
        transaminase
Egyptian splenomegaly

EH
  essential hypertension
EHBF
  estimated hepatic blood flow
  exercise hyperemia blood flow
EHEC
  enterohemorrhagic *Escherichia coli*
EHF
  exophthalmos-hyperthyroid factor
EHL
  endogenous hyperlipidemia
Ehlers-Danlos syndrome (EDS)
EHO
  extrahepatic obstruction
EHP
  excessive heat production
Ehrlich
  E. acid hematoxylin stain
  E. anemia
  E. aniline crystal violet stain
  E. ascites carcinoma (EAC)
  E. benzaldehyde reaction
  E. diazo reaction
  E. diazo reagent
  E. inner body
  E. phenomenon
  E. postulate
  E. side-chain theory
  E. test
  E. triacid stain
  E. triple stain
  E. unit (EU)
Ehrlichia
ehrlichiosis
EI
  enzyme inhibitor
  eosinophilic index
EIA
  enzyme immunoassay
  EIA interface
Eichhorst corpuscle
EID
  electroimmunodiffusion
EIEC
  enteroinvasive *Escherichia coli*
eighth nerve tumor
Eijkman lactose broth
Eikenella
  E. corrodens
Eimeria
Eimeriidae
Einarson gallocyanin-chrome alum stain

einsteinium
Einthoven law
Eisenlohr syndrome
Eisenmenger
  E. syndrome
  tetralogy of E.
ejection murmur (EM)
EK
  erythrokinase
Ekbom syndrome
EKC
  epidemic keratoconjunctivitis
ekiri
Ektachem
EL
  electroluminescence
Elaeophora schneideri
elaidic acid
E-LAM
  endothelial-leukocyte adhesion molecule
elastance
elastase
elastic
  e. fiber
  e. fiber stain
  e. lamellae
  e. scattering
  e. skin
elastica
  cutis e.
elastica-van Gieson stain
elasticity
elasticum
  pseudoxanthoma e. (PXE)
elastin stain
elastofibroma
  e. dorsi
  mediastinal e.
elastoid degeneration
elastoma
  juvenile e.
  Miescher e.
elastomer envelope
elastorrhexis
elastosis
  e. colloidalis conglomerata
  e. perforans serpiginosa
  senile e.
  solar e.
elastotic degeneration
Elavil
elective culture

E

NOTES

electric
 e. field vector
 e. potential
 e. potential difference
 e. susceptibility
electrical artifact
electroblot analysis
electrocardiogram
 fetal e. (FECG)
electrochemical cell
electrochemistry
electrocorticogram (ECoG)
electrocorticography (ECoG)
electrode
 active e.
 bipolar needle e.
 calomel e.
 carbon dioxide e.
 Clark oxygen e.
 e. of first kind
 glass e.
 hydrogen e.
 e. impedance
 indicator e.
 indifferent e.
 inert e.
 ion-selective e. (ISE)
 P_{CO_2} e.
 P_{O_2}e.
 pH e.
 e. potential
 quinhydrone e.
 recording e.
 reference e.
 e. response time
 e. of second kind
 e. sensitivity
 Severinghaus e.
 silver/silver chloride e.
 standard hydrogen e.
electroendosmosis
electrogenerated chemiluminescence (ECL)
electroimmunoassay
electroimmunodiffusion (EID)
electroluminescence (EL)
electrolysis
electrolyte
 amphoteric e.
 e. balance and homeostasis
 colloidal e.
 e. imbalance
 protein e.
electrolytic
 e. capacitor
 e. cell
 e. stripping
electromagnet

electromagnetic
 e. flowmeter (EMF)
 e. radiation
 e. unit (emu)
electrometer amplifier
electromotance
electromotive force (EMF)
electron
 Auger e.
 e. beam
 e. capture (EC)
 e. capture detector
 conduction e.
 conversion e.
 free e.
 e. lens
 e. micrograph
 e. microprobe
 e. microscope (EM)
 e. microscopy (EM)
 e. pair
 e. pair bond
 e. paramagnetic resonance
 paramagnetic resonance of e.'s
 e. spin resonance (ESR, esr)
 e. transport chain
 e. transport inhibitor
 valence e.
 e. volt (ev)
electron-dense droplet
electronegative
electronegativity
electronic
 e. cell counter
 e. focal spot
electroosmosis
electroparacentesis
electropathology
electropherogram
electrophile
electrophoresis (EP)
 acrylamide gel e.
 agarose gel e.
 alkaline phosphatase isoenzyme e.
 cerebrospinal fluid e.
 citrate agar gel e.
 creatine kinase isoenzyme e.
 denaturing gradient gel e. (DGGE)
 disk e.
 hemoglobin e.
 high-voltage e. (HVE)
 immunofixation e.
 isoenzyme e.
 lipoprotein e. (LPE)
 polyacrylamide gel e. (PAGE)
 protein e.
 pulsed-field gel e.
 SDS-gel e.

serum protein e. (SPE)
sodium dodecyl sulfate-polyacrylamide gel e. (SDS-PAGE)
e. test
thin-layer e. (TLE)
electrophoretic
e. mobility
electrophoretogram
electropositive
electroscope
electrostatic unit (ESU)
electrotransfer test
elegans
Cunninghamella e.
eleidin
Elek test
element
e. disorder
rare earth e.
symmetry e.
trace e.
transposable e.
elementary
e. body
e. charge
e. granule
e. particle
eleoma
elephantiac, elephantiasic
elephantiasis
e. congenita angiomatosa
congenital e.
e. neuromatosa
nevoid e.
e. nostras
e. scroti
e. telangiectodes
e. vulvae
elephant leg
elfin facies
elimination
e. diet
immune e.
e. reaction
elinin
ELISA
enzyme-linked immunosorbent assay
ELISA titer assay
elizabethae
Bartonella e.
ellipse

ellipsoid
ellipsoidal
elliptical
elliptocyte
elliptocytic anemia
elliptocytosis
hereditary e. (HE)
Ellis
E. type 1, 2 glomerulonephritis
E. types 1 and 2 nephritis
Ellis-van Creveld syndrome
Ellsworth-Howard test
elongated cell
elongation factor
ELT
euglobulin lysis time
El Tor vibrio
eluant
eluate
eluent
elusive ulcer
elute
elution
elutriate
elutriation
EM
ejection murmur
electron microscope
electron microscopy
erythrocyte mass
EMA
epithelial membrane antigen
EMA antibody
emaciation
EMB
eosin-methylene blue
EMB agar
Embadomonas
Embden-Meyerhof pathway
embed
embedding agents
embolemia
emboli (*pl. of* embolus)
embolic
e. abscess
e. aneurysm
e. gangrene
e. glomerulonephritis
e. infarct
embolism
air e.
amniotic fluid e.

E

NOTES

embolism *(continued)*
    arterial e.
    atheroma e.
    bacillary e.
    bland e.
    bone marrow e.
    capillary e.
    cellular e.
    cerebral e.
    cholesterol e.
    coronary e.
    cotton-fiber e.
    fat e.
    gas e.
    infective e.
    lipid e.
    lymph e.
    lymphogenous e.
    miliary e.
    obturating e.
    oil e.
    pantaloon e.
    paradoxical e.
    plasmodium e.
    pulmonary e. (PE)
    pyemic e.
    retinal e.
    retrograde e.
    riding e.
    saddle e.
    spinal e.
    straddling e.
    trichinous e.
    tumor e.
    venous e.
embolomycotic
    e. aneurysm
embolus, pl. **emboli**
    air e.
    amniotic fluid e.
    atheromatous e.
    bland e.
    bone marrow e.
    fat e.
    foreign body e.
    massive e.
    paradoxical e.
    parasitic e.
    recent e.
    septic e.
    tumor e.
    valvular tissue e.
embryo
    cylindrical e.
    nodular e.
    stunted e.
embryocardia

embryoma
    e. of the kidney
embryonal
    e. adenoma
    e. carcinosarcoma
    e. cell carcinoma
    e. duct cyst
    e. leukemia
    e. nephroma
    e. rest
    e. rhabdomyosasrcoma
    e. teratoma
    e. tumor
embryonate
embryonic
    e. competence
    e. hemoglobin
    e. sphere
    e. tumor
embryoniform
embryonization
embryonum
    smegma e.
embryophore
embryotoxicity
EMC
    encephalomyocarditis
    EMC virus
emerging virus
emetine
EMF
    electromagnetic flowmeter
    electromotive force
    endomyocardial fibrosis
    erythrocyte maturation factor
EMG
    exophthalmos, macroglossia, gigantism
    EMG syndrome
emigration
    e. theory
    e. of white cells
emission
    e. line
    e. spectroscopy
    e. spectrum
    thermionic e.
EMIT
    enzyme-multiplied immunoassay
    technique
emitter
    beta e.
emitter-coupled logic (ECL)
Emmens S/L test
EMMM
    epidermotropic metastatic malignant
    melanoma
**Emmon modification of Sabouraud
dextrose agar**

Emmonsia
Emmonsiella capsulata
emotional leukocytosis
EMP
    extramedullary solitary plasmacytoma
emperipolesis
    megakaryocytic e.
emphraxis
emphysema
    blue bloater e.
    bullous e.
    centri-acinar e.
    centrilobular e.
    chronic pulmonary e. (CPE)
    compensatory e.
    congenital lobar e.
    cutaneous e.
    diffuse e.
    familial e.
    gangrenous e.
    generalized e.
    interstitial e.
    intestinal e.
    obstructive e.
    panacinar e.
    panlobular e.
    pulmonary e.
    pulmonary interstitial e. (PIE)
    subcutaneous e.
    surgical e.
    vesicular e.
emphysematous
    e. asthma
    e. bleb
    e. cholecystitis
    e. gangrene
    e. phlegmon
    e. vaginitis
empirical
Empirin
empty
    e. sella
    e. sella syndrome
empyema
    e. articuli
    e. benignum
    latent e.
    loculated e.
    e. necessitatis
    e. of the pericardium
    e. of pericardium

    pulsating e.
    subdural e.
empyemic
empyocele
emu
    electromagnetic unit
emulsify
emulsion
EN
    erythema nodosum
en
    e. bloc
    e. grappe
    e. thyrse
ENA
    extractable nuclear antigen
enalapril
enamel
    e. hypoplasia
    mottled e.
enamelogenesis imperfecta
enantiobiosis
enantiomer
enantiomerism
enantiomorph
enantiomorphism
encainide
encapsulated
encarditis
encelitis, enceliitis
encephalemia
encephalitis, pl. **encephalitides**
    acute hemorrhagic e.
    acute necrotizing e.
    allergic e.
    arthropod-borne virus e.
    Australian X e.
    bacterial e.
    bunyavirus e.
    California e. (CE)
    Coxsackievirus e.
    Dawson e.
    eastern equine e.
    eastern equine e.
    epidemic e.
    equine e.
    experimental allergic e.
    Far East Russian e.
    fox e.
    e. hemorrhagica
    herpes simplex e.
    hyperergic e.

E

NOTES

encephalitis *(continued)*
    Ilhéus e.
    inclusion body e.
    Japanese B e. (JBE)
    e. japonica
    lead e.
    lethargic e.
    e. lethargica
    Mengo e.
    Murray Valley e.
    necrotizing e.
    e. neonatorum
    e. periaxialis concentrica
    postinfectious allergic e.
    postvaccinal e.
    postvaccination allergic e.
    Powassan e.
    purulent e.
    e. pyogenica
    Russian autumn e.
    Russian spring-summer e. (Eastern subtype)
    Russian spring-summer e. (Western subtype)
    Russian tick-borne e.
    secondary e.
    St. Louis e. (SLE)
    subacute inclusion body e.
    e. subcorticalis chronica
    suppurative e.
    tick-borne e. (Central European subtype)
    tick-borne e. (Eastern subtype)
    varicella e.
    Venezuelan equine e.
    Venezuelan equine e.
    vernal e.
    e. virus
    western e. (WE)
    western equine e.
    western equine e.
    woodcutter's e.
encephalitogen
encephalitogenic
    e. factor (EF)
Encephalitozoon
encephalocele
encephaloclastic microcephaly
encephalocraniocutaneous lipomatosis
encephalocystocele
encephalodysplasia
encephaloid
    e. cancer
encephaloma
encephalomalacia
encephalomeningitis
encephalomeningocele
encephalomeningopathy

encephalomyelitis
    acute disseminated e. (ADEM)
    acute necrotizing hemorrhagic e.
    allergic e.
    autoimmune e.
    avian infectious e.
    benign myalgic e.
    eastern equine e. (EEE)
    enzootic e.
    epidemic myalgic e.
    equine e.
    experimental allergic e. (EAE)
    granulomatous e.
    herpes B e.
    infectious porcine e.
    mouse e.
    postinfectious e.
    Venezuelan equine e. (VEE)
    viral e.
    western e. (WE)
    western equine e. (WEE)
    zoster e.
encephalomyelocele
encephalomyeloneuropathy
encephalomyelopathy
    carcinomatous e.
    epidemic myalgic e.
    infantile necrotizing e. (INE)
    necrotizing e.
    paracarcinomatous e.
    paraneoplastic e.
encephalomyeloradiculitis
encephalomyeloradiculopathy
encephalomyocarditis (EMC)
    e. virus
encephalopathia
    e. addisonia
encephalopathy
    anoxic e.
    bilirubin e.
    Binswanger e.
    bovine spongiform e.
    demyelinating e.
    hepatic e.
    HIV e.
    hypercapnic e.
    hypernatremic e.
    hypertensive e.
    hypoglycemic e.
    lead e.
    metabolic e.
    palindromic e.
    pancreatic e.
    portal-systemic e. (PSE)
    progressive subcortical e.
    recurrent e.
    saturnine e.
    spongiform e.

subacute necrotizing e.
subacute spongiform e.
subcortical arteriosclerotic e.
thyrotoxic e.
transmissible mink e.
traumatic progressive e.
uremic e.
Wernicke e.
Wernicke-Korsakoff e.
encephalotrigeminal angiomatosis
enchondroma
enchondromatosis
enchondromatous
enchondrosarcoma
encode
encoder
encoding
encysted
e. calculus
e. pleurisy
encystment
end
e. artery
blunt e.
e. cell
e. piece of spermatozoon
e. point
e. product
e. stage
e. of tape
end
endoreduplication
endadelphos
Endamoeba
endangiitis, endangeitis
e. obliterans
endaortitis
bacterial e.
endarteritis
bacterial e.
e. deformans
e. obliterans
obliterating e.
e. proliferans
proliferating e.
endemia
endemic
e. colic
e. disease
e. fluorosis
e. funiculitis
e. goiter

e. hemoptysis
e. hypertrophy
e. index
e. murine typhus
e. nonbacterial infantile gastroenteritis
e. typhus
endemoepidemic
endergonic reaction
endermosis
endoamylase
endoangiitis
endo-aortitis
endoappendicitis
endoarteritis
endobiotic
endobronchial
e. tuberculosis
e. tumor
endocardial
e. cushion defect
e. fibroelastosis (EFE)
e. sclerosis
endocarditic
endocarditis
abacterial thrombotic e.
acute bacterial e.
acute infective e.
atypical verrucous e.
bacteria-free stage of bacterial e.
bacterial e. (BE)
cachectic e.
e. chordalis
constrictive e.
infectious e.
infective e.
isolated parietal e.
Libman-Sacks e.
malignant e.
marantic e.
mural e.
nonbacterial thrombotic e. (NBTE)
nonbacterial verrucous e.
polypous e.
rheumatic e.
septic e.
subacute bacterial e. (SBE)
subacute infective e.
terminal e.
thrombotic nonbacterial e.
valvular e.
vegetative e.

E

NOTES

endocarditis *(continued)*
    verrucal atypical e.
    verrucal nonbacterial e.
    verrucous e.
endocellular complement
endocervical smear
endocervicitis
endocervicosis
endocervix
    vagina, ectocervix, and e. (VCE)
endochondromatous myxoma
endocrine
    e. adenomatosis
    e. disease
    e. ductal carcinoma in situ (E-DCIS)
    e. granule
    e. granule constituent (EGC)
    e. marker
    e. myopathy
    e. polyglandular syndrome
endocrinoma
    multiple e.
endocrinopathy
    multiple e.
endocyst
endocystitis
endocytosis
endodeoxyribonuclease
endodermal sinus tumor
Endodermophyton
endodyocyte
endodyogeny
endoenteritis
endoenzyme
endoesophagitis
endogamy
endogastritis
endogenote
endogenous
    e. aneurysm
    e. antigen-cell-bound antibody reaction
    e. antigen-circulating antibody reaction
    e. antigen-transferred antibody reaction
    e. antigen-transferred cell-bound antibody reaction
    e. bacterium
    e. creatinine clearance
    e. fecal calcium (EFC)
    e. hemosiderosis
    e. hyperglyceridemia
    e. hyperlipidemia (EHL)
    e. infection
    e. peroxidase

    e. pigments and deposits
    e. variable
endoglobular, endoglobar
endointoxication
Endolimax
    E. nana
endolymphatic
    e. dye
    e. hydrops
    e. stromal myosis
endomerogony
endometria (*pl. of* endometrium)
endometrial
    e. adenocarcinoma
    e. atrophy
    e. brush
    e. carcinoma
    e. carcinoma in situ (ECIS)
    e. cast
    e. cavity
    e. curettage
    e. cyst
    e. cytology
    e. gestational alteration
    e. hyperplasia
    e. polyp
    e. smear
    e. stromal sarcoma (ESS)
    e. stromatosis
endometrioid
    e. carcinoma
    e. tumor
endometrioma
endometriosis
    stromal e.
endometritis
    decidual e.
    e. dissecans
    syncytial e.
endometrium, pl. endometria
    e. anaerobic culture
    atrophic e.
    cystic hyperplasia of e.
    FIGO adenocarcinoma of e.
    regenerative e.
    Swiss cheese e.
endomitosis
Endomyces
    E. albicans
    E. capsulatus
    E. epidermatidis
    E. epidermidis
    E. geotrichum
Endomycetales
endomyocardial
    e. fibroelastosis
    e. fibrosis (EMF)
    e. sclerosis

endomyocarditis
endomyometritis
endomysial antibodies
endonuclease
    restriction e.
endonucleolus
endoparasite
endoparasitism
endopeptidase
endoperiarteritis
endopericarditis
endoperimyocarditis
endoperitonitis
endoperoxide
    prostaglandin e.
endophlebitis
endophthalmitis
endophyte
endophytic
endoplasm
endoplasmic recticulum
endoplast
endoplastic
endopolygeny
endopolyploidy
endoreduplication (end)
endoribonuclease
endorphin
    e. assay
    β-e.
    beta e.
endosalpingiosis
endosalpingitis
endosalpinx
endosarc
endosmosis
endosome
endosperm
endospore
endosteitis, endostitis
endosteoma
endosteum
endostitis (*var. of* endosteitis)
endostoma
endosulfan
endothelia (*pl. of* endothelium)
endothelial
    e. cell
    e. cyst
    e. differentiation
    e. leukocyte
    e. metaplasia

    e. myeloma
    e. phagocyte
    e. relaxing factor
    e. sarcoma
endothelial-leukocyte adhesion molecule (E-LAM)
endotheliocyte
endotheliolytic serum
endothelioma
endotheliosis
endothelium, pl. endothelia
    continuous e.
    discontinuous e.
    fenestrated e.
endothelium-derived relaxing factor (EDRF)
endothermic
endothrix
endotoxemia
endotoxicosis
endotoxic shock
endotoxin
    e. shock
endotracheal insufflation
endotrachelitis
endovasculitis
    hemorrhagic e.
end-point measurement
end-product repression
endrin
end-systolic pressure (ESP)
end-tidal CO_2 tension
energetics
    biochemical e.
energy
    activation e.
    binding e.
    bond e.
    e. dispersive x-ray microanalysis
    free e.
    kinetic e. (KE)
    potential e.
    radiant e.
    e. resolution
    standard free e.
enflagellation
Engelmann disease
Engel-von Recklinghausen disease
engineering
    biomedical e.
    genetic e.
    human e.

E

NOTES

English disease
englobe
englobement
Engman disease
engulfment
    cytologic e.
enhancement
    immunologic e.
    immunological e.
enhancer
enhematospore
enkephalin
ENL
    erythema nodosum leprosum
enlargement
    cardiac e. (CE)
    left atrial e. (LAE)
    left ventricular e. (LVE)
    right atrial e. (RAE)
    right ventricular e. (RVE)
enol
enolase
    neuron-specific e. (NSA, NSE)
enostosis
enoyl-coenzyme A hydratase
enrichment
    e. culture
    e. medium
    POES growth promoting e.
ensheathing callus
entamebiasis
Entamoeba
    E. buccalis
    E. coli
    E. gingivalis
    E. hartmanni
    E. histolytica
    E. histolytica serological test
    E. nana
    E. polecki
    E. tetragena
    E. tropicalis
Entemopoxvirus
enteramine
enterectasis
enterelcosis
enteric
    e. bacillus
    e. cytopathogenic bovine orphan
      virus (ECBO virus)
    e. cytopathogenic human orphan
      virus (ECHO virus)
    e. cytopathogenic monkey orphan
      virus (ECMO virus)
    e. cytopathogenic swine orphan
      virus (ECSO virus)
    e. helminthic zoonosis

    e. orphan virus
    e. tularemia
enteric-coated (EC)
Enteritidis
    E. salmonella
enteritis
    e. anaphylactica
    bovine e. (BE)
    chronic cicatrizing e.
    diphtheritic e.
    eosinophilic e.
    feline infectious e.
    granulomatous e.
    e. of mink
    e. necroticans
    phlegmonous e.
    e. polyposa
    regional e. (RE)
    staphylococcal e.
    transmissible e.
Enterobacter
    E. aerogenes
    E. agglomerans
    E. alvei
    E. cloacae
    E. gergoviae
    E. hafniae
    E. liquefaciens
    E. sakazakii
    E. subgroup C.
Enterobacteriaceae
enterobiasis
Enterobius
    E. vermicularis
enterobrosia
enterobrosis
enterocele
enterocholecystostomy
enterochromaffin
    e. cell
    e. staining
enterochromaffin-cell hyperplasia (EC)
enterochromaffin-like (ECL)
enterochromaffin-like-cell hyperplasia
Enterococcus
enterococcus, pl. enterococci
enterocolitis
    acute necrotizing e.
    antibiotic e.
    cicatrizing e.
    necrotizing e.
    neonatal necrotizing e.
    pericrypt eosinophilic e.
    pseudomembranous e.
    regional e.
enterocutaneous fistula
enterocyst
enterocystoma

enterocyte
enterocytopathogenic dog orphan
Enterocytozoon
 E. bieneusi
enterogastritis
enterogastrone
enterogenous
 e. cyanosis
 e. cyst
 e. methemoglobinemia
enteroglucagon
enterohemorrhagic
 e. *Escherichia coli* (EHEC)
enterohepatitis
enteroinvasive
 e. *Escherichia coli* (EIEC)
enterokinase
enterolith
enterolithiasis
enteromegalia
enteromegaly
Enteromonas
 E. hominis
enteromycosis
enteronitis
enteropathogen
enteropathogenic
 e. *Escherichia coli* (EPEC)
enteropathy
 gluten-sensitive e. (GSE)
 protein-losing e.
enteropathy-associated T-cell lymphoma
 (ETCL)
enteropeptidase
enteroptosia
enteroptosis
enteroptotic
enterosepsis
enterostenosis
enterotoxigenic
enterotoxin
 Escherichia coli e.
 staphylococcal e.
enterovaginal fistula
enterovesical fistula
Enterovirus
enterovirus
 e. culture
enterozoic
enterozoon, pl. enterozoa
enthalpy of reaction
enthesitis

enthesopathic
enthesopathy
enthetic
Entner-Doudoroff pathway
Entoloma sinuatum
entomology
Entomophthora
 E. coronata
entomophthoramycosis
 e. basidiobolae
 e. conidiobolae
entomophthoromycosis
entomopox virus
entopic
entosarc
Entozoa
entozoal
entozoic
entozoon
entrapment neuropathy
entropion
entropy
enucleate
enucleated
enucleation
envelope
 cell e.
 elastomer e.
 nuclear e.
 viral e.
envenomation
environment
environmental
 e. illness
 e. stress
 e. toxicology
enz.
 enzymatic
Enzinger tumor classification
enzootic
 e. bovine leukosis
 e. encephalomyelitis
 e. encephalomyelitis virus
enzymatic (enz.)
 e. adaptation
 e. digestion method
enzyme
 activating e.
 adaptive e.
 allosteric e.
 1,4-alpha glucan branching e.
 amino acid-activating e.

E

NOTES

enzyme *(continued)*
 amylolytic e.
 e. analyzer
 angiotensin I-converting e.
 e. antagonist
 antitumor e.
 e. assay
 autolytic e.
 bacterial e.
 e. balance
 BamH1 e.
 brancher e.
 branching e.
 catheptic e.
 citrate condensing e.
 coagulating e.
 constitutive e.
 converting e.
 cryptic e.
 debranching e.
 e. demonstration method
 EcoR1 e.
 1,4-α-glucan branching e.
 glycogen branching e.
 glycolytic e.
 hydrolytic e.
 immobilized e.
 e. immunoassay (EIA)
 inducible e.
 e. induction
 e. inhibition
 e. inhibitor (EI)
 inhibitory e.
 inverting e.
 lipolytic e.
 e. marker
 microsomal e.
 proteolytic e.
 receptor-destroying e. (RDE)
 e. repression
 restriction e.
 serum e.
 steatolytic e.
 terminal addition e.
 topoisomerase II e.
 e. unit (EU)
enzyme-assisted immunoassay technique
enzyme-linked
 e.-l. antibody test
 e.-l. immunosorbent assay (ELISA)
enzyme-multiplied
 e.-m. immunoassay
 e.-m. immunoassay technique
  (EMIT)
enzymic fat necrosis
enzymolysis
eo, eos
 eosinophil

eosin
 alcohol-soluble e.
 e. B
 ethyl e.
 hematoxylin and e. (H&E)
 e. I bluish
 e.-methylene blue (EMB)
 e. stain
 e. Y
 e. y
 e. yellowish
 e. Ys
eosin-methylene blue agar
eosinocyte
Eosinofix reagent
eosinopenia
eosinophil, eosinophile (eo, eos)
 e. adenoma
 e. chemotactic factor
 e. chemotactic factor of
  anaphylaxis (ECF-A)
 e. count
 e. granule
 e. leukocytic infiltrate
 polymorphonuclear e. (PME)
 e. smear
 e. stimulation promoter (ESP)
eosinophilia
 granulomatous angiitis with e.
 pulmonary e.
 pulmonary infiltration and e. (PIE)
 simple pulmonary e.
eosinophilia-myalgia syndrome
eosinophilic
 e. cellulitis
 e. endomyocardial disease
 e. enteritis
 e. fasciitis
 e. gastroenteritis (EGE)
 e. granule
 e. granuloma
 e. granuloma of lung (EGL)
 e. hyperplasia
 e. index (EI)
 e. leukemia
 e. leukocyte
 e. leukocytosis
 e. leukopenia
 e. lung
 e. macronucleoli
 e. marrow
 e. meningoencephalitis
 e. metamyelocyte
 e. myelocyte
 e. pneumonia
 e. promyelocyte
eosinophilocytic leukemia
eosinophiluria

eosinotactic
EOT
    effective oxygen transport
EP
    ectopic pregnancy
    electrophoresis
    erythrocyte protoporphyrin
        EP test
        EP toxicity
EPC
    epilepsia partialis continua
EPEC
    enteropathogenic *Escherichia coli*
ependyma
ependymal
        e. cell
        e. cyst
        e. layer
ependymitis
ependymoblastoma
ependymoma
        epithelial e.
        Grades I-IV e.
        malignant e.
        myxopapillary e.
        papillary e.
Eperythrozoon
EPF
    exophthalmos-producing factor
ephedrine
ephelis, pl. **ephelides**
ephemeral
        e. fever of cattle
        e. fever virus
epiallopregnanolone (EAP)
epiboly, epibole
epicarcinogen
epicardium
epichlorohydrin
epicondylitis
Epics
        E. C flow cytometer
        E. Profile flow cytometer
epicystitis
epicyte
epidemic
        e. benign dry pleurisy
        e. cerebrospinal meningitis
        e. curve
        e. diaphragmatic pleurisy
        e. disease
        e. dysentery

        e. encephalitis
        e. exanthema
        e. gastroenteritis virus
        e. hemoglobinuria
        e. hemorrhagic fever
        hemorrhagic fever e.
        e. hepatitis
        e. keratoconjunctivitis (EKC)
        e. keratoconjunctivitis virus
        e. louse-borne typhus
        e. myalgia
        e. myalgia virus
        e. myalgic encephalomyelitis
        e. myalgic encephalomyelopathy
        e. myositis
        e. nausea
        e. nonbacterial gastroenteritis
        e. parotiditis
        e. parotitis virus
        parotitis virus e.
        e. pleurodynia
        e. pleurodynia virus
        e. polyarthritis
        e. roseola
        e. transient diaphragmatic spasm
        e. tremor
        typhus e.
        e. vomiting
epidemica
    nephropathia e.
epidemicity
epidemiography
epidemiology
epidermal
        e. dermal nevus
        e. growth factor
        e. growth factor receptor (EGFR)
        e. inclusion cyst
epidermalization
epidermic-dermic nevus
epidermides (*pl. of* epidermis)
epidermidization
        e. of cervix
epidermidosis
epidermis, pl. **epidermides**
    keratohyalin granule of e.
epidermitis
epidermodysplasia
        e. verruciformis
epidermoid
        e. cancer
        e. carcinoma

E

NOTES

epidermoid *(continued)*
    e. carcinoma in situ
    e. inclusion cyst
    e. metaplasia
epidermolysin
epidermolysis
    e. bullosa (EB)
    e. bullosa acquista
    e. bullosa dystrophica
    e. bullosa lethalis
    e. bullosa simplex
epidermolytic hyperkeratosis
epidermophytid
Epidermophyton
    E. floccosum
    E. inguinale
    E. rubrum
epidermophytosis
epidermosis
epidermotropic metastatic malignant melanoma (EMMM)
epidermotropism
epididymal cyst
epididymitis
epididymo-orchitis
epidural
    e. abscess
    e. hematoma
    e. meningitis
epifluorescence microscopy
epigastric hernia
epigastrius parasiticus
epigenesis
epigenetics
epigenotype
epiglottiditis
epiglottitis
epignathus
epihyal bone
epilating dose
epilepidoma
epilepsia partialis continua (EPC)
epilepsy
    familial myoclonic e.
    focal cortical e.
    grand mal e.
    jacksonian e.
    minor e.
    myoclonic e.
    petit mal e.
    posttraumatic e.
    psychomotor e.
    rolandic e.
    temporal lobe e.
    uncinate e.
epilepticus
    status e.

epileptiform
    e. discharge (ED)
epileptogenic zone
epiloia
epimastical fever
epimastigote
epimer
epimerase
epimerite
epimerization
epimorphic regeneration
epimyoepithelial carcinoma
epinephrine and norepinephrine assays
epiphenotype
epiphrenic diverticulum
epiphyseal
    e. arrest
    e. giant cell tumor
    e. plate
epiphysial aseptic necrosis
epiphysis, pl. epiphyses
    stippled e.
epiphysitis
epiphyte
episcleritis
    rheumatoid e.
episode
    transient cerebral ischemic e. (TCIE)
    transient ischemic e. (TIE)
episomal
episome
    resistance-transferring e.
epispadias
episplenitis
epistasis
epistasy
epistatic
epitaxy
epitestosterone
epithalaxia
epithelia (*pl. of* epithelium)
epithelial
    e. basement membrane
    e. cancer
    e. cast
    e. cell
    e. cell disease
    e. cell urinary cast
    e. differentiation
    e. dysplasia
    e. ependymoma
    e. hyperplasia
    e. inclusion cyst
    e. membrane antigen (EMA)
    e. neoplasm
    e. nest
    e. pearl

e. pigment
e. rest
e. thymoma
e. tumor
epithelialization
epitheliocyte
epithelioid
    e. cell
    e. cell melanoma
    e. cell nevus
    e. hemangioendothelioma
    e. sarcoma
    e. soft-tissue neoplasm (ESTN)
epitheliolytic
epithelioma
    e. adenoides cysticum
    basal cell e.
    benign e.
    Borst-Jadassohn type
      intraepidermal e.
    calcifying e. of Malherbe
    chorionic e.
    e. contagiosum
    e. cuniculatum
    Malherbe calcifying e.
    multiple self-healing squamous e.
    sebaceous e.
epitheliomatous
epitheliopathy
epitheliosis
epitheliotropism
epithelium, pl. epithelia
    Barrett e.
    columnar e.
    crypt e.
    foveolar e.
    glandular e.
    metaplastic columnar e.
    seminiferous e.
epithelization
epitope
    phosphorylation-
      dependent/independent
      neurofilament e.
    phosphorylation-independent NF-
      H/M e.
epitoxoid
epituberculous infiltration
epizoic
epizoon
epizootic
    e. cellulitis

    e. hemorrhagic disease of deer
    e. lymphangitis
Epon-Araldite resin
Epon tissue embedding media
epoxide
    heptachlor e.
epoxy resin
EPP
    erythropoietic protoporphyria
Eppendorf
    E. centrifuge
    E. tube
EPS
    exophthalmos-producing substance
epsilon, ε
    e. acid
    e. staphylolysin
Epstein
    E. disease
    E. syndrome
Epstein-Barr
    E.-B. nuclear antigen (EBNA)
    E.-B. virus (EBV)
    E.-B. virus antibody assay
    E.-B. virus culture
    E.-B. virus serology
epulis, pl. epulides
    pigmented e.
eq
    equivalent
equal
    bilateral, symmetrical, and e. (BSE)
Equanil
equation
    alveolar air e.
    Bohr e.
    chemical e.
    Eadie-Hofstee e.
    Friedewald e.
    Hanes e.
    Hasselbalch e.
    Henderson-Hasselbalch e.
    Hill e.
    Hüfner e.
    Lineweaver-Burk e.
    Michaelis-Menten e.
    Nernst e.
    Scatchard e.
    Svedberg e.
    van der Waals e.
equational division
equatorial plate

E

NOTES

equi
　　Rhodococcus e.
equilibration
equilibrium
　　chemical e.
　　e. constant
　　e. dialysis
　　dynamic e.
　　physiologic e.
　　radioactive e.
　　secular e.
　　sedimentation e.
　　thermal e.
　　thermodynamic e.
　　transient e.
equine
　　e. abortion virus
　　e. antihuman lymphoblast globulin
　　　(EAHLG)
　　e. antihuman lymphoblast serum
　　　(EAHLS)
　　e. arteritis virus
　　e. coital exanthema virus
　　e. encephalitis
　　e. encephalomyelitis
　　e. encephalomyelitis virus
　　e. gonadotropin unit
　　e. infectious anemia
　　e. infectious anemia virus
　　e. influenza
　　e. influenza virus
　　e. rhinopneumonitis (ERP)
　　e. rhinopneumonitis virus
　　e. rhinovirus
　　e. serum hepatitis
　　e. viral arteritis
　　e. virus abortion
equinus
equipment
　　eyewash e.
equipotential line
equivalence
　　e. point
　　e. relation
　　e. zone
equivalent (eq)
　　age e. (AEq)
　　Joule e. (J)
　　lethal e.
　　metabolic e. (MET)
　　nitrogen e.
　　toxic e.
equorum
　　Parascaris e.
ER
　　estrogen receptor
ERA
　　estrogen receptor assay

Eranko fluorescence stain
erase
Erb
　　E. disease
　　E. syndrome
Erb-Charcot disease
ERBF
　　effective renal blood flow
Erb-Goldflam disease
erbium
ERC
　　erythropoietin-responsive cell
Erdheim
　　E. disease
　　E. rest
　　E. tumor
erectile myxoma
ergastoplasm
ergocalciferol
ergoloid mesylate
ergometer
ergosterol
ergot
　　corn e.
ergothioneine
ergotism
ergotoxine
Erlanger and Gasser peripheral nerve
　　assay
Erlenmeyer
　　E. flask
　　E. flask-like
erode
E-rosette test
erosion
erosive
　　e. adenomatosis of nipple
　　e. aneurysm
　　e. esophagitis
　　e. gastritis
　　e. inflammation
ERP
　　effective refractory period
　　equine rhinopneumonitis
error
　　coincidence e.
　　e. detector
　　machine e.
　　probable e.
　　random e.
　　e. rate
　　standard e. (SE)
　　syntax e.
　　systematic e.
　　type I, II e.
ERRT
　　extrarenal rhabdoid tumor

eruption
  bullous e.
  creeping e.
  Kaposi varicelliform e.
  macular e.
  maculopapular e.
  polymorphic light e.
  polymorphous e.
  varicelliform e.
eruptive fever
Erwinia
  E. amylovora
  E. herbicola
Erwinieae
erysipelas
erysipeloid
Erysipelothrix
  E. insidiosa
  E. rhusiopathiae
erythema
  e. ab igne
  e. annulare centrifugum
  e. chronicum migrans (ECM)
  e. dose
  e. dyschromicum perstans
  e. elevatum diutinum
  e. exfoliativa
  e. figuratum
  e. induratum
  e. infectiosum
  e. iris
  e. keratodes
  macular e.
  e. marginatum rheumaticum
  e. multiforme
  e. multiforme bullosum
  e. multiforme exudativum
  e. neonatorum
  e. nodosum (EN)
  e. nodosum leprosum (ENL)
  Osler e.
  palmar e.
  e. pernio
  e. perstans
  e. polymorphe
  toxic e.
  e. toxicum
erythematosum
  anetoderma e.
erythematosus
  acute dissseminated lupus e.

  lupus e. (LE)
  systemic lupus e. (SLE)
erythrasma
erythremia
erythremic myelosis
erythritol
Erythrobacillus
Erythrobacter longus
erythroblast
  basophilic e.
  definitive e.
  primitive e.
erythroblastemia
erythroblastic
  e. anemia
  e. island
erythroblastoma
erythroblastomatosis
erythroblastopenia
erythroblastosis
  fetal e.
  e. fetalis
  e. neonatorum
erythroblastotic
erythrocatalysis
erythrochromia
erythroclasis
erythroclastic
erythrocuprein
erythrocytapheresis
erythrocyte (E)
  e. adherence phenomenon
  e. adherence test
  e., antibody, complement (EAC)
  e., antibody, complement rosette
  assay
  e. antigen
  e. fragility
  e. fragility test
  e. glutamic oxaloacetic transaminase
  (EGOT)
  e. indices
  e. mass (EM)
  e. maturation factor (EMF)
  e. membrane
  e. protoporphyrin (EP)
  e. rosette
  e. sedimentation
  e. sedimentation rate (ESR)
erythrocyte-sensitizing substance (ESS)
erythrocythemia

E

NOTES

225

erythrocytic
    e. blood cell
    e. marrow
    e. series
erythrocytoblast
erythrocytolysin
erythrocytolysis
erythrocytometer
erythrocytopenia
erythrocytophagy
erythrocytopoiesis
erythrocytorrhexis
erythrocytoschisis
erythrocytosis
    absolute e.
    leukemic e.
    e. megalosplenica
    relative e.
erythrocyturia
erythrodegenerative
erythroderma
    e. exfoliativa
    Sézary e.
erythrodextrin
erythrodysesthesia syndrome
erythrogenesis imperfecta
erythrogenic
    e. toxin
erythroglutinin
    Phaseolus vulgaris e. (PHA-E)
erythrogonium, pl. **erythrogonia**
erythrohepatic porphyria
erythroid
    e. aplasia
    e. cell
    e. hyperplasia
    e. hypoplasia
erythrokeratoderma
    e. variabilis
erythrokeratodermia
    e. variabilis
erythrokinase (EK)
erythrokinetics
erythrokinetic study
erythroleukemia
erythroleukosis
erythrolysin
erythrolysis
erythromelia
erythromycin
erythromyeloblastic leukemia
erythron
erythroneocytosis
erythropenia
erythrophagia
erythrophagocytosis
erythrophil
erythrophilic

erythroplakia
erythroplasia
    e. of Queyrat
erythropoiesis
    extramedullary e.
    ineffective e.
    megaloblastic e.
erythropoietic
    e. hormone
    e. porphyria
    e. protoporphyria (EPP)
erythropoietic-stimulating factor (ESF)
erythropoietin
    e. test
erythropoietin-responsive cell (ERC)
erythropyknosis
erythrorrhexis
erythrose
erythrosin B
erythruria
ES
    Ewing sarcoma
Esbach reagent
Esch.
    Escherichia
Escherich bacillus
Escherichia **(Esch.)**
    E. aurescens
    E. coli (EC, *E. coli*)
    E. coli enterotoxin
    E. dispar var. *ceylonensis*
    E. dispar var. *madampensis*
    enterohemorrhagic *E. coli* (EHEC)
    enteroinvasive *E. coli* (EIEC)
    enteropathogenic *E. coli* (EPEC)
esculenta
    Gyromitra e.
    Helvella e.
esculin hydrolysis test
ESF
    erythropoietic-stimulating factor
esoethmoiditis
esogastritis
esophageal
    e. achalasia
    e. acid infusion test
    e. atresia
    e. hernia
    e. smear
    e. tumor
    e. varices
    e. web
esophagectasia
esophagectasis
esophagi (*pl. of* esophagus)
esophagitis
    corrosive e.
    erosive e.

infectious e.
monilial e.
peptic e.
reflux e.

esophagomalacia
esophagomycosis
esophagoptosia
esophagoptosis
esophagosalivary reflex
esophagostenosis
esophagostomiasis
esophagus, pl. **esophagi**
Barrett e.

esosphenoiditis
ESP
end-systolic pressure
eosinophil stimulation promoter

espundia
ESR
electron spin resonance
erythrocyte sedimentation rate
ESR assay

esr
electron spin resonance

ESS
endometrial stromal sarcoma
erythrocyte-sensitizing substance

essential
e. albuminuria
e. asthma
e. atrophy
e. fatty acids (EFA)
e. fever
e. fructosuria
e. hematuria
e. hypercholesterolemia
e. hyperlipemia
e. hypertension (EH)
e. oil
e. pentosuria
e. telangiectasia
e. thrombocythemia
e. thrombocytopenia

established
e. cell line

ester
cholesterol e. (ChE)
hexosephosphoric e.'s

esterase
C1 e.
e. staining method
e. test

esterification
estetrol (E$_4$)
esthesioneuroblastoma
olfactory e.

esthesioneurocytoma
esthiomene
esthiomenous
estimate
biased e.
consistent e.
dose e.
interval e.
median unbiased e.
point e.
pooled e.
standard error of e. (SEE)
unbiased e.

estimated
e. blood loss (EBL)
e. hepatic blood flow (EHBF)

ESTN
epithelioid soft-tissue neoplasm

estradiol (E$_2$)
17β-e.
e. assay
e. benzoate (EB)
e. benzoate unit
17 beta e.
e. receptor
e. test

Estren-Dameshek anemia
estriol (E$_3$)
e. assay
conjugated e.
free e.
serum e.
total e.
unconjugated e.
urinary e.

estrogen
e. receptor (ER)
e. receptor assay (ERA)
e. withdrawal bleeding (EWB)

estrogenic
e. hormone

estrone (E$_1$)
e. unit

ESU
electrostatic unit

ET
effective temperature
etiology

E

NOTES

eta
état
    e. mamelonné
ETCL
    enteropathy-associated T-cell lymphoma
ethacrynic acid (ECA)
ethambutol
ethane
ethanedial
ethanoic acid
ethanol
    e. assay
    e. gelation test
    e. level
ethanolamine
ethchlorvynol
    e. assay
ethene
ether
    dimethyl e.
    ethyl e.
    petroleum e.
    e. storage
ethidium
    e. bromide
    e. bromide stain
ethidium bromide
ethion
ethionamide
ethionine
ethmoiditis
ethosuximide
    e. assay
ethoxazene hydrochloride
ethyl
    e. acetate
    e. alcohol
    e. alcohol poisoning
    e. cyanide
    e. eosin
    e. ether
    e. green
    e. orange
    e. violet azide broth
ethylcocaine
ethylene
    e. chlorohydrin
    e. dibromide
    e. dichloride
    e. glycol
    e. glycol assay
    e. glycol dinitrate
    e. oxide
    e. tetraacetic acid
ethylenediaminetetraacetic acid (EDTA)
ethylidene dichloride
ethyne
etiocholanolone

etiocobalamine
etiol
    etiology
etiologic
    e. agent
etiology (ET, etiol)
    genetic e.
    pyrexia of unknown e. (PUE)
    unknown e.
etoposide
EU
    Ehrlich unit
    enzyme unit
eubacteria
Eubacteriales
Eubacterium
        E. aerofaciens
        E. alactolyticum
        E. contortum
        E. endocarditis
        E. lentum
        E. limosum
        E. parvum
        E. rectale
        E. ventriosum
eucalyptus oil
eucapnia
eucaryote
eucaryotic
Eucestoda
eucholia
euchromatic
euchromatin
Euflagellata
Euglena
        E. gracilis
Euglenidae
euglenoid movement
euglobulin
    e. clot lysis
    e. clot lysis time (ECLT)
    e. clot test (ECT)
    e. lysis test
    e. lysis time (ELT)
euglycemia
euglycemic
eugnosia
eugonic
Eugregarinida
eukaryon
eukaryosis
Eukaryotae
eukaryote
eukaryotic
    e. cell cycle
Eulenburg disease
eumelanin
eumetria

eumycetes
Eumycetozoea
eumycotic mycetoma
eunuchoidism
euosmia
euparal
Euparyphium
euplastic lymph
euploid
euploidy
eupraxia
europaeus
  Ulex e.
European
  E. blastomycosis
  E. hookworm
  E. rat flea
europium
Eurotium
  E. malignum
eurythermal
Eusimulium
eustachianography
eustachian tube
Eustrongylus
eutectic temperature
euthyroid
euthyroidism
eutonic
Eutriatoma
Eutrombicula
  E. alfreddugesi
eutrophic
EV
  extravascular
ev
  electron volt
evacuation procedure
evagination
Evans
  E. blue
  E. syndrome
evaporation
eventration
  e. of diaphragm
  e. of the diaphragm
eversion
evil
  king's e.
evisceration
evisceroneurotomy

EWB
  estrogen withdrawal bleeding
Ewing
  E. sarcoma (ES)
  E. tumor
EWL
  egg-white lysozyme
ex
  excision
  exophthalmos
ExacTech blood glucose meter test
examination
  cytologic e.
  double-contrast e.
  duodenal contents e.
  full blood e. (FBE)
  gastric residue e.
  Papanicolaou e.
  pericardial fluid e.
  peritoneal fluid e.
  pleural fluid e.
  postmortem e.
  semen e.
  sputum e.
  synovial fluid e.
exanthem
  Boston e.
  e. subitum
  e. subitum virus
exanthema
  Boston e.
  epidemic e.
  e. subitum
  vesicular e.
exanthematous
  e. disease
  e. fever
  e. inflammation
exanthesis
  e. arthrosia
excavation
excavatum
  pectus e.
excess (XS)
  antibody e.
  antigen e.
  base e. (BE)
  negative base e.
excessive
  e. cornification
  e. fatigue
  e. heat production (EHP)

NOTES

E

excessive *(continued)*
  e. lacrimation
  e. sweating
  e. tearing
  e. weakness
  e. weight gain
  e. weight loss
exchange
  e. pairing
  plasma e.
  e. transfusion
exchangeable mass
excipient
excision (ex)
excisional biopsy
excitation spectrum
excited
  e. skin syndrome
  e. state
exciter filter
excitomotor
exclusion
  allelic e.
exconjugant
excoriation
excrescence
excretion
  pseudouridine e.
excretory
  e. urogram (XU)
excystation
execute
execution time
exencephalia
exencephalic
exencephalocele
exencephalous
exencephaly
exenteration
exenteritis
exercise hyperemia blood flow (EHBF)
exergonic reaction
exflagellation
exfoliatin
exfoliation
exfoliative
  e. cytodiagnosis
  e. cytologic alteration
  e. cytology
  e. dermatitis
  e. gastritis
  e. psoriasis
exhaust
  slot e.
exhaustion atrophy
existence proof
exit
  e. access

  e. discharge
  e. dose
exoantigen
exocellular
exocervix
exocrine
exocytosis
exodus
exoenzyme
exoerythrocytic plasmodium
exogamy
exogenetic
exogenote
exogenous
  e. aneurysm
  e. anticoagulant coagulation
  e. antigen cell-bound antibody
    reaction
  e. antigen-circulating antibody
    reaction
  e. bacterium
  e. creatinine clearance
  e. creatinine clinoscope
  e. growth factor
  e. hemochromatosis
  e. hemosiderosis
  e. hyperglyceridemia
  e. infection
  e. pigmentation
  e. pigment and deposits
  e. variable
exon
exonuclease
exopeptidase
Exophiala
  E. jeanselmei
  E. mycetoma
  E. werneckii
exophthalmica
  cachexia e.
exophthalmic goiter
exophthalmos (ex)
  e., macroglossia, gigantism (EMG)
exophthalmos-hyperthyroid factor (EHF)
exophthalmos-producing
  e.-p. factor (EPF)
  e.-p. substance (EPS)
exophyte
exophytic
  e. growth
  e. papilla
exoribonuclease
exoskeleton
exosmosis
exospore
exosporium
exostosis, pl. exostoses
  e. bursata

e. cartilaginea
chondromatous e.
diaphysial juxtaepiphysial e.
hereditary multiple exostoses
ivory e.
multiple e.
osteocartilaginous e.
solitary osteocartilaginous e.
exothermic
exotoxic
exotoxin
exotropia (XT)
expander
plasma volume e.
expansa
Moniezia e.
expansion
clonal e.
expectation
expectoration
prune-juice e.
experiment
control e.
double blind e.
double-masked e.
experimental
e. allergic encephalitis
e. allergic encephalomyelitis (EAE)
e. allergic neuritis (EAN)
e. pathology
explant
explantation
explode
explosion
explosion-proof
explosive
e. atmosphere
e. limit
e. material
exponent
hydrogen e.
exponential
e. decay
e. function
e. phase
exposure
expression
latent membrane protein-1 e. (LMP-1)
e. vector
expressivity
exsanguinate

exsanguination
exsanguine
Exserohilum longirostratum
exsiccant
exsiccate
exsiccation
exstrophy
e. of the bladder
e. of the cloaca
externa
otitis e.
external
e. elastic lamellae
e. fistula
e. hemorrhoid
e. meningitis
e. pyocephalus
e. storage
extinction coefficient
extinguishing
extra-abdominal
e.-a. desmoid
e.-a. fibromatosis
extracapillary lesion (ECL)
extracapsular ankylosis
extracellular (EC)
e. aggregate alteration lipid
e. cholesterolosis
e. fibril alteration
e. fluid
e. fluid volume (ECFV, EFV)
e. granule
e. ground substance
e. lipid aggregate
e. macromolecule aggregate
e. material (ECM)
e. matrix
e. matrix alteration
e. parasite
e. plasma
e. structural alteration
e. toxin
e. vacuole
e. volume (ECV)
e. water (ECW)
extrachromosomal inheritance
extracorporeal
e. dialysis
e. photophoresis
e. photophoresis technique
extract
adipose tissue e. (ATE)

NOTES

231

extract *(continued)*
    adrenocortical e. (ACE)
    allergenic e.
    allergic e.
    anterior pituitary e. (APE)
    ceanothus e.
    parathyroid e. (PTE)
    pollen e.
    whole ragweed e. (WRE)
extractable nuclear antigen (ENA)
extraction
    Baker pyridine e.
    e. coefficient
    countercurrent e.
    e. fraction (E)
    solvent e.
extracystic
extradural hematorrhachis
extraembryonic mesoblast
extrafective
extraglomerular mesangium
extragonadal germ cell tumor
extrahepatic obstruction (EHO)
extramammary Paget disease
extramedullary
    e. erythropoiesis
    e. hematopoiesis
    e. myelopoiesis
    e. solitary plasmacytoma (EMP)
extraneural
extranodal lymphoma
extranuchal nuchal fibroma
extrapineal pinealoma
extrapolation
extraprostatitis
extrapulmonary tuberculosis
extrapyramidal disease
extrarenal
    e. azotemia
    e. rhabdoid tumor (ERRT)
extraskeletal chondroma
extrauterine pregnancy
extravasate
extravasation
    bile e.
    blood e.
    e. cyst

    e. feces
    e. gas
    mucus e.
extravascular (EV)
    e. hemolysis
extreme capsule
extrinsic
    e. allergic alveolitis
    e. asthma
    e. factor
    e. hemolysis
    e. pathway
    e. semiconductor
extrude
extrusion
exuberant
exudate
    acute inflammatory e.
    inflammatory e.
    mucopurulent e.
exudation
    e. cell
    e. corpuscle
    e. cyst
exudative
    e. arthritis
    e. bronchiolitis
    e. glomerulonephritis
    e. granulomatous inflammation
exude
exulcerans
exuviae
eye
    e. tumor
    e. tumor localization
eyepiece
    comparison e.
    compensated e.
    high eyepoint e.
    huygenian e.
    Ramsden e.
    wide field e.
eyepoint
eyespot
eyewash equipment
eyeworm

F
Fahrenheit
Fahrenheit temperature scale
farad
feces
female
force
gilbert (unit of magnetomotive force)
hydrocortisone (compound F)
    F agent
    F body
    F distribution
    F donor
    F factor
    F genote
    F pilus
    F plasmid
    F thalassemia
F₂
second filial generation
F₁
first filial generation
FA
fatty acid
fluorescent antibody
free acid
    FA technique
    FA virus
FAB
French-American-British
    FAB leukemia classification
    FAB tumor staging
Fab
    F. fragment
    F. piece
Faber
    F. anemia
    F. syndrome
fabism
Fabry disease
face
    adenoid f.
    cleft f.
    hippocratic f.
    f. velocity of laboratory hood
facial
    f. diprosopus duplication
    f. eczema
    f. hemiatrophy
    f. myiasis
    f. trophoneurosis
facies, pl. **facies**
    adenoid f.
    cherubic f.
    cushingoid f.

elfin f.
f. hepatica
hippocratic f.
hound-dog f.
hurloid f.
leonine f.
leprechaun f.
Parkinson f.
Potter f.
scaphoid f.
facilitated diffusion
faciodigitogenital dysplasia
facioscapulohumeral-type
    f.-t. progressive muscular dystrophy
Facklam classification scheme
FACS
    fluorescence-activated cell sorter
FACscan
    fluorescence-activated cell sorter scan
factitia
    thyrotoxicosis f.
factitious
    f. dermatitis
    f. melanin
    f. urticaria
factor
    f. A
    ABO f.
    accelerator f.
    adrenocorticotropic hormone-
        releasing f. (ACTH-RF)
    AHG f.
    amplification f.
    anabolism-promoting f. (APF)
    angiogenesis f.
    animal protein f. (APF)
    antialopecia f.
    antianemic f.
    anticomplementary f.
    antigen-specific helper f.
    antigen-specific suppressor f.
    antihemophilic f.
    antihemophilic f. A (AHF)
    antihemophilic f. B
    antiheparin f.
    antinuclear f. (ANF)
    antipernicious anemia f. (APA)
    f. assay
    autocrine growth f.
    autocrine motility f.
    automated motility f. (AMF)
    f. B
    bacteriocin f.
    basophil chemotactic f. (BCF)
    B-cell differentiating f.

F

factor *(continued)*
    B-cell differentiation/growth f.
    B-cell growth f. I, II
    B-cell stimulating f.
    Bittner milk f.
    blastogenic f. (BF)
    blood f.
    B-lymphocyte stimulatory f. (BSF)
    CAMP f.
    Castle f.
    chemotactic f. (CF)
    Christie-Atkins-Munch-Petersen f.
    Christmas f.
    citrovorum f. (CF)
    clearing f.
    clone-inhibiting f. (CIF)
    cloning inhibitory f.
    clotting f.
    coagulation f.
    coagulation f.'s I, II, III, IV, V,
      VII, VIII, IX, X, XI, XII, XIII
    cobra venom f.
    colony-stimulating f. (CSF)
    complement chemotactic f.
    conglutinogen-activating f.
    cord f.
    corticotropin-releasing f. (CRF)
    cryoprecipitated antihemophilic f.
    crystal-induced chemotactic f.
    f. D
    decay antibody-accelerating f.
    deficiency f. (DF)
    f. deficiency anemia
    deficiency f.'s I, II, V, VII, VIII,
      IX, X, XI
    dose-reduction f. (DRF)
    Duran-Reynals permeability f.
    f. E
    elongation f.
    encephalitogenic f. (EF)
    endothelial relaxing f.
    endothelium-derived relaxing f.
      (EDRF)
    eosinophil chemotactic f.
    eosinophil chemotactic f. of
      anaphylaxis (ECF-A)
    epidermal growth f.
    erythrocyte maturation f. (EMF)
    erythropoietic-stimulating f. (ESF)
    exogenous growth f.
    exophthalmos-hyperthyroid f. (EHF)
    exophthalmos-producing f. (EPF)
    extrinsic f.
    F f.
    Fc f.
    fertility f.
    fibrin-stabilization f. (FSF)
    fibrin-stabilizing f. (FSF)

    Fitzgerald f.
    Flaujeac f.
    Fletcher f.
    G f.
    g f.
    glass f.
    f. Gm
    gonadotropin-releasing f. (GRF)
    granulocyte colony-stimulating f.
      (G-CSF)
    granulocyte-macrophage colony-
      stimulating f. (GM-CSF)
    growth hormone-releasing f. (GH-
      RF, GRF)
    growth inhibitory f.
    Hageman f. (HF)
    hemophilic f. A
    high-molecular-weight neutrophil
      chemotactic f.
    histamine-releasing f.
    human antihemophilic f.
    humoral thymic f. (THF)
    hydrazine-sensitive f.
    hyperglycemic-glycogenolytic f.
      (HGF)
    f. I, II, III, IV, IX, IX complex,
      V, VII, VIII, VIII:C, VIII:R,
      VIII concentrate, X, XI, XII,
      XIII, XIIIa
    immunoglobulin-binding f. (IBF)
    inhibiting f.
    inhibition f.
    initiation f.
    insulin-like growth f.
    intrinsic f. (IF)
    labile f.
    Lactobacillus bulgaricus f. (LBF)
    Laki-Lorand f. (LLF)
    LE f.
    leukocyte inhibitory f.
    leukocytosis-promoting f. (LPF)
    leukopenic f.
    L-L f.
    load f.
    luteinizing hormone-releasing f.
      (LH-RF)
    lymph node permeability f. (LNPF)
    lymphocyte-activating f.
    lymphocyte blastogenic f.
    lymphocyte mitogenic f.
    lymphocyte-transforming f.
    lymphocytosis-promoting f. (LPF)
    macrophage-activating f.
    macrophage activation f. (MAF)
    macrophage agglutination f.
      (MAggF)
    macrophage chemotactic f. (MCF)
    macrophage colony-stimulating f.

macrophage-derived growth f.
macrophage growth f.
macrophage-inhibiting f. (MIF)
macrophage migration inhibition f.
melanocyte-stimulating hormone-inhibiting f. (MIF)
melanocyte-stimulating hormone-releasing f. (MRF)
migration inhibition f. (MIF)
migration-inhibitory f.
milk f.
mitogenic f.
monocyte-derived neutrophil chemotactic f. (MDNCF)
myocardial depressant f. (MDF)
natural killer cell-stimulating f. (NKSF)
necrotizing f.
nephritic f.
nerve growth f. (NGF)
neutrophil activating f. (NAF)
neutrophil chemotactant f.
neutrophilic chemotactic f.
osteoclast activating f. (OAF)
Ovenstone f. (OF)
Passovoy f.
plasma clotting f.
plasma labile f.
plasma thromboplastin f. (PTF)
plasma thromboplastin f. B
plasma f. X
plasmin prothrombins conversion f. (PPCF)
platelet f. (PF)
platelet f. 1, 2, 3, 4
platelet-activating f. (PAF)
platelet-aggregating f. (PAF)
platelet-derived growth f. (PDGF)
platelet tissue f.
polymorphonuclear neutrophil chemotactic f.
prognostic f.
prolactin-inhibiting f. (PIF)
prolactin-releasing f.
proliferation inhibitory f. (PIF)
properdin f. A, B, D, E
prothrombokinase f.
Prower f.
Prower-Stuart f.
quality f. (QF)
R f.
recognition f.

releasing f. (RF)
renal erythropoietic f. (REF)
resistance f.
resistance-inducing f. (RIF)
resistance transfer f. (RTF)
Rh f.
Rhesus f. (Rh)
rheumatoid f. (RF)
rheumatoid arthritis f. (RAF)
rho f.
ripple f.
risk f.
rough f.
secretor f.
serum prothrombin conversion accelerator f.
sex f.
Simon septic f.
skin-reactive f. (SRF)
slow-reacting f. of anaphylaxis (SRF-A)
somatotropin-releasing f. (SRF)
SPCA f.
specific macrophage-arming f. (SMAF)
spreading f.
stable f.
Stuart f.
Stuart-Prower f.
sulfation f.
T-cell growth f.
T-cell growth f.-1
T-cell growth f.-2
T cell-replacing f. (TRF)
termination f.
thymic humoral f.
thymic lymphopoietic f.
thymic replacing f.
thyroid stimulating hormone-releasing f. (TSH-RF)
thyrotoxic complement-fixation f.
thyrotropin-releasing f. (TRF)
tissue f.
tissue-coding f. (TSF)
tissue-damaging f. (TF)
transfer f. (TF)
transforming growth f.
transforming growth f. α (TGFα)
transforming growth f. β (TGFβ)
transforming growth f. alpha
transforming growth f. beta
translocation f.

NOTES

F

factor *(continued)*
 tumor angiogenic f. (TAF)
 tumor necrosis f. (TNF)
 tumor necrosis f.-beta
 undegraded insulin f. (UIF)
 uterine relaxing f. (URF)
 V f.
 f. V
 f. VI
 f. VIII-crossed
  immunoelectrophoresis
 f. VIII inhibitor
 f. VIII-related antigen test
 von Willebrand f.
 Williams f.
 X f.
 f. X
 f. Xa inhibitor
 f. XI
 f. XII
 f. XIII
 f. XIIIa
factorial
facultative
 f. anaerobe
 f. autotroph
 f. bacterium
 f. heterochromatin
 f. histiocyte
 f. organisms
 f. parasite
FAD
 flavin adenine dinucleotide
FADF
 fluorescent antibody darkfield
Fahr disease
Fahrenheit (F)
 F. temperature scale (F)
 F. thermometer
failure
 acute renal f. (ARF)
 f. of all vital forces (FOAVF)
 cardiac f. (CF)
 chronic renal f. (CRF)
 circulatory f.
 congestive cardiac f. (CCF)
 congestive heart f. (CHF)
 fulminant hepatic f. (FHF)
 heart f. (HF)
 left ventricular f. (LVF)
 mean time between f.'s
 peripheral circulatory f.
 pituitary gonadotropic f.
 f. rate
 respiratory f.
falciform

falciparum
 f. fever
 f. malaria
fallopian tube tumor
Fallot
 F. syndrome
 tetralogy of F. (Tet, TF)
false
 f. agglutination
 f. albuminuria
 f. anemia
 f. aneurysm
 f. cast
 f. cyanosis
 f. cyst
 f. dextrocardia
 f. diphtheria
 f. diverticulum
 f. hematuria
 f. hypertrophy
 f. knot (umbilical cord)
 f. membrane
 f. mole
 f. negative
 f. neuroma
 f. positive
false-negative (FN)
 f. reaction
false-positive (FP)
 biologic f.-p. (BFP)
 chronic f.-p. (CFP)
 f.-p. reaction
familial
 f. benign pemphigus
 f. cancer
 f. cardiomyopathy
 f. cerebellar ataxia
 f. cystinuria
 f. dysautonomia
 f. dysbetalipoproteinemia
 f. emphysema
 f. erythroblastic anemia
 f. erythrophagocytic
  lymphohistiocytosis (FEL)
 f. fibrous dysplasia of jaws
 f. goiter
 f. gonadal dysgenesis
 f. hemolytic anemia
 f. hypercholesterolemia
 f. hypertriglyceridemia
 f. hypocalciuric hypercalcemia
 f. hypoplastic anemia
 f. intestinal polyposis
 f. juvenile nephrophthisis (FJN)
 f. juvenile polyp (FJP)
 f. Mediterranean fever (FMF)
 f. microcytic anemia

f. multiple endocrine adenomatosis, type 1, 2
f. myoclonic epilepsy
f. nephritis
f. nephronophthisis
f. nephrosis
f. nonhemolytic jaundice
f. paroxysmal polyserositis
f. paroxysmal rhabdomyolysis
f. periodic paralysis
f. polyposis
f. primary systemic amyloidosis
f. pyridoxine-responsive anemia
f. recurrent polyserositis
f. splenic anemia

family
cancer f.

FAN
fuchsin, amido black, and naphthol yellow

FANA
fluorescent antinuclear antibody
FANA test

Fanconi
F. anemia
F. pancytopenia
F. syndrome

Fanconi-Zinsser syndrome
fan-in
Fannia
F. *canicularis*
F. *scalaris*
fan-out
farad (F)
Faraday
F. constant
F. effect
F. law of electrolysis
faradic shock
Farber
F. disease
F. lipogranulomatosis
F. syndrome
F. test
Farber-Uzman syndrome
farcy
Far East Russian encephalitis
farmer's
f. lung
f. skin

Farr
F. law
F. test
Farrant
F. medium
F. mounting fluid
fascial fibrosarcoma
fascicles
fascicular sarcoma
fasciculate bladder
fasciitis, fascitis
eosinophilic f.
infiltrative f.
necrotizing f.
nodular f.
parosteal f.
proliferative f.
pseudosarcomatous f.
Fasciola
F. *gigantica*
F. *hepatica*
fascioliasis
fasciolid
Fascioloides magna
fasciolopsiasis
Fasciolopsis
F. *buski*
fascitis (*var. of* fasciitis)
fast
acid f. (AF)
f. green FCF
f. hemoglobin
low-voltage f. (LVF)
f. smear
f. yellow
fastidious
fasting blood sugar (FBS)
fastness
FAT
fluorescent antibody test
fat
f. absorption
f. absorption study
f. absorption test
f. assay
brown f.
f. cell
f. depot
f. embolism
f. embolus
f. free (FF)
f. necrosis

NOTES

F

fat *(continued)*
  f. necrosis of pancreas
  f. staining
  subcutaneous f.
  f. tide
  total body f. (TBF)
  yellow f.
fatal
  f. dose (FD)
  f. granulomatous disease (FGD)
fat-deficiency disease
fat-free
  f.-f. dry weight (FFDW)
  f.-f. mass (FFM)
  f.-f. wet weight (FFWW)
fat-induced hyperlipidemia
fat-mobilizing
  f.-m. hormone
  f.-m. substance (FMS)
fatty
  f. acid (FA)
  f. acid assay
  f. acid oxidation
  f. acid profile
  f. acid synthesis
  f. ascites
  f. atrophy
  f. cast
  f. change
  f. cirrhosis
  f. degeneration
  f. deposition
  f. heart
  f. infiltration
  f. kidney
  f. liver
  f. metamorphosis
  f. oil
  f. urinary cast
fauces
Fauchard disease
faucial
faucitis
faulty union
faun tail nevus
FAV
  feline ataxia virus
favic chandeliers
favid
favism
favosa
  trichomycosis f.
Favre-Racouchot disease
favus
Faxitron x-ray machine
FB
  foreign body

FBE
  fibrinogen breakdown product
  full blood examination
FBS
  fasting blood sugar
  fetal bovine serum
Fc
  Fc fragment
  Fc piece
  Fc receptor
FCA
  ferritin-conjugated antibody
FCAP
  Fellow of the College of American
   Pathologists
FCC
  follicular center cell
F$^+$ cell
FCF
  fast green FCF
FCM
  flow cytometry
FD
  fatal dose
FD$_{50}$
  median fatal dose
FDC
  follicular dendritic cell
FDNB
  fluoro-2,4-dinitrobenzene
FDP
  fibrin degradation product
  fibrin/fibrinogen degradation product
F-duction
feathery degeneration
febrile
  f. agglutination test
  f. agglutinins
  f. albuminuria
  f. nonhemolytic transfusion reaction
  f. urine
febrilis
  calor f.
FEC
  free erythrocyte coproporphyrin
fecal
  f. abscess
  f. fat
  f. fat test
  f. fistula
  f. impaction
  f. incontinence
  f. leukocyte count
  f. marker
  f. occult blood test
  f. tumor
  f. urobilinogen (FU)
  f. vomitus

fecalith
fecaloma
feces (F)
    extravasation f.
    impacted f.
FECG
    fetal electrocardiogram
Fechner tumor
FECP
    free erythrocyte coproporphyria
Fede disease
feedback
    f. inhibition mutation
    f. loop
Feer disease
feet
    basal f.
Fehleisen streptococcus
Fehling
    F. solution
    F. test
FEL
    familial erythrophagocytic
    lymphohistiocytosis
feline
    f. agranulocytosis
    f. ataxia virus (FAV)
    f. distemper
    f. infectious enteritis
    f. infectious peritonitis
    f. leukemia
    f. leukemia-sarcoma virus complex
    f. leukemia virus (FeLV)
    f. panleukopenia virus
    f. rhinotracheitis virus
    f. viral rhinotracheitis
felis
    Afipia f.
Felix-Weil (FW)
    F. reaction (FWR)
Fellow of the College of American
Pathologists (FCAP)
felon
Felton phenomenon
Felty syndrome
FeLV
    feline leukemia virus
female (F)
    f. carrier
    f. castration
    f. genital tract (FGT)
    f. genital tract cytologic smear

    f. hormone
    f. pseudohermaphroditism
    f. sex chromatin pattern
feminization
    f. syndrome, adrenal
    testicular f.
feminizing tumor
femoral
    f. hernia
    f. puncture
femorocele
femoropopliteal occlusive disease
femtoliter (fL, fl)
femtometer (fm)
femtomole (fmol)
fenac
fenestra
    alveolar f.
fenestrata
    placenta f.
fenestrated endothelium
fenestration
    atrophic f.
Fenwick disease
Fenwick-Hunner ulcer
FEP, FEPP
    free erythrocyte protoporphyrin
FEPP-B
    vindesine, etoposide, procarbazine,
    prednisone, bleomycin
ferment
fermentation
    mannitol f.
    mixed acid f.
    f. test
fermi
fermium
Fernandez reaction
Fernbach flask
ferning
fern test
Ferrata
    F. cell
ferredoxin
Ferribacterium
ferric
    f. ammonium sulfate stain
    f. chloride reaction of epinephrine
    f. chloride test
    f. ferricyanide reduction test
    f. ferrocyanide
    f. oxide

F

NOTES

ferricyanide
  ferrous f.
ferrihemoglobin
ferrimagnetic
ferriprotoporphyrin (FPP)
ferrite
ferritin
  f. assay
ferritin-conjugated antibody (FCA)
ferritin-coupled antibody
ferrocalcinosis
ferrocalcinotic deposition
ferrochelatase
ferrocyanide
  ferric f.
  potassium f.
ferroflocculation
ferrohemoglobin
ferrokinetic
ferrokinetics
  f. study
ferromagnetic
ferrous
  f. citrate Fe 59
  f. ferricyanide
ferroxidase
ferrugination
ferruginous
  f. body
  f. micelles
fertile eunuch syndrome
fertility
  f. agent
  f. factor
  f. inhibition
fertilization
fervens
  calor f.
FES
  flame emission spectroscopy
  forced expiratory spirogram
fester
festoon
festooning
fetal
  f. abnormality
  f. adenoma
  f. alcohol syndrome
  f. antigen
  f. bovine serum (FBS)
  f. death
  f. duplication
  f. electrocardiogram (FECG)
  f. erythroblastosis
  f. face syndrome
  f. fat cell lipoma
  f. hemoglobin (HbF)
  f. hemoglobin test

  f. hydantoin syndrome
  f. lobulation
  f. lung maturity (FLM)
  f. trimethadione syndrome
fetid rhinitis
α-fetoglobin
fetoglobulin
  α_1-f.
  alpha-1 f.
fetoplacental anasarca
fetoprotein
  α-f. (AFP)
  α_1-f.
  alpha f.
  alpha-1 f.
  beta fetoprotein
  β-fetoprotein
  γ-f.
  gamma f.
α_1-fetoprotein assay
α-fetoprotein test
fetotoxicity
fetus, pl. fetuses
  f. acardiacus
  f. amorphus
  f. compressus
  f. in fetu
  harlequin f.
  macerated f.
  f. papyraceus
  parasitic f.
  stunted f.
Feuerstein-Mims syndrome
Feulgen
  F. reaction
  F. stain
  F. test
fever
  abortus f.
  Aden f.
  aestivoautumnal f.
  African hemorrhagic f.
  African swine f.
  African tick-borne f.
  aphthous f.
  Argentinean hemorrhagic f.
  f. blister
  Bolivian hemorrhagic f.
  bouquet f.
  boutonneuse f.
  bovine ephemeral f.
  breakbone f.
  Bullis f.
  Bunyamwera f.
  Bwamba f.
  camp f.
  cat-bite f.
  f. caused by infection (FI)

Central European tick-borne f.
cerebrospinal f.
chikungunya f.
childbed f.
Colorado tick f.
continued f.
Crimean-Congo hemorrhagic f.
dandy f.
date f.
death f.
dengue hemorrhagic f.
desert f.
diphasic milk f.
dumdum f.
Dutton relapsing f.
Ebola hemorrhagic f.
eczema, asthma, hay f. (EAHF)
ephemeral f. of cattle
epidemic hemorrhagic f.
epimastical f.
eruptive f.
essential f.
exanthematous f.
falciparum f.
familial Mediterranean f. (FMF)
flood f.
food f.
glandular f.
Haverhill f.
hay f.
hematuric bilious f.
hcmoglobinuric f.
hemorrhagic f. (HF)
hemorrhagic f. with renal syndrome
herpetic f.
hospital f.
Ilhéus f.
intermittent malarial f.
inundation f.
island f.
jail f.
Japanese river f.
jungle yellow f.
kedani f.
Korean hemorrhagic f.
Lassa hemorrhagic f.
laurel f.
malarial f.
malignant catarrhal f.
malignant tertian f.
Malta f.
Manchurian hemorrhagic f.

Marseilles f.
marsh f.
Mediterranean f.
miliary f.
miniature scarlet f.
monoleptic f.
mud f.
Omsk hemorrhagic f.
o'nyong-nyong f.
Oroya f.
paludal f.
pappataci f.
paratyphoid f. (types A, B, and
  C)
parrot f.
Pel-Ebstein f.
pharyngoconjunctival f.
phlebotomus f.
polka f.
polyleptic f.
Pontiac f.
protein f.
puerperal f.
Pym f.
pyogenic f.
Q f.
quartan f.
quotidian f.
rat-bite f.
recrudescent typhus f.
relapsing f.
remittent malarial f.
rheumatic f. (RF)
Rift Valley f.
Rocky Mountain spotted f. (RMSF)
Ross River f.
sandfly f.
San Joaquin f.
San Joaquin Valley f.
scarlet f. (SF)
septic f.
ship f.
shipping f.
Sindbis f.
slow f.
solar f.
spotted f.
steroid f.
swamp f.
swine f.
symptomatic f.
syphilitic f.

F

NOTES

fever *(continued)*
    tertian f.
    three-day f.
    tick f.
    traumatic f.
    trench f.
    tsutsugamushi f.
    typhoid f.
    f. of undetermined origin (FUO)
    undifferentiated type f.
    undulant f.
    f. of unknown origin (FUO)
    uveoparotid f.
    valley f.
    viral hemorrhagic f.
    vivax f.
    Wesselsbron f.
    West African f.
    West Nile f.
    wound f.
    yellow f. (YF)
    Zika f.
feverish
    f. urine
Fevold test
FF
    fat free
FFA
    free fatty acids
FFDW
    fat-free dry weight
FFL
    floral variant of follicular lymphoma
FFM
    fat-free mass
FFP
    fresh frozen plasma
FFWW
    fat-free wet weight
FG
    fibrinogen
FGD
    fatal granulomatous disease
FGT
    female genital tract
      FGT cytologic smear
FH
    follicular hyperplasia
FH$_4$
    N_5-formyl F.
FHF
    fulminant hepatic failure
FI
    fever caused by infection
    fibrinogen
FI$_{O2}$, FIO$_2$
    forced inspiratory oxygen
    fraction of inspired oxygen

FIA
    fluorescent immunoassay
fib
    fibrinogen
fiber
    argyrophilic f.
    collagenous f.
    f. density
    elastic f.
    meat f.
    oxytalan f.
    reticulin f.
    Rosenthal f.
    skeinoid f.
    skeinoid f.
    f. spectrum
    U f.'s
fiberoptic
fibremia
fibril
fibrillar astrocyte
fibrillary
    f. astrocyte
    f. astrocytoma
    f. neuroma
fibrillated
fibrin
    f. body
    f. breakdown product
    f. calculus
    f. degradation product (FDP)
    f. degradation products method
    f. monomer
    f. plate lysis
    reptilase f.
    f. stain
    f. staining
    f. thrombus
    f. titer
    f. titer test
fibrinase
fibrin/fibrinogen degradation product (FDP)
fibrinocellular
fibrinogen (FG, FI, fib)
    f. breakdown product (FBE)
    f. deficiency
    f. I-125
    f. method
    f. split product (FSP)
    f. titer test
fibrinogenase
fibrinogenemia
fibrinogen-fibrin conversion syndrome
fibrinogenic
fibrinogenolysis
fibrinogenopenia
fibrinogenous

fibrinoid
    f. degeneration
    f. necrosis
    f. necrotizing inflammation
fibrinokinase
fibrinolysin
    f. coagulation
    seminal f.
    streptococcal f.
fibrinolysis
    primary f.
fibrinolysokinase
fibrinolytic
    f. protein
    f. purpura
    f. split product (FSP)
fibrinopenia
fibrinopeptide
fibrinopurulent
    f. inflammation
fibrinoscopy
fibrinous
    f. acute lobar pneumonia
    f. acute pleuritis
    f. adhesion
    f. bronchitis
    f. cast
    f. degeneration
    f. exudation
    f. inflammation
    f. lymph
    f. pericarditis
    f. peritonitis
    f. pleurisy
    f. pleuritis
    f. polyp
fibrin-split product
fibrin-stabilization factor (FSF)
fibrin-stabilizing
    f.-s. factor (FSF)
    f.-s. factor test
fibrinuria
fibroadenoma
    f. of breast
    giant f.
    intracanalicular f.
    juvenile f.
    pericanalicular f.
fibroadenosis
fibroameloblastic
    f. dentinoma
    f. odontoma

fibroblast
    chick embryo f. (CEF)
    f. interferon
    pericryptal f.
fibroblastic
    f. meningioma
fibroblastoma
    giant cell f. (GCF)
    perineural f.
fibrocalcific
    f. nodule
fibrocarcinoma
fibrocartilage
    degenerated intervertebral f.
    f. matrix alteration
fibrocaseous
    f. inflammation
    f. peritonitis
fibrochondritis
fibrochondroma
fibrocollagenous stroma
fibrocongestive
    f. hypertrophy
    f. splenomegaly
fibrocyst
fibrocystic
    f. condition of the breast
    f. disease of the breast
    f. disease of the pancreas
    f. mastitis
    f. mastopathy
fibrocystoma
fibrodysplasia
    f. ossificans progressiva
fibroelastic
fibroelastogenesis
fibroelastosis
    endocardial f. (EFE)
    endomyocardial f.
fibroenchondroma
fibroepithelial
    f. papilloma
    f. polyp
fibroepithelioma
fibrofolliculoma
fibrogenesis
    f. imperfecta ossium
fibrogliosis
fibrohistiocytic lesion
fibroid
    f. adenoma
    f. inflammation

F

NOTES

fibroid *(continued)*
    f. tumor
    f. uterus
fibroin
fibrokeratoma
fibrolamellar liver cell carcinoma
fibroleiomyoma
fibrolipoma
fibroliposarcoma
fibroma
    ameloblastic f.
    aponeurotic f.
    cementifying f.
    cemento-ossifying f. (COF)
    chondromyxoid f. (CMF)
    concentric f.
    desmoplastic f.
    extranuchal nuchal f.
    giant cell f.
    irritation f.
    f. molle
    f. molle gravidarum
    myxoid f.
    f. myxomatodes
    nonossifying f.
    nuchal f.
    odontogenic f.
    ossifying f.
    periosteal f.
    peripheral odontogenic f.
    periungual f.
    pleural f.
    rabbit f.
    recurring digital f.'s of childhood
    senile f.
    Shope f.
    telangiectatic f.
fibromatoid
fibromatosis
    abdominal f.
    aggressive infantile f.
    f. colli
    congenital generalized f.
    Dupuytren f.
    extra-abdominal f.
    inclusion body f.
    infantile digital f.
    juvenile hyalin f.
    juvenile palmo-plantar f.
    musculoaponeurotic f.
    palmar f.
    penile f.
    plantar f.
    retroperitoneal f.
    f. virus of rabbits
fibromatous
fibrometer

fibromuscular
    f. dysplasia
    f. hyperplasia
fibromyoma
fibromyositis
fibromyxoid
fibromyxolipoma
fibromyxoma
fibromyxosarcoma
fibronectin
    large, external transformation-sensitive f. (LETS)
    plasma f.
fibroneuroma
fibro-osteoma
fibropapilloma
fibroplasia
    retrolental f. (RLF)
fibroplastic
fibropolypus
fibrosa
    periosteitis f.
fibrosarcoma
    Earle L f.
    fascial f.
    infantile f.
    medullary f.
    odontogenic f.
    periosteal f.
fibrose
fibrosiderotic nodule
fibrosing
    f. adenomatosis
    f. adenosis
    f. alveolitis
fibrosis
    bridging f.
    condensation f.
    cystic f. (CF)
    diffuse interstitial f.
    endomyocardial f. (EMF)
    focal f.
    hepatic f.
    idiopathic pulmonary f. (IPF)
    idiopathic retroperitoneal f.
    inflammation with f.
    interstitial f.
    leptomeningeal f.
    mediastinal f.
    multifocal f.
    nodular subepidermal f.
    pericentral f.
    perimuscular f.
    periportal f.
    pipestem f.
    progressive massive f. (PMF)
    pulmonary f.
    replacement f.

retroperitoneal f.
septal f., liver
subadventitial f.
subepidermal f.
subsinusoidal f.
Symmers clay pipestem f.
fibrositis
fibrothorax
fibrotic
fibrous
f. adhesion
f. ankylosis
f. astrocyte
f. astrocytoma
f. bacterial virus
f. body
f. cavernitis
f. cortical defect
f. degeneration
f. dysplasia of bone
f. dysplasia of jaws
f. dysplasia protuberans
f. familial dysplasia
f. goiter
f. hamartoma of infancy
f. histiocytoma
f. hypertrophic pachymeningitis
f. layer
f. mesothelioma
f. monostotic dysplasia
f. nodule
f. obliteration
f. osteoma
f. polyp
f. protein
f. repair
f. replacement
f. tendon sheath
f. thyroiditis
f. tissue (FT)
f. tubercle
f. union
f. xanthoma
fibrous long-spacing (collagen) (FLS)
fibroxanthoma
atypical f.
ficin
Fick
F. bacillus
F. law
F. principle
Ficoll-Hypaque technique

FID
flame ionization detector
Fiedler
F. disease
F. myocarditis
field
depth of f.
f. effect transistor
high power f. (hpf)
high-power f. (HPF)
low-power f. (LPF, lpf)
magnetic f.
f. method
f. of microscope
oil immersion f. (OIF)
F. rapid stain
red blood cells per high power f.
(RBC/hpf)
f. of view
white blood cells per high
power f. (WBC/hpf)
field-vole
Fiessinger-Leroy-Reiter syndrome
fifth
f. disease
f. disease virus
FIGLU
formiminoglutamic acid
formiminoglutamic acid test
FIGLU excretion test
FIGO
International Federation of Gynecology
and Obstetrics
FIGO adenocarcinoma of
endometrium
FIGO classification of tumor
staging
Figueira syndrome
figure
flame f.
mitotic f.
myelin f. (MF)
fig wart
filament
cytoskeletal f.
f. polymorphonuclear leukocyte
filamented neutrophil
filament-nonfilament count
filamentous
f. bacterial virus
f. bacteriophage

F

NOTES

filar
  f. mass
  f. substance
Filaria
  F. bancrofti
  F. conjunctivae
  F. demarquayi
  F. hominis oris
  F. juncea
  F. labialis
  F. lentis
  F. loa
  F. lymphatica
  F. medinensis
  F. ozzardi
  F. palpebralis
  F. philippinensis
  F. sanguinis
  F. tucumana
  F. volvulus
filaria, pl. **filariae**
  Ozzards f.
  persistent f.
filarial
  f. arthritis
  f. funiculitis
filariasis
  Bancroft f.
  Malayan f.
  f. peripheral blood preparation
  f. serological test
filaricidal
filaricide
filariform
Filariicae
Filarioidea
Filaroides
Filatov, Filatow
  F. disease
file
  Indian f.
  master f.
  Rare Donor F.
filiform
  f. hyperkeratosis
  f. process
  f. wart
filling defect
film
  blood f.
  f. density calibration
  fixed blood f.
  gelatin f.
  spot f.
  f. stripping autoradiography
  sulfa f.

Filobasidiella
  F. bacillisporus
  F. neoformans
filopodia
filopodium
Filoviridae
Filovirus
filter
  bacterial f.
  barrier f.
  Berkefeld f.
  blocking f.
  f. capacitor
  Centriflo f.
  Chamberland f.
  collodion f.
  exciter f.
  gelatin f.
  Gelman f.
  glass fiber f.
  HEPA f.
  high-pass f.
  f. hybridization
  inherent f.
  interference f.
  line f.
  low-pass f.
  membrane f.
  microaggregate f.
  MILLEX-GS plasma f.
  Millipore f.
  Nuclepore f.
  f. paper microscopic (FPM)
  f. paper microscopic test
  f. photometer
  Seitz f.
  Selas f.
  Wratten f.
filterable virus
filtering
filtrable
  f. virus
Filtracheck-UTI
  F.-U. disposable colormetric
    bacteriuria detection system
  F.-U. test
filtrate
  tuberculin f. (TF)
filtration
  gel f.
  glomerular f.
fimbria, pl. **fimbriae**
fimbriated
finder
fine-needle aspiration biopsy (FNAB)
fine structure
finger
  clubbed f.

dead f.
drumstick f.
hippocratic f.
mallet f.
rudimentary f.
sausage f.
spade f.
waxy f.
webbed f.
fingerprint
    DNA f.
    genetic f.
fingerprinting
    DNA f.
finite
Fink-Heimer stain
Finn chamber patch test
FIO$_2$ (*var. of* FI$_{O2}$)
fire
    f. ant
    Saint Anthony f.
firmware
first
    f. arch syndrome
    f. filial generation (F$_1$)
first degree
    f. d. burn
    f. d. frostbite
    f. d. heart block
    f. d. radiation injury
first-order reaction
first-set
    f.-s. graft rejection
    f.-s. rejection
Fischer
    F. exact test
    F. projection
FISH
    fluorescence in situ hybridization
fish
    f. skin
    f. tapeworm
    f. tapeworm anemia
Fishberg concentration test
Fisher
    F. exact test
    F. syndrome
Fisher-Race (notation) (FR)
Fishman-Lerner unit
fish-slime disease
fission
    binary f.

f. fungus
f. product
fissiparity
fissiparous
fissural cyst
fissure
    f. in ano
fissured nucleus
fist.
    fistula
fistula, pl. fistulae, fistulas (fist.)
    abdominal f.
    amphibolic f.
    amphibolous f.
    anal f.
    f. in ano
    arteriovenous f. (AVF)
    biliary f.
    f. bimucosa
    blind f.
    branchial f.
    bronchoesophageal f.
    bronchopleural f.
    carotid-cavernous f.
    cervical f.
    cholecystoduodenal f.
    coccygeal f.
    colocutaneous f.
    coloileal f.
    colonic f.
    colovaginal f.
    colovesical f.
    complete f.
    duodenal f.
    enterocutaneous f.
    enterovaginal f.
    enterovesical f.
    external f.
    fecal f.
    gastric f.
    gastrocolic f.
    gastrocutaneous f.
    gastroduodenal f.
    gastrointestinal f.
    genitourinary f.
    hepatic f.
    hepatopleural f.
    horseshoe f.
    incomplete f.
    inflammatory f.
    internal f.
    intestinal f.

F

NOTES

fistula *(continued)*
    lacteal f.
    mammary f.
    metroperitoneal f.
    parietal f.
    perineovaginal f.
    pilonidal f.
    pulmonary f.
    pulmonary arteriovenous f. (PAF)
    rectolabial f.
    rectourethral f.
    rectovaginal f.
    rectovesical f.
    rectovestibular f.
    rectovulvar f.
    sigmoidovesical f.
    spermatic f.
    stercoral f.
    thoracic f.
    thoracic duct f. (TDF)
    thyroglossal f.
    tracheobiliary f.
    tracheoesophageal f. (TEF)
    umbilical f.
    urachal f.
    ureterocutaneous f.
    ureterovaginal f.
    urethrovaginal f.
    urinary f.
    urogenital f.
    uteroperitoneal f.
    vesical f.
    vesicocolic f.
    vesicocutaneous f.
    vesicointestinal f.
    vesicouterine f.
    vesicovaginal f.
    vesicovaginorectal f.
fistulation
fistulization
fistulous
fit
FITC
    fluorescein isothiocyanate
Fite
    F. method
    F. stain
Fite-Faraco stain
fitness
"fitter" cell theory
fitting
    curve f.
Fitzgerald factor
Fitz-Hugh and Curtis syndrome
Fitz syndrome
fix
fixation
    alcohol f.

    f. artifact
    autotrophic f.
    carbon dioxide f.
    complement f. (CF)
    microwave f.
    f. reaction
    secondary f.
fixative
    acetone f.
    aldehyde f.
    Altmann f.
    B5 f.
    Bouin picroformol-acetic f.
    Brasil f.
    buffered formalin f.
    Carnoy f.
    Champy f.
    chlorpalladium f.
    chromic acid f.
    coating f.
    CytoLyt f.
    Flemming f.
    formaldehyde f.
    formalin f.
    formol-calcium f.
    formol-Müller f.
    formol-saline f.
    formol-Zenker f.
    Gendre f.
    glacial acetic acid f.
    glutaraldehyde f.
    Golgi osmiobichromate f.
    Helly f.
    Hermann f.
    Jores f.
    Kaiserling f.
    Karnovsky f.
    lead f.
    Luft potassium permanganate f.
    Marchi f.
    mercuric f.
    methanol f.
    Millonig phosphate-buffered
      formalin f.
    Müller f.
    neutral buffered formalin f.
    Newcomer f.
    Orth f.
    osmic acid f.
    Park-Williams f.
    periodate-lysing-paraformaldehyde f.
    Permount slide f.
    picric acid f.
    picroformol f.
    PreservCyt f.
    Regaud f.
    Saccomanno f.
    Schaudinn f.

Shandon f.
Spray-Cyte slide f.
Supermount slide f.
Thoma f.
Zenker f.
fixed
f. blood film
f. oil
f. sediment method
f. virus
fixed-point variable
FJN
familial juvenile nephrophthisis
FJP
familial juvenile polyp
FK506
Fl
follicle lysis
fL, fl
femtoliter
flaccid
flaccidity
flag
flagella (*pl. of* flagellum)
flagellar
f. agglutinin
f. antigen
Flagellata
flagellate
f. dysentery
flagellated
flagellin
flagellosis
flagellum, pl. **flagella**
Flajani disease
flame
f. background
capillary f.
f. cell
f. emission spectrophotometry
f. emission spectroscopy (FES)
f. figure
f. intensity zone
f. ionization detector (FID)
manometric f.
f. nevus
f. photometer
f. photometry
flammability
flammable
flash-point temperature

flask
f. culture
Dewar f.
Erlenmeyer f.
Fernbach f.
Florence f.
vacuum f.
volumetric f.
flask-like
Erlenmeyer f.
flat
f. condyloma
f. substrate method
f. wart
Flatau-Schilder disease
flat-field objective
flatworm
Flaujeac factor
flavianic acid
flavin
f. adenine dinucleotide (FAD)
f. mononucleotide (FMN)
Flaviviridae
Flavivirus
flavivirus
Flavobacterium
F. meningosepticum
flavoenzyme
flavoprotein
flaxseed oil
flea
American rat f.
dog f.
European rat f.
human f.
Indian rat f.
flea-bitten kidney
flecainide
Flegel disease
Fleischner syndrome
Fleitmann test
Flemming
F. fixative
F. triple stain
flesh
proud f.
fleshflies
fleshy
f. mole
f. polyp
Fletcher factor
Flexner dysentery

F

NOTES

Flexner-Strong bacillus
flight
    time of f.
flint
    f. disease
    f. glass
flip-flop
FLM
    fetal lung maturity
floating
    f. beta disease
    f. organ
floating-point variable
floc
    flocculation
floccose
flocculable
floccular degeneration
flocculate
flocculation (floc)
    cephalin f.
    cephalin-cholesterol f. (CCF)
    limes f. (Lf)
    limit f. (LF)
    Ramon f.
    f. reaction (FR)
    f. test
    thymol f. (TF)
floccule
    toxoid-antitoxin f.'s (TAF)
flocculence
flocculent
flocculoreaction
flocculus
flood
    f. fever
    f. plate
    f. source
flora
    intestinal f.
    oral f.
floral
    f. variant
    f. variant of follicular lymphoma
    (FFL)
Florence
    F. crystal
    F. flask
Florey unit
florid oral papillomatosis
Florisil
flotation
    f. bath
    centrifugal f.
    direct centrifugal f. (DCF)
    f. rate
    f. technique

flow
    abnormal f.
    f. birefringence
    cerebral blood f. (CBF)
    f. chart
    coronary blood f. (CBF)
    f. cytometer
    f. cytometric reticulocyte analysis
    f. cytometry (FCM)
    f. cytophotometry
    effective renal blood f. (ERBF)
    effective renal plasma f.
    estimated hepatic blood f. (EHBF)
    exercise hyperemia blood f.
    (EHBF)
    gene f.
    hepatic blood f. (HBF)
    high f. (HF)
    f. meter
    pulmonary blood f.
    f. rate (FR)
    reactive hyperemia blood f.
    (RHBF)
    renal plasma f. (RPF)
    splanchnic blood f. (SBF)
    uterine blood f. (UBF)
flowing hyperostosis
flowmeter (FM)
    electromagnetic f. (EMF)
FLS
    fibrous long-spacing (collagen)
FLSA
    follicular lymphosarcoma
flu
    influenza
fluctuation
flucytosine
fludrocortisone
fluid (fl)
    amniotic f.
    ascitic f.
    f. balance
    f. balance and homeostasis
    Bensley osmic dichromate f.
    body f.'s
    Bouin f.
    Callison f.
    cerebrospinal f. (CSF)
    Ciaccio f.
    Clarke f.
    De Castro f.
    dentinal f.
    extracellular f.
    Farrant mounting f.
    gastric f. (GF)
    Gendre f.
    Helly f.
    interstitial f.

intracellular f. (ICF)
Orth f.
pleural f.
Rees-Ecker f.
respiratory tract f. (RTF)
f. retention
seminal f.
serous f.
spinal f.
subretinal f. (SRF)
synovial f.
tubular f. (TF)
f. volume (FV)
Zamboni f.
Zenker f.
fluke
blood f.
cat liver f.
Chinese liver f.
giant intestinal f.
giant liver f.
lancet f.
liver f.
lung f.
Oriental blood f.
Oriental lung f.
sheep liver f.
vesical blood f.
Yokogawa f.
fluor
fluorescein
f. isothiocyanate (FITC)
f. mercuric acetate
f. sodium
fluorescence
f. microscopy
f. plus Giemsa stain
f. quenching
relative f. (RF)
resonance f.
f. in situ hybridization (FISH)
f. spectrum
fluorescence-activated
f.-a. cell sorter (FACS)
f.-a. cell sorter scan (FACscan)
fluorescent
f. antibody (FA)
f. antibody darkfield (FADF)
f. antibody technique
f. antibody test (FAT)
f. antinuclear antibody (FANA)
f. antinuclear antibody test

f. cytoprint assay
f. dye
f. immunoassay (FIA)
f. material
f. microscope
f. probe
f. stain
f. staining
f. treponemal antibody (FTA)
f. treponemal antibody-absorption
(FTA-ABS, FTA-AB)
f. treponemal antibody-absorption
test
**fluorescent-treponemal antibody
absorption test (FTA-AB)**
fluorescin
fluoride
f. assay
hydrogen f.
f. number
fluorine
f. 18
fluorite objective
fluoroacetamide
fluoroacetate
f. assay
sodium f.
fluorocarbon assay
fluorochrome
fluorochroming
fluorocyte
5-fluorocytosine
fluorodeoxyuridine (FUDR)
fluoro-2,4-dinitrobenzene (FDNB)
fluorometer
fluorometry
fluorosilicate
sodium f.
fluorosis
dental f.
endemic f.
fluosol-DA
fluoxetine
fluphenazine
flurazepam
Flury
F. strain rabies virus
F. strain vaccine
flutamide
flux
luminous f.
magnetic f.

F

NOTES

fly
- f. agaric
- black f.
- deer f.
- dog f.
- fruit f.
- f. larva
- larva f.
- stable f.
- tsetse f.
- warble f.

Flynn-Aird syndrome

FM
- flowmeter

fm
- femtometer

FMD
- foot-and-mouth disease
  - FMD virus

FMF
- familial Mediterranean fever

FMN
- flavin mononucleotide

fmol
- femtomole

FMS
- fat-mobilizing substance

FN
- false-negative

FNAB
- fine-needle aspiration biopsy

foam
- f. cell
- f. stability test

foamy
- f. agent
- f. degeneration
- f. degeneration of hepatocytes
- f. histiocyte
- f. virus

FOAVF
- failure of all vital forces

focal
- f. amyloidosis
- f. appendicitis
- f. atrophy
- f. bronchopneumonia
- f. calcification
- f. cortical epilepsy
- f. dermal hypoplasia
- f. dermal hypoplasia syndrome
- f. disease
- f. distance
- f. embolic glomerulonephritis
- f. fibrosis
- f. granulomatous inflammation
- f. hyperplasia
- f. hypertrophy

- f. infarct
- f. infection
- f. length
- f. lymphocytic thyroiditis
- f. necrosis
- f. nephritis
- f. plane
- f. pneumonia
- f. reaction
- f. sclerosing glomerulopathy
- f. segmental glomerulosclerosis
- f. ulcer
- f. zone

focus, pl. **foci**
- conjugate f.
- depth of f.
- disseminated foci (DF)
- ectopic f. (EF)
- Ghon f.
- low-voltage foci (LVF)
- natural f. of infection
- principal f.

focused grid

focusing
- isoelectric f.

foil
- air f.

Foix-Alajouanine myelitis

Foix syndrome

folate
- f. deficiency
- f. deficiency anemia
- red cell f. (RCF)
- f. reductase
- whole-blood f. (WBF)

fold
- giant gastric f.'s

folded
- f. cell
- f. nucleus

folded-cell index

folded-lung syndrome

foliaceous, foliacious

folic
- f. acid
- f. acid anemia
- f. acid assay
- f. acid receptor

Folin
- F. test
- F. and Wu method (FW)

Folin-Ciocalteu reagent

folinic acid

Folin-Looney test

follicle
- atretic f.
- f. cyst
- cystic ovarian f.

f. hormone
f. lysis (Fl)
nabothian f.
thyroid f.

follicle-stimulating
f.-s. hormone (FSH)
f.-s. hormone assay
f.-s. hormone-releasing
f.-s. hormone-releasing hormone (FSH-RH)
f.-s. principle

follicular
f. abscess
f. adenocarcinoma
f. adenoma
f. atresia
f. carcinoma
f. center f. (FCC)
f. center
f. cholecystitis
f. conjunctivitis
f. cyst
f. cystitis
f. dendritic cell (FDC)
f. dendritic cell sarcoma
f. dermatitis
f. goiter
f. hyperplasia (FH)
f. inflammation
f. inverted keratosis
f. lymphosarcoma (FLSA)
f. mucinosis
f. and papillary adenocarcinoma
f. pharyngitis
f. predominantly large cell lymphoma
f. predominantly small cleaved cell lymphoma
f. salpingitis
f. urethritis

follicularis keratosis
folliculitis
f. abscedens et suffodiens
f. barbae
f. decalvans
f. keloidalis
f. ulerythematosa reticulata

folliculoma
folliculorum
Simonea *f.*
folliculosis

Folling disease
fomes, pl. **fomites**
Fonio solution
Fonsecaea
F. *compactum*
F. *dermatitidis*
F. *jeanselmei*
F. *pedrosoi*
Fontana-Masson
F.-M. silver stain
F.-M. staining method
Fontana methenamine silver stain
food
f. ball
f. deprivation
f. fever
f. intolerance
f. poisoning
foot
athlete's f.
fungous f.
Hong Kong f.
Madura f.
Morand f.
mossy f.
f. process
F. reticulin impregnation stain
F. reticulin method
sandal f.
trench f.
foot-and-mouth
f.-a.-m. disease (FMD)
f.-a.-m. disease virus
f.-a.-m. disease virus vaccine
foramen ovale
anatomically patent f. o.
functionally patent f. o.
incompetent valve f. o.
patent f. o.
prematurely closed f. o.
probe patent f. o.
Foraminifera
foraminiferous
Forbes-Albright syndrome
Forbes disease
force (F)
centrifugal f.
centripetal f.
electromotive f. (EMF)
failure of all vital f.'s (FOAVF)
London f.

F

NOTES

force *(continued)*
    relative centrifugal f. (RCF)
    van der Waals f.'s
forced
    f. expiratory spirogram (FES)
    f. inspiratory oxygen (FI_{O2}, FIO_2)
forceps
Fordyce
    F. angiokeratoma
    F. disease
    F. granule
    F. spot
forehead
    olympian f.
foreign
    f. body (FB)
    f. body aspiration
    f. body embolus
    f. body giant cell
    f. body granuloma
    f. body reaction
    f. body salpingitis
    f. body tumorigenesis
    f. material deposition
    f. protein
    f. protein therapy
    f. serum
forensic
    f. medicine
    f. toxicology
forespore
Forestier disease
forest yaws
fork
    replication f.
form
    appliqué f.
    band f.
    f. birefringence
    cell wall-deficient bacterial f.'s
     (CWDF)
    involution f.
    replicative f.
    spore f.
Formad kidney
formaldehyde
    f. fixative
    f. solution
formaldehyde-induced fluorescence
  method
formalin
    alcoholic f.
    f. ammonium bromide
    B-5 sodium acetate-sublimate f.
    buffered neutral f.
    calcium acetate f.
    f. fixative
    phosphate buffered f.

    f. pigment
    f. solution
    zinc f.
formalin-ether sedimentation method
formalin-fixed tissue section
formalinize
format
formation
    ketone body f.
    localized plaque f. (LPF)
    mesencephalic reticular f. (MRF)
    rouleaux f.
    standard enthalpy of f.
formazan
forme
    f. fruste
    f. tardive
formic
    f. acid
    f. aldehyde
formication
formiminoglutamic
    f. acid (FIGLU)
    f. acid test (FIGLU)
formol ammonium bromide solution
formol-calcium fixative
formol-gel test
formol-Müller fixative
formol-saline fixative
formol-Zenker fixative
forms
    accolé f.
formula, pl. **formulas, formulae**
    Arneth f.
    Christison f.
    Häser f.
    Haworth f.
    Long f.
    Poisson-Pearson f.
    Ranke f.
    Reuss f.
    Runeberg f.
    f. translation (FORTRAN)
    Trapp f.
    Trapp-Häser f.
    Van Slyke f.
formulary
Forney syndrome
Forssman
    F. antibody
    F. antigen
    F. antigen-antibody reaction
Förster disease
FORTRAN
    formula translation
forward
    f. bias
    f. mutation

fosfomycin
Foshay test
fossula
Foster Kennedy syndrome
Fothergill disease
Fouchet
    F. reagent
    F. stain
    F. test
founder effect
Fourier analysis
four locus
Fournier
    F. disease
    F. gangrene
fourth
    f. venereal disease
fourth degree
    f. d. burn
    f. d. frostbite
    f. d. radiation injury
foveate
foveated chest
foveolar
    f. epithelium
    f. hyperplasia
Foville syndrome
fowl
    f. diphtheria
    f. erythroblastosis virus
    f. leukosis
    f. lymphomatosis
    f. lymphomatosis virus
    f. myeloblastosis virus
    f. neurolymphomatosis virus
    f. paralysis
    f. pest
    f. plague
    f. plague virus
Fowler solution
fowlpox
    f. virus
fox
    f. encephalitis
    f. encephalitis virus
Fox-Fordyce disease
FP
    false-positive
    freezing point
    frozen plasma
FPM
    filter paper microscopic

FPN reagent
FPP
    ferriprotoporphyrin
FR
    Fisher-Race (notation)
    flocculation reaction
    flow rate
fract
    fracture
fraction
    amorphous f. of adrenal cortex
    blood plasma f.
    branching f.
    extraction f. (E)
    growth f.
    heparin-precipitable f. (HPF)
    f. of inspired oxygen (FI_{O2}, FIO_2)
    mole f.
    plasma protein f. (PPF)
    saponifiable f.
fractional
    f. distillation
    f. sterilization
    f. uptake of carbon monoxide
    f. urinalysis
fractionated alkaline phosphatase
fractionation
fracture (fract)
    chip f.
    closed f.
    comminuted f.
    compound f.
    compound comminuted f. (CCF)
    compound multiple f.'s
    compressed f.
    depressed f.
    f. dislocation
    Frykman hand f.
    greenstick f.
    healed f.
    Hunt and Hess hand f.
    impacted f.
    incomplete f.
    Judet epiphyseal f.
    linear f.
    Neer shoulder f. I, II, III
    nonunion f.
    oblique f.
    pathologic f.
    Pauwel femoral neck f.
    simple f.
    spiral f.

F

NOTES

fracture *(continued)*
  stellate f.
  transverse f.
  ununited f.
frag
  fragility
fragile X syndrome
fragilis
  Dientamoeba f.
fragilitas
  f. ossium
  f. sanguinis
fragility (frag)
  f. of the blood
  capillary f.
  erythrocyte f.
  mechanical f.
  osmotic f.
  red cell f.
  f. test
fragillograph
fragilocyte
fragilocytosis
fragment
  Fab f.
  Fc f.
  Klenow f.
  P-radiolabeled DNA probe f.
  retained placental f.
  f. Y
fragmentation
  f. myocarditis
  f. of the myocardium
fragmentography
  mass f.
Fraley syndrome
frambesia
frame
  main f.
  reading f.
  f. shift mutation
frame-shift mutagen
Franceschetti-Jadassohn syndrome
Franceschetti syndrome
Francis
  F. disease
  F. skin test
Francisella
  F. (Pasteurella) tularensis
  F. tularensis
francium
François syndrome
Frankl-Hochwart disease
franklin
Franklin disease
Frank-Starling mechanism
Fraser-Lendrum stain for fibrin
Fraser syndrome

fraternal twins
FRC
  frozen red cell
freckle
  Hutchinson melanotic f.
  melanotic f.
Fredrickson dyslipoproteinemia classification
free
  f. acid (FA)
  f. catecholamine fractionation
  f. electron
  f. energy
  f. erythrocyte coproporphyria (FECP)
  f. erythrocyte coproporphyrin (FEC)
  f. erythrocyte protoporphyrin (FEP, FEPP)
  f. estriol
  fat f. (FF)
  f. fatty acids (FFA)
  f. radical
  f. T_4
  f. T_3
  f. thyroxine index (FTI)
  f. toxicology
  f. T_4 ratio
  f. triiodothyronine index (FT_3I)
  f. (unbound) thyroxine (FT_4)
  f. water clearance
freedom
  degrees of f. (df)
Freeman-Sheldon syndrome
freeze-clamp
freeze-cleave method
freeze-drying
freeze-etch method
freeze-fracture-etch method
Freezer
  Gentle Jane Snap F.
freeze-substitution
freezing
  f. injury
  f. microtome
  f. point (FP)
  f. point depression osmometer
Frei
  F. disease
  F. test
Freiberg disease
Frei-Hoffmann reaction
French-American-British (FAB)
French proof agar
Frenkel anterior ocular traumatic syndrome
frenulum
  f. linguae

frequency
    angular f.
    f. counter
    crossover f.
    cutoff f.
    discharge f.
    f. distribution
    gene f.
    high f. (HF)
    mean dominant f. (MDF)
    medium f. (MF)
    f. polygon
    recombination f.
    very high f.
Frerichs theory
fresh frozen plasma (FFP)
Fresnel fringe
Freund
    F. anomaly
    F. complete adjuvant
    F. incomplete adjuvant
Frey syndrome
friable
friction
Friderichsen-Waterhouse syndrome
Friedewald equation
Friedländer
    F. bacillus
    F. disease
    F. pneumobacillus
    F. pneumonia
    F. stain for capsules
Friedmann
    F. disease
    F. vasomotor syndrome
Friedman test
Friedreich disease
Friend
    F. disease
    F. leukemia virus
frigidity
frigorism
fringe
    Fresnel f.
frog test
Fröhlich
    F. dwarfism
    F. syndrome
Frohn reagent
Froin syndrome
Frommel-Chiari syndrome
Frommel disease

front-end processor
Froriep induration
frost
frostbite
    second degree f.
    third degree f.
frosted
    f. heart
    f. liver
frozen
    f. blood
    f. pelvis
    f. plasma (FP)
    f. red blood cells
    f. red cell (FRC)
    f. section (FZ)
    f. section method
fructofuranose
fructokinase
fructopyranose
fructosamine
fructose
    f. assay
    f. bisphosphate
    f. diphosphate
    f. intolerance
    f. test
fructose-bisphosphate aldolase
fructosemia
fructosuria
    essential f.
fructosyl
fruit fly
fruiting body
Frykman hand fracture
FSF
    fibrin-stabilization factor
    fibrin-stabilizing factor
FSH
    follicle-stimulating hormone
        FSH assay
FSH-RH
    follicle-stimulating hormone-releasing
      hormone
        FSH-RH assay
FSP
    fibrinogen split product
    fibrinolytic split product
FSR
    fusiform skin revision
FT
    fibrous tissue

F

NOTES

FT₄
    free (unbound) thyroxine
FT₃
    free triiodothyroxine
FTA
    fluorescent treponemal antibody
FTA-ABS, FTA-AB
    fluorescent treponemal antibody-
      absorption
        FTA-ABS test
FTI
    free thyroxine index
FT₃I
    free triiodothyronine index
FT₄index
FT₃index
FU
    fecal urobilinogen
FU-48 Zenker fixative solution
Fuchs
        F. adenoma
        F. syndrome
fuchsin
        acid f.
        aldehyde f. (AF)
        f., amido black, and naphthol
          yellow (FAN)
        aniline f.
        basic f.
        f. body
        diamond f.
        new f.
        f. stain
fuchsinophil
        f. cell
        f. granule
        f. reaction
fuchsinophilia
fuchsinophilic
L-fucose
fucosidosis
FUDR
    fluorodeoxyuridine
fugacity
fugitive swelling
Fuhrman system
Fujiwara reaction
full
        f. blood examination (FBE)
        f. scale
full-thickness burn
full-wave rectifier
full-width half-maximum
fulminant
        f. dysentery
        f. hepatic failure (FHF)

fulminating
        f. anoxia
        f. smallpox
fumagillin
fumarase
fumarate hydratase
fumaric acid
fume hood
fumigation
functio laesa
function
        autocorrelation f.
        Boolean f.
        continuous f.
        density f.
        detector transfer f. (DTF)
        discriminant f.
        distribution f.
        exponential f.
        line-spread f.
        modulation transfer f.
        split renal f. (SRF)
        step f.
        transfer f.
functional
        f. aerobic impairment
        f. albuminuria
        f. bleeding
        f. death
        f. disease
        f. disorder
        f. group
        f. group isomerism
        f. hypertrophy
        f. pathology
functionally patent foramen ovale
fundic mucosa
fungal
        f. antibody screen
        f. pericarditis
        f. pneumonia
        f. spore
        f. stain
Fungalase-F stain
fungate
fungating sore
fungemia
fungi (*pl. of* fungus)
fungicidal
fungicide
fungiform
fungistatic
fungitoxic
fungitoxicity
Fungizone
fungoid
fungoides
        mycosis f. (MF)

fungoma
fungosity
fungous
    f. foot
fungus, pl. **fungi**
    ascospore-forming f.
    f. ball
    f. cerebri
    f. culture
    cutaneous f.
    dematiaceous fungi
    dimorphic pathogenic fungi
    fission f.
    imperfect f.
    Fungi Imperfecti
    mosaic f.
    mycelial f.
    perfect f.
    fungi smear
    fungi staining
    thrush f.
    yeast f.
funicular
    f. myelitis
    f. myelosis
funiculitis
    endemic f.
    filarial f.
funnel
    f. breast
    f. chest
    separatory f.
FUO
    fever of undetermined origin
    fever of unknown origin
furan
furanose
furanoside
furazolidone
furcal
furcate
furfural reagent
furfurol reaction
Furstner disease
Furst-Ostrum syndrome
furuncle
furunculoid
furunculosis
fusariomycosis
Fusarium
    F. moniliforme

    F. oxysporum
    F. solanae
fuse alarm
fuseau
fused kidney
fusible calculus
fusiform
    f. aneurysm
    f. bacillus
    f. bronchiectasis
    f. cell
    f. skin revision (FSR)
Fusiformis
    F. necrophorus
fusion
    cell f.
    centric f.
    critical flicker f. (CFF)
    protoplast f.
    splenogonadal f.
    whole-arm f.
Fusobacterium
    F. aquatile
    F. fusiforme
    F. glutinosum
    F. gonidiaformans
    F. mortiferum
    F. naviforme
    F. necrophorum
    F. nucleatum
    F. plauti-vincentii
    F. prausnitzii
    F. symbiosum
    F. varium
fusocellular
fusospirillary
fusospirillosis
fusospirochetal
fusospirochetosis
fusostreptococcicosis
fustic
fuzzy coat
FV
    fluid volume
FW
    Felix-Weil
    Folin and Wu method
FWR
    Felix-Weil reaction
Fy antigen
FZ
    frozen section

F

NOTES

γ (*var. of* gamma)
    γ hemolysis
    γ metachromasia
    γ ray
    γ staphylolysin

G
  gauss
  giga
  gonidial (colony)
    G antigen
    G factor
    G syndrome
    G unit of streptomycin

g
  gram
    g factor

G₀ phase

G_0 phase

G_1 phase

G_2 phase

GA
  gastric analysis
  gestational age
  gut-associated

GABA
  γ-aminobutyric acid
  gamma-aminobutyric acid

GAD
  glutamic acid decarboxylase

Gaddum and Schild test

gadfly

gadolinium

Gadus

Gaffky
    G. scale
    G. table

Gaffkya
    G. *tetragena*

gag
    g. reflex

gage

Gailliard syndrome

gain
  antigen g.
  current g.

Gairdner disease

Gaisböck
    G. disease
    G. syndrome

galactan

galactic

galactitol

galactoblast

galactocele

galactocerebroside β-galactosidase

galactokinase
    g. deficiency

galactolipid

galactolipin

galactophoritis

galactopoietic hormone

galactorrhea

galactosamine

galactose
    g. assay
    g. breath test
    g. tolerance test

galactosemia

galactose-1-phosphate

galactosidase
    beta g.

β-galactosidase
    cerebroside β-g.
    galactocerebroside β-g.

galactoside

galactosuria

galactosylceramidase

galactosylhydrolase
    beta g.

β-galactosylhydrolase

galacturia

gall

gallbladder
    g. hydrops
    sandpaper g.
    strawberry g.

Gall body

Gallego differentiating solution

gallein

gallinacea
    Echidnophaga g.

gallinae
    Dermanyssus g.

gallinatum
    pectus g.

gallium
    g. citrate
    g. scan

gallium-67

gallocyanin, gallocyanine

gallop
    atrial g. (AG)

gallstone
    g. ileus

gallus adeno-like virus

Gallyas method

galoche chin

GALT
  gut-associated lymphoid tissue

G

GaLV
　　gibbon ape lymphosarcoma virus
galvanic
　　g. cell
　　g. skin response (GSR)
galvanism
galvanometer
GAL virus
Gambian trypanosomiasis
gametangium
gamete
gametic chromosome
gametocide
gametocyst
gametocyte
gametocytemia
gametogenesis
gametogonia
gametogony
gametoid
　　g. theory
gametokinetic
gametophagia
gamma, γ (Gm)
　　g. camera
　　g. cell
　　g. chain disease
　　g. fetoprotein
　　g. globulin (GG)
　　g. heavy-chain disease
　　g. hemolysis
　　g. metachromasia
　　g. ray
　　g. spectrometer
　　g. spectrometry
　　g. staphylolysin
　　g. streptococcus
gamma-aminobutyric acid (GABA)
gammaglobulin
　　human g. (hGG)
gammaglobulinopathy
gamma glutamyl transferase
gammaphoto
gamma-ray spectrum
gamma-well counter
gammopathy
　　benign monoclonal g. (BMG)
　　biclonal g.
　　monoclonal g.
　　polyclonal g.
Gamna disease
Gamna-Favre body
Gamna-Gandy nodule
gamogony
gamont
gamophagia
Gamstorp syndrome

Gandy-Gamna
　　G.-G. body
Gandy-Nanta disease
ganglia (*pl. of* ganglion)
gangliitis
gangliocytoma
ganglioglioma
　　desmoplastic infantile g.
gangliolysis
　　percutaneous radiofrequency g.
ganglioma
ganglion, pl. ganglia, ganglions
　　aberrant g.
　　Acrel g.
　　g. cell (GC)
　　g. cyst
　　diffuse g.
　　nodose g.
　　periosteal g.
　　Troisier g.
ganglioneuroblastoma (GNBL)
ganglioneuroma (GN)
　　central g.
　　dumbbell g.
ganglioneuromatosis
ganglionic blocking agent (GBA)
ganglionitis
ganglionopathy
ganglions (*pl. of* ganglion)
ganglioside
　　g. GM_1
　　g. GM_2
gangliosidosis
　　generalized g.
　　GM_1g.
　　GM_2g.
gangosa
gangrene
　　arteriosclerotic g.
　　cold g.
　　diabetic g.
　　dry g.
　　embolic g.
　　emphysematous g.
　　Fournier g.
　　gas g.
　　hemorrhagic g.
　　hot g.
　　Meleney g.
　　moist g.
　　presenile spontaneous g.
　　progressive bacterial synergistic g.
　　static g.
　　symmetrical g.
　　thrombotic g.
　　trophic g.
　　venous g.

wet g.
white g.
gangrenous
g. appendicitis
g. emphysema
g. granulomatous inflammation
g. necrosis
g. pharyngitis
g. pneumonia
g. stomatitis
gannister disease
Ganser syndrome
gap
anion g.
auscultatory g.
chromatid g.
isochromatid g.
g. junction
osmolar g.
GAPD, GAPDH
glyceraldehyde phosphate dehydrogenase
gapes
gapeworm
Gardner-Diamond syndrome
Gardnerella
G. vaginalis
Gardner syndrome
gargantuan mastitis
gargoylism type of histiocyte
Garré
G. disease
G. sclerosing osteomyelitis
Gartner
G. cyst
Gärtner bacillus
gas
g. abscess
g. amplification
arterial blood g. (ABG)
blood g.
BTPS conditions of g.
carrier g.
g. chromatograph
g. chromatography (GC)
g. chromatography-mass
spectrometry (GC-MS)
combustible g.
g. constant
g. cyst
g. embolism
extravasation g.
g. gangrene

g. gangrene antitoxin
hemolytic g.
hepatic portal venous g. (HPVG)
ideal g.
g. law
g.-liquid chromatography (GLC)
mustard g.
oxidizing g.
g. peritonitis
g. phlegmon
g. retention
g.-solid chromatography (GSC)
g. sterilizer
g. storage limit
STPD conditions of g.
g. thermometer
water g.
gaseous
gas-liquid chromatography (GLC)
gasoline
gasometry
gasping disease
Gasser syndrome
gas-solid chromatography (GSC)
Gasteromycetes
Gasterophilidae
Gasterophilus
gastradenitis
gastrectasia
gastrectasis
gastric
g. algid malaria
g. analysis (GA)
g. argentaffin cell
g. aspirate cell count
g. atrophy
g. calculus
g. emptying halftime (GET1/2)
g. emptying time (GET)
g. fistula
g. fluid (GF)
g. function test
g. inhibitory polypeptide (GIP)
g. lavage
g. myiasis
g. parietal cell (GPC)
g. parietography
g. polyp
g. residue examination
g. smear
g. ulcer (GU)

G

NOTES

gastric *(continued)*
    g. volvulus
    g. zymogenic cell
gastrin
    g. assay
gastrin-calcium infusion stimulation test
gastrinoma
gastrin-protein stimulation test
gastrin-secretin stimulation test
gastritis
    acute g.
    antral g.
    atrophic chronic g.
    catarrhal g.
    chronic atrophic g. (CAG)
    chronic hypertrophic g.
    g. cystica polyposa
    erosive g.
    exfoliative g.
    g. fibroplastica
    giant hypertrophic g.
    hemorrhagic g.
    hypertrophic g.
    interstitial g.
    phlegmonous g.
    polypous g.
    pseudomembranous g.
    sclerotic g.
gastroadenitis
Gastroccult test
gastrocele
gastrocolic fistula
gastrocolitis
gastrocoloptosis
gastrocolostomy
gastrocutaneous fistula
gastrodisciasis
Gastrodiscoides hominis
Gastrodiscus hominis
gastroduodenal fistula
gastroduodenitis
gastroduodenostomy
gastroenteritis
    acute infectious nonbacterial g.
    endemic nonbacterial infantile g.
    eosinophilic g. (EGE)
    epidemic nonbacterial g.
    infantile g.
    porcine transmissible g.
    transmissible g. (TGE)
    transmissible g. of swine
    viral g.
    g. virus type A
    g. virus type B
gastroenterocolitis
gastroenterocolostomy
gastroenteroptosis
gastroesophageal reflux disease (GERD)

gastroesophagitis
gastroileitis
gastrointestinal (GI)
    g. adsorbent
    g. autonomic nerve tumor
    g. blood loss test
    g. contents
    g. disease
    g. fistula
    g. hormone
    g. protein loss test
    g. series (GI series)
    g. stromal tumor (GIST)
    g. tuberculosis
gastrolith
gastrolithiasis
gastromalacia
gastromegaly
gastropathy
    hypertrophic hypersecretory g.
gastropexy
Gastrophilidae
Gastrophilus
gastropod
Gastropoda
gastroptosia
gastroptosis
gastrorrhagia
gastrorrhexis
gastroschisis
gastrosia
    g. fungosa
gastrostaxis
gastrostenosis
gastrotoxin
gate
    AND g.
    OR g.
gating
Gaucher
    G. cell
    G. disease
    G. type of histiocyte
gauge
    vacuum g.
gauss (G)
gaussian distribution
Gay-Lussac law
gay lymph node syndrome
gay-related immunodeficiency disease
GB
    Guillain-Barré syndrome
GBA
    ganglionic blocking agent
G-banding
    G.-b. stain
GBIA
    Guthrie bacterial inhibition assay

GBM
glomerular basement membrane
GC
ganglion cell
gas chromatography
gonococcus
gonorrhea culture
granular cast
guanine cytosine
GC value
g-cal
gram-calorie
GCF
giant cell fibroblastoma
GCH
giant cell hepatitis
GCIS
isolated gland carcinoma in situ
g-cm
gram-centimeter
GC-MS
gas chromatography-mass spectrometry
G-CSF
granulocyte colony-stimulating factor
GCT
germ cell tumor
granulosa cell tumor
GCTTS
giant cell tumor of tendon sheath
GDP
guanosine 5′-diphosphate
GDP-L-fucose
GDP-D-mannose
G/E
granulocyte-erythroid ratio
Ge antigen
Gedoelstia
gedoelstiosis
Gee disease
Gee-Herter disease
Gee-Herter-Heubner disease
Gee-Thaysen disease
Gehrig
Geiger-Müller counter
gel
aluminum hydroxide g.
denaturing g.'s
g. diffusion
g. diffusion precipitin test
g. diffusion precipitin test in one
dimension

g. diffusion precipitin test in two
dimensions
g. diffusion reaction
g. electrophoresis pattern
g. filtration
g.-filtration chromatography
hydrophilic g.
hydrophobic g.
polyacrylamide g.
silica g.
gelatin
Arlex g.
g. film
g. filter
g. slide adhesive
gelatinous
g. acute inflammation
g. acute pneumonia
g. adenocarcinoma
g. ascites
g. atrophy
g. carcinoma
g. infiltration
g. inflammation
g. polyp
gelation
gel-filtration chromatography
Gélineau syndrome
Gell
G. and Coombs classification
G. and Coombs reaction
Gelman filter
gelosis
gel-permeation chromatography
gem-**diol**
geminal
geminate
gemistocyte
gemistocytic
g. astrocyte
g. astrocytoma
g. cell
g. tumor
gemistocytoma
gemma
gemmation
gemmule
Hoboken g.
genavense
Mycobacterium g.

G

NOTES

265

Gendre
    G. fixative
    G. fluid
gene
    allelic g.
    g. amplification
    c-Ki-*ras* g.
    g. cloning
    complementary g.
    cyclin D1 g.
    g. deletions
    derepressed g.
    dominant g.
    g. dosage
    g. flow
    g. frequency
    H g.
    HER-2 g.
    HER-2/neu g.
    histocompatibility g.
    holandric g.
    holgynic g.
    immune response g.
    Ir g.
    Is g.
    jumping g.
    g. library
    major g.
    g. mapping
    mobile g.
    modifying g.
    mutant g.
    MyoD1 regulatory g.
    nonstructural g.
    operator g.
    p53 g.
    g. pool
    g. product
    g. rearrangement
    recessive g.
    regulator g.
    regulatory g.
    repressor g.
    secretor g.
    sex-linked g.
    g. splicing
    split g.
    structural g.
    supplementary g.
    suppressor g.
    transfer g.
    transforming g.
    tumor suppressor g.
    wild-type g.
    X-linked g.
gene-arrangement study
genera (*pl. of* genus)

general
    g. gonadotropic activity (GGA)
    g. immunity
    g. paresis (GP)
    g. pathology
    g. peritonitis
    g. radiation
    g. transduction
    g. tuberculosis
generalized
    g. anaphylaxis
    g. chondromalacia
    g. cortical hyperostosis
    g. emphysema
    g. eruptive histiocytoma
    g. gangliosidosis
    g. pustular psoriasis of Zambusch
    g. Sanarelli-Shwartzman reaction (GSSR)
    g. Shwartzman phenomenon
    g. Shwartzman reaction (GSR)
    g. transduction
    g. vaccinia
    g. xanthelasma
generation
    alternation of g.'s
    first filial g. (F_1)
    parental g. (P_1)
    second filial g. (F_2)
    spontaneous g.
    g. time
generative
generator
    aerosol g.
    diazomethane g.
    random number g.
generic name
genesistasis
genestatic
genetic
    g. abnormality
    g. abnormality analysis
    g. adaptation
    g. anemia
    g. balance
    g. code
    g. counseling
    g. determinant
    g. drift
    g. engineering
    g. etiology
    g. fingerprint
    g. linkage analysis
    g. map
    g. mapping
    g. marker
    g. recombination
    g. regulation

g. screening
g. susceptibility
genetically significant dose (GSD)
genetics
    bacterial g.
    bacteriophage g.
    behavior g.
    biochemical g.
    clinical g.
    immunogenetics
    mathematical g.
    medical g.
    mendelian g.
    microbial g.
    molecular g.
    phage g.
    population g.
    reverse g.
    somatic cell g.
Gengou phenomenon
genic balance
genicula (*pl. of* geniculum)
geniculocalcarine tract
geniculotemporal tract
geniculum, pl. **genicula**
genioglossus muscle
geniohyoid
genital
    g. condyloma
    g. culture
    g. disorder
    g. mycoplasma
    g. tubercle
    g. wart
genitalia
    ambiguous external g.
genitourinary
    g. fistula
    g. myiasis
genoblast
genocopy
genome
genomic
    g. DNA clone (chromosomal)
genospecies
genote
    F g.
genotype
genotypic blot hybridization
Gensoul disease
gentamicin

gentian
    g. aniline water
    g. orange stain
    g. violet (GV)
    g. violet stain
gentianophil, gentianophile
gentianophilous
gentianophobic
gentiobiase
Gentle Jane Snap Freezer
genu, pl. **genua**
    g. recurvatum
    g. valgum
    g. varum
genus, pl. **genera**
Geodermatophilus
geographic
    g. pathology
    g. tongue
geometric
    G. Data Miniprep slide maker
    g. efficiency
    g. isomerism
    g. optics
geophilic
Geophilus
geotrichosis
geotrichum
    G. candidum
    Endomyces g.
    G. immite
geotropism
Geraghty test
geranyl geranyl diphosphate
Gerbode defect
GERD
    gastroesophageal reflux disease
Gerhardt
    G. disease
    G. reaction
    G. syndrome
    G. test for acetoacetic acid
    G. test for urobilin in the urine
Gerlier disease
germ
    g. cell
    g. cell tumor (GCT)
    g. layer
    g. theory
    g. tube
    g. tube test

G

NOTES

German
G. measles
G. measles virus
germanium
germ-free (GF)
germicidal
germicide
germinal
g. aplasia
g. center
g. center of lymph node
g. epithelial inclusion cyst
g. vesicle
germinoblast
germinoma
pineal g.
Germiston virus
germline configuration
geroderma
g. osteodysplastica
geromarasmus
gerontine
Gerstmann syndrome
gestagen
gestational
g. age (GA)
g. alteration
g. proteinuria
g. trophoblastic disease (GTD)
gestosis
GET
gastric emptying time
GET1/2
gastric emptying halftime
GF
gastric fluid
germ-free
gluten-free
G factor
GFAP
glial fibrillary acidic protein
GFR
glomerular filtration rate
GG
gamma globulin
GGA
general gonadotropic activity
GGT
glutamyltransferase
GGT assay
GH
growth hormone
GHD
growth hormone deficiency
Ghon
G. complex
G. focus

G. primary lesion
G. tubercle
Ghon-Sachs bacillus
ghost
blood g.
g. cell
g. corpuscle
ghoul hand
GH-RF
growth hormone-releasing factor
GH-RH
growth hormone-releasing hormone
GH-RIH
growth hormone-release-inhibiting
hormone
GHz
gigahertz
GI
gastrointestinal
globin insulin
Gianotti-Crosti syndrome
giant
g. baby
g. blue nevus
g. cell
g. cell aortitis
g. cell arteritis
g. cell carcinoma
g. cell carcinoma of thyroid gland
g. cell fibroblastoma (GCF)
g. cell fibroma
g. cell hepatitis (GCH)
g. cell interstitial pneumonia (GIP)
g. cell monstrocellular sarcoma of
Zülch
g. cell myeloma
g. cell myocarditis
g. cell pneumonia
g. cell reaction
g. cell reparative granuloma
g. cell sarcoma
g. cell thyroiditis
g. cell tumor
g. cell tumor of bone
g. cell tumor of lung
g. cell tumor of tendon sheath
(GCTTS)
g. colon
g. condyloma
g. condyloma of Buschke-
Löwenstein
g. fibroadenoma
g. follicle lymphoma
g. follicular lymphoblastoma
g. follicular lymphoma
g. gastric folds
g. hairy nevus
g. hives

g. hypertrophic gastritis
g. hypertrophy of gastric mucosa
g. intestinal fluke
g. intracanalicular fibro-adenoma
g. liver fluke
g. melanosome
g. neutrophil
g. neutrophilia
g. osteoid osteoma
g. pigmented nevus
g. platelet disease
g. platelets
g. rugal hypertrophy
g. urticaria

giantism

Giardia

G. *intestinalis*
G. *lamblia*

giardiasis

g. dysentery

gibbon ape lymphosarcoma virus (GaLV)

Gibney disease

Gibson-Cooke sweat test

Giemsa chromosome banding stain

Gierke disease

giga (G)

g. electron volt

gigahertz (GHz)

gigantism

exophthalmos, macroglossia, g. (EMG)

gigantocellular glioma

gigantomastia

Gigantorhynchus

gigohm

GIK

glucose, insulin, and potassium

Gilbert

G. disease
G. syndrome

gilbert (unit of magnetomotive force) (F)

Gilchrist

G. disease
G. mycosis

Gilles de la Tourette syndrome

Gill #2 hematoxylin blue stain

GIM

gonadotropin-inhibitory material

Gimenez stain

gingival

g. hyperplasia

gingivitis

diphenylhydantoin g.
hypertrophic g.
necrotizing ulcerative g. (NUG)
scorbutic g.

gingivosis

gingivostomatitis

herpetic g.
necrotizing ulcerative g.

GIP

gastric inhibitory polypeptide
giant cell interstitial pneumonia

Girard reagent

GI series

gastrointestinal series

GIST

gastrointestinal stromal tumor

gitalin

gitaloxin

gitoxin

GITT

glucose insulin tolerance test

gitter cell

gitterzelle

GL

greatest length

glabrosa

glabrous

g. skin

glacial

g. acetic acid
g. acetic acid fixative

gland

acinic cell tumor of salivary g.
adrenal g.
Bartholin, urethral, Skene g.'s (BUS)
Brunner g.
jugular g.
Philip g.
sentinel g.

glanders bacillus

glandular

g. cancer
g. carcinoma
g. epithelium
g. fever
g. hyperplasia
g. mastitis

NOTES

G

glandular *(continued)*
  g. metaplasia
  g. pharyngitis
glandularis
  g. proliferans cholecystitis
  pyelitis g.
  ureteritis g.
Glanzmann
  G. disease
  G. thrombasthenia
Glanzmann-Naegeli thrombasthenia
Glanzmann-Riniker syndrome
glass
  g. body
  cover g.
  g. electrode
  g. factor
  g. fiber filter
  flint g.
  ground g.
  heat-resistant g.
  low-actinic g.
  optical g.
  Wood g.
glass-bead retention method
glass-ceramic
glasses
  safety g.
glassy
  g. cell carcinoma
  g. membrane
glaucoma
  angle closure g.
  congenital g.
  infantile g.
  open angle g.
  primary g.
  secondary g.
glaucosuria
GLC
  gas-liquid chromatography
Gleason
  G. score
  G. tumor grade
Glénard disease
Glenner-Lillie stain for pituitary
glia
gliadin
glial fibrillary acidic protein (GFAP)
glioblast
glioblastoma
  g. cell line
  g. multiforme
glioma
  brainstem g.
  gigantocellular g.
  lipidized g.
  malignant g.

mixed g.
nasal g.
g. of optic chiasm
optic nerve g.
g. of the spinal cord
subependymal g.
telangiectatic g.
gliomatosis
  g. cerebri
gliomatous
gliomyxoma
glioneuroma
gliosarcoma
gliosis
  isomorphous g.
  g. uteri
gliotoxin
Glisson
  G. cirrhosis
  G. disease
glissonitis
glitter cell
glob.
  globulin
globe cell anemia
globi (*pl. of* globus)
Globidium
globin insulin (GI)
Globocephalus
globoid
  g. cell
  g. leukodystrophy
globose
globoside
globular
  g. leukocyte
  g. protein
  g. sputum
  g. thrombus
  g. value
globular-fibrous transformation
globule
  hyaline g.
globuliferous
  g. phagocyte
globulin (glob.)
  α_1 g.'s
  α_2 g.'s
  α_1-g.
  α_2-g.
  accelerator g. (AcG, ac-g)
  alpha g.'s
  alpha-1 g.
  alpha-2 g.
  α-g. antibody
  antidiphtheritic g.
  antihemophilic g. (AHG)
  antihemophilic g. A

antihemophilic g. B
antihuman g. (AHG)
antilymphocyte g. (ALG)
antilymphocytic g.
antimacrophage g. (AMG)
beta-1F g.
beta-1E g.
beta-1A g.
beta-1C g.
β_{1A}-g.
β_{1C}-g.
β_{1E}-g.
β_{1F}-g.
β-g.
beta g.
bovine gamma g. (BGG)
chickenpox immune g. (human)
corticosteroid-binding g. (CBG)
cortisol-binding g. (CBG)
equine antihuman lymphoblast g. (EAHLG)
gamma g. (GG)
hepatitis B immune g. (HBIG)
horse antihuman thymus g. (HAHTG)
human gamma g.
human rabies immune g. (HRIG)
immune g. (IG)
immune serum g. (ISG)
measles immune g. (human)
pertussis immune g.
plasma accelerator g.
poliomyelitis immune g. (human)
rabies immune g.
$Rh_o(D)$ immune g.
serum g. (SG)
serum accelerator g.
specific immune g. (human)
testosterone-estradiol-binding g. (TeBG)
tetanus immune g.
thyroxine-binding g. (TBG)
unbound thyroxine-binding g. (UTBG)
vaccinia-immune g. (VIG)
g. X
zoster immune g. (ZIG)
globulinuria
globulomaxillary cyst
globus, pl. **globi**
glomangioma

glomangiomatous osseous malformation syndrome
glomangiosis
pulmonary g.
glomera
g. aortica
glomerular
g. basal lamina
g. basement membrane (GBM)
g. basement membrane antibody
g. basement membrane disease
g. crescent
g. cyst
g. filtration
g. filtration rate (GFR)
g. nephritis
g. sclerosis
glomerulitis
glomerulocystic disease
glomerulonephritis (GN)
acute g. (AGN)
acute crescentic g.
acute exudative g.
acute hemorrhagic g.
acute post-streptococcal g.
anti-basement membrane g.
Berger focal g.
chronic g. (CG, CGN)
chronic membranous g. (CMGN)
diffuse g.
Ellis type 1, 2 g.
embolic g.
exudative g.
focal embolic g.
healed g.
hemorrhagic g.
hypocomplementemic g.
idiopathic pauci-immune necrotizing crescentic g.
immune complex g.
induced g.
lobular g.
local g.
membranoproliferative g. (MPGN)
membranous g. (MGN)
membranous-proliferative g.
mesangial proliferative g.
mesangiocapillary g.
mesangioproliferative g.
necrotizing g.
postinfectious g.
poststreptococcal g. (PSGN)

G

NOTES

glomerulonephritis *(continued)*
> proliferative g.
> rapidly progressive g. (RPGN)
> segmental g.
> subacute g.

glomerulopathy
> crescentic g.
> focal sclerosing g.
> immune complex g.
> proliferative g.

glomerulosclerosis
> cirrhotic g.
> diabetic g.
> focal segmental g.
> intercapillary g.
> nodular g.

glomus
> g. coccygeum
> g. jugulare tumor

Glossina

glossitis
> atrophic g.
> Hunter g.
> median rhomboid g.

glottis, pl. **glottides**

glow modulator tube

Glu
> glutamic acid

glucagon
> gut g.
> immunoreactive g. (IRG)
> g. test

glucagonoma

glucan
> g. branching enzyme
> g. branching glycosyltransferase

1,4-α-glucan branching enzyme

α-glucan-branching glycosyltransferase

glucemia

glucitol

glucocerebrosidase

glucocerebroside

glucocorticoid therapy

glucocorticosteroid

glucofuranose

glucogenesis

glucogenic amino acid

glucohemia

glucokinase

gluconeogenesis

gluconeogenetic

glucopenia

glucopyranose

glucosamine

glucose
> g. assay
> blood g. (BG)
> buffered desoxycholate g. (BDG)

> cerebral metabolic rate of g. (CMRG)
> g. insulin tolerance test (GITT)
> maximal tubular reabsorption of g. (T_{mg})
> g. metabolism
> g. nitrogen ratio (GN)
> g. oxidase
> g. oxidase method
> g. oxidase paper strip test
> g. 6-phosphatase hepatorenal deficiency glycogenosis
> renal threshold for g.
> g. tolerance (GT)
> g. tolerance test (GTT)

glucose-format broth

glucose, insulin, and potassium (GIK)

glucose-6-phosphatase

glucosephosphate
> g. isomerase
> g. isomerase assay
> g. isomerase deficiency

glucose-1-phosphate

glucose-6-phosphate
> g.-p. dehydrogenase (G-6-PD)
> g.-p. dehydrogenase deficiency
> g.-p. dehydrogenase deficiency anemia
> g.-p. dehydrogenase screen
> g.-p. dehydrogenase test

glucosidase
> beta g.

β-glucosidase
> cerebroside β-g.

glucoside

glucosuria

glucosyl

glucosylceramidase assay

glucuronate

glucuronic acid

glucuronide

glucuronosyltransferase
> UDP-bilirubin g.

glucuronyl-transferase

Gluge corpuscle

glutamate
> arginine g.
> g. decarboxylase
> g. dehydrogenase
> monosodium g.
> g. semialdehyde

glutamate-pyruvate transaminase

glutamic
> g. acid (Glu)
> g. acid decarboxylase (GAD)

glutamic-oxaloacetic transaminase

glutaminase

glutamine

glutaminyl
glutaminyl-peptide gamma glutamyltransferase
glutaminyl-peptide-γ-glutamyltransferase
glutamyl
    g. transfer cycle
    g. transpeptidase
glutamyltransferase (GGT)
glutaral
glutaraldehyde
    g. fixative
glutaric acid
glutathione
    g. peroxidase
    reduced g. (GSH)
    g. reductase
    g. reductase assay
    g. reductase deficiency
    g. stability test
    g. synthetase
    g. synthetase deficiency
glutathionemia
glutathionuria
gluten
gluten-free (GF)
glutenin
gluten-sensitive enteropathy (GSE)
glutethimide
    g. assay
glutin
glutinous
glutitis
Gly
glycan
glycemia
glyceraldehyde phosphate dehydrogenase (GAPD, GAPDH)
glyceride
glycerin
    g. broth
    g. method
glycerinated lymph
glycerin-potato broth
glycerol
    g. gelatin medium
glycerolization
glycerolize
glycerophosphate
glycerophosphatide
glyceryl
    g. triacetate
glycine-arginine reaction

glycine assay
glycinemia
glycine-rich
    g.-r. β-glycoprotein
    g.-r. β-glycoproteinase
glycinuria
Glyciphagus
    G. buski
    G. domesticus
glycocalyx
glycochenodeoxycholate
glycochenodeoxycholic acid
glycocholate
glycocholic acid
glycodeoxycholic acid
glycogen
    g. acanthosis
    accumulation of g.
    g. branching enzyme
    cytoplasmic g.
    g. digestion
    hepatic g.
    g. infiltration
    g. phosphorylase
    g. stain
    g. staining
    g. (starch) synthase
    g. storage disease
    g. storage test
    g. synthesis
    tissue g.
glycogenesis
glycogenic acanthosis
glycogenolysis
glycogenolytic
glycogenosis, pl. glycogenosis
    glucose 6-phosphatase hepatorenal deficiency g.
    hepatophosphorylase deficiency g.
    hepatorenal g.
    idiopathic generalized g.
    myophosphorylase deficiency g.
glycogen-rich squamous cell carcinoma
glycoglycinuria
glycol
    ethylene g.
    g. methacrylate
    polyethylene g.
glycolic
    g. acid test
    g. aciduria
glycolic aciduria

G

NOTES

glycolipid
- g. lipidosis
- g. stain
- g. staining

glycolithocholic acid
glycolysis
glycolytic enzyme
glycone
glyconeogenesis
glycopenia
glycopeptide
Glycophagus
glycophorin
glycoprotein
- acid g.
- α-acid g.
- α₁-acid g.
- alpha acid g.
- alpha-1-acid g.
- beta g.
- g. hormone
- platelet membrane g.
- g. stain
- g. staining
- submaxillary g.
- tumor-associated g. (TAG)

β-glycoprotein
- glycine-rich β-g.

glycoprotein-1
- lysosomal membrane g. (LAMP-1)

glycoprotein-2
- lysosomal membrane g. (LAMP-2)

glycoproteinase
- beta g.

β-glycoproteinase
- glycine-rich β-g.

β₂-glycoprotein II
glycoptyalism
glycopyrrolate
glycopyrronium bromide
glycorrhachia
glycorrhea
glycosaminoglycan
glycosaminolipid
glycosialia
glycosidase
glycoside
- cardiac g.
- cyanophoric g.
- digitalis g.
- sterol g.

glycosphingolipid
glycosuria
- alimentary g.
- benign g.
- digestive g.
- normoglycemic g.
- pathologic g.

- phloridzin g.
- renal g.
- toxic g.

glycosuric melituria
glycosylated
- g. hemoglobin
- g. hemoglobin test

glycosylated hemoglobin
glycosylation
glycosyl ceramide
glycosyltransferase
- alpha glucan-branching g.
- glucan branching g.
- α-glucan-branching g.

glycuresis
glycuronuria
glycyl
glycyl-glycine dipeptidase
glycyl-leucine dipeptidase
glycyltryptophan test
Glycyphagus
- *G. domesticus*

glyodin
glyoxalase
glyoxylate reductase
glyoxylic acid test
Gm
- gamma
- Gm allotype
- Gm antigen

g-m
- gram-meter

GM₁ gangliosidosis
GM₂ gangliosidosis
GM-CSF
- granulocyte-macrophage colony-stimulating factor

Gmelin test
GMP
- cyclic G.

3′:5′-GMP
GMS
- Gomori methenamine-silver stain
- GMS stain

GMW
- gram-molecular weight

GN
- ganglioneuroma
- glomerulonephritis
- glucose nitrogen ratio
- gram-negative
- GN broth

gnat
Gnathostoma
- *G. spinigerum*

gnathostomiasis
GNBL
- ganglioneuroblastoma

GNID
  Gram-negative intracellular diplococci
gnotobiology
gnotobiota
gnotobiote
gnotobiotic
gnotophoresis
GnRH
  gonadotropin-releasing hormone
goatpox
  g. virus
goat's milk anemia
goblet cell
Godwin tumor
Gofman test
goiter
  aberrant g.
  acute g.
  adenomatous g.
  colloid g.
  congenital g.
  cystic g.
  diffuse g.
  diving g.
  dyshormonogenic g.
  endemic g.
  exophthalmic g.
  familial g.
  fibrous g.
  follicular g.
  hyperplastic g.
  lingual g.
  lymphadenoid g.
  microfollicular g.
  multinodular g.
  nodular colloid g.
  nodular hyperplastic g.
  nontoxic g. (NTG)
  parenchymatous g.
  simple g.
  sporadic diffuse g.
  sporadic nodular g.
  substernal g.
  suffocative g.
  thoracic g.
  toxic g. (TG)
  wandering g.
goitrous
gold
  g. assay
  g. chloride
  g. chloride reagent

colloidal g. (CG)
  g. sol test
  g. toning
gold-198
Goldberg-Maxwell syndrome
Goldblatt
  G. hypertension
  G. kidney
Goldenhar syndrome
Goldflam disease
Goldflam-Erb disease
Goldscheider disease
Goldstein disease
Goldz-Gorlin syndrome
golf-hole ureteral orifice
Golgi
  G. apparatus
  G. cavity alteration
  G. complex
  G. membrane alteration
  G. osmiobichromate fixative
  G. stain
  G. vacuole alteration
  G. vesicle alteration
  G. zone
Goltz syndrome
Gomori
  G. aldehyde fuchsin stain
  G. chrome alum hematoxylin-
    phloxine stain
  G. methenamine-silver stain (GMS)
  G. method for chromaffin
  G. nonspecific acid phosphatase
    stain
  G. nonspecific alkaline phosphatase
    stain
  G. one-step trichrome stain
  G. silver impregnation stain
**Gomori-Jones periodic acid-
  methenamine-silver stain**
Gomori-Takamatsu stain
gonad
  streak g.
gonadal
  g. agenesis
  g. aplasia
  g. dysgenesis
  g. endocrine disorder
  g. shield
  g. streak
  g. stromal tumor
gonadoblastoma

G

NOTES

gonadotrope
gonadotropic hormone (GTH)
gonadotropin
    chorionic g. (CG, CGT)
    g. hormone-releasing hormone
    human chorionic g. (hCG)
    human menopausal g. (HMG)
    human pituitary g. (hPG)
    menopausal g. (MG)
    pituitary g.
    pregnant mare serum g. (PMSG)
    g. test
    total urinary g. (TUG)
    urinary chorionic g. (UCG)
gonadotropin-inhibitory material (GIM)
gonadotropin-producing adenoma
gonadotropin-releasing
    g.-r. agent (GRA)
    g.-r. factor (GRF)
    g.-r. hormone (GnRH)
gonarthritis
gonatagra
gonatocele
gondii
    Toxoplasma g.
gonecystolith
Gongylonema
    G. pulchrum
gongylonemiasis
gonidial (colony) (G)
gonioma
gonitis
gonocele
gonococcal
    g. arthritis-dermatitis syndrome
    g. conjunctivitis
    g. ophthalmia
    g. peritonitis
gonococcemia
gonococcus, pl. gonococci (GC)
gonohemia
gono-opsonin
gonophage
gonorrhea
    g. culture (GC)
    venereal disease-g. (VDG)
gonorrheal
    g. ophthalmia
    g. rheumatism
    g. salpingitis
gonotoxemia
gonotoxin
gonotyl
Gonyaulax catanella
Good
    G. antigen
    G. syndrome

Goodpasture
    G. stain
    G. syndrome
Gopalan syndrome
Gordius
    G. aquaticus
    G. robustus
Gordon
    G. agent
    G. body
    G. and Sweet stain
    G. test
Gorham disease
Goriaew rule
Gorlin-Chaudhry-Moss syndrome
Gorlin-Goltz syndrome
Gorlin-Psaume syndrome
Gorlin syndrome
Gorman syndrome
gorondou
Göthlin capillary fragility test
Gougerot-Blum
    G.-B. disease
    G.-B. syndrome
Gougerot-Blum disease
Gougerot-Carteaud syndrome
gougerotii
    Sporotrichum g.
Gougerot-Ruiter disease
Gougerot-Sjögren disease
goundou
gout
    abarticular g.
    articular g.
    calcium g.
    lead g.
    saturnine g.
    tophaceous g.
gouty
    g. arthritis
    g. nephropathy
    g. tophus
    g. urine
Gowers
    G. solution
    G. syndrome
GP
    general paresis
GPAIS
    guinea pig anti-insulin serum
GPC
    gastric parietal cell
G-6-PD
    glucose-6-phosphate dehydrogenase
    G-6-PD test
GPI
    Gram-positive identification
    Vitek GPI

GPIIb/IIIa
platelet G.
GPIPID
guinea pig intraperitoneal infectious dose
GPK
guinea pig kidney (antigen)
GPKA
guinea pig kidney absorption (test)
G. protein
GPS
guinea pig serum
GRA
gonadotropin-releasing agent
gracilis syndrome
grade
ACS g.
analytical reagent g. (AR)
AR g.
Gleason tumor g.
g. I, II, III, IV astrocytoma
g.'s I-IV ependymoma
reagent g.
Gradenigo syndrome
gradient
average g.
grading
histologic g.
tumor g.
graduate
graduated
g. cylinder
g. pipette
Graefe disease
Graffi virus
graft
allogenic g.
autogeneic g.
autogenic g.
autologous g.
autoplastic g.
bone g. (BG)
coronary artery bypass g. (CABG)
heterologous g.
heteroplastic g.
heterospecific g.
homologous g.
homoplastic g.
interspecific g.
isogeneic g.
isogenic g.
isologous g.
isoplastic g.

material g.
g. rejection
serum chemistry g. (SCG)
skin g. (SG)
split-thickness skin g. (STSG)
syngeneic g.
white g.
xenogeneic g.
graft-versus-host (GVH)
g.-v.-h. disease (GVHD)
g.-v.-h. disease reaction
g.-v.-h. reaction (GVHR)
Graham
G. law
G. Little syndrome
Graham-Cole test
grain
g. count halving time
g. itch
g. itch mite
Gram
G. iodine
G. method
G. stain
G. stain of stool
gram (g)
g. ion
gram-calorie (g-cal)
gram-centimeter (g-cm)
gramicidin
gram-meter (g-m)
gram-molecular weight (GMW)
Gram-negative, gram-negative
G.-n. bacilli
G.-n. bacterium
G.-n. broth
G.-n. cocci
G.-n. intracellular diplococci (GNID)
Gram-positive, gram-positive
G.-p. bacilli
G.-p. bacterium
G.-p. cocci
G.-p. identification (GPI)
Gram-Sure reagent
Gram-Weigert stain
granddaughter cyst
grand mal
g. m. epilepsy
Granger method
Gr antigen

NOTES

granular
g. atrophy
g. cast (GC)
g. cell myoblastoma
g. cell tumor
g. conjunctivitis
g. degeneration
g. endoplasmic reticulum
g. kidney
g. leukoblast
g. leukocyte
g. pharyngitis
g. pneumocyte
g. urethritis
g. urinary cast
g. vaginitis
granulation
arachnoid g.
pacchionian g.
g. tissue
toxic g.
granule
acidophil g.
acrosomal g.
alpha g.
Altmann g.
amphophil g.
argentaffin g.
azurophil g.
azurophilic g.
Babes-Ernst g.
basal g.
basophil g.
basophilic g.
beta g.
Birbeck g.
Bollinger g.
chromatophilic g.
chromophil g.
chromophobe g.
Crooke g.
dense-core neurosecretory g.
g.'s of developing neutrophils
elementary g.
endocrine g.
eosinophil g.
eosinophilic g.
Fordyce g.
fuchsinophil g.
Grawitz g.
iodophil g.
juxtaglomerular g.
κ-g.
kappa g.
keratohyalin g.
Langerhans g.
metachromatic g.
mucigen g.'s

neurosecretory g.'s
Neusser g.
neutrophil g.
oxyphil g.
pigment g.
primary g.
sand g.
Schüffner g.
secondary g.
secretory g.
siderocytic g.
siderotic g.
specific g.
sulfur g.
toxic g.
Zimmermann g.
zymogen g.
granuloblast
granulocyte
band-form g.
g. colony-stimulating factor (G-CSF)
g. concentrate
immature g.
segmented g.
granulocyte-erythroid ratio (G/E)
granulocyte-macrophage colony-stimulating factor (GM-CSF)
granulocytic
g. g.
g. aplasia
g. blood cell
g. hyperplasia
g. hypoplasia
g. leukemia
g. sarcoma
g. series
granulocytopenia
granulocytopoiesis
granulocytopoietic
granulocytosis
granulogenesis
granuloma
amebic g.
g. annulare
apical g.
beryllium g.
bilharzial g.
calcified g.
caseating g.
coccidioidal g.
dental g.
g. endemicum
eosinophilic g.
g. faciale
foreign body g.
g. gangrenescens
giant cell reparative g.

histiocytic g.
Hodgkin g.
infectious g.
g. inguinale
g. inguinale tropicum
laryngeal g.
lethal midline g.
lipoid g.
lipophagic g.
Majocchi g.
malignant g.
midline lethal g.
mineral oil g.
multifocal eosinophilic g.
noncaseating g.
non-necrotizing g.
oily g.
palisading g.
paracoccidioidal g.
parasitic g.
periapical g.
plasma cell g.
pyogenic g.
g. pyogenicum
reparative giant cell g.
reticulohistiocytic g.
sarcoid g.
g. sarcoid
sarcoidal g.
schistosome g.
sea urchin g.
silica g.
silicon g.
spermatogenic g.
suture g.
swimming pool g.
g. telangiectaticum
tuberculoid g.
unifocal eosinophilic g.
zirconium g.

granulomatosis
allergic g.
angiitic g.
bronchocentric g.
g. disciformis chronica et
   progressiva
Langerhans cell g. (LCG)
lipophagic intestinal g.
lymphomatoid g. (LYG)
Miescher g.
g. siderotica
Wegener g.

granulomatous
g. angiitis with eosinophilia
g. colitis
g. disease
g. encephalomyelitis
g. enteritis
g. hepatitis
g. inflammation
g. mastitis
g. orchitis
g. polyp
g. thyroiditis
granulomere
granulopenia
granulophthisis
granuloplasm
granulopoiesis
granulopoietic
granulopoietin
granulosa
g. cell
g. cell carcinoma
g. cell tumor (GCT)
granulosa-lutein cell
granulosa-theca cell tumor
granulosis
g. rubra nasi
granulosity
granulovacuolar degeneration
granzymes
grape mole
graph
Davenport g.
g. tablet
graphanesthesia
graphesthesia
graphic
g. analysis
g. terminal
Graphium
graphomotor
graphospasm
grappe
en g.
grating
diffraction g.
replica g.
gravel
Graves disease
grave wax
gravimetric
Gravindex pregnancy test

NOTES

G

gravis
    myasthenia g. (MG, MyG)
gravitation abscess
gravity
    specific g. (SG, sp gr)
gravity-settling culture (GSC)
Gravlee jet wash
Grawitz
    G. basophilia
    G. granule
    G. tumor
gray
    g. degeneration
    g. hepatization
    g. induration
    g. infiltration
    g. patch
    g. platelet syndrome
    g. scale
gray-patch ringworm
greatest length (GL)
green
    brilliant g.
    bromcresol g.
    bromocresol g. (BCG)
    g. cancer
    ethyl g.
    g. hemoglobin
    indocyanine g. (ICG)
    malachite g.
    methyl g.
    g. monkey virus
    Paris g.
    g. pus
    g. sickness
    g. sputum
Greenfield disease
Greenhow disease
greenstick fracture
gregaloid
Gregarina
gregarine
Gregarinia
gregarinosis
Gregg syndrome
Greig syndrome
grenz ray
GRF
    gonadotropin-releasing factor
    growth hormone-releasing factor
GRH
    growth hormone-releasing hormone
grid
    aligned g.
    Bucky g.
    crossed g.
    focused g.
    g. index

    g. line
    parallel g.
    Potter-Bucky g.
    g. ratio
Gridley stain for fungi
Griesinger disease
griffin claw
Grimelius
    G. argyrophil reaction
    G. argyrophil stain method
    G. stain
grinders' asthma
grip
    devil's g.
grippe
Griscelli syndrome
griseofulvin
Grisonella ratellina
Grocott-Gomori
    G.-G. methenamine-silver method
    G.-G. methenamine-silver stain
groin ulcer
Grönblad-Strandberg syndrome
groove
    Harrison g.
    g. sign
Gross
    G. disease
    G. leukemia virus
    G. virus antigen (GSA)
gross
    g. hematuria
    g. lesion
ground
    g. glass
    g. itch anemia
    g. state
    g. substance
grounded
ground-glass
    g.-g. cytoplasm
    g.-g. hepatocyte
group
    g. A beta hemolytic streptococci throat culture
    ABO blood g.
    acyloxy g.
    g. agglutination
    g. agglutinin
    g. A hapten
    g. A β-hemolytic streptococci throat culture
    alkyl g.
    g. antigens
    arbovirus g. A
    aryl g.
    g. A *Streptococcus*
    blood g.

Bombay blood g.
g. B *Streptococcus*
coli-aerogenes g.
control g.
coryneform g.
cytophil g.
determinant g.
g. D *Streptococcus*
functional g.
guanidinium g.
hydroxyl g.
g. I-IV mycobacteria
g. immunity
Kell blood g. (K)
keto g.
Lewis blood g.
Lutheran Blood G.
MNS blood g.
g. N *Streptococcus*
P blood g.
peptide g.
platinum g.
prenyl g.
prosthetic g.
proteus g.
g. reaction
Rh blood g.
salmonella g.
sulfhydryl g.
symmetry g.
thiocarbonyl g.
g. transfer
grouping
    antigenic structural g.
    blood g.
    haptenic g.
    Lancefield g.
    reverse g.
Grover disease
grower
    rapid g.
growing point
growth
    g. acceleration
    g. alteration
    appositional g.
    g. arrest
    g. disorder
    exophytic g.
    g. fraction
    g. hormone (GH)
    g. hormone deficiency (GHD)

g. hormone-producing adenoma
g. hormone-release-inhibiting
    hormone (GH-RIH)
g. hormone-releasing factor (GH-
    RF, GRF)
g. hormone-releasing hormone (GH-
    RH, GRH)
g. inhibitory factor
interstitial g.
new g.
g. retardation
grub
Gruber syndrome
Gruber-Widal reaction
grumous
gryochrome
GSA
    Gross virus antigen
GSC
    gas-solid chromatography
    gravity-settling culture
GSD
    genetically significant dose
GSE
    gluten-sensitive enteropathy
GSH
    reduced glutathione
GSR
    galvanic skin response
    generalized Shwartzman reaction
GSSR
    generalized Sanarelli-Shwartzman
    reaction
GT
    glucose tolerance
GTD
    gestational trophoblastic disease
GTH
    gonadotropic hormone
GTP
    guanosine triphosphate
GTT
    glucose tolerance test
GU
    gastric ulcer
guaiacin
guaiac test
Guama virus
guanase
guanidinemia
guanidinium group
guanidino-aminovaleric acid

G

NOTES

guanine
> g. cytosine (GC)
> g. deaminase
> g. deaminase assay

guanosine
> g. 3′:5′-cyclic phosphate
> g. diphosphate
> g. 5′-diphosphate (GDP)
> g. monophosphate
> g. triphosphate (GTP)

guanosine-′5-phosphate
guanylic acid
guanylyl
guarding
Guarnieri body
Guaroa virus
Gubler
> G. line
> G. syndrome
> G. tumor

Guillain-Barré syndrome (GB)
guinea
> g. green B
> g. worm infection

guinea pig
> g. p. anti-insulin serum (GPAIS)
> g. p. intraperitoneal infectious dose (GPIPID)
> g. p. kidney absorption (test) (GPKA)
> g. p. kidney (antigen) (GPK)
> g. p. serum (GPS)

Guinon disease
Gulf War syndrome
Gull disease
Gull-Sutton syndrome
gumma, pl. gummata, gummas
gummatous
> g. abscess
> g. syphilid
> g. ulcer

gummosa
> periarteritis g.

gummy
Gumprecht shadow
gums
> strawberry g.

Gunning-Lieben test
Gunn syndrome
gunshot wound
Günther disease
Günzberg
> G. reagent
> G. test

gustation
gustin
gut-associated (GA)
> g. lymphoid tissue (GALT)

gut glucagon
Guthrie
> G. bacterial inhibition assay (GBIA)
> G. test

Gutman unit
gutturotetany
Gutzeit test
GV
> gentian violet

GVH
> graft-versus-host
> GVH disease
> GVH reaction

GVHD
> graft-versus-host disease

GVHR
> graft-versus-host reaction

Gymnamoebida
Gymnoascaceae
Gymnoascus
gymnobacterium
Gymnodinium
gymnothecium
gynandrism
gynandroblastoma
gynandromorphism
gynecogen
gynecoid
gynecomastia
gynecomasty
gyrectomy
Gyromitra esculenta

H
Hauch (motile microorganism)
henry
Holzknecht unit
Hounsfield unit
hypermetropia
 H agglutination
 H agglutinin
 H antigen
 H band
 H chain
 H colony
 cytolipin H
 H and E staining
 H gene
 H substance
H-2
 H-2 antigen
 H-2 complex
H-2^b mouse cell
HA
 hemagglutinating antibody
HA1 virus
HA2 virus
HAA
 hepatitis-associated antigen
Haagensen test
Habermann disease
Haber syndrome
habitual abortion
habituation
Habronema
habronemiasis
Hadfield-Clarke syndrome
Hadrurus
Haemadipsa ceylonica
Haemagogus
Haemamoeba
Haemaphysalis
 H. concinna
 H. leporis-palustris
 H. spinigera
Haematopinus
Haemobartonella
Haemococcidium
Haemodipsus ventricosus
Haemogregarina
Haemonchus
 H. contortus
 H. placei
Haemophilus
 H. aegyptius
 H. ducreyi
 H. influenzae
 H. parainfluenzae

 H. pertussis vaccine (HPV)
 H. suis
 H. vaginalis
Haemoproteus
Haemosporidia
Haemosporina
Haemostrongylus vasorum
Haenszel test
Haff disease
Haffkine vaccine
Hafnia
 H. alvei
hafnium
Hageman factor (HF)
Haglund disease
Hagner disease
Hahn oxine reagent
HAHTG
 horse antihuman thymus globulin
HAI
 hemagglutination inhibition
 hemagglutinin inhibition
Hailey-Hailey disease
hair
 h. analysis
 h. ball
 beaded h.
 h. cell (HC)
 ingrown h.
 lanugo h.
 Schridde cancer h.'s
 telogen h.
hairpin loop
hairworm
hairy
 h. cell
 h. cell leukemia (HCL)
 h. heart
 h. mole
Hakim syndrome
Halberstaedter-Prowazek body
Haldane effect
Haldol
Hale colloidal iron stain
half-bandwidth
half-cell
half-Gram
half-life
 biologic h.
 effective h.
 physical h.
 terminal h. (T½, T 1/2, t½)
half-maximum
 full-width h.

H

283

half-moon
    red h.-m.
half-reaction
halftime
    gastric emptying h. (GET1/2)
half-value layer (HVL)
half-wave
    h.-w. potential
    h.-w. rectifier
halide
halisteresis
halisteretic
Hall
    H. disease
    H. method
Hallermann-Streiff-François syndrome
Hallermann-Streiff syndrome
Hallervorden-Spatz
    H.-S. disease
    H.-S. syndrome
Hallervorden syndrome
Hallgren syndrome
Hallopeau disease
Hallopeau-Siemens syndrome
hallucinogen
halo
    anemic h.
    h. melanoma
    h. nevus
halogen
halogenated hydrocarbon assay
halogenation
halometer
Halon system
haloperidol
    h. assay
halophile
haloprogin
halosteresis
halothane
    h. assay
    h. hepatitis
Halsted law
Halteridium
halzoun
HAM-56
    human alveolar macrophage-56
    HAM-56 antibody
hamartia
hamartoblastoma
hamartochondromatosis
hamartoma
    fibrous h. of infancy
    mesenchymal h.
    neurocristic h.
    neurovascular h.
    peribiliary gland h.
    pulmonary h.

hamartomatous polyp
Hamburger
    H. law
    H. phenomenon
Hamel test
Hamilton
    H. pseudophlegmon
    H. Rating Scale (HRS)
Hamman
    H. disease
    H. syndrome
Hamman-Rich syndrome
Hammarsten
    H. reagent
    H. test
Hammerschlag method
Hammond disease
hamster
    h. egg penetration assay
    h. egg penetration test
Ham test
hand
    crab h.
    H. disease
    ghoul h.
    opera-glass h.
    skeleton h.
    spade h.
    trident h.
hand-foot-and-mouth
    h.-f.-a.-m. disease
    h.-f.-a.-m. disease virus
hand-foot syndrome
handling
    toxic chemical h.
Hand-Schüller-Christian
    H.-S.-C. disease
    H.-S.-C. type of histiocyte
HANE
    hereditary angioneurotic edema
Hanes equation
Hanger test
hanging-block culture
hanging-drop
    h. d. culture
Hanhart syndrome
Hanker-Yates reagent
Hanot
    H. cirrhosis
    H. disease
Hanot-Chauffard syndrome
Hansel stain
Hansemann macrophage
Hansen
    H. bacillus
    H. disease
Hansenula
Hantaan virus

Hantavirus
    H. pulmonary syndrome
HAP
    heredopathia atactia polyneuritiformis
HAPA
    hemagglutinating anti-penicillin antibody
hapalonychia
haploid
    h. genome ("n")
    h. number
haploidy
Haplorchis
haplosomic
Haplosporidia
haplotype
    h. association study
hapten
    conjugated h.
    group A h.
    h. inhibition of precipitation
haptenic grouping
haptoglobin (hp)
    h. assay
    h., Hp^1 and Hp^2
    h. test
Harada syndrome
hard
    h. chancre
    h. pad disease
    h. pad virus
    h. papilloma
    h. sore
    h. tissue
    h. tubercle
    h. ulcer
hardened pelvis
Harding-Passey melanoma
hardness
Hardy-Weinberg law
Hare syndrome
Hargraves cell
haricot broth
Harleco synthetic resin
harlequin
    h. color change
    h. fetus
Harley disease
harmaline
harmine
harmonic
Harris
    H. alum hematoxylin

    H. and Ray test
    H. syndrome
Harrison
    H. groove
    H. test
Hartmannella
Hartmann solution
Hartnup
    H. disease
    H. syndrome
Harvard criteria of irreversible coma
harvest
    h. bug
    h. mite
Häser formula
HASHD
    hypertensive arteriosclerotic heart disease
Hashimoto
    H. disease
    H. struma
    H. thyroiditis
Hassall corpuscle
Hasselbalch equation
Hassin syndrome
hatchetti
    Acanthamoeba h.
HATTS
    hemagglutination treponemal test for
    syphilis
Hauch
    ohne H.
Hauch (motile microorganism) (H)
haupt-agglutinin
HAV
    hepatitis A virus
Haverhill fever
Haverhillia
    H. moniliformis
    H. multiformis
Hawaii agent
hawkinsin
hawkinsinuria
Haworth formula
hay
    h. asthma
    h. fever
Hayem
    H. hematoblast
    H. solution
Hayem-Widal
    H.-W. anemia
    H.-W. syndrome

NOTES

H

Haygarth node
hazard
    h. identification
    radiation h.
    h. symbol
hazardous
    h. concentration
    h. material
    h. materials labeling
    h. substance
HB
    heart block
Hb
    hemoglobin
      Hb D
HBA71 antigen
HB$_c$Ab
    antibody to the hepatitis B core antigen
HB$_c$Ag
    hepatitis B core antigen
HbCO
    carboxyhemoglobin
HBe
    hepatitis B$_e$ antigen
HB$_e$Ab
HBF
    hepatic blood flow
HbF
    fetal hemoglobin
HBI
    high serum-bound iron
HBIG
    hepatitis B immune globulin
HbO$_2$
    oxyhemoglobin
Hb S
    sickle cell hemoglobin
    sulfhemoglobin
HB$_s$Ab
    antibody to the hepatitis B surface
      antigen
HB$_s$Ag
    hepatitis B surface antigen
HBV
    hepatitis B virus
HBW
    high birth weight
HC
    hair cell
    Huntington chorea
    hyaline cast
    hydroxycorticoid
HCC
    hepatocellular carcinoma
    hydroxycholecalciferol
HCCC
    hyalinizing clear cell carcinoma

hCG
    human chorionic gonadotropin
      hCG-alpha subunit
      hCG-beta subunit
hCG-α
    h. subunit
hCG-β
    h. subunit
hCG-alpha
hCG-beta
H chain
HCL
    hairy cell leukemia
HCO$_3$ concentrations
HCP
    hepatocatalase peroxidase
    hereditary coproporphyria
HCr
    hemoglobin content of reticulocytes
hCS, hCSM
    human chorionic somatomammotropin
HCT
    hematocrit
    homocytotrophic
    hydrochlorothiazide
Hct
    hematocrit
HCU
    homocystinuria
HCV
    hepatitis C virus
HCVD
    hypertensive cardiovascular disease
HD
    heart disease
    high dosage
    Hirschsprung disease
    Hodgkin disease
    hydatid disease
HDC
    histidine decarboxylase
HDCV
    human diploid cell rabies vaccine
HDH
    heart disease history
HDL, HDLP
    high-density lipoprotein
      HDL cholesterol assay
HDL-C
    high-density lipoprotein-cholesterol
HDN
    hemolytic disease of newborn
HDRA assay
HDS
    herniated disk syndrome
HDV
    hepatitis delta virus

HDW
    reticulocyte hemoglobin distribution
      width
HE
    hereditary elliptocytosis
    human enteric (virus)
H&E
    hematoxylin and eosin
      H&E stain
head
    angle h.
    bulldog h.
    H. line
    h. louse
    Medusa h.
    h. space analysis
healed
    h. appendicitis
    h. fracture
    h. glomerulonephritis
    h. infarct
    h. tuberculosis
    h. ulcer
healing appendicitis
health physics
He antigen
heart
    h. antigen
    armored h.
    athletic h.
    h. block (HB)
    bony h.
    h. disease (HD)
    h. disease history (HDH)
    disordered action of h. (DAH)
    drop h.
    h. failure (HF)
    h. failure cell
    fatty h.
    frosted h.
    hairy h.
    hypoplastic h.
    icing h.
    luxus h.
    movable h.
    myxedema h.
    parchment h.
    pendulous h.
    tiger h.
    trilocular h.
    h. tumor
    valvular disease of h. (VDH)

heart-hand syndrome
heart-lung preparation
heartwater
heartworm
HEAT
    human erythrocyte agglutination test
heat
    h. capacity
    h. coagulation test
    h. of combustion
    h. content
    h. edema
    h. of formation
    h. of fusion
    h. instability test
    h. killed (HK)
    h. labile
    h. labile test
    latent h.
    molar h. capacity
    h. precipitation test
    h. of reaction
    h. sink
    h. of solution
    specific h.
    specific h. capacity
    h. of sublimation
    h. unit (HU)
    h. of vaporization
**heat-killed *Listeria monocytogenes*
(HKLM)**
heat-resistant glass
heat-shock protein
heat-stable (HS)
    h.-s. alkaline phosphatase
    h.-s. lactic dehydrogenase (HLDH)
heavy
    h. chain
    h.-chain disease
    h. metal
    h.-metal poisoning
    h.-metal screen
    h.-metal screening test
α-heavy-chain disease
γ-heavy-chain disease
μ-heavy-chain disease
Hebeloma
Heberden
    H. disease
    H. node
Hebra disease
Hecht pneumonia

NOTES

H

hectogram
hectometer
heel
    cracked h.
Heerfordt
    H. disease
    H. syndrome
Hegglin
    H. anomaly
    H. syndrome
Heidenhain
    H. azan stain
    H. iron hematoxylin
    H. iron hematoxylin stain
    H. syndrome
height (ht)
    peak h.
Heine-Medin disease
Heinz
    H. body stain
    H. body test
Heinz-body hemolytic anemia
Heinz-Ehrlich body
HEK
    human embryo kidney
    human embryonic kidney
Hektoen enteric agar
HEL
    human embryo lung
HeLa cell
Heleidae
helenine
helianthine
helical
helicis
    chondrodermatitis nodularis
        chronica h.
Helicobacter
    H. pylori serology
    H. pylori urease
    H. pylori urease test and culture
helicotrema
heliencephalitis
Heliozoea
Helisal rapid blood test
helium equilibration time (HET)
helix
    alpha h.
    double h.
    right-handed alpha h.
α-helix
    right-handed α-h.
Heller-Döhle disease
helle Zellen
Helly
    H. fixative
    H. fluid
helmet cell

helminth
    h. identification procedure
helminthagogue
helmintheca
    Neorickettsia h.
helminthemesis
helminthiasis
helminthic
    h. disease
helminthism
helminthoid
helminthology
helminthoma
Helminthosporium
helmintic
Heloderma
Helophilus
helper
    h. cell
    h. T lymphocyte
    h. virus
Helvella
    H. esculenta
Helweg-Larssen syndrome
hemachromatosis
hemachrome
hemachrosis
hemacytometer
hemacytozoon
hemadsorption
    mixed h. (MHA)
    h. virus test
    h. virus, type 1, 2
hemafacient
hemagglutinating
    h. antibody (HA)
    h. anti-penicillin antibody (HAPA)
    h. cold autoantibody
    h. unit (HU)
hemagglutination
    indirect h. (IHA)
    h. inhibition (HAI, HI)
    h. inhibition assay
    passive h. (PHA)
    reverse passive h.
    h. test
    h. titer (HT)
    h. treponemal test for syphilis
        (HATTS)
    Treponema pallidum h. (TPH)
    viral h.
hemagglutination-inhibition
    h.-i. antibody (HIA)
    h.-i. test (HIT)
hemagglutinin
    autologous h.
    cold h.
    heterologous h.

homologous h.
h. inhibition (HAI)
warm h.
hemalum
Hemalumeosin
hemamebiasis
hemanalysis
hemangiectatic hypertrophy
hemangioblast
hemangioblastoma
hemangioendothelial sarcoma
hemangioendothelioblastoma
hemangioendothelioma
epithelioid h.
h. tuberosum multiplex
hemangiofibroma
juvenile h.
hemangiolipoma
hemangioma
ameloblastic h.
arterial h.
capillary h.
cavernous h.
h. congenitalle
infantile h.
nuchal h.
h. planum extensum
racemose h.
sclerosing h.
senile h.
h. simplex
hemangioma-thrombocytopenia syndrome
hemangiomatosis
hemangioperic-like
hemangiopericytic
hemangiopericytoma
lipomatous h. (LHPC)
hemangiosarcoma
splenic h.
hemapheic
hemaphein
hemapheism
hemapheresis
hemarthrosis
hemastrontium
hematapostema
hematein
Baker acid h.
h. test
hematemesis
hematencephalon
Hematest

hematherapy
hemathidrosis
hemathorax
hematic
hematid
hematidrosis
hematimeter
hematin
acid formaldehyde h.
h. albumin
h. pigmentation
reduced h.
hematinemia
hematinic
h. principle
hematobilia
hematobium
hematoblast
Hayem h.
hematocele
hematocelia
hematocephaly
hematochezia
hematochlorin
hematochyluria
hematoclasis
hematoclastic
hematocrit (HCT, Hct)
large vessel h. (LVH)
mean circulatory h.
total body h. (TBH)
venous h. (VH)
whole-blood h. (WBH)
hematocrystallin
hematocyst
hematocystis
hematocyte
hematocytoblast
hematocytolysis
hematocytometer
hematocytozoon
hematocyturia
hematodyscrasia
hematodystrophy
hematogen
hematogenesis
hematogenic
hematogenous
h. abscess
h. hyalin
h. jaundice
h. metastasis

NOTES

H

hematogenous *(continued)*
    h. osteitis
    h. pigment
    h. theory of endometriosis
hematogone
hematohistioblast
hematohyaloid
hematoid
hematoidin
    h. crystal
    h. pigmentation
hematologist
hematology
hematolymphangioma
hematolymphoid chimerism
hematolysis
hematolytic
hematoma
    chronic subdural h. (CSH)
    corpus luteum h.
    epidural h.
    intracranial h.
    intramural h.
    organized h.
    subdural h.
hematometra
hematometry
hematomyelia
hematomyelopore
hematonic
hematopathology
hematopathy
hematopenia
hematophagia
hematophagous
hematophagus
hematophilia
hematoplastic
hematopneic index
hematopoiesis
    extramedullary h.
hematopoietic
    h. aplasia
    h. cell cytoplasmic alteration
    h. hyperplasia
    h. hypoplasia
    h. maturation
    h. maturation alteration
    h. maturation arrest
    h. progenitor cell
    h. stem cell
    h. system
    h. tissue
hematopoietin
hematoporphyrinemia
hematoporphyrinuria
hematorrhachis
    h. externa

    extradural h.
    h. interna
    subdural h.
hematosalpinx
hematosepsis
hematoside
hematosis
hematospectroscope
hematospectroscopy
hematospermatocele
hematospermia
hematostatic
hematostaxis
hematotoxic
hematotoxin
hematotropic
hematoxic
hematoxin
hematoxylin
    h. body
    Boehmer h.
    Carazzi h.
    Clara h.
    Cole h.
    Delafield h.
    h. and eosin (H&E)
    h. and eosin staining
    Harris alum h.
    Heidenhain iron h.
    iron h.
    Lillie h.
    Mayer h.
    phosphotungstic acid h. (PTAH)
    Weigert iron h.
hematoxylin-eosin stain
hematoxylin-malachite green-basic
    fuchsin stain
hematoxylin-phloxine B stain
hematozoic
hematozoon
hematuresis
hematuria
    essential h.
    false h.
    gross h.
    initial h.
    microscopic h.
    renal h.
    terminal h.
    total h.
    urethral h.
    vesical h.
hematuric bilious fever
heme
    h. synthetase (HS)
hemendothelioma
hemerythrins
hemiacardius

hemiacetal
hemianopsia
    binasal h.
    bitemporal h.
hemiaplasia
hemiatrophy
    facial h.
hemiballismus
hemiblock
hemic
    h. calculus
Hemichorda
Hemichordata
hemidesmosome
hemidiaphoresis
hemidrosis
hemiglobin
hemihidrosis
hemihyperhidrosis
hemihyperidrosis
hemilesion
hemimetabolous
hemin
Hemiptera
hemipyonephrosis
Hemispora stellata
hemisyndrome
hemizygosity
hemizygous
hemoagglutination
hemoagglutinin
hemoantitoxin
Hemobartonella
hemobilia
hemoblast
    lymphoid h. of Pappenheim
hemoblastosis
hemocatharsis
hemocatheresis
hemocatheretic
hemoccult test
hemocele
hemocholecyst
hemocholecystitis
hemochromatosis
    exogenous h.
hemochromogen
hemochromometry
hemoclasia
hemoclasis

hemoclastic
    h. reaction
    h. shock
hemoconcentration
hemoconia
hemoconiosis
hemocryoscopy
HemoCue glucose meter
hemocyanin
    keyhole-limpet h. (KLH)
hemocystinuria
hemocyt.
    hemocytometer
hemocyte
hemocytoblast
hemocytocatheresis
hemocytolysis
hemocytometer (hemocyt.)
hemocytometry
hemocytotripsis
hemocytozoon
hemodiagnosis
hemodialysis
    peritoneal h.
hemodialyzer
    ultrafiltration h.
hemodilution
hemodyscrasia
hemodystrophy
hemofiltration
hemoflagellate
hemofuscin
    h. pigmentation
hemogenesis
hemogenic
hemoglobin (Hb, Hg, Hgb)
    h. A
    h. A_2
    h. A_{1c}
    aberrant h.
    adult h.
    h. Bart
    bile pigment h.
    h. C
    h. C_{Harlem}
    h. $C_{Georgetown}$
    h. carbamate
    carbon monoxide h.
    h. cast
    h. C disease
    h. Chesapeake
    h. content of reticulocytes (HCr)

NOTES

H

hemoglobin *(continued)*
  h. D$_{Punjab}$
  h. demonstration in tissue
  deoxygenated h.
  h. E
  h. electrophoresis
  embryonic h.
  h. E-thalassemia disease
  h. F
  h. F assay
  fast h.
  fetal h. (HbF)
  h. F (hereditary persistence of)
  glycosylated h.
  h. Gower-1, -2
  green h.
  h. H
  h. H assay
  Hb D
  h. H disease
  hereditary persistence of fetal h. (HPFH)
  h. I
  h. identification
  h. J$_{Capetown}$
  h. Kansas
  h. Lepore
  h. M
  mean cell h. (MCH)
  mean corpuscular h. (MCH)
  muscle h.
  oxygenated h.
  oxygen half-saturation pressure of h.
  h. pigmentation
  h. Rainier
  reduced h.
  h. S
  sickle cell h. (Hb S)
  "slow" h.
  h. thalassemia
  total circulating h. (TCH)
  un-ionized h. (HHb)
  unstable h.
  variant h.
  h. Yakima
hemoglobinated
hemoglobinemia
hemoglobinocholia
hemoglobinolysis
hemoglobinometer
hemoglobinometry
hemoglobinopathy
  heterozygous h.
  homozygous h.
  mixed h.
hemoglobinopepsia
hemoglobinophilic

hemoglobinorrhea
hemoglobin-polyoxyethylene
  pyridoxylated h.-p. (PHP)
hemoglobinuria
  bacillary h.
  cold h.
  epidemic h.
  intermittent h.
  malarial h.
  march h.
  paroxysmal cold h. (PCH)
  paroxysmal nocturnal h. (PNH)
  toxic h.
hemoglobinuric
  h. fever
  h. nephropathy
  h. nephrosis
hemogram
hemohistioblast
hemokinesis
hemolamella
hemoleukocyte
hemolith
hemology
hemolymph
  h. heteroagglutinin
  h. node
hemolysate
hemolysin
  α h.
  alpha h.
  β h.
  bacterial h.
  beta h.
  cold h.
  D-L h.
  heterophil h.
  immune h.
  natural h.
  h. saponin
  specific h.
  h. unit
  warm-cold h.
hemolysinogen
hemolysis
  α h.
  alpha h.
  β h.
  beta h.
  colloid osmotic h.
  extravascular h.
  extrinsic h.
  γ h.
  gamma h.
  immune h.
  h. interference
  intramedullary h.
  intravascular h.

osmotic h.
passive h.
traumatic h.

hemolytic
h. amboceptor
h. anemia
h. anemia of newborn
h. chain
h. disease of newborn (HDN)
h. gas
h. index
h. jaundice
h. malaria
h. plaque assay
h. reaction
h. splenomegaly
h. streptococcus
h. substance
h. transfusion reaction
h. unit
h. uremic syndrome
β-hemolytic streptococcus (BHS)
hemolytic-uremic syndrome (HUS)
hemolyzable
hemolyzation
hemolyze
hemometry
hemonchosis
hemonephrosis
hemopathology
hemopathy
hemoperfusion
hemopericardium
hemoperitoneum
hemopexin
hemophagia
hemophagocytosis
hemophil
hemophilia
h. A
h. B
h. B Leyden
h. Bm
h. C
classical h.
vascular h.
hemophiliac
hemophilic
h. factor A
hemophilus
h. of Koch-Weeks
h. of Morax-Axenfeld

hemophoresis
hemophthalmia
hemophthisis
hemoplastic
hemoplasty
hemopneumopericardium
hemopneumothorax
hemopoiesic diuretic
hemopoiesis
hemopoietic
hemopoietin
hemoprecipitin
hemoprotein
hemoptysis
cardiac h.
endemic h.
oriental h.
parasitic h.
vicarious h.
hemopyelectasia
hemopyelectasis
HemoQuant fecal blood test
hemorepellant
hemorrhage
antepartum h. (APH)
cerebral h.
intraventricular h. (IVH)
petechial h.
postpartum h. (PPH)
renal h.
subarachnoid h. (SAH)
transplacental h. (TPH)
hemorrhagic
acute h. bronchopneumonia
acute h. cholecystitis
acute h. cystitis
acute h. glomerulonephritis
acute h. inflammation
acute h. ulcer
acute h. ulceration
h. anemia
h. ascites
h. bronchopneumonia
h. colitis
h. cyst
h. cystitis
h. dengue
h. diathesis
h. disease of deer
h. disease of the newborn
h. diverticulitis
h. endovasculitis

NOTES

H

hemorrhagic *(continued)*
  h. fever (HF)
  h. fever epidemic
  h. fever with renal syndrome
  h. gangrene
  h. gastritis
  h. glomerulonephritis
  h. infarct
  h. inflammation
  h. lobar pneumonia
  h. malaria
  h. nephritis
  h. pachymeningitis
  h. pancreatitis
  h. pericarditis
  h. plague
  h. pleurisy
  h. pneumonia
  h. rickets
  h. shock
  h. smallpox
  h. thrombocythemia
  h. ulcer
hemorrhagicum
  cystic corpus h.
hemorrhagin
hemorrhoid
  cutaneous h.
  external h.
  internal h.
  thrombosed h.
hemorrhoidal
  h. artery
  h. nerve
  h. vein
  h. zone
hemosiderin
  h. deposition
  h. stain
  h. staining
hemosiderinuria test
hemosiderosis
  endogenous h.
  exogenous h.
  idiopathic pulmonary h. (IPH)
  pulmonary h.
  secondary pulmonary h. (SPH)
hemospermia
  h. spuria
  h. vera
Hemosporidia
hemosporidium
hemosporines
hemostasia
hemostasis
hemostatic
hemotherapeutics
hemotherapy

hemothorax
hemotoxic
  h. anemia
hemotoxin
  cobra h.
hemotropic
hemozoic
hemozoin
hemozoon
HEMPAS
  hereditary erythrocytic multinuclearity
    with positive acidified serum
  HEMPAS cell
hemuresis
Hench-Rosenberg syndrome
Henderson-Hasselbalch equation
Henderson-Jones disease
Hendersonula toruloidea
Henle
  loop of H.
  H. reaction
Henoch purpura
Henoch-Schönlein purpura
Henoch-Schonlein syndrome
henpuye
Henry
  H. fructose test
  H. law
henry (H)
henselae
  Bartonella h.
  Rochalimaea h.
Hensen node
HEPA
  high-efficiency particulate air (filter)
  HEPA filter
Hepadnaviridae
hepar, gen. **hepatis**
  h. lobatum
heparan-*N*-sulfatase
heparan sulfate
heparin
  h. cofactor
  h. unit
heparinase
  Dade Hepzyme h.
heparinate
heparinemia
heparinic acid
heparin-induced thrombocytopenia (HIT)
heparinize
heparin-precipitable fraction (HPF)
heparitinsulphate lyase
hepatatrophia
hepatatrophy
hepatic
  h. abscess
  h. adenoma

h. blood flow (HBF)
h. capsulitis
h. coma
h. cyst
h. docimasia
h. encephalopathy
h. failure
h. fibrosis
h. fistula
h. function test
h. glycogen
h. porphyria
h. portal venous gas (HPVG)
h. steatosis
h. transaminase
h. veno-occlusive disease

hepatica
adiposis h.
hepatis (*gen. of* hepar)
hepatitic
hepatitis, pl. **hepatitides**
h. A
h. A antibody
active chronic h.
acute focal h.
acute parenchymatous h.
acute viral h. (AVH)
alcoholic h.
anicteric virus h.
h. antibody
h. antigen
autoimmune h.
h. A virus (HAV)
A virus h.
h. B
h. B$_e$ antigen (HBe)
h. B core antibody
h. B core antigen (HB$_c$Ag)
h. B e antibody
h. B immune globulin (HBIG)
h. B surface antibody
h. B surface antigen (HB$_s$Ag)
h. B surface antigen test
h. B vaccine
B virus h.
h. B virus (HBV)
h. C
cholangiolitic h.
cholestatic h.
chronic active h. (CAH)
chronic interstitial h.
chronic lobular h. (CLH)

chronic viral h.
h. contagiosa canis
h. C serology
h. C virus (HCV)
δ h.
h. D
delta h.
h. delta virus (HDV)
drug-induced h.
h. D serology
h. D virus
h. E
epidemic h.
equine serum h.
h. E virus (HEV)
h. externa
giant cell h. (GCH)
granulomatous h.
halothane h.
icteric serum h. (ISH)
infectious h. (IH)
infectious canine h.
long incubation h.
lupoid h.
mouse h.
murine h.
NANB h.
neonatal h.
non-A h.
non-A, non-B h.
non-B h.
peliosis h.
persistent chronic h.
plasma cell h.
posttransfusion h. (PTH)
serum h. (SH)
short incubation h.
Simbu h.
subacute h.
suppurative h.
transfusion h.
unresolved h.
viral h. (VH)
viral h. type A, B, C, D, E
h. virus
virus A, B h.
virus h. of ducks
hepatitis-associated antigen (HAA)
hepatization
gray h.
red h.
yellow h.

NOTES

H

hepatobiliary cystadenoma
hepatoblastoma
hepatocarcinogenesis model
hepatocarcinoma
hepatocatalase peroxidase (HCP)
hepatocele
hepatocellular
    h. adenoma
    h. bile duct carcinoma
    h. carcinoma (HCC)
    h. jaundice
hepatocholangitis
hepatocuprein
Hepatocystis
hepatocyte
    foamy degeneration of h.'s
hepatogenic
hepatogenous
    h. jaundice
    h. pigment
hepatohemia
hepatoid
hepatojugular reflux
hepatolenticular
    h. degeneration
    h. disease
hepatolienomegaly
hepatolith
hepatolithiasis
hepatolysin
hepatoma
    malignant h.
hepatomalacia
hepatomegalia
hepatomegaly
hepatomelanosis
hepatonecrosis
hepatonephromegaly
hepatoperitonitis
hepatophosphorylase deficiency
  glycogenosis
hepatophyma
hepatopleural fistula
hepatoptosis
hepatorenal
    h. glycogenosis
    h. glycogen storage disease
    h. syndrome
hepatorrhexis
hepatosplenitis
hepatosplenomegaly
hepatotoxemia
hepatotoxic
hepatotoxicity
hepatotoxin
Hepatozoon
heptabarbital
heptachlor epoxide

heptane
HER-2
    HER-2 gene
    HER-2 protein
herald patch
herbicide
    chlorophenoxy h.
herd
    h. immunity
hereditary
    h. adynamia
    h. angioneurotic edema (HANE)
    h. benign intraepithelial dyskeratosis
    h. clubbing
    h. coproporphyria (HCP)
    h. deforming chondrodysplasia
    h. deforming chondrodystrophy
    h. disease
    h. elliptocytosis (HE)
    h. enzymatic-type
    methemoglobinemia
    h. erythroblastic multinuclearity
    h. erythroblastic multinuclearity
    with a positive acidified serum
    h. erythrocytic multinuclearity with
    positive acidified serum
    (HEMPAS)
    h. fructose intolerance (HFI)
    h. hemolytic anemia (HHA)
    h. hemorrhagic telangiectasia (HHT)
    h. hemorrhagic thrombasthenia
    h. hypersegmentation of neutrophils
    h. lymphedema
    h. methemoglobinemic cyanosis
    h. multiple exostoses
    h. multiple trichoepithelioma
    h. nephritis (HN)
    h. nonhemolytic bilirubinemia
    h. nonspherocytic hemolytic anemia
    (HNSHA)
    h. osteo-onychodysplasia (HOOD)
    h. persistence of fetal hemoglobin
    (HPFH)
    h. plasmathromboplastin component
    deficiency
    h. progressive arthro-ophthalmopathy
    h. renal-retinal dysplasia
    h. sensory radicular neuropathy
    h. spherocytosis (HS)
heredity
    autosomal h.
    sex-linked h.
    X-linked h.
heredodegenerative disease
heredopathia atactia polyneuritiformis
  (HAP)
Herlitz syndrome
Hermann fixative

Hermansky-Pudlak syndrome
hermaphrodism
hermaphroditism
Hermetia
    H. illucens
hermetic seal
HER-2/neu
    HER-2/neu gene
    HER-2/neu oncogene
    HER-2/neu protein
hernia
    cerebral h.
    diaphragmatic h.
    epigastric h.
    esophageal h.
    femoral h.
    hiatal h.
    incarcerated h.
    inguinal h.
    irreducible h.
    meningeal h.
    Morgagni h.
    peritoneal h.
    retrocolic h.
    retrosternal h.
    Richter h.
    strangulated h.
    umbilical h.
hernial aneurysm
herniated
    h. disk syndrome (HDS)
    h. nucleus pulposus (HNP)
herniation
    cerebral h.
herniorrhaphy
heroin
herpangina
    h. virus
herpes
    h. B encephalomyelitis
    h. catarrhalis
    h. corneae
    h. cytology
    h. desquamans
    h. digitalis
    h. facialis
    h. febrilis
    h. generalisatus
    h. genitalis
    h. gestationis
    h. gladiatorum
    h. iris

    h. labialis
    neonatal h.
    h. progenitalis
    h. simplex (HS)
    h. simplex antibody
    h. simplex encephalitis
    h. simplex virus (HSV)
    h. simplex virus culture
    h. simplex virus I (HSV-I)
    h. simplex virus II (HSV-II)
    h. simplex virus isolation
    traumatic h.
    h. virus
    h. whitlow
    h. zoster
    h. zoster ophthalmicus
    h. zoster varicellosus
    h. zoster virus
herpes-like virus (HLV)
herpes-type virus (HTV)
Herpesviridae
Herpesvirus (HV)
    H. hominis (HVH)
herpesvirus (HV)
    h. antigen
    canine h.
    caprine h.
    human h. (HHV)
    human h. 1, 2, 3, 4, 5, 6, 7
    suid h.
herpetic
    h. fever
    h. gingivostomatitis
    h. keratitis
    h. keratoconjunctivitis
    h. meningoencephalitis
    h. paronychia
    h. stomatitis
    h. ulcer
    h. viral disease
    h. whitlow
Herpetomonas
    H. donovani
    H. furunculosa
    H. tropica
Herpetoviridae
herpetovirus
    canine h.
    caprine h.
Herring body
herringbone
herring-worm disease

NOTES

H

Herrmann syndrome
Hers disease
Herter disease
Herter-Heubner disease
hertz (Hz)
Herxheimer
    H. reaction
    H. spiral
HET
   helium equilibration time
hetastarch
heterakid
Heterakis
heterauxesis
heterecious
heterecism
heteroagglutination
heteroagglutinin
    hemolymph h.
heteroallele
heteroantibody
heteroantigen
heteroantiserum
heteroatom
Heterobilharzia
heteroblastic
heterobrachial inversion
heterochromatic
heterochromatin
    constitutive h.
    facultative h.
heterochromatinization
heterochromia
heterochromic iridocyclitis
heterochromous
heterochthonous
heterocycle
heterocyclic compound
heterocytotropic
    h. antibody
Heterodera
    H. radicicola
heterodermic
heterodimer
Heterodoxus spiniger
heteroduplex
heterodyne
heterofermentation
heterogametic sex
heterogamy
heterogeneic antigen
heterogeneity
heterogeneous
    h. nuclear RNA (hnRNA)
    h. nucleation
heterogenetic
    h. antibody
    h. antigen

heterogenic
    h. enterobacterial antigen
heterogenote
heterogenous
    h. nuclear RNA
    h. vaccine
heterogony
heterograft
heterokaryon
heterokaryotic twins
heterokeratoplasty
heterolactic
heterologous
    h. antiserum
    h. bone
    h. chimera
    h. desensitization
    h. graft
    h. hemagglutinin
    h. protein
    h. serotype
    h. serum
    h. tumor
heterology
heterolysin
heterolysis
heterolysosome
heterolytic
    h. cleavage
heteromastigote
heterometabolous
heterometaplasia
heteromorphic
    h. bivalent
    h. chromosome
hetero-osteoplasty
heteropathy
heterophagic vacuole
heterophagosome
heterophagy
heterophil
    h. agglutinin
    h. antibody
    h. antibody test
    h. antigen
    h. antigen reaction
    h. hemolysin
heterophilic leukocyte
Heterophyes
    H. heterophyes
    H. katsuradai
heterophyiasis
heterophyid
Heterophyidae
heterophyidiasis
heteroplasia
heteroplastic
    h. graft

heteroplastid
heteroplasty
heteroploid
heteroploidy
heteropolymer
heteropolysaccharide
heteropyknotic chromatin
heteroscedasticity
heterosis
heterosomal aberration
heterosome
heterospecific
    h. graft
heterotaxia
    cardiac h.
heterotaxic
heterotaxis
heterotaxy
heterothallic
heterothallism
heterotopia
heterotopic
    h. transplantation
heterotopous
heterotransplantation
heterotroph
heterotrophic
    h. bacterium
heterovaccine therapy
heteroxenous
heterozygosity
heterozygote
    manifesting h.
heterozygous
    h. hemoglobinopathy
    h. thalassemia
    h. type of hemoglobin disorder
Heublein method
Heubner disease
heuristic
    h. method
HEV
    hepatitis E virus
hexacanth
hexachloride
    benzene h. (BHC)
hexachlorobenzene
1,2,3,4,5,6-hexachlorocyclohexane
hexachlorophene assay
hexadecimal
Hexadnovirus

hexafluorosilicate
    sodium h.
hexamer
hexamethonium bromide
hexamethylenetetramine
hexamethylpararosanilin
hexamethyl violet
Hexamita
hexamitiasis
hexane
hexanoic acid
hexaphosphate
    inositol h.
Hexapoda
hexavalent
hexazonium salts
hexokinase method
hexon
    h. antigen
hexosamine
hexosaminidase
    h. A.
hexose
    h. diphosphate
    h. monophosphate (HMP)
    h. monophosphate pathway (HMP)
    h. monophosphate shunt (HMPS)
hexose-1-phosphate uridyltransferase
hexosephosphate
    h. dehydrogenase
    h. isomerase
hexosephosphoric esters
hexoside
    ceramide h.
hexuronate
hexuronic acid
HF
    Hageman factor
    heart failure
    hemorrhagic fever
    high flow
    high frequency
HFI
    hereditary fructose intolerance
Hfr
    high-frequency recombination
    Hfr mutant
HFR strain
Hg, Hgb
    hemoglobin
    mercury

NOTES

H

HGA
homogentisic acid
HGF
hyperglycemic-glycogenolytic factor
hGG
human gammaglobulin
hGH
human growth hormone
HGPRT
hypoxanthine guanine phosphoribosyl transferase
HHA
hereditary hemolytic anemia
HHb
un-ionized hemoglobin
HHD
hypertensive heart disease
HHF-35
muscle-specific actin
HHF-35 stain
HHLL
histocytoid hemangioma-like lesion
HHT
hereditary hemorrhagic telangiectasia
HHV
human herpesvirus
HI
hemagglutination inhibition
HIA
hemagglutination-inhibition antibody
hiatal hernia
hiatus
h. hernia
hibernoma
Hicks-Pitney thromboplastin generation test
hidebound disease
hidradenitis
h. axillaris of Verneuil
h. suppurativa
hidradenoma
clear cell h.
nodular h.
papillary h.
hidroa
hidrocystoma
apocrine h.
hidrosadenitis
hidrotic ectodermal dysplasia
high
h. birth weight (HBW)
h. dosage (HD)
h. dose tolerance
h. eyepoint eyepiece
h. flow (HF)
h. frequency (HF)
h. frequency transduction
h. level

h. molecular weight (HMW)
h. molecular weight kininogen
h. power field (hpf)
h. protein (HP)
h. serum-bound iron (HBI)
h. vacuum
h. voltage
high-density
h.-d. lipoprotein (HDL, HDLP)
h.-d. lipoprotein-cholesterol (HDL-C)
high-efficiency particulate air (filter) (HEPA)
high-egg-passage vaccine
high-energy
h.-e. bond
h.-e. phosphate
higher bacteria
high-frequency
h.-f. recombination (Hfr)
h.-f. recombination mutant
high-level language
Highman
H. Congo red technique
H. method
H. method for amyloid
high-molecular-weight neutrophil chemotactic factor
high-order
high-pass filter
high-performance liquid chromatography
high-power field (HPF)
high-pressure liquid chromatography (HPLC)
high-resolution banding
high-voltage
h.-v. electrophoresis (HVE)
h.-v. transformer
Higoumenakia sign
hilar
h. cell
h. cell tumor of ovary
h. node (HN)
Hildenbrand disease
hilitis
Hill equation
hilus cell
hindrance
steric h.
Hine-Duley phantom
Hines-Bannick syndrome
Hinfl solution
hinge region
Hinton test
hip
congenital dislocation of h. (CDH)
Hippelates
Hippel disease
Hippel-Lindau disease

Hippeutis
Hippobosca
Hippoboscidae
hippocampal sclerosis
hippocratic
    h. face
    h. facies
    h. finger
hippurate broth
hippuria
hippuric
    h. acid
    h. acid excretion test
Hirschfeld disease
Hirschowitz syndrome
Hirsch-Peiffer stain
Hirschsprung disease (HD)
hirsutism
    amenorrhea and h. (AH)
hirud
hirudin
Hirudinea
hirudiniasis
hirudinization
Hirudo
    H. aegyptiaca
    H. medicinalis
His disease
Hiss stain
histadyl
Histalog test
histamine
    h. flare test
    h. liberator
    h. shock
histaminemia
histamine-releasing factor
histaminuria
histidase
histidinase
histidine
    h. alpha deaminase
    analog of h. (AHH)
    h. α-deaminase
    h. decarboxylase (HDC)
histidinemia
histidinuria
histiocyte
    cardiac h.
    facultative h.
    foamy h.
    gargoylism type of h.

    Gaucher type of h.
    Hand-Schüller-Christian type of h.
    Niemann-Pick type of h.
    phagocytic h.
    sea-blue h.
histiocytic
    h. granuloma
    h. leukemia
    h. lymphoma (HL)
    h. medullary reticulosis
histiocytoid carcinoma
histiocytoma
    atypical fibrous h.
    fibrous h.
    generalized eruptive h.
    malignant fibrous h. (MFH)
    malignant fibrous h. (MFH)
histiocytosis
    kerasin h.
    kerasin-type h.
    Langerhans cell h.
    lipid h.
    localized h.
    malignant h.
    nodular non-X h.
    nonlipid h.
    phosphatid h.
    phosphatid-type h.
    regressing atypical h.
    sinus h. (SH)
    sinus h. with massive
      lymphadenopathy (SHML)
    systemic h.
    h. X
    h. Y
histioid
histioma
histochemical stain
histochemistry
Histoclad
Histoclear slide processing solution
histocompatibility
    h. complex
    h. gene
    h. locus (HL)
    h. testing
histocompatibility antigen
    major h. a.
    minor h. a.
histoculture drug response assay
    (HDRA assay)

NOTES

H

histocyte
histocytoid hemangioma-like lesion
  (HHLL)
histocytosis
histodifferentiation
Histofine staining method
histofluorescence
histogenesis
histogram mode
histoid
   h. leprosy
   h. neoplasm
   h. tumor
histoincompatibility
histologic
   h. grading
   h. lesion
   h. staining
   h. technician
histologist
histology
   pathologic h.
histolysis
histolytic
histoma
histometaplastic
Histomonas meleagridis
histomoniasis
histomorphology
histone
histonuria
histopathogenesis
histopathology
Histoplasma
   H. antibody assay
   H. capsulatum
   H. farciminosus
histoplasmin
histoplasmin-latex test
histoplasmoma
histoplasmosis
   African h.
   h. serology
historadiography
history
   case h.
   heart disease h. (HDH)
histotechnologist
histotechnology
histotope
histotoxic
   h. anoxia
   h. hypoxia
histotropic
histozoic
His-Werner disease
HIT
   hemagglutination-inhibition test

   heparin-induced thrombocytopenia
   hypertrophic infiltrative tendinitis
Hitachi 704 analyzer
hitchhiker thumb
HIV
   human immunodeficiency virus
   HIV culture
   HIV encephalopathy
   HIV I serology
HIV-1
HIV-2
HIVAGEN test
HIV-antibody test
hives
   giant h.
HJ
   Howell-Jolly body
Hjärre disease
HK
   heat killed
HKLM
   heat-killed *Listeria monocytogenes*
HL
   histiocytic lymphoma
   histocompatibility locus
   hypermetropia, latent
HLA
   human leukocyte antigen
   HLA antigen
   HLA complex
   HLA typing
HLA-B27
HLA-D antigen
HLA-DR antigen
HLA-type II antigen
HLDH
   heat-stable lactic dehydrogenase
hLH
   human luteinizing hormone
hLT
   human lymphocyte transformation
HLV
   herpes-like virus
HM
   hydatidiform mole
Hm
   manifest hyperopia
HMB-45
   H. antibody
   H. antigen
   H. marker
HMD
   hyaline membrane disease
HMG
   human menopausal gonadotropin
   hydroxymethylglutaryl
HML
   human milk lysozyme

HMO
hypothetical mean organism
HMP
hexose monophosphate
hexose monophosphate pathway
HMPS
hexose monophosphate shunt
HMS
hypothetical mean strain
HMSAS
hypertrophic muscular subaortic stenosis
HMW
high molecular weight
HN
hereditary nephritis
hilar node
HNP
herniated nucleus pulposus
hnRNA
heterogeneous nuclear RNA
HNSHA
hereditary nonspherocytic hemolytic
anemia
Ho antigen
hobnail
h. cell
h. liver
Hoboken
H. gemmule
H. nodule
HOC
hydroxycorticoid
hock disease
HOCM
hypertrophic obstructive cardiomyopathy
Hodara disease
Hodgkin
H. disease (HD)
H. granuloma
H. lymphoma
H. sarcoma
Hodgson disease
HOECHST 33258
Hofbauer cell
Hoffa disease
Hoffman
H. test
H. violet
Hoffmann-Werdnig syndrome
Hofmann bacillus
Hofmeister test

hog
h. cholera
h. cholera serum
h. cholera vaccine
h. cholera virus
Hogben test
holandric
h. gene
h. inheritance
holarthritic
holarthritis
holgynic gene
Hollander test
Hollenhorst plaque
Hollerith code
hollow cathode lamp
Holmes
H. alkaline buffer
H. method
H. stain
Holmes-Adie syndrome
holmium
holoacardius
h. acephalus
h. acormus
h. amorphus
holocord
holocrine
holoendemic disease
holoenzyme
hologynic inheritance
holomastigote
holometabolous
Holophyra coli
holophytic
holoprosencephaly
holorachischisis
holotelencephaly
holotrichous
holotype
holozoic
Holt-Oram syndrome
Holzer method
Holzknecht unit (H)
Homalomyia
Homén syndrome
**homeopathic symbol for decimal scale
of potencies (X)**
homeoplasia
homeoplastic
homeostasis
electrolyte balance and h.

NOTES

H

homeostasis *(continued)*
 fluid balance and h.
 immunologic h.
homeostatic
homeotherapy
Homer-Wright rosette
hominis
 Gastrodiscoides h.
 Gastrodiscus h.
 Herpesvirus h. (HVH)
 Octomitus h.
 poliovirus h.
homme rouge
homoallele
homobiotin
homobrachial inversion
homocarnosine
homochronous inheritance
homocyclic
homocysteine
 h. desulfhydrase
homocystine
homocystinemia
homocystinuria (HCU)
 h. test
homocytotrophic (HCT)
homocytotropic
 h. antibody
homofermentation
homogametic sex
homogenate
homogeneity
homogeneous immersion
homogeneously staining region
homogenize
homogenote
homogenous
 h. immersion
homogentisate
 h. dioxygenase
 h. 1,2-dioxygenase
 h. oxidase
 h. oxygenase
homogentisic
 h. acid (HGA)
 h. acid test
homogentisuria
homograft
 h. rejection
homoioplasia
homolactic
homolog, homologue
homologous
 h. antigen
 h. antiserum
 h. artificial insemination (AIH)
 h. chimera
 h. chromosome

 h. desensitization
 h. graft
 h. hemagglutinin
 h. series
 h. serotype
 h. serum
 h. serum jaundice
 h. structure
 h. tumor
homology
 h. of chains
 DNA h.
 h. of strands
homolysin
homolysis
homolytic cleavage
homomorphic bivalent
homophil
homoplastic graft
homopolymer
homoscedasticity
homosomal aberration
homothallic
homothallism
homotopic transplantation
homotransplantation
homovanillic
 h. acid (HVA)
 h. acid test
homozygote
homozygous
 h. achondroplasia
 h. hemoglobinopathy
 h. thalassemia
 h.-type hemoglobin disorder
hone
 automatic h.
honeycomb
 h. lung
 h. macula
 h. ringworm
 h. tetter
honey urine
Hong
 H. Kong foot
 H. Kong influenza
 H. Kong toe
honing
HOOD
 hereditary osteo-onychodysplasia
hood
 fume h.
 laboratory h.
hoof-and-mouth disease
Hooke law
Hooker-Forbes test
hooklets

hookworm
    American h.
    h. anemia
    h. disease
    dog h.
    European h.
    New World h.
    Old World h.
Hopkins-Cole test
Hoplopsyllus anomalus
Hoppe-Goldflam disease
Hoppe-Seyler test
hordeolum
Horie tumor classification
horizontal transmission
HORM collagen reagent
hormonal
    h. evaluation
hormone
    adaptive h.
    adenohypophyseal h.
    adipokinetic h.
    adrenocortical h. (ACH)
    adrenocorticotropic h. (ACTH)
    adrenomedullary h.
    androgenic h.
    anterior pituitary h. (APH)
    antidiuretic h. (ADH)
    anti-müllerian h. (AMH)
    Aschheim-Zondek h.
    bovine growth h. (BGH)
    chondrotropic h.
    chromaffin h.
    chromatophorotropic h.
    corpus luteum h.
    cortical h.
    h. demonstration in tissue
    diabetogenic h.
    ectopic h.
    erythropoietic h.
    estrogenic h.
    fat-mobilizing h.
    female h.
    follicle h.
    follicle-stimulating h. (FSH)
    follicle-stimulating hormone-
      releasing h. (FSH-RH)
    galactopoietic h.
    gastrointestinal h.
    glycoprotein h.
    gonadotropic h. (GTH)
    gonadotropin hormone-releasing h.

    gonadotropin-releasing h. (GnRH)
    growth h. (GH)
    growth hormone-release-inhibiting h.
      (GH-RIH)
    growth h.-releasing hormone (GH-
      RH, GRH)
    human growth h. (hGH)
    human luteinizing h. (hLH)
    human pituitary follicle-
      stimulating h. (hPFSH)
    hypophysiotropic h.
    immunoreactive human growth h.
      (IRhGH)
    inappropriate antidiuretic h. (IADH)
    inhibiting h.
    inhibitory h.
    interstitial cell-stimulating h. (ICSH)
    juvenile h.
    ketogenic h.
    lactogenic h.
    langerhansian h.
    lipolytic h.
    luteal h.
    luteinizing h. (LH)
    luteinizing hormone-releasing h.
      (LH-RH)
    luteotropic h. (LTH)
    lymphocyte-stimulating h.
    male h.
    mammotropic h. (MH)
    melanocyte-inhibiting h.
    melanocyte-stimulating h. (MSH)
    melanocyte-stimulating hormone-
      release-inhibiting h.
    melanocyte-stimulating hormone-
      releasing h.
    melanophore-stimulating h. (MSH)
    neurohypophyseal h.
    orchidic h.
    ovarian h.
    ovine lactogenic h. (OLH)
    parathyroid h. (PTH)
    peptide h.
    pituitary h.
    pituitary growth h. (PGH)
    placental h.
    posterior pituitary h.
    progestational h.
    prolactin release-inhibiting h.
    prolactin-releasing h. (PRH)
    proparathyroid h.
    prothoracicotropic h.

NOTES

H

hormone *(continued)*
    h. receptor
    releasing h. (RH)
    sex h. (SH)
    somatotropic h. (STH)
    steroid h.
    syndrome of inappropriate
      antidiuretic h. (SIADH)
    testicular h.
    thyroid-stimulating h. (TSH)
    thyrotropic h. (TTH)
    thyrotropin-releasing h. (TRH)
    TSH-releasing h.
hormone-releasing
    follicle-stimulating h.-r.
horn
    cicatricial h.
    cutaneous h.
    iliac h.
    nail h.
    sebaceous h.
    warty h.
Horner syndrome
hornification
horny
horror
    h. autotoxicus
horse
    h. antihuman thymus globulin
      (HAHTG)
    h. red blood cell (HRBC)
    h. serum (HS)
horsefly
horsepox
    h. virus
horseradish
    h. peroxidase
horseshoe
    h. fistula
    h. kidney
Hortega neuroglia stain
Horton
    H. disease
    H. syndrome
hose
    drench h.
Hospidex microtiter plate
hospital-acquired penetration contact
hospital fever
host
    accidental h.
    alternate h.
    amplifier h.
    dead-end h.
    h. defenses
    definitive h.
    intermediate h.
    h.-parasite relationship

    paratenic h.
    h. of predilection
    reservoir h.
    h. response
    transfer h.
host-parasite relationship
host-range mutation
hot
    h. abscess
    h. antigen suicide
    h. gangrene
    h. lesion
    h. nodule
Hotchkiss-McManus PAS technique
Hottentot apron
hound-dog facies
Hounsfield unit (H)
hourglass
    h. gallbladder
    h. stomach
housefly
housekeeping
Houssay
    H. animal
    H. phenomenon
    H. syndrome
Howard test
Howell
    H. prothrombin test
    H. unit
Howell-Jolly body (HJ)
Howship lacuna
HP
    high protein
hp
    haptoglobin
HPF
    heparin-precipitable fraction
    high-power field
hpf
    high power field
HPFH
    hereditary persistence of fetal
      hemoglobin
hPFSH
    human pituitary follicle-stimulating
      hormone
hPG
    human pituitary gonadotropin
hPL
    human placental lactogen
HPLC
    high-pressure liquid chromatography
HPS
    hypertrophic pyloric stenosis
HPT
    hyperparathyroidism

HPV
Haemophilus pertussis vaccine
human papillomavirus
HPVD
hypertensive pulmonary vascular disease
HPVG
hepatic portal venous gas
H.P. Wright method
HRBC
horse red blood cell
HRIG
human rabies immune globulin
HRS
Hamilton Rating Scale
HRS4 MAb immunoperoxidase stain
HS
heat-stable
heme synthetase
hereditary spherocytosis
herpes simplex
horse serum
Hurler syndrome
HSA
human serum albumin
HSU method
HSV
herpes simplex virus
HSV culture
HSV isolation
HSV-I
herpes simplex virus I
HSV-II
herpes simplex virus II
HT
hemagglutination titer
hypertension
5-HT
5-hydroxytryptamine
ht
height
H-tetanase
HTHD
hypertensive heart disease
HTLV
human T cell leukemia-lymphoma virus
HTLV-I
human T-cell lymphotropic virus type I
HTLV-I antibody
HTLV-II
human T-cell lymphotropic virus type II
HTLV-III
human T-cell lymphotropic virus type III

HTV
herpes-type virus
HU
heat unit
hemagglutinating unit
Hu antigens
Huchard disease
Hucker-Conn
H.-C. crystal violet solution
H.-C. stain
Huddleston agglutination test
**Huebener-Thomsen-Friedenreich
phenomenon**
Hüfner equation
Huhner test
hum
human
h. alpha-1 proteinase inhibitor
h. alveolar macrophage-56 (HAM-56)
h. antihemophilic factor
h. chorionic gonadotropin (hCG)
h. chorionic gonadotropin injection test
h. chorionic somatomammotropin (hCS, hCSM)
h. diploid cell rabies vaccine (HDCV)
h. embryo kidney (HEK)
h. embryo lung (HEL)
h. embryonic kidney (HEK)
h. engineering
h. enteric (virus) (HE)
h. erythrocyte agglutination test (HEAT)
h. flea
h. gammaglobulin (hGG)
h. gamma globulin
h. growth hormone (hGH)
h. herpesvirus (HHV)
h. herpesvirus 1, 2, 3, 4, 5, 6, 7
h. immunodeficiency virus (HIV)
h. immunodeficiency virus culture
h. leukemia-associated antigen
h. leukocyte antigen (HLA)
h. luteinizing hormone (hLH)
h. lymphocyte antigen
h. lymphocyte transformation (hLT)
h. lymphoproliferative diseases
h. measles immune serum
h. menopausal gonadotropin (HMG)
h. milk lysozyme (HML)

NOTES

H

human (*continued*)
   h. normal immunoglobulin
   h. papilloma virus
   h. papillomavirus (HPV)
   h. papillomavirus DNA probe test
   h. pertussis immune serum
   h. pituitary follicle-stimulating
     hormone (hPFSH)
   h. pituitary gonadotropin (hPG)
   h. placental lactogen (hPL)
   h. α_1-proteinase inhibitor
   h. rabies immune globulin (HRIG)
   h. scarlet fever immune serum
   h. serum albumin (HSA)
   h. T cell leukemia-lymphoma virus
     (HTLV)
   h. T-cell lymphoma/leukemia virus
   h. T-cell lymphotropic virus
   h. T-cell lymphotropic virus type I
     (HTLV-I)
   h. T-cell lymphotropic virus type
     II (HTLV-II)
   h. T-cell lymphotropic virus type
     III (HTLV-III)
   h. thymus antiserum (HUTHAS)
   h. T lymphotrophic virus
   h. tubercle bacillus
HUMARA
   X-linked human androgen receptor
humectant
humor, pl. **humores**
   aqueous h.
   plasmoid h.
   vitreous h.
humoral
   h. immunity
   h. pathology
   h. thymic factor (THF)
Hünermann syndrome
Hunner
   H. cystitis
   H. stricture
   H. ulcer
Hunt
   H. disease
   H. and Hess hand fracture
   H. syndrome
Hunter
   H. glossitis
   H. syndrome
Hunter-Hurler syndrome
Hunter-Schreger line
Huntington
   H. chorea (HC)
   H. disease
Hurler
   H. disease
   H. syndrome (HS)

hurloid facies
Hürthle
   H. cell
   H. cell adenocarcinoma
   H. cell adenoma
   H. cell carcinoma
   H. cell metaplasia
   H. cell tumor
HUS
   hemolytic-uremic syndrome
   hyaluronidase unit for semen
Hutchinson
   H. melanotic freckle
   H. triad
Hutchinson-Boeck disease
Hutchinson-Gilford
   H.-G. disease
   H.-G. syndrome
Hutchison syndrome
HUTHAS
   human thymus antiserum
Hutinel disease
huygenian eyepiece
HV
   Herpesvirus
   herpesvirus
HVA
   homovanillic acid
   HVA test
HVD
   hypertensive vascular disease
HVE
   high-voltage electrophoresis
HVH
   Herpesvirus hominis
HVL
   half-value layer
HVSD
   hydrogen-detected ventricular septal
     defect
hyalin
   alcoholic h.
   hematogenous h.
hyaline
   alcoholic h.
   h. arteriolosclerosis
   h. body
   h. capsule
   h. cast (HC)
   h. cell
   h. core
   h. degeneration
   h. globule
   h. leukocyte
   Mallory h.
   h. membrane
   h. membrane disease (HMD)

h. membrane disease of the newborn
h. necrosis
h. nephrosclerosis
h. perisplenitis
h. sclerosis
h. thickening
h. thrombus
h. tubercle
h. urinary cast
hyalinization
hyalinized stroma
hyalinizing clear cell carcinoma (HCCC)
hyalinosis
systemic h.
hyalinuria
hyalohyphomycosis
hyaloid
hyalomere
Hyalomma
H. variegatum
hyaloplasm
hyaloplasmic
hyaloserositis
hyalosome
hyaluronate
hyaluronic acid
hyaluronidase
h. digestion
h. unit for semen (HUS)
hyaluronoglucosaminidase
hyaluronoglucuronidase
H-Y antigen
Hybond-N-filter
Hybond N+ nylon membrane
hybrid
h. cell
h. orbital
SV40-adenovirus h.
hybridization
cellular h.
competition h.
cross h.
DNA h.
DNA-DNA h.
DNA-RNA h.
filter h.
fluorescence in situ h. (FISH)
genotypic blot h.
liquid (solution) h.
RNA-driven h.

RNA-RNA h.
saturation h.
in situ h. (ISH)
solution h.
hybridoma
Hybritech PSA determination system
hydantoin
hydatid
alveolar h.
alveolar h. disease
h. cyst
h. degeneration
h. disease (HD)
h. mole
h. of Morgagni
osseous h.
h. polyp
h. rash
sessile h.
unilocular h.
Virchow h.
hydatidiform
h. mole (HM)
hydatidocele
hydatidoma
hydatidosis
hydatiduria
Hydatigera
H. infantis
H. taeniaeformis
Hyde disease
hydradenitis
hydradenoma
hydralazine lupus
hydranencephaly
hydrargyromania
hydrarthrosis
hydratase
aconitate h.
fumarate h.
hydrate
chloral h.
hydrated alumina
hydration
hydrazide
isonicotinic acid h. (INH)
hydrazine
α-h.
h. yellow
hydrazine-sensitive factor
hydremia
hydrencephalocele

NOTES

H

hydrencephalomeningocele
hydrencephalus
hydride
hydroa
   h. aestivale
   h. febrile
   h. vesiculosum
hydroappendix
hydrocalycosis
hydrocarbon
   alicyclic h.
   aliphatic saturated h.
   aliphatic unsaturated h.
   aromatic h.
   carcinogenic h.
   cyclic h.
   saturated h.
   unsaturated h.
hydrocele
   h. sac
   h. spinalis
hydrocephalic
hydrocephalocele
hydrocephaloid
   h. disease
hydrocephalus
   communicating h.
   noncommunicating h.
hydrochloric acid
hydrochloride
   adiphenine h.
   5-aminoacridine h.
   9-aminoacridine h.
   arginine h.
   chloroguanide h.
   colestipol h.
   cyproheptadine h.
   diphenhydramine h.
   ethoxazene h.
   hydromorphone h.
   meperidine h.
   phenazopyridine h.
   prazosin h.
   procaine h.
   quinacrine h.
   semicarbazide h.
hydrochlorothiazide (HCT)
hydrocholecystis
hydrocholeresis
hydrocholeretic
hydrocirsocele
hydrocortisone
   h. (compound F) (F)
hydrocyanic acid
hydrocyst
hydrocystoma
hydrocytosis
hydroencephalocele

hydrofluoric acid
hydrogen
   h. acceptor
   h. bacterium
   h. bond
   h. chloride
   h. cyanide
   h. electrode
   h. exponent
   h. fluoride
   h. ion
   h. ion concentration (pH)
   h. peroxide
   h. peroxide solution
   h. sulfide
hydrogenase
hydrogenate
hydrogenation
hydrogen-detected ventricular septal
   defect (HVSD)
hydrogenolysis
hydrolase
   acetyl-CoA h.
   acid h.
   aminoacyl-tRNA h.
   aryl-ester h.
   phosphoric monoester h.
hydro-lyase
hydrolysate
   casein h.
   lactalbumin h. (LAH)
   protein h.
hydrolysis
hydrolytic enzyme
hydrolyze
hydroma
hydromeningocele
hydrometer scale
hydromicrocephaly
hydromorphone hydrochloride
hydromphalus
hydromyelia
hydromyelocele
hydromyoma
hydronephrosis
hydronephrotic
hydronium ion
hydropericardium
hydroperitoneum
hydroperitonia
hydroperoxide
hydrophilic gel
hydrophobia
hydrophobic
   h. gel
hydrophthalmos
hydropic
   h. degeneration

hydropneumatosis
hydropneumopericardium
hydropneumoperitoneum
hydropneumothorax
hydrops
    h. abdominis
    h. amnii
    h. articuli
    cochlear h.
    endolymphatic h.
    h. fetalis
    h. folliculi
    gallbladder h.
    immune fetal h.
    labyrinthine h.
    nonimmune fetal h.
    h. tubae profluens
hydropyonephrosis
hydroquinone
hydrorchis
hydrosalpinx
hydrosarca
hydrosarcocele
hydrostatic
hydrosyringomyelia
Hydrotaea
hydrotaxis
hydrothionemia
hydrothionuria
hydrothorax
    chylous h.
hydrotropism
hydrotympanum
hydroureter
hydroxide
    aluminum h.
    h. ion
    potassium h. (KOH)
hydroxyapatite
hydroxybenzene
hydroxybutyrate
    β-h. (BHBA)
    beta h.
    3-h. dehydrogenase
hydroxybutyric test
hydroxycholecalciferol (HCC)
hydroxycorticoid (HC, HOC)
hydroxycorticosteroid
    17-hydroxycorticosteroid test
17-hydroxycorticosteroid
    17-h. assay
17-hydroxycorticosterone

18-hydroxycorticosterone
hydroxyethyl starch
5-hydroxyindoleacetic
    5-h. acid
    5-h. acid assay
    5-h. test
hydroxyketone dye
hydroxyl
    h. concentration (pOH)
    h. group
hydroxylase
    phenylalanine h.
    proline h.
    pyroglutamate h.
hydroxymethylglutaryl (HMG)
p-**hydroxyphenylpyruvate**
    p-h. dioxygenase
    p-h. oxidase
hydroxyphenyluria
hydroxyprogesterone
    17 alpha h.
17-hydroxyprogesterone (17-OHP)
    17-h. test
17α-hydroxyprogesterone
hydroxyproline
    h. assay
    h. index
    h. oxidase
hydroxyprolinemia
hydroxyprolinuria
hydroxystilbamidine isethionate
5-hydroxytryptamine (5-HT)
hydroxytryptophan decarboxylase
hydroxyurea
25-hydroxyvitamin D assay
Hydrozoa
hygienic laboratory coefficient
hygroma, pl. hygromata
    h. axillare
    cervical h.
    h. colli cysticum
    cystic h.
    subdural h.
hygrometer
hygrophilous
hygroscopic
Hylemyia
hylic
    h. tumor
hyloma
    mesenchymal h.
    mesothelial h.

NOTES

hymen
    imperforate h.
hymenal tag
hymenolepiasis
hymenolepidid
Hymenolepididae
Hymenolepis
    H. diminuta
    H. nana
Hymenomycetes
Hymenoptera
Hymorphan
Hyostrongylus rubidus
hypalbuminemia
Hypaque
hypazoturia
hyperacanthosis
hyperacidity
hyperacute rejection
hyperadenosis
hyperadiposis
hyperadiposity
hyperadrenalism
hyperadrenocorticism
hyper-β-alaninemia
hyper-β-alaninemia
hyperalbuminemia
hyperalbuminosa
    polyemia h.
hyperaldosteronemia
hyperaldosteronism
    primary h.
    secondary h.
hyperallantoinuria
hyperalphaglobulinemia
hyperaminoacidemia
hyperaminoaciduria
hyperammonemia
    h. I, II
hyperamylasemia
hyperamylasuria
hyperbaric chamber
hyperbeta-alaninemia
hyperbetaglobulinemia
hyperbetalipoproteinemia
hyperbilirubinemia
    conjugated h., type III
    constitutional h.
    h. I, II
hyperbilirubinuria
    obstructive h.
hyperbola
hyperbradykinism
hypercalcemia
    familial hypocalciuric h.
    idiopathic infantile h.
    idiopathic h. of infants

hypercalcemic
    h. sarcoidosis
    h. uremia
hypercalcinuria
hypercalcitoninemia
hypercalcitoninism
hypercalciuria
    idiopathic h. (IHC)
hypercalcuria
hypercapnia
hypercapnic
    h. acidosis
    h. encephalopathy
hypercarbia
hypercardia
hypercellular
hypercellularity
hyperchloremia
hyperchloremic
hyperchlorhydria
hyperchloruria
hypercholesteremia
hypercholesterinemia
hypercholesterolemia
    essential h.
    familial h.
hypercholesterolia
hypercholia
hyperchromasia
    nuclear h.
hyperchromatic
    h. anemia
    h. macrocythemia
    h. nuclei
hyperchromatism
hyperchromemia
hyperchromia
    macrocytic h.
hyperchromic
    h. anemia
    h. shift
hyperchylomicronemia
hypercoagulability
hypercoagulable
    h. state
    h. state coagulation screen
hypercorticism
hypercorticosolism
hypercortisolism
hypercupremia
hypercupruria
hypercyanotic
hypercythemia
hypercytochromia
hypercytosis
hyperdiploid
hyperdistention
hyperdiuresis

hyperechoic
hyperelastosis cutis
hyperemesis
    h. gravidarum
hyperemia
    peristatic h.
    rat ovarian h. (ROH)
    reactive h. (RH)
hyperemic
hyperendemic disease
hypereosinophilia
hypereosinophilic syndrome
hyperergia
hyperergic
    h. encephalitis
hypererythrocythemia
hyperesthetic zone
hyperestrogenism
hyperferremia
hyperfibrinogenemia
hyperfibrinolysis
hyperflexion
hypergammaglobulinemia
    monoclonal h.
    polyclonal h.
hyperganglionosis
hypergastrinemia
hypergenesis
hypergenetic
hypergenitalism
hypergia
hypergic
hyperglobulia
hyperglobulinemia
hyperglobulinemic purpura
hyperglobulism
hyperglycemia
    nonketotic h.
hyperglycemic
hyperglycemic-glycogenolytic factor
  (HGF)
hyperglyceridemia
    endogenous h.
    exogenous h.
hyperglycinemia
    ketotic h.
    nonketotic h.
hyperglycinuria
hyperglycosemia
hyperglycosuria
hyperglyoxylemia
hypergonadism

hypergonadotropic
hypergranulosis
hyperguanidinemia
hyperhemoglobinemia
hyperheparinemia
hyperhydropexis
hyperhydropexy
hyper-IgE syndrome
hyperimmune
    h. serum
hyperimmunity
hyperimmunization
hyperimmunoglobulin
    h. E syndrome
    h. M syndrome
hyperimmunoglobulinemia
hyperindicanemia
hyperinfection
hyperinosemia
hyperinosis
hyperinsulinemia
hyperinsulinism
hyperirritability
hyperisotonic
hyperkalemia
hyperkaliemia
hyperkaluresis
hyperkaluria
hyperkeratinization
hyperkeratomycosis
hyperkeratosis
    h. congenita
    h. eccentrica
    epidermolytic h.
    h. figurata centrifuga atrophica
    h. filiform
    h. follicularis et parafollicularis
    h. lenticularis perstans
    h. penetrans
hyperkeratotic papilloma
hyperketonemia
hyperketonuria
hyperkinesis
hyperleukocytosis
hyperlipemia
hyperlipidemia
    carbohydrate-induced h.
    endogenous h. (EHL)
    fat-induced h.
hyperlipoidemia
hyperlipoproteinemia
hyperliposis

NOTES

H

hyperlithuria
hyperlucency
    h. of bone
hyperlucent lung
hyperlysinemia
    h. type I
    h. type II
hyperlysinuria
hypermagnesemia
hypermature
hypermelanosis
hypermenorrhea
hypermetropia (H)
    h., latent (HL)
hypermobility
hypermyotrophy
hypernatremia
hypernatremic encephalopathy
hyperneocytosis
hypernephroid
hypernephroma
hyperoncotic
hyperonychia
hyperopia
    manifest h. (Hm)
hyperorchidism
hyperornithinemia
hyperorthocytosis
hyperorthokeratosis
hyperosmolality
hyperosmolar diabetic coma
hyperosmolarity
hyperosmotic
    nonketotic h. (NKH)
hyperostosis
    h. corticalis deformans
    h. corticalis deformans juvenilis
    h. corticalis generalisata
    flowing h.
    h. frontalis interna
    generalized cortical h.
    infantile cortical h.
    streak h.
hyperostotic spondylosis
hyperoxaluria
hyperparakeratosis
hyperparasite
hyperparasitism
hyperparathyroidism (HPT)
    primary h. (PHP)
hyperperistalsis
    ureteral h.
hyperphenylalaninemia
hyperphosphatasemia
hyperphosphatasia
hyperphosphatemia
hyperphosphaturia
hyperpigmentation

hyperpituitarism
    postpubertal h.
    prepubertal h.
hyperplasia
    adenomatous h.
    adrenal cortical h.
    alveolar pneumocyte h.
    angiofollicular mediastinal lymph
      node h.
    angiolymphoid h. with eosinophilia
    atypical adenomatous h. (AAH)
    atypical melanocytic h.
    basal cell h.
    basophilic h.
    benign giant lymph node h.
    benign mediastinal lymph node h.
    benign prostatic h.
    capsular synovial-like h. (CSH)
    C-cell h.
    congenital adrenal h. (CAH)
    congenital sebaceous h.
    cortical stromal h. (CSH)
    cutaneous lymphoid h. (CLH)
    cystic h.
    cystic h. of the breast
    cystic endometrial h.
    diffuse h.
    ductal h.
    endometrial h.
    enterochromaffin-cell h. (EC)
    enterochromaffin-like-cell h.
    eosinophilic h.
    erythroid h.
    fibromuscular h.
    focal h.
    follicular h. (FH)
    foveolar h.
    glandular h.
    granulocytic h.
    hematopoietic h.
    intracystic h.
    intraductal h.
    intravascular papillary endothelial h.
    Leydig cell h.
    lipomelanotic reticuloendothelial
      cell h.
    lymphoid h.
    mast cell h.
    megakaryocytic h.
    microglandular h. (MGH, mgh)
    myeloid h.
    myointimal h.
    neuronal h.
    neutrophilic h.
    nodular mesothelial h.
    nodular h. of prostate
    nodular regenerative h.
    papillar villous h.

papillary h.
plasma cell h.
polypoid h.
postatrophic h. (PAH)
primary h.
pseudoangiomatous stromal h.
  (PASH)
pseudocarcinomatous h.
pseudoepitheliomatous h.
pulmonary lymphoid h. (PLH)
reactive follicular h.
reserve cell h.
reticuloendothelial cell h.
reticulum cell h.
secondary h.
senile sebaceous h.
stromal h.
Swiss cheese h.
verrucous h.
wasserhelle h.
water-clear-cell h.

hyperplasia/metaplasia
complex atypical h. (CAHM)

hyperplastic
h. arteriosclerosis
h. bone marrow
h. cholecystosis
h. goiter
h. inflammation
h. nephrosclerosis
h. nodular goiter
h. osteoarthritis
h. polyp

hyperploid
hyperploidy
hyperpolarization
hyperpotassemia
hyperprebetalipoproteinemia
hyperproinsulinemia
hyperprolactinemia
hyperprolinemia
hyperproteinemia
hyperreninemia
hypersalemia
hypersarcosinemia
hypersecretion
hypersegmentation
hereditary h. of neutrophils
leukocytic h.

hypersegmented neutrophil
hypersensitive
hypersensitiveness

hypersensitivity
h. angiitis
contact h.
delayed h.
delayed-type h. (DTH)
immediate h.
h. pneumonitis
h. pneumonitis serology
h. reaction
tuberculin-type h.
h. vasculitis

hypersensitization
hyperserotonemia
hyperskeocytosis
hypersomia
hypersplenism
hypersplenosis
hypersthenuria
hypersusceptibility
hypertelorism
ocular h.

hypertension (HT)
arterial h. (AH)
benign intracranial h. (BIH)
diastolic h.
essential h. (EH)
Goldblatt h.
idiopathic h.
malignant h.
mineralocorticoid h.
orthostatic h.
paroxysmal h.
portal h.
primary pulmonary h. (PPH)
pulmonary h. (PII)
pulmonary artery h. (PAH)
renal h.
renovascular h.
systolic h.

hypertensive
h. arteriopathy
h. arteriosclerosis
h. arteriosclerotic heart disease
  (HASHD)
h. cardiovascular disease (HCVD)
h. encephalopathy
h. heart disease (HHD, HTHD)
h. pulmonary vascular disease
  (HPVD)
h. vascular disease (HVD)

hyperthecosis
testoid h.

NOTES

H

hyperthelia
hyperthermia
hyperthrombinemia
hyperthymic
hyperthymism
hyperthymization
hyperthyroidism
hyperthyroiditis
hyperthyroxinemia
hypertonia
    h. polycythemica
hypertonic
hypertonicity
hypertrichosis
    h. lanuginosa acquisita
    nevoid h.
hypertriglyceridemia
    familial h.
hypertrophia
hypertrophic
    h. amphophil cell
    h. arthritis
    h. cervical pachymeningitis
    h. chronic vulvitis
    h. fibrous pachymeningitis
    h. gastritis
    h. gingivitis
    h. hypersecretory gastropathy
    h. infiltrative tendinitis (HIT)
    h. interstitial neuropathy
    h. lichen planus
    h. muscular subaortic stenosis
    (HMSAS)
    h. obstructive cardiomyopathy
    (HOCM)
    h. osteoarthropathy
    h. pulmonary osteoarthropathy
    h. pyloric stenosis (HPS)
    h. scar
hypertrophy
    adaptive h.
    asymmetrical septal h. (ASH)
    asymmetric septal h.
    benign prostatic h. (BPH)
    combined ventricular h. (CVH)
    compensatory h.
    compensatory h. of the heart
    complementary h.
    concentric h.
    diffuse h.
    eccentric h.
    endemic h.
    false h.
    fibrocongestive h.
    focal h.
    functional h.
    giant h. of gastric mucosa
    giant rugal h.

    hemangiectatic h.
    idiopathic myocardial h. (IMH)
    Kupffer cell h.
    left atrial h. (LAH)
    left ventricular h. (LVH)
    lipomatous h.
    numerical h.
    physiologic h.
    prostatic h. (PH)
    quantitative h.
    right atrial h. (RAH)
    right ventricular h. (RVH)
    simple h.
    simulated h.
    true h.
    ventricular h.
    vicarious h.
hypertropic polyneuritic-type muscular
  atrophy
hypertyrosinemia
hypertyrosinemia, Oregon type
hyperuremia
hyperuresis
hyperuricemia
hyperuricemic
hyperuricosuria
hyperuricuria
hyperurobilinogenemia
hypervaccination
hypervalinemia
hypervariable region
hypervascular
hyperviscosity syndrome
hypervitaminosis
hypervolemia
hypha, pl. hyphae
    racquet h.
    spiral hyphae
hyphemia
Hyphomyces destruens
Hyphomycetes
hyphomycosis
hypnocyst
hypnotic
hypnozoite
hypoacidity
hypoadrenalism
hypoadrenocorticism
    primary h.
    secondary h.
hypoalbuminemia
hypoaldosteronism
hypoaldosteronuria
hypoalphaglobulinemia
hypoazoturia
hypobaric
hypobetalipoproteinemia
hypocalcemia

hypocalcification
hypocalciuria
hypocapnia
hypocapnic
hypocarbia
hypocellular
hypocellularity
hypochloremia
hypochloremic
    h. azotemia
hypochlorhydria
hypochlorite
hypochlorous acid
hypochloruria
hypocholesteremia
hypocholesterinemia
hypocholesterolemia
hypochondriac region
hypochondriasis
hypochondroplasia
hypochromasia
hypochromatic
hypochromatism
hypochromemia
    idiopathic h.
hypochromia
hypochromic
    h. microcytic anemia
    h. shift
hypochrosis
hypocitraturia
hypocomplementemia
hypocomplementemic glomerulonephritis
hypocorticoidism
hypocythemia
    progressive h.
hypocytosis
Hypoderma
    H. bovis
hypodermatosis
hypodermic implantation
hypodermolithiasis
hypodiploid
hypoeosinophilia
hypoestrogenism
hypoferremia
hypoferric anemia
hypofibrinogenemia
hypogaea
    Arachis h. (AH)
hypogammaglobinemia

hypogammaglobulinemia
    acquired h.
    common variable h. (CVH)
    physiologic h.
    primary h.
    secondary h.
    Swiss-type h.
    transient h.
    transient h. of infancy
    X-linked h.
    X-linked infantile h.
hypoganglionosis
hypogenesis
hypoglobulia
hypoglobulinemia
hypoglycemia
    leucine h.
    neonatal h.
hypoglycemic
    h. encephalopathy
    h. shock
hypogonadism
hypogonadotropic
hypogranulocytosis
hypohidrotic ectodermal dysplasia
hypohydremia
hypohydrochloria
hypohyloma
hypoinsulinism
hypoisotonic
hypokalemia
hypokalemic
    h. alkalosis
    h. nephropathy
    h. nephrosis
hypokaluria
hypolepidoma
hypoleukemia
hypoleydigism
hypolipoproteinemia
hypoliposis
hypolymphemia
hypomagnesemia
hypomelanosis
    h. of Ito
hyponatremia
hyponatrurla
hyponeocytosis
hypooncotic
hypoorthocytosis
hypoparathyroidism
hypopharyngeal diverticulum

NOTES

H

hypophosphatasemia
hypophosphatasia
    congenital h.
hypophosphatemia
    X-linked familial h.
hypophosphaturia
hypophysial syndrome
hypophysiopriva
    cachexia h.
hypophysio-sphenoidal syndrome
hypophysiotropic
    h. hormone
hypophysis staining procedure
hypophysitis
    lymphocytic h.
    lymphoid h.
hypopigmentation
hypopigmentation-immunodeficiency
  disease
hypopituitarism
hypoplasia
    cartilage-hair h. (CHH)
    erythroid h.
    focal dermal h.
    granulocytic h.
    hematopoietic h.
    lymphoid h.
    megakaryocytic h.
    renal h.
    right ventricular h.
    thymic h.
hypoplastic
    h. anemia
    h. bone marrow
    h. heart
hypoploid
hypoploidy
hypopotassemia
hypoproaccelerinemia
hypoproconvertinemia
hypoproteinemia
    prehepatic h.
hypoprothrombinemia
hypopyon
hyporeninemia
hyporeninemic
hyposalemia
hyposarca
hyposecretion
hyposegmentation
    leukocytic nuclear h.
hyposensitivity
hyposensitization
hyposialadenitis
hyposkeocytosis
hyposmotic
hypospadias
hyposplenism

hypostasis
    postmortem h.
    pulmonary h.
hypostatic
    h. abscess
    h. congestion
    h. ectasia
    h. pneumonia
hyposthenuria
hypostome
hypotension
    orthostatic h.
hypotensive
hypothermia
hypothesis
    alternative h.
    autocrine h.
    Benditt h.
    biogenic amine h.
    cardionector h.
    chemiosmotic h.
    Lyon h.
    omnibus h.
    proton-motive h.
    h. testing
    unitarian h.
    wobble h.
hypothetical
    h. mean organism (HMO)
    h. mean strain (HMS)
hypothrombinemia
hypothromboplastinemia
hypothyroid
hypothyroidism
hypothyroxinemia
hypotonia
    vasomotor h.
hypotonic
hypotonicity
hypotonus
hypotransferrinemia
hypotriploid
hypouricemia
hypouricuria
hypovitaminosis
hypovolemia
hypovolemic
    h. shock
hypoxanthine
    h. guanine phosphoribosyltransferase
    h. guanine phosphoribosyl
      transferase (HGPRT)
hypoxemia
hypoxia
    anemic h.
    histotoxic h.
    hypoxic h.
    ischemic h.

oxygen affinity h.
stagnant h.
hypoxic
  h. anoxia
  h. hypoxia
  h. nephrosis
hypsochrome
hypsochromic shift

hysteratresia
hysteresis
  h. loop
hysterolith
hysteromyoma
hysterotonin
Hz
  hertz

NOTES

H

I
> I antigen
> I band
> I cell
> I pilus
> I region

¹³¹I
> radioactive iodine
> ¹³¹I uptake test
> ¹³¹I uptake test

Ia antigen
IADH
> inappropriate antidiuretic hormone

IADHS
> inappropriate antidiuretic hormone
> syndrome

IAP
> International Academy of Pathology

IASD
> interatrial septal defect

IAT
> invasive activity test
> iodine-azide test

iatrogenic
> i. agent
> i. anemia

IB
> inclusion body

Ibaraki virus
IBC
> iron-binding capacity

IBF
> immunoglobulin-binding factor

IBR
> infectious bovine rhinotracheitis
> IBR virus

IBU
> international benzoate unit

IBV
> infectious bronchitis virus

IBW
> ideal body weight

IC
> intermittent claudication
> irritable colon
> isovolumic contraction

ICA
> intracranial aneurysm
> islet cell antibody

ICAM-1
> intercellular adhesion molecule-1

ICAO
> internal carotid artery occlusion

ICC
> immunocompetent cell
> Indian childhood cirrhosis

ICD
> International Classification of Diseases

ice
> i. point
> i. water calorics test

I-cell disease
ICF
> intracellular fluid

ICG
> indocyanine green
> ICG excretion test

ichorous pus
ichorrhea
ichthyoacanthotoxism
ichthyohemotoxism
ichthyosarcotoxism
ichthyosis
> acquired i.
> i. congenita
> i. congenita neonatorum
> i. fetalis
> i. hystrix
> i. intrauterina
> lamellar i.
> i. linguae
> nacreous i.
> i. palmaris et plantaris
> i. sauroderma
> i. scutulata
> i. sebacea
> i. sebacea cornea
> i. simplex
> i. spinosa
> i. uteri
> i. vulgaris
> X-linked i.

ichthyotic
ichthyotoxin
icing
> i. heart
> i. liver

icosahedral
> i. symmetry

ICSH
> International Committee for
> Standardization in Hematology
> interstitial cell-stimulating hormone

ICT
> inflammation of connective tissue
> insulin coma therapy

icteric
>   i. index
>   i. serum hepatitis (ISH)

icteroanemia

icterogenic
>   i. spirochetosis

icterohematuric

icterohemoglobinuria

icterohemolytic anemia

icterohepatitis

icteroid

icterus
>   acquired hemolytic i.
>   benign familial i.
>   chronic familial i.
>   congenital familial i.
>   congenital hemolytic i.
>   cythemolytic i.
>   i. gravis
>   i. gravis of newborn
>   i. index (ict ind)
>   i. index test
>   i. interference
>   i. melas
>   i. neonatorum
>   i. praecox

ict ind
>   icterus index

ICW
>   intracellular water

ID
>   identification
>   immunodiffusion
>   infecting dose
>   infective dose

ID$_{50}$
>   median infectious dose

IDA
>   image display and analysis
>   iron deficiency anemia

IDC
>   infiltrating ductal carcinoma
>   intraductal carcinoma

IDDM
>   insulin-dependent diabetes mellitus

ideal
>   i. body weight (IBW)
>   i. gas
>   i. gas law
>   i. solution

identical twins

identification (ID)
>   antibody i.
>   arthropod i.
>   Gram-positive i. (GPI)
>   hazard i.
>   hemoglobin i.

identifier

identity pattern

Ide test

idioagglutinin

idiocy
>   amaurotic familial i.
>   late infantile amaurotic familial i.
>   (LIAFI)

idiogram

idioheteroagglutinin

idioheterolysin

idioisoagglutinin

idioisolysin

idiolysin

idiopathic
>   i. Bamberger-Marie disease
>   i. bone cavity
>   i. cardiomyopathy
>   i. etiology
>   i. fibrous mediastinitis
>   i. fibrous retroperitonitis
>   i. generalized glycogenosis
>   i. hemosiderosis
>   i. hypercalcemia of infants
>   i. hypercalcemic sclerosis of infants
>   i. hypercalciuria (IHC)
>   i. hypertension
>   i. hypertrophic osteoarthropathy
>   (IHO)
>   i. hypertrophic subaortic stenosis
>   (IHSS)
>   i. hypochromemia
>   i. infantile hypercalcemia
>   i. megacolon
>   i. myocardial hypertrophy (IMH)
>   i. nephrotic syndrome (INS)
>   i. paroxysmal rhabdomyolysis
>   i. pauci-immune necrotizing
>   crescentic glomerulonephritis
>   i. pentosuria
>   i. pericarditis
>   i. proctitis
>   i. pulmonary fibrosis (IPF)
>   i. pulmonary hemosiderosis (IPH)
>   i. respiratory distress syndrome
>   (IRDS)
>   i. retroperitoneal fibrosis
>   i. thrombocytopenic purpura (ITP)

idiopathy
>   toxic i.

idiosyncrasy

idiosyncratic sensitivity

idiotope

idiotoxin

idiotype
>   i. antibody
>   i. autoantibody
>   set of i.'s

idiotypic antigenic determinant

iditol
    i. dehydrogenase
    i. dehydrogenase assay
IDL
    intermediate-density lipoprotein
idoxuridine (IDU)
IDR
    intradermal reaction
id reaction
IDS
    immunity deficiency state
IDU
    idoxuridine
    iododeoxyuridine
iduronic
    i. acid
    i. sulfatase
iduronidase
L-iduronidase
IE
    immunoelectrophoresis
IEOP
    immunoelectro-osmophoresis
IEP
    immunoelectrophoresis
IF
    immunofluorescence
    intrinsic factor
IFA
    indirect fluorescent antibody
IFC
    intrinsic factor concentrate
IFCC
    International Federation of Clinical
      Chemistry
IFN
    interferon
IFN-α
    interferon alpha
IFN-β
    interferon beta
IFN-γ
    interferon gamma
ifosfamide
IFRA
    indirect fluorescent rabies antibody (test)
IFV
    intracellular fluid volume
IG
    immune globulin
Ig
    immunoglobulin

IgA
    immunoglobulin A
      IgA antibodies
      IgA endomysial antibody
      IgA immunodeficiency
      IgA nephropathy
      secretory IgA
IgD
    immunoglobulin D
IgE
    immunoglobulin E
IgG
    immunoglobulin G
      IgG desmoplakin antibody
      IgG index
      IgG ratios
IGGNU
    intratubular germ cell neoplasia of the
      unclassified type
IgM
    immunoglobulin M
      IgM nephropathy
ignitability
ignition
    i. point
    i. source control
    i. temperature
IGV
    intrathoracic gas volume
IH
    infectious hepatitis
IHA
    indirect hemagglutination
IHBTD
    incompatible hemolytic blood transfusion
      disease
IHC
    idiopathic hypercalciuria
IHD
    ischemic heart disease
IHO
    idiopathic hypertrophic osteoarthropathy
IHSA
    iodinated human serum albumin
IHSS
    idiopathic hypertrophic subaortic stenosis
IIF
    indirect immunofluorescent
Ikegami videocamera
IL
    interleukin
      IL-1 through -15

NOTES

ILA
insulin-like activity
ILC
infiltrating lobular carcinoma
ILD
ischemic leg disease
ischemic limb disease
ileal
i. intussusception
i. pouch-anal anastomosis (IPAA)
ileitis
backwash i.
distal i.
regional i. (RI)
terminal i.
ileocecal intussusception
ileocolic intussusception
ileocolitis
i. ulcerosa chronica
ileojejunitis
ileum
i. duplex
duplex i.
ileus
adynamic i.
dynamic i.
gallstone i.
mechanical i.
meconium i.
paralytic i.
spastic i.
i. subparta
ureteral i.
Ilhéus
I. encephalitis
I. fever
I. virus
iliac
i. horn
i. roll
ill
louping i.
ill-defined
illness
environmental i.
respiratory i. (RI)
illuminance
illumination
critical i.
diffuse i.
Köhler i.
Ilosvay reagent
IM
infectious mononucleosis
IMAA
iodinated macroaggregated albumin
image
i. analysis

i. cytology
i. cytometry
i. display and analysis (IDA)
imaginary number
imago
imbalance
electrolyte i.
sympathetic i.
imbed
imbibition
imbricata
IMC
immunohistochemical
Imerslund-Grasbeck syndrome
IMH
idiopathic myocardial hypertrophy
imidazolepyruvic acid
imide
imine
imino acid
iminoacidopathies
iminoglycinuria
imipramine
i. and desipramine assays
immature
i. granulocyte
i. neutrophil
immediate
i. allergy
i. contagion
i. hypersensitivity
i. hypersensitivity reaction
i. principle
immersion
i. foot
homogeneous i.
homogenous i.
i. objective
oil i.
i. syndrome
water i.
immersion-submersion
imminent abortion
immiscible
immobilization
Treponema pallidum i. (TPI)
immobilized enzyme
immobilizing antibody
immortalization
immotile cilia syndrome
immotility
IMMU-MARK immunostaining kit
immune
i. adherence
i. adherence hemagglutination assay
i. adherence phenomenon
i. adhesion test
i. adsorption

i. agglutination
i. agglutinin
i. clearance
i. complex
i. complex assay
i. complex disease
i. complex disorder
i. complex glomerulonephritis
i. complex glomerulopathy
i. complex nephritis
i. complex nephropathy
i. cytolysis
i. deficiency
i. deviation
i. electron microscopy
i. elimination
i. fetal hydrops
i. globulin (IG)
i. hemolysin
i. hemolysis
i. inflammation
i. interferon
i. lactoglobulin
i. opsonin
i. paralysis
i. precipitation
i. protein
i. reaction
i. response (Ir)
i. response gene
i. serum
i. serum globulin (ISG)
i. surveillance
i. system
i. thrombocytopenia
i. thrombocytopenic purpura
immunifacient
immunity
acquired i.
active i.
adoptive i.
antiviral i.
artificial active i.
artificial passive i.
bacteriophage i.
cell-mediated i. (CMI)
cellular i.
concomitant i.
i. deficiency
i. deficiency state (IDS)
general i.
group i.

herd i.
humoral i.
infection i.
innate i.
local i.
maternal i.
natural i.
passive i.
relative i.
specific active i.
specific passive i.
i. substance
immunization
active i.
paratyphoid i.
passive i.
i. reaction poliomyelitis
smallpox i.
immunize
immunizing unit (IU)
immunoadjuvant
immunoadsorbent
immunoagglutination
immunoassay
double antibody i.
enzyme i. (EIA)
enzyme-multiplied i.
enzyme-multiplied i. technique (EMIT)
fluorescent i. (FIA)
light-scattering i.
nonradioisotopic i.
radioisotopic i.
solid phase i.
thin-layer i.
turbidimetric i.
immunobiology
immunoblast
immunoblastic
i. lymphadenopathy
i. lymphoma
i. sarcoma
immunoblot
i. test
immunoblotting
immunocatalysis
immunochemical assay
immunochemistry
immunocompetence
immunocompetent
i. cell (ICC)
immunocomplex

NOTES

immunocompromised
immunoconcentration assay
immunoconglutinin
immunocyte
immunocytoadherence
immunocytochemistry
immunodeficiency
    cellular i. with abnormal
      immunoglobulin synthesis
    combined i.
    common variable i.
    i. disease
    IgA i.
    phagocytic dysfunction disorders i.
    secondary i.
    severe combined i. (SCID)
    i. syndrome
    i. with hypoparathyroidism
immunodeficient
immunodepressant
immunodepression
immunodepressor
immunodiagnosis
immunodiffusion (ID)
    double i.
    Ouchterlony i.
    Oudin i.
    radial i. (RID)
    single i.
immunodominance
immunoelectro-osmophoresis (IEOP)
immunoelectrophoresis (IE, IEP)
    countercurrent i. (CIE)
    crossed i.
    factor VIII-crossed i.
    radio-i.
    reverse i.
    rocket i.
    two-dimensional i.
immunoenhancement
immunoenhancer
immunoenzymometric assay
immunoferritin
immunofiltration
    analytical i.
    preparative i.
immunofixation electrophoresis
immunofluorescence (IF)
    adenovirus i.
    i. method
    i. microscopy
    mixed i. (MIF)
    i. technique
    i. test
immunofluorescent
    i. assay
    indirect i. (IIF)
    i. stain

immunogen
immunogenetics
immunogenic
    i. determinant
immunogenicity
immunogenotyping
immunoglobulin (Ig)
    i. A (IgA)
    i. A, D, G, M test
    anti-D i.
    chickenpox i.
    i. class
    i. D (IgD)
    i. domains
    i. E (IgE)
    i. G (IgG)
    i. gene rearrangement
    human normal i.
    i. M (IgM)
    measles i.
    monoclonal i.
    pertussis i.
    poliomyelitis i.
    rabies i.
    $Rh_o(D)$ i.
    secretory i.
    secretory i. A
    i. subclass
    tetanus i.
    thyroid-stimulating i. (TSI)
    TSH-binding inhibitory i. (TBII)
immunoglobulin-binding factor (IBF)
immunoglobulinopathy
immunohematology
immunohistochemical (IMC)
    i. marker
    i. stain
    i. staining
    i. technique
immunohistochemistry
immunohistofluorescence
immunoincompetent
immunolabeling
    double i.
immunologic
    i. competence
    i. enhancement
    i. high dose tolerance
    i. homeostasis
    i. memory
    i. paralysis
    i. pregnancy test
    i. tolerance
    i. unresponsiveness
immunological
    i. competence
    i. deficiency
    i. enhancement

i. mechanism
i. paralysis
i. surveillance
i. tolerance
immunologically
i. activated cell
i. competent cell
i. privileged site
immunologist
immunology
immunomodulation
immunomodulator
immunomodulatory
immunomorphology
immunoparalysis
immunopathogenesis
immunopathology
immunoperoxidase
paraffin i. (PIP)
i. stain
i. staining method
i. technique
i. test
immunophenotype
immunophenotypic
i. study
immunophenotypical
immunophenotyping
leukemia i.
lymphoma i.
immunopotency
immunopotentiation
immunopotentiator
immunoprecipitation
automated i. (AIP)
immunoprofile
immunoproliferative
i. disorder
i. small intestinal disease (IPSID)
immunoprophylaxis
immunoradioassayable human chorionic somatomammotropin (IRHCS)
immunoradiometric assay (IRMA)
immunoradiometry
immunoreaction
immunoreactive (IR)
i. glucagon (IRG)
i. human growth hormone (IRhGH)
i. insulin (IRI)
immunoreactivity
immunoregulation
immunoselection

immunosenescence
immunosorbent
immunostain
TdT i.
immunostainer
Shandon Candenza i.
Techmate 1000 i.
immunostaining
immunostimulant
immunostimulation
immunosuppressant
immunosuppression
immunosuppressive
immunosurveillance
immunosympathectomy
immunotherapy
adoptive i.
biological i.
immunotolerance
immunotransfusion
impacted
i. feces
i. fracture
i. tooth
impaction
fecal i.
i. lesion
impaired clot retraction
impairment
functional aerobic i.
impalpable
impatent
impedance
electrode i.
output i.
imperfect
i. fungus
i. stage
i. state
i. yeast
imperfecta
amelogenesis i.
erythrogenesis i.
Imperfecti
Fungi I.
imperforate
i. anus
i. hymen
imperforation
impermeable
impetiginized

NOTES

impetigo
    bullous i.
    bullous i. of newborn
    i. contagiosa
    i. neonatorum
    i. vulgaris
implant
    carcinomatous i.
    silicone i.
implantation
    i. bleeding
    circumferential i.
    i. cyst
    i. dermoid
    hypodermic i.
    interstitial i.
    periosteal i.
    i. site
    superficial i.
    i. test (IT)
imprecision
impregnation
    silver i.
impression preparation
improvement
    quality i. (QI)
impulse sealing
impurity
IMR
    infant mortality rate
IMT
    inflammatory myofibroblastic tumor
IMViC tests
    indole, methyl red, Voges-Proskauer, and
    citrate test
in
    i. situ
    i. situ DNA nick end labeling
    (TUNEL)
    i. situ hybridization (ISH)
    i. vacuo
    i. vivo adhesive platelet (IVAP)
    i. vivo compatibility test
inactivate
inactivated
    i. leukocytolytic serum
    i. poliovaccine (IPV)
    i. poliovirus vaccine
inactivation
    complement i.
inactivator
    anaphylatoxin i.
inactive tuberculosis
INAD
    infantile neuroaxonal dystrophy
inanition
inapparent infection

inappropriate
    i. antidiuretic hormone (IADH)
    i. antidiuretic hormone syndrome
    (IADHS)
inborn
    i. error of metabolism
    i. lysosomal disease
inbreeding
    coefficient of i.
    i. coefficient
incarcerated
    i. hernia
inch
    pounds per square i. (p.s.i.)
incidence
    angle of i.
    i. rate
incident light
incineration
incised
    i. wound
incision
incisional biopsy
inclusion
    blennorrhea i.
    i. blennorrhea
    i. body (IB)
    i. body disease
    i. body encephalitis
    i. body fibromatosis
    i. cell
    cell i.
    i. cell disease
    i. conjunctivitis
    i. conjunctivitis virus
    i. cyst
    cytoplasmic i.
    i. dermoid
    Döhle i.
    Döhle i. body
    epidermal i. cyst
    epidermoid i. cyst
    epithelial i. cyst
    germinal epithelial i. cyst
    leukocyte i.
    viral i.
inclusive
incompatibility
    ABO i.
    chemical i.
    physiologic i.
    Rh i.
incompatible
    i. blood transfusion reaction
    i. chemicals
    i. hemolytic blood transfusion
    disease (IHBTD)

incompetence
  aortic i. (AI)
  mitral i. (MI)
  pulmonary i. (PI)
  tricuspid i. (TI)
  valvular i.
incompetent
  i. aortic valve
  i. cervix
  i. foramen ovale valve
  i. mitral valve
  i. pulmonic valve
  i. tricuspid valve
  i. valve foramen ovale
incomplete
  i. abortion
  i. agglutinin
  i. amnion
  i. amputation
  i. antibody
  i. antigen
  i. compound fracture
  i. conjoined twins
  i. differentiation (cardiac valve)
  i. dislocation
  i. dominance
  i. fistula
  i. fracture
  i. hernia
  i. neurofibromatosis
  i. penetrance
  i. regeneration
  i. right bundle-branch block
    (IRBBB)
  i. transposition
incontinence
  i. of pigment
incontinentia
  i. pigmenti
  i. pigmenti achromians
increase
  absolute cell i.
increased
  i. basal metabolism
  i. capillary fragility
  i. flow
  i. metabolism
  i. pressure
  i. specific gravity
  i. turbidity
  i. viscosity
  i. volume

increment
increta
  placenta i.
incrustation
incubate
incubation
  i. period (IP)
incubative stage
incubator
incubatory carrier
incurable
indamine dye
indenization
independence
  anchorage i.
independent
  i. assortment
  i. variable
Inderal
indeterminate
  indeterminate leprosy
  i. pattern
index, gen. and pl. **indicis**, pl. **indexes**
  absorbency i.
  acidophilic i.
  antitryptic i.
  Arneth i.
  bacteriological i. (BI)
  Broders tumor i.
  burn i. (BI)
  carbohydrate metabolism i. (CMI)
  cardiac i.
  i. case
  cephalic i.
  chemotherapeutic i. (CI)
  color i. (CI)
  Colour I. (CI)
  coronary prognostic i. (CPI)
  crowded cell i.
  degenerative i.
  development-at-birth i. (DBI)
  endemic i.
  eosinophilic i. (EI)
  eosinophilic i. (EI)
  erythrocyte indices
  folded-cell i.
  free thyroxine i. (FTI)
  hematopneic i.
  hemolytic i.
  hydroxyproline i.
  icteric i.
  icterus i. (ict ind)

NOTES

index *(continued)*
 IgG i.
 International Sensitivity I. (ISI)
 iron i.
 juxtaglomerular granulation i. (JGI)
 karyopyknotic i. (KI)
 karyopyknotic i. (KI)
 Knodell histological activity i.
 Kovats i.
 Krebs leukocyte i.
 labeling i.
 leukopenic i.
 maturation i.
 maturation i.
 metacarpal i.
 mitosis-karyorrhexis i. (MKI)
 mitotic i.
 nucleoplasmic i. (NP)
 O'Grady prognostic indices
 opsonic i.
 phagocytic i.
 phenylalanine tolerance i.
 phosphate excretion i. (PEI)
 proliferative i. (PI)
 pyknotic i.
 red cell indices
 i. of refraction
 refractive i. (RI)
 i. register
 Reid i.
 relative value i. (RVI)
 retention i.
 reticulocytic production i. (RPI)
 saturation i. (SI)
 Schilling i.
 sedimentation i.
 splenic i.
 squamous cell i.
 staphylo-opsonic i.
 steroid protein activity i. (SPAI)
 thoracic i. (TI)
 thyroxine-binding i. (TBI)
 time-tension i. (TTI)
 tuberculo-opsonic i.
 uricolytic i.
 volume i.
India
 I. ink capsule stain
 I. ink mount
 I. ink preparation
Indian
 I. childhood cirrhosis (ICC)
 I. file
 I. rat flea
indican
 metabolic i.
 plant i.
 i. test

indicanidrosis
indicanuria
indicator
 acid-base i.
 alizarin i.
 i. electrode
 i. organism
 oxidation-reduction i.
 pH i.
 redox i.
 i. system
 i. tube
indicator-dilution curve
indices
indicis (*gen. and pl. of* index)
Indiella
indifferent
 i. electrode
 i. neutrotaxis
indigenous
 i. bacterium
indigo
 i. blue
 i. calculus
 i. carmine
indigo-carmine test
indigoid dye
indigotin
indigouria
indiguria
indirect
 i. addressing
 i. agglutination
 i. assay
 i. bilirubin test
 i. Coombs test
 i. fluorescent antibody (IFA)
 i. fluorescent antibody test
 i. fluorescent rabies antibody (test) (IFRA)
 i. hemagglutination (IHA)
 i. hemagglutination test
 i. hernia
 i. immunofluorescent (IIF)
 i. maternal death
 i. reacting bilirubin
 i. transport
indiscriminate lesion
indium
indium-111
 i. chloride
 i. trichloride
Indocin
indocyanine green (ICG)
indolacetic acid
indolaceturia
indolaceturic acid

indole, methyl red, Voges-Proskauer, and citrate test (IMViC tests)
indole-nitrate broth
indolent ulcer
indole test
indollactic acid
indoluria
indomethacin
indophenol
    i. dye
    i. method
    i. test
indoxyl
    i. sulfate
indoxyluria
induced
    i. abortion
    i. allergic encephalomyelitis
    i. allergic neuritis
    i. aspermatogenesis
    i. glomerulonephritis
    i. phagocytosis
    i. sensitivity
    i. thyroiditis
    i. uveitis
inducer cell
inducible
    i. enzyme
inductance
induction
    enzyme i.
    lysogenic i.
    magnetic i.
    negative control enzyme i.
    i. period
    positive control enzyme i.
inductive
    i. phase
    i. reactance
inductor
indulin
indulinophil, indulinophile
indurated
induration
    brown i. of the lung
    cyanotic i.
    Froriep i.
    gray i.
    pigment i. of the lung
    plastic i.
    red i.

indurative
    i. myocarditis
industrial
    i. poison
    i. toxicology
INE
    infantile necrotizing encephalomyelopathy
ineffective erythropoiesis
inelastic scattering
Inermicapsifer
    I. madagascariensis
inert electrode
inertia
inevitable abortion
inf
    infusion
infancy
    chronic pneumonitis of i. (CPI)
infant
    i. death
    low birth weight i. (LBWI)
    i. mortality rate (IMR)
    premature i.
    splenic anemia of i.'s
infantile
    i. amaurotic familial idiocy
    i. celiac disease
    i. cortical hyperostosis
    i. digital fibromatosis
    i. fibrosarcoma
    i. gastroenteritis
    i. gastroenteritis virus
    i. glaucoma
    i. hemangioma
    i. muscular atrophy
    i. myofibromatosis
    i. myxedema
    i. necrotizing encephalomyelopathy (INE)
    i. neuroaxonal dystrophy (INAD)
    i. paralysis
    i. progressive spinal muscular dystrophy
    i. purulent conjunctivitis
    i. respiratory distress syndrome
    i. spasm
    i. type coarctation
    i. uterus
infantilism
    tubal i.

NOTES

infarct
    acute i.
    anemic i.
    anterior lateral myocardial i. (ALMI)
    anteroseptal myocardial i. (ASMI)
    bile i.
    bland i.
    bone i.
    Brewer i.
    cerebral i.
    embolic i.
    focal i.
    healed i.
    hemorrhagic i.
    microscopic i.
    old i.
    pale i.
    posterior wall i. (PWI)
    pulmonary i.
    recent i.
    red i.
    ruptured myocardial i.
    septic i.
    thrombotic i.
    uric acid i.
    white i.
    Zahn i.

infarction
    acute myocardial i. (AMI)
    anterior wall i. (AWI)
    anterior wall myocardial i. (AWMI)
    atrial i.
    cerebral i. (CI)
    inferior wall myocardial i. (IWMI)
    intestinal i.
    mesenteric i.
    myocardial i. (MI)
    myocardial i. in dumbbell form
    myocardial i. in H-form
    nontransmural myocardial i.
    old myocardial i. (OMI)
    pulmonary i. (PI)
    renal i.
    silent myocardial i.
    subendocardial myocardial i.
    through-and-through myocardial i.
    transmural myocardial i.

infect
infected abortion
infecting dose (ID)
infection
    abortive i.
    airborne i.
    colonization i.
    cross i.
    cryptogenic i.

    dragon worm i.
    droplet i.
    ectothrix i.
    endogenous i.
    exogenous i.
    fever caused by i. (FI)
    focal i.
    guinea worm i.
    i. immunity
    inapparent i.
    latent i.
    mass i.
    medina i.
    mixed i.
    nosocomial i.
    opportunistic i.
    persistent tolerant i. (PTI)
    pyogenic i.
    recurrent upper respiratory tract i. (RURTI)
    secondary i.
    serpent i.
    upper respiratory i. (URI)
    upper respiratory tract i. (URTI)
    urinary tract i. (UTI)
    viral respiratory i. (VRI)
    whipworm i.
    zoonotic i.

infection-immunity
infectiosity
infectious
    i. agent
    i. anemia
    i. arteritis
    i. arteritis virus of horses
    i. avian bronchitis
    i. bovine rhinotracheitis (IBR)
    i. bovine rhinotracheitis virus
    i. bronchitis virus (IBV)
    i. bulbar paralysis
    i. canine hepatitis
    i. disease
    i. ectromelia virus
    i. eczematoid dermatitis
    i. endocarditis
    i. esophagitis
    i. granuloma
    i. hepatitis (IH)
    i. hepatitis virus
    i. mononucleosis (IM)
    i. mononucleosis screening test
    i. myositis
    i. myxoma
    i. nucleic acid
    i. papilloma of cattle
    i. papilloma virus
    i. parotitis
    i. plasmid

i. polyneuritis
i. porcine encephalomyelitis
i. porcine encephalomyelitis virus
i. wart
i. waste
infectiousness
infective
i. dose (ID)
i. embolism
i. endocarditis
i. thrombus
infectivity
inferior
i. complete closed dislocation
i. complete compound dislocation
i. dislocation
i. displacement
i. lipodystrophy
i. wall myocardial infarction (IWMI)
infertility
i. screen
infest
infestation
infidelity
lineage i.
infiltrate
acute inflammatory i.
Assmann tuberculous i.
eosinophil leukocytic i.
eosinophil leukocytic i.
inflammatory i.
infraclavicular i.
leukocytic i.
lymphocytic inflammatory i.
lymphoplasmacytic i.
monocytic inflammatory i.
neutrophilic i.
plasma cell i.
polymorphonuclear leukocytic i.
polymorphonuclear leukocytic i.
polymorphous lymphoid i.
infiltrating
i. comedocarcinoma
i. duct adenocarcinoma
i. ductal carcinoma (IDC)
i. duct carcinoma
i. lipoma
i. lobular carcinoma (ILC)
infiltration
adipose i.
calcareous i.

cellular i.
epituberculous i.
fatty i.
gelatinous i.
glycogen i.
gray i.
lipomatous i.
lymphocytic i. of skin
sanguineous i.
tuberculous i.
infiltrative
i. fasciitis
i. ophthalmopathy
infinite
infinitely miscible
infinitesimal
infinity
inflamed ulcer
inflammable
inflammation
active chronic i.
acute and chronic i.
adhesive i.
allergic i.
alterative i.
atrophic i.
blennorrhagic i.
bullous granulomatous i.
calcified granulomatous i.
caseating granulomatous i.
caseous i.
catarrhal i.
cavitating i.
chronic active i.
circumscribed i.
confluent i.
i. of connective tissue (ICT)
croupous i.
cystic acute i.
cystic chronic i.
cystic granulomatous i.
degenerative i.
diffuse i.
disseminated i.
erosive i.
exanthematous i.
exudative granulomatous i.
fibrinoid necrotizing i.
fibrinopurulent i.
fibrinous i.
fibrocaseous i.
fibroid i.

NOTES

inflammation *(continued)*
    focal granulomatous i.
    follicular i.
    gangrenous granulomatous i.
    gelatinous i.
    granulomatous i.
    hemorrhagic i.
    hyperplastic i.
    immune i.
    interstitial i.
    localized i.
    membranous acute i.
    miliary granulomatous i.
    multifocal i.
    necrotic i.
    necrotizing granulomatous i.
    non-necrotizing granulomatous i.
    obliterative i.
    organizing i.
    ossifying i.
    productive i.
    proliferative i.
    pseudomembranous acute i.
    purulent i.
    pustular i.
    recurrent i.
    sclerosing i.
    serofibrinous i.
    serous acute i.
    sinusoidal i.
    subacute i.
    suppurative acute i.
    suppurative chronic i.
    suppurative granulomatous i.
    transudative i.
    ulcerative i.
    uremic i.
    vesicular acute i.
    vesicular granulomatous i.
    i. with fibrosis
inflammatory
    i. adenocarcinoma
    i. bowel disease
    i. carcinoma
    i. cavity
    i. corpuscle
    i. cyst
    i. edema
    i. exudate
    i. fistula
    i. infiltrate
    i. lymph
    lymphocytic i. infiltrate
    i. macrophage
    i. membrane
    monocytic i. infiltrate
    i. myofibroblastic tumor (IMT)
    i. necrosis

    i. pelvic disease (IPD)
    i. perforation
    i. polyp
    i. pseudomembrane
    i. pseudotumor
    i. reaction
    i. rheumatism
    i. rupture
    i. sinus
    i. sinus tract
    i. transudate
inflation
inflection
    point of i.
influenza (flu)
    i. A, B, C
    i. A and B titer
    avian i.
    equine i.
    Hong Kong i.
    Spanish i.
    swine i.
    i. virus
    i. virus culture
    i. virus, types A, B, C
    i. virus vaccine
Influenzavirus
infolding
    papillary i.
information
    i. retrieval
    i. theory
infraclavicular infiltrate
infrared
    infrared CO_2 analyzer
    i. microscope
    i. spectrophotometry (IRS)
    i. spectroscopy
infrasubspecific
infundibular stenosis
infundibuloma
infundibulum
    Choanotaenia i.
infusion (inf)
    brain-heart i. (BHI)
    peripheral blood stem cell i.
    total-dose i. (TDI)
Infusoria
infusorian
ingestion
ingestive
ingrown
    i. hair
    i. toenail
inguinal hernia
INH
    isoniazid
    isonicotinic acid hydrazide

inhalation pneumonia
inherent
    i. filter
inheritance
    alternative i.
    amphigonous i.
    autosomal dominant i.
    autosomal recessive i.
    biparental i.
    codominant i.
    complemental i.
    cytoplasmic i.
    dominant i.
    extrachromosomal i.
    holandric i.
    hologynic i.
    homochronous i.
    intermediate i.
    maternal i.
    mendelian i.
    multifactorial i.
    polygenic i.
    quantitative i.
    quasicontinuous i.
    quasidominant i.
    recessive i.
    sex-linked i.
    supplemental i.
    unit i.
    X-linked dominant i.
    X-linked recessive i.
inherited
    i. albumin variant
    i. disease
inhibin
inhibit
inhibiting
    i. antibody
    i. factor
    i. hormone
inhibition
    allogenic i.
    allosteric i.
    competitive i.
    contact i.
    enzyme i.
    i. factor
    fertility i.
    hapten i. of precipitation
    hemagglutination i. (HAI, HI)
    hemagglutinin i. (HAI)

    i. test
    tetrazolium reduction i. (TRI)
inhibitor
    α_1-i.
    alpha-1 i.
    alpha-2 macroglobulin i.
    alpha-1 protease inhibitor
    alpha-1 trypsin i.
    i. assay
    carbonic anhydrase i.
    cell-cycle i.
    C1 esterase i.
    C_1 esterase i.
    cholinesterase i.
    coagulation factor i.
    electron transport i.
    enzyme i. (EI)
    factor VIII i.
    factor Xa i.
    human alpha-1 proteinase i.
    human α_1-proteinase i.
    inter alpha trypsin i.
    inter-α-trypsin i.
    lupus erythematosus i.
    α_2-macroglobulin i.
    monoamine oxidase i.
    oxidative phosphorylation i.
    protease i. (PI)
    α_1-protease inhibitor (α_1PI)
    soybean trypsin i. (SBTI)
    tissue factor pathway i. (TFPI)
    i.'s of transcription
    Trojan Horse i.
    trypsin i.
    α_1-trypsin i.
inhibitory
    i. enzyme
    i. hormone
    i. mold agar
iniasis
iniencephaly
initial
    i. hematuria
    i. prognostic score (IPS)
    i. syphilitic lesion
initialization
initiating agent
initiation
    i. codon
    i. factor
initis

NOTES

injection
    i. mass
    sensitizing i.
injury
    birth i.
    blast i.
    cold i.
    compression i.
    crush i.
    decompensation i.
    decompression i.
    radiation i.
    second degree radiation i.
    third degree radiation i.
    torsion i.
innate
    i. immunity
innatus
    calor i.
innidiation
innocent
    i. bystander cell
    i. tumor
innocuous
innoxious
inochondritis
inoculability
inoculable
inoculate
inoculation
    i. smallpox
inoculum
Inocybe
inopectic
inopexia
inorganic
    i. acid
    i. chemistry
    i. phosphate
    i. pyrophosphatase
    i. pyrophosphate
inoscopy
inosemia
inosinase
inosine
    i. cyclohydrolase
    i. dehydrogenase
    i. diphosphate
    i. monophosphate
    i. phosphate
    i. phosphorylase
    i. pyrophosphorylase
    i. triphosphate
inosine-5′-phosphate
inosinic acid
inosita
    melituria i.
inosite-free broth

inosithin
inositol
    i. dehydrogenase
    i. hexanitrate
    i. hexaphosphate
    i. niacinate
myo-**inositol**
inosituria
inosuria
inotropic
Inoviridae
inquiline
inquiry
INR
    International Normalized Ratio
INS
    idiopathic nephrotic syndrome
insect
    i. bite
    i. virus
Insecta
insectarium
insecticides
    organochlorine i.
    organophosphate i.
insemination
    homologous artificial i. (AIH)
insertion
    i. mutation
    i. sequence
insertional
    i. activity
    i. translocation
insheathed
insidiosum
    Pythium i.
insipidus
    nephrogenic diabetes i. (NDI)
insol
    insoluble
insoluble (insol)
inspissate
inspissated
inspissation
inspissator
instability
instant thin-layer chromatography (ITLC)
instar
instillation
instructive theory
instrumentation
insudate
insufficiency
    adrenal i.
    adrenocortical i.
    aortic i. (AI)
    circulatory i.

coronary i. (CI)
metabolic i.
mitral i. (MI)
primary adrenal i.
pulmonary i.
renal i.
respiratory i.
tricuspid i. (TI)
uteroplacental i. (UPI)
velopharyngeal i.
venous i.
insufficient signal (IS)
insufflation
cranial i.
endotracheal i.
perirenal i.
presacral i.
retroperitoneal gas i.
insular sclerosis
insulated gate field effect transistor
insulator
insulin
i. antagonist
i. antibody
atypical i.
i. clearance (C/in/)
i. clearance test
i. coma therapy (ICT)
crystalline i. (CI)
globin i. (GI)
i. hypoglycemia test
immunoreactive i. (IRI)
i. lipoatrophy
i. lipodystrophy
potassium, glucose, and i. (PGI)
protamine i. (PI)
protamine zinc i. (PZI)
i. resistance
i. sensitivity test (IST)
i. shock
i. shock therapy (IST)
soluble i. (SI)
i. tolerance test (ITT)
i. unit
insulinase
insulin-dependent
i.-d. diabetes mellitus (IDDM)
insulin-dependent diabetes mellitus (IDDM)
insulinemia

insulin-like
i.-l. activity (ILA)
i.-l. growth factor
insulinoma
insulinopenic
insulitis
insuloma
insusceptibility
intake and output (I/O)
integral
i. dose
i. protein
integrating microscope
integration
large-scale i.
medium-scale i.
very large scale i. (VLSI)
integrator
integrin
intensity
luminous i.
interaction
drug i.
i. of radiation with matter
sample i.
interactive processing
inter alpha trypsin inhibitor
interatrial septal defect (IASD)
interband
intercalary
i. deletion
intercalate
intercalated disk
intercapillary
i. glomerulosclerosis
i. nephrosclerosis
intercellular
i. adhesion molecule-1 (ICAM-1)
i. bridge
i. canaliculus
i. cement
i. lymph
y-intercept
interchange
interchromosomal aberration
intercoronary anastomosis
i. anastomosis
intercristal space
intercurrent disease
interdigitating
i. dendritic cell tumor

NOTES

interdigitating *(continued)*
    i. papillary neoplasm
    i. reticulum cell
interdigitation
interelectrode distance
interface
    EIA i.
interfacial canal
interference
    anion i.
    background i.
    bacterial i.
    cation i.
    centromere i.
    chemical i.
    chromatid i.
    constructive i.
    destructive i.
    drug i.
    i. filter
    hemolysis i.
    icterus i.
    ionization i.
    i. microscope
    spectral i.
    i. test
interferon (IFN)
    i. α
    i. alpha (IFN-α)
    antigen i.
    i. β
    i. beta (IFN-β)
    fibroblast i.
    i. γ
    i. gamma (IFN-γ)
    immune i.
    leukocyte i.
α-interferon therapy
inter-α-globulin
interkinesis
interleukin (IL)
interleukin-1 through -15
interlobitis
interlobular pleurisy
intermediary metabolism
intermediate
    i. carcinoma
    i. coliform bacteria
    i. filament protein
    i. host
    i. inheritance
    malignant teratoma i. (MTI)
    i. normoblast
    reaction i.
intermediate-density lipoprotein (IDL)
intermedin
intermittent
    i. albuminuria

    i. claudication (IC)
    i. hemoglobinuria
    i. malaria
    i. malarial fever
    i. parasite
    i. sterilization
internal
    i. adhesive pericarditis
    i. carotid artery occlusion (ICAO)
    i. conversion
    i. elastic lamellae
    i. fistula
    i. hemorrhoid
    i. meningitis
    i. pathology
    i. pyocephalus
    i. resistance (IR)
    i. standard
    i. storage
international
    I. Academy of Pathology (IAP)
    I. Association of Geographic Pathology
    i. benzoate unit (IBU)
    I. Classification of Diseases (ICD)
    I. Committee for Standardization in Hematology (ICSH)
    I. Council of Societies of Pathology
    I. Federation of Clinical Chemistry (IFCC)
    I. Federation of Gynecology and Obstetrics (FIGO)
    I. Federation of Gynecology and Obstetrics classification of tumor staging
    I. Normalized Ratio (INR)
    I. Sensitivity Index (ISI)
    I. Society for Clinical Laboratory Technology (ISCLT)
    I. Society of Comparative Pathology (ISCP)
    I. Society of Hematology (ISH)
    I. Society of Microbiologists (ISM)
    I. Standards Organization (ISO)
    I. System of Units (SI)
    I. Union of Pure and Applied Chemistry (IUPAC)
    i. unit (IU)
interocclusal clearance
interpapillary ridge
interphase
interphyletic
interplant
interplanting
interpolation
interpreter
interrupt

interspecific graft
interspersed repeats
interstice
interstitial
    i. cell
    i. cell of Leydig
    i. cell-stimulating hormone (ICSH)
    i. cell tumor
    i. cell tumor of testis
    i. cystitis
    i. deletion
    i. emphysema
    i. fibrosis
    i. fluid
    i. gastritis
    i. giant cell pneumonia
    i. growth
    i. implantation
    i. inflammation
    i. keratitis
    i. lung disease
    i. mastitis
    i. myositis
    i. nephritis
    i. plasma cell pneumonia
    i. pneumonitis
    i. water (ISW)
interstitium
intertrigo
intertropical anemia
inter-α-trypsin inhibitor
interval
    confidence i.
    i. estimate
    rupture-delivery i. (RDI)
    i. scale
    systolic time i. (STI)
    time i. (TI)
    tolerance i.
intervening sequence
interventricular septal defect (IVSD)
intestinal
    i. atresia
    i. calculus
    i. colic
    i. emphysema
    i. fistula
    i. flora
    i. flow disorder
    i. infarction
    i. lipodystrophy

    i. lymphangiectasis
    i. malrotation
    i. metaplasia
    i. myiasis
    i. obstruction (IO)
    i. sand
    i. sepsis
intestinalis
    Lamblia i.
    Septata i.
intestinotoxin
intima
    aortic tunica i.
intimal cell
intimitis
    proliferative i.
intolerance
    cold i.
    fructose i.
    hereditary fructose i. (HFI)
    lysine i.
    lysinuric protein i. (LPI)
    sucrose i.
intoxication
    acid i.
    alkaline i.
    anaphylactic i.
    citrate i.
    septic i.
    serum i.
    vitamin D i.
    water i.
intra-arterial
intracanalicular fibroadenoma
intracapsular ankylosis
intracavernous aneurysm
intracavitary
intracellular
    i. accumulation(s)
    i. fluid (ICF)
    i. fluid volume (IFV)
    i. parasite
    i. toxin
    i. water (ICW)
intrachange
intrachromosomal aberration
intracranial
    i. aneurysm (ICA)
    i. hematoma
intracristal space
intracutaneous reaction

NOTES

339

intracystic
    i. hyperplasia
    i. papilloma
intradermal
    i. nevus
    i. reaction (IDR)
    i. test (IT)
intraductal
    i. carcinoma (IDC)
    i. hyperplasia
    i. papillary carcinoma (IPC)
    i. papilloma
    i. papillomatosis
intraepidermal
    i. basal cell epithelioma, Borst-Jadassohn type
    i. carcinoma
    i. squamous cell carcinoma
intraepidermic bulla
intraepithelial
    i. carcinoma
    i. dyskeratosis
intraesophageal pH test
intralesional
intramedullary hemolysis
intramembranous space
intramural hematoma
intraocular foreign body (IOFB)
intraoperative cell salvage
intraosseous
intraosteal
intrapulmonary spindle cell thymoma
intrathoracic gas volume (IGV)
intratubular
    i. germ cell neoplasia
    i. germ cell neoplasia of the unclassified type (IGGNU)
intratumoral (IT)
intrauterine
    i. death (IUD)
    i. fetally malnourished (IUM)
    i. foreign body (IUFB)
    i. growth rate (IUGR)
    i. transfusion
intravasation
intravascular
    i. agglutination
    i. coagulation screen
    i. consumption coagulopathy (IVCC)
    i. hemolysis
    i. lymph
    i. mass (IVM)
    i. papillary endothelial hyperplasia
intravenous
    i. glucose tolerance test (IVGTT)
    i. leiomyomatosis (IVL)

    i. tolbutamide tolerance test (IVTTT)
intraventricular
    i. conduction defect (IVCD)
    i. hemorrhage (IVH)
intravital stain
intrinsic
    i. asthma
    i. factor (IF)
    i. factor antibody
    i. factor concentrate (IFC)
    i. pathway
    i. semiconductor
intron
introsusception
introversion
intumesce
intumescence
intumescent
intussusception
    colic i.
    double i.
    ileal i.
    ileocecal i.
    ileocolic i.
    jejunogastric i.
    retrograde i.
intussusceptive
intussusceptum
intussuscipiens
inulin clearance
inundation fever
InV
    InV allotype
    InV group antigen
invaccination
invagination
invasin
invasion
    angiolymphatic i.
    perineural i.
invasive
    i. activity test (IAT)
    i. aspergillosis
    i. carcinoma
    i. fibrous thyroiditis
    i. mole
invasiveness
invermination
inverse anaphylaxis
inverse-square law
inversion
    carbohydrate i.
    chromosomal i.
    heterobrachial i.
    homobrachial i.
    overlapping i.

i. of uterus
visceral i.
invertase
inverted
i. follicular keratosis
i. papilloma
i. repeat
i. testis
inverter
inverting enzyme
invert sugar
investigation
involucre
involucrum, pl. involucra
involution
i. cyst
i. form
senile i.
IO
intestinal obstruction
I/O
intake and output
I/O device
Iodamoeba
I. bütschlii
iodate reaction of epinephrine
iodemia
iodic acid
iodide
i. assay
saturated solution of potasium i.
(SSKI)
i. transport defect
iodimetry
iodinated
i. human serum albumin (IHSA)
i. I-125 serum albumin (human)
i. I-131 serum albumin (human)
i. macroaggregated albumin (IMAA)
iodine
butanol-extractable i. (BEI)
i. cyst
i. escape peak
Gram i.
i. mumps
i. number
plasma inorganic i. (PII)
protein-bound i.
radioactive i. (^{131}I, RAI)
i. reaction of epinephrine
serum precipitable i. (SPI)
serum protein-bound i. (SPBI)

i. solution
i. stain
i. staining
i. test
tincture of i.
i. value
iodine-123
iodine-125
iodine-131 uptake test
iodine-azide test (IAT)
iodine-131-6 beta iodomethyl-19-norcholesterol
iodine-131-6β-iodomethyl-19-norcholesterol
iodinophil, iodinophile
iodinophilous
iodobismuthate
iodochlorhydroxyquin
iodocholesterol I-131
iododeoxyuridine (IDU, IUDR)
5-iododeoxyuridine
iodometric
iodometry
iodophil granule
iodophilia
iodophor
iodoplatinate
iodotyrosine deiodinase defect
ioduria
IOFB
intraocular foreign body
iometer
ion
alkoxide i.
carbonium i.
carboxylate i.
i. counter
dipolar i.
i. disorder
gram i.
hydrogen i.
hydronium i.
hydroxide i.
oxonium i.
i. pair
ion-exchange
i.-e. chromatography
i.-e. resin
ionic
i. bond
i. charge
i. concentration
i. strength

NOTES

ionization
 avalanche i.
 i. chamber
 i. constant
 i. interference
 specific i.
ionize
ionized
 i. calcium
 i. calcium assay
ionizing radiation
ionogram
ionopherogram
ionophore
ion-selective electrode (ISE)
iontophoresis
IP
 incubation period
IPAA
 ileal pouch-anal anastomosis
IPC
 intraductal papillary carcinoma
IPD
 inflammatory pelvic disease
IPF
 idiopathic pulmonary fibrosis
IPH
 idiopathic pulmonary hemosiderosis
Ipomoea
iproniazid
IPS
 initial prognostic score
ipsefact
IPSID
 immunoproliferative small intestinal
 disease
ipsilateral intraductal carcinoma
IPV
 inactivated poliovaccine
IR
 immunoreactive
 internal resistance
Ir
 immune response
 Ir gene
IRBBB
 incomplete right bundle-branch block
IRDS
 idiopathic respiratory distress syndrome
IRG
 immunoreactive glucagon
IRHCS
 immunoradioassayable human chorionic
 somatomammotropin
IRhGH
 immunoreactive human growth hormone
IRI
 immunoreactive insulin

iridescent
 i. virus
iridium
iridocapsulitis
iridochoroiditis
iridocyclitis
 heterochromic i.
 i. septica
iridokeratitis
Iridoviridae
Iridovirus
IRI/G ratio
iritis
IRMA
 immunoradiometric assay
iron
 i. absorption
 i. assay
 bound serum i. (BSI)
 i. broth
 i. deficiency anemia (IDA)
 i. hematoxylin
 i. hematoxylin stain
 high serum-bound i. (HBI)
 i. index
 low serum-bound i. (LBI)
 i. plasma clearance
 serum i. (SI)
 i. stain
 i. storage disease
iron-binding
 i.-b. capacity (IBC)
 i.-b. capacity test
 total i.-b. capacity (TIBC)
 unsaturated i.-b. capacity (UIBC)
iron-positive pigment demonstration
iron-sulfide protein
irovirus
irradiation
 i. damage
 ultraviolet blood i. (UBI)
irreducible hernia
irreversible
 i. coma
 i. reaction
irreversibly sickled cell (ISC)
irrigation
irritability
irritable
 i. bowel syndrome
 i. colon (IC)
irritans
 Siphona i.
irritant
 primary i.
irritation
 i. cell
 i. fibroma

I

irritative lesion
irruption
irruptive
IRS
    infrared spectrophotometry
Irvine syndrome
IS
    insufficient signal
Isambert disease
Isamine blue
ISC
    irreversibly sickled cell
ischemia
    mucosal i.
    myocardial i.
    i. retinae
    transient cerebral i. (TCI)
ischemic
    i. bowel disease
    i. colitis
    i. contracture
    i. heart disease (IHD)
    i. hypoxia
    i. leg disease (ILD)
    i. limb disease (ILD)
    i. muscular atrophy
    i. necrosis
ischial tuberosity
ischiopagus
ischiorectal abscess
ISCLT
    International Society for Clinical
    Laboratory Technology
ISCP
    International Society of Comparative
    Pathology
ISE
    ion-selective electrode
isethionate
    hydroxystilbamidine i.
ISG
    immune serum globulin
Is gene
ISH
    icteric serum hepatitis
    International Society of Hematology
    in situ hybridization
ISI
    International Sensitivity Index
island
    blood i.
    i. disease

    erythroblastic i.
    i. fever
islet
    i. beta cell
    i. α cell, i. alpha cell
    i. β cell
    i. δ cell
    δ cell i.
    i. cell adenoma
    i. cell antibody (ICA)
    i. cell antibody screening test
    i. cell carcinoma
    i. cell hyperinsulinism
    i. cell hyperplasia
    i. cell tumor
    delta cell i.
    i. delta cell
    i. hormones
    i.'s of Langerhans
ISM
    International Society of Microbiologists
ISO
    International Standards Organization
isoagglutination
isoagglutinin
isoagglutinogen
isoallele
isoallelism
isoallotypic determinant
isoanaphylaxis
isoantibody
    platelet i.
isoantigen
isobar
isobaric
isobuteine
isobutyl alcohol
isobutyric acid
isochromatic
isochromatid
    i. break
    i. gap
isochromatophil, isochromatophile
isochromic anemia
isochromosome
isochronal rhythm
isochronous
isochroous
isocitrate
    i. dehydrogenase
    i. dehydrogenase assay
    i. dehydrogenase test

NOTES

isocitric
    i. acid
    i. dehydrogenase
isocyanate
isocytolysin
isodactylism
isodesmosine
isoelectric
    i. focusing
    i. level
    i. point
isoenzyme
    alkaline phosphatase i.
    creatine kinase i.
    i. electrophoresis
    lactate dehydrogenase i.
    Regan i.
isoerythrolysis
    neonatal i.
isogamy
isogeneic
    i. graft
isogenic graft
isogenous chondrocytes
isograft
isohemagglutination
isohemagglutinin
isohemolysin
isohemolysis
isohydric shift
isohydruria
isohypercytosis
isohypocytosis
isoimmune
    i. hemolytic anemia
    i. neonatal thrombocytopenia
isoimmunization
    Rh i. syndrome
isoiodeikon test
isolate
isolated
    i. dextrocardia
    i. dyskeratosis follicularis
    i. gland carcinoma in situ (GCIS)
    i. levocardia
    i. parietal endocarditis
    i. proteinuria
    i. sinistrocardia
isolation
    CMV i.
    cytomegalovirus i.
    herpes simplex virus i.
    HSV i.
Isolator
    I. blood culture system
    I. lysis-centrifugation tube
isoleucine
isoleucyl

isoleucyl-RNA synthetase
isoleukoagglutinin
isologous
    i. chimera
    i. graft
isolysin
isolysis
isolytic
isomaltase
isomastigote
isomer
    optical i.
isomerase
    glucosephosphate i.
    hexosephosphate i.
    triosephosphate i.
isomeric transition (IT)
isomerism
    chain i.
    dynamic i.
    functional group i.
    geometric i.
    nuclear i.
    optical i.
    position i.
    spatial i.
    stereochemical i.
    structural i.
isomerization
isometric
isomicrogamete
isomorphic response
isomorphous
    i. gliosis
isomuscarine
isoniazid (INH)
    i. assay
    i. phenotype test
isonicotinic acid hydrazide (INH)
isonormocytosis
iso-osmolar
iso-osmotic, isoosmotic
Isopaque
Isoparorchis
    I. trisimilitubis
isopathy
Δ^2**-isopentenyl diphosphate**
Δ^3**-isopentenyl diphosphate**
isophagy
isoplastic
    i. graft
isopleth
isoprecipitin
isoprene
isoprenoid
isopropanol
    i. assay
    i. precipitation test

isopyknic
isopyknotic
isosbestic point
isosensitize
isoserum treatment
isosexual
isosmotic
Isospora
    I. belli
    I. hominis
isosporiasis
isosthenuria
isosulfan blue
isothermal
isothiocyanate
    fluorescein i. (FITC)
isotone
isotonic
    i. coefficient
    i. sodium chloride solution
isotope dilution-mass spectrometry
isotransplantation
isotropic
isotype
isotypic
isovaleric acid
isovalericacidemia
isovaleryl-CoA dehydrogenase
isovolumic contraction (IC)
isozyme
Israels familial jaundice
IST
    insulin sensitivity test
    insulin shock therapy
ISW
    interstitial water
IT
    implantation test
    intradermal test
    intratumoral
    isomeric transition
Itai-Itai disease
Itaqui virus
itch
    barber's i.
    Cuban i.
    dhobie i.
    grain i.
    jock i.
    mad i.
    Malabar i.
    prairie i.

    swimmer's i.
    winter i.
iteration
iterative process
ITLC
    instant thin-layer chromatography
Ito nevus
Ito-Reenstierna test
ITP
    idiopathic thrombocytopenic purpura
ITT
    insulin tolerance test
IU
    immunizing unit
    international unit
IUD
    intrauterine death
IUDR
    iododeoxyuridine
IUFB
    intrauterine foreign body
IUGR
    intrauterine growth rate
IUM
    intrauterine fetally malnourished
IUPAC
    International Union of Pure and Applied
      Chemistry
IVAP
    in vivo adhesive platelet
IVCC
    intravascular consumption coagulopathy
IVCD
    intraventricular conduction defect
Ivemark syndrome
IVGTT
    intravenous glucose tolerance test
IVH
    intraventricular hemorrhage
IVL
    intravenous leiomyomatosis
IVM
    intravascular mass
ivory exostosis
IVSD
    interventricular septal defect
IVTTT
    intravenous tolbutamide tolerance test
Ivy
    I. bleeding time test
    I. method

NOTES

Ivy *(continued)*
  I. method of bleeding time
  I. template bleeding time
IWMI
 inferior wall myocardial infarction
Ixodes
  I. bicornis
  I. cavipalpus
  I. cookei
  I. dammini
  I. frequens
  I. holocyclus
  I. pacificus
  I. persulcatus
  I. rasus
  I. ricinus
  I. scapularis
  I. spinipalpis
ixodiasis
ixodic
ixodid
Ixodidae
Ixodoidea

J

joule
Joule equivalent
juxtapulmonary-capillary
J chain
J receptor
jaagsiekte
Jaccoud
J. arthritis
J. arthropathy
J. syndrome
jacksonian epilepsy
Jackson syndrome
Jacobsson method
Jacod syndrome
Jacquemin test
Jadassohn-Lewandowski syndrome
Jadassohn nevus
Jadassohn-Tièche nevus
Jaffe
J. assay
J. reaction
J. test
Jaffe-Lichtenstein disease
Jahnke syndrome
jail fever
Jakob-Creutzfeldt
J.-C. disease
J.-C. pseudosclerosis
Jakob disease
Jaksch disease
Jamaican vomiting sickness
Jamestown Canyon virus
Janet disease
Janeway lesion
janiceps
Jansen disease
Jansky-Bielschowsky disease
Jansky human blood group classification
Janus green B
Japanese
J. B encephalitis (JBE)
J. B encephalitis virus
J. river fever
jar
anaerobic j.
Coplin j.
Jarisch-Herxheimer reaction
Jass staging system
Jatlow-Nadim procedure
Jatropha
jaundice
acholuric j.

acute febrile j.
black j.
catarrhal j.
cholestatic j.
chronic acholuric j.
chronic familial j.
chronic idiopathic j.
congenital familial non-hemolytic j.
congenital hemolytic j.
familial nonhemolytic j.
hematogenous j.
hemolytic j.
hepatocellular j.
hepatogenous j.
homologous serum j.
Israels familial j.
leptospiral j.
malignant j.
mechanical j.
nonhemolytic j.
nonobstructive j.
obstructive j.
painless j.
regurgitation j.
retention j.
spherocytic j.
toxemic j.
jaw
lumpy j.
JBE
Japanese B encephalitis
JCT
juxtaglomerular cell tumor
JC virus
Jeanselme nodule
Jeghers-Peutz syndrome
jejunitis
jejunogastric intussusception
jejunoileitis
Jendrassik-Grof method
Jenner
J. method
J. stain
Jenner-Giemsa stain
Jenner-Kay unit
Jensen
J. classification
J. disease
J. sarcoma
JEOL
J. 100 S transmission electron microscope
J. 1200 transmission electron microscope

Jerne
  J. plaque assay
  J. technique
Jervell and Lange-Nielsen syndrome
jet lesion
Jeune syndrome
Jewett
  J. bladder carcinoma
  J. and Strong staging
JG
  juxtaglomerular cell
JGCT
  juvenile granulosa cell tumor
JGI
  juxtaglomerular granulation index
JH virus
jigger
Jk antigen
Jobbins antigen
Job syndrome
jock itch
Jod-Basedow phenomenon
Joest body
Johne
  J. bacillus
  J. disease
johnin
Johnson-Dubin syndrome
Johnson-Steven disease
joint
  j. calculus
  Clutton j.
Jolles test
Jones-Cantarow test
Jones method
Jones-Mote reaction
Jores fixative
Joseph syndrome
Joule
  J. equivalent (J)
  J. law
joule (J)
Jourdain disease
JRA
  juvenile rheumatoid arthritis
Js antigen
J-sella deformity
juccuya
Judet epiphyseal fracture
jugular gland
juice
  cancer j.
  pancreatic j.
jump
  conditional j.
  unconditional j.

jumping
  j. disease
  j. gene
junction
  j. capacitor
  cell j.
  j. field effect transistor
  gap j.
  j. nevus
  j. potential
  squamocolumnar j.
junctional
  j. complex
  j. cyst
  j. nevus
Jung
  J. Autostainer XL
  J. CV 5000 Robotic Coverslipper
jungle yellow fever
Jüngling disease
Junin virus
justifiable abortion
justify
juvenile
  j. angiofibroma
  j. carcinoma
  j. cell
  j. cerebellar astrocytoma
  j. cirrhosis
  j. diabetes mellitus
  j. elastoma
  j. fibroadenoma
  j. granulosa cell tumor (JGCT)
  j. hemangiofibroma
  j. hormone
  j. hyalin fibromatosis
  j. kyphosis
  j. melanoma
  j. neutrophil
  j. osteoporosis
  j. Paget disease
  j. palmo-plantar fibromatosis
  j. papillomatosis
  j. pernicious anemia
  j. pilocytic astrocytoma
  j. polyp
  j. polyposis syndrome
  j. rheumatoid arthritis (JRA)
  j. xanthogranuloma (JXG)
  j. xanthoma
juvenile-onset diabetes
juxta-articular nodule
juxtacortical
  j. chondroma
  j. osteogenic sarcoma
juxtaglomerular
  j. apparatus
  j. cell (JG)

j. cell tumor (JCT)
j. granulation index (JGI)
j. granule
juxtanuclear
juxtapulmonary-capillary (J)
j.-c. receptor

juvenile xanthogranuloma

NOTES

J

κ (*var. of* kappa)
K
    Kell blood group
    kelvin
        K antigen
        K capture
        K cell
        K virus
k
    constant
KA
    ketoacidosis
    King-Armstrong
kabure
Kaffir pox
Kahlbaum disease
Kahler disease
Kahn test
Kaiserling fixative
kala azar
kalemia
kaliopenia
kaliopenic
Kalischer disease
kalium
kaliuresis
kaliuretic
kallidin
kallikrein-inhibiting unit (KIU)
kallikrein system
Kallmann syndrome
kaluresis
kaluretic
Kanagawa phenomenon
kanamycin
Kandinskii-Clerambault syndrome
kang cancer
kangri
        k. burn carcinoma
        k. cancer
Kanner syndrome
kaodzera
Kaolin-clotting time
kaolinosis
kaolin partial thromboplastin time (KPTT)
Kaplan-Meier staining method
Kaposi
        K. sarcoma
        K. varicelliform eruption
kappa, κ
        k. chain
        k. granule
Karmen unit (KU)
Karnofsky status

Karnovsky
    K. fixative
    K. II solution
Kartagener syndrome
karyochrome
karyoclasis
karyocyte
karyogamy
karyogonad
karyokinesis
karyology
karyolysis
karyolytic
karyomere
karyomitome
karyomorphism
karyon
karyophage
karyoplasmolysis
karyoplast
karyoplastin
karyopyknosis
karyopyknotic
        k. index (KI)
karyorrhectic
karyorrhexis
karyotype
        k. aberration
        numerical k.
        X k.
        XO k.
        XX k.
        XXX k.
        XXY k.
        XY k.
        XYY k.
karyotyping
karyozoic
Kasabach-Merritt syndrome
kasai
Kashin-Bek disease
Kasten
    K. fluorescent Feulgen stain
    K. fluorescent PAS stain
    K. fluorescent Schiff reagent
Kast syndrome
kat
    katal
katal (kat)
Katayama test
katharometer
Kato thick smear technique
Katzenstein and Peiper criteria
KAU
    King-Armstrong unit

Kauffman-White classification
Kawasaki disease
Kayser disease
Kayser-Fleischer ring
KB
  ketone body
kb
  kilobase
kbp
  kilobase pair
kc
  kilocycle
kcal
  kilocalorie
K capture
kcps
  kilocycles per second
KE
  kinetic energy
Kearns syndrome
ked
kedani
  k. disease
  k. fever
  k. mite
Keflex
Keith-Wagener (KW)
  K.-W. classification
Keith-Wagener-Barker (KWB)
  K.-W.-B. classification
Kelev strain rabies virus
kelis
Kell
  K. antigens
  K. blood group (K)
  K. blood group system
keloid
  Addison k.
keloidosis
kelosomia
Kelvin
  K. temperature scale
  K. thermometer
kelvin (K)
Kennedy syndrome
Kenyon stain
kerasin histiocytosis
kerasin-type histiocytosis
keratan sulfate
keratiasis
keratic
keratin
  k. pearl
  k. stain
  k. staining
keratinization
  metaplastic k.
keratinize

keratinized
keratinocyte
keratinophilic
keratinous
  k. cyst
keratitic precipitate (KP)
keratitis
  acne rosacea k.
  k. bullosa
  k. disciformis
  herpetic k.
  interstitial k.
  mycotic k.
  parenchymatous k.
  reticular k.
  sclerosing k.
  serpiginous k.
  suppurative k.
  vascular k.
  vesicular k.
  zonular k.
keratoacanthoma
keratoangioma
keratoatrophoderma
keratoconjuctivitis
  phlyctenular k.
keratoconjunctivitis
  epidemic k. (EKC)
  herpetic k.
  superior limbic k. (SLKC)
  virus k.
keratoconus
keratocyst
keratocyte
keratoderma
  k. acquisitum
  k. blennorrhagica
  k. climactericum
  k. eccentrica
  lymphedematous k.
  mutilating k.
  k. palmaris et plantaris
  palmoplantar k.
  k. plantare sulcatum
  punctate k.
  senile k.
  k. symmetrica
keratodermatitis
keratohyalin
  k. granule
  k. granule of epidermis
keratohyaline alteration
keratoid
keratolysis
  k. exfoliativa
keratolytic
keratoma
  k. disseminatum

k. hereditarium mutilans
k. plantare sulcatum
senile k.
keratomalacia
keratomycosis
keratonosis
keratopathy
band k.
keratoplasia
keratose
keratosis, pl. **keratoses**
actinic k.
arsenic k.
arsenical k.
k. blennorrhagica
k. diffusa fetalis
follicularis k.
k. follicularis
inverted follicular k.
lichenoid k.
k. nigricans
k. palmaris et plantaris
pilaris k.
k. punctata
k. rubra figurata
seborrheic k.
k. seborrheica
senile k.
k. senilis
solar k.
tar k.
k. vegetans
keratotic
k. papilloma
k. precipitate
kerion
Celsus k.
kernicterus
keroid
Keshan disease
ketal
ketimine
keto
k. acid
k. group
ketoacidosis (KA)
ketoaciduria
branched-chain k.
ketoconazole
keto-enol tautomer
ketogenesis

ketogenic
k. amino acid
k. corticoids test
k. hormone
k. steroid (KGS)
17-ketogenic
17-k. steroid assay test
17-k. steroids
17-k. steroids assay
ketogenic-antiketogenic ratio
ketohexokinase
ketohexose
ketone
k. body (KB)
k. body formation
k. body test
k. body utilization
dimethyl k.
methyl butyl k.
methyl ethyl k. (MEK)
methyl isobutyl k.
ketonemia
ketonimine dye
ketonuria
branched-chain k.
ketopentose
ketose
ketosis
ketosteroid (KS)
17-ketosteroid
17-k. assay
17-k. assay test
17-k.'s fractionation
Ketostix
ketosuria
ketotic hyperglycinemia
ketotransferase
ketotriose
Kety-Schmidt method
kev
kilo electron volt
keyhole-limpet hemocyanin (KLH)
key vein
KFAb
kidney-fixing antibody
KFS
Klippel-Feil syndrome
kg
kilogram
kg-cal
kilogram-calorie

K

NOTES

KGS
    ketogenic steroid
kHz
    kilohertz
KI
    karyopyknotic index
Ki-67
    K. antibody
    K. antigen
    K. oncogene
Ki-1 antigen
Ki-1+ lymphoma
KIA
    Kliger iron agar
Kidd blood group system
kidney
    amyloid k.
    Armanni-Ebstein k.
    arteriolosclerotic k.
    arteriosclerotic k.
    artificial k.
    Ask-Upmark k.
    atrophic k.
    k. biopsy
    cake k.
    k. carbuncle
    contracted k.
    cow k.
    crush k.
    cystic k.
    diseased k. (DK)
    disk k.
    duplex k.
    fatty k.
    flea-bitten k.
    Formad k.
    fused k.
    Goldblatt k.
    granular k.
    horseshoe k.
    human embryo k. (HEK)
    human embryonic k. (HEK)
    maximal tubular excretory capacity
      of k.'s (T_m)
    medullary sponge k.
    monkey k. (MK)
    mortar k.
    multilocular cystic k.
    pancake k.
    pelvic k.
    polycystic k.
    primary African green monkey k.
      (PAGMK)
    k. profile
    putty k.
    pyelonephritic k.
    rabbit k. (RK)
    rhesus monkey k. (RMK)

    Rose-Bradford k.
    sclerotic k.
    k. stone analysis
    supernumerary k.
    waxy k.
kidney-fixing antibody (KFAb)
Kiel classification
Kienböck
    K. atrophy
    K. disease
kieselguhr
Ki-FDC1p antibody
Kikuchi
    K. disease
    K. lymphadenitis
Kikuchi-Fujimoto disease
Kilham rat virus
killed
    heat k. (HK)
    k. measles virus vaccine (KMV)
    k. vaccine (KV)
killer
    k. cell
    k. lymphocyte
    natural k. (NK)
kilobase (kb)
    k. pair (kbp)
kilocalorie (kcal)
kilocycle (kc)
kilocycles per second (kcps)
kilo electron volt (kev)
kilogram (kg)
kilogram-calorie (kg-cal)
kilohertz (kHz)
kilohm
Kiloh-Nevin syndrome
kilojoule (kJ)
kilometer
kilopascal (kPa)
kilovolt (kV)
    k. ampere (kVa)
    k. peak (kvp)
kilovoltage
    peak k. (pkV)
kilowatt (kW)
kilowatt-hour (kW-hr)
KIM1P antibody
Ki-M4p antibody
Kimex
Kimmelstiel-Wilson
    K.-W. disease
    K.-W. lesion
    K.-W. syndrome
Kimura disease
kinase
    adenylate k.
    aspartate k.
    creatine k. (CK)

phosphoglycerate k.
phosphorylase k.
pyruvate k.
serum creatine k. (SCK)
kindred
kinematic viscosity
kinetic
k. analyzer
cell k.'s
cellular k.
k. energy (KE)
k. measurement
tumor cell k.'s
kinetochore
kinetocyte
kinetoplasm
kinetoplast
kinetosome
Kinevac
KINEX anatomic specimen stand
King-Armstrong (KA)
K.-A. unit (KAU)
kingdom
Kingella
K. denitrificans
K. kingae
king's evil
King unit
kininogen
high molecular weight k.
low molecular weight k.
kinin system
kink
kinky hair disease
Kinnier Wilson disease
kinocilium
Kinsbourne syndrome
Kinyoun carbol fuchsin stain
Kirby-Bauer test
Kirchoff law
Kirkland disease
Kisenyi sheep disease virus
kissing disease
kit
ABC Elite staining k.
IMMU-MARK immunostaining k.
spill control k.
Staclot Protein S test k.
Vecta-Stain Universal Elite ABC k.
Vecta-Stain Universal Quick k.
Wako NEFA test k.
Kitasato broth

Kittrich stain
KIU
kallikrein-inhibiting unit
kJ
kilojoule
Kjeldahl method
Klauder syndrome
Klebs disease
Klebsiella
K. friedländeri
K. oxytoca
K. ozaenae
K. pneumoniae
K. rhinoscleromatis
Klebsielleae
Klebs-Löffler bacillus
Kleihauer
K. acid elution test
K. stain
Kleihauer-Betke
K. test
Klein bacillus
Kleine-Levin syndrome
Klein-Gumprecht shadow nuclei
Klemperer disease
Klenow fragment
KLH
keyhole-limpet hemocyanin
Kliger iron agar (KIA)
Klinefelter syndrome (KS)
Klinger-Ludwig
K.-L. acid-thionin stain for sex
chromatin
Klippel disease
Klippel-Feil
K.-F. deformity
K.-F. syndrome (KFS)
Klippel-Trenaunay syndrome
Klippel-Trenaunay-Weber syndrome
Klump and Bieth method
Klumpke-Dejerine syndrome
Klüver-Barrera Luxol fast blue stain
Klüver-Bucy syndrome
Km
K. allotype
K. antigen
KMV
killed measles virus vaccine
knee
Brodie k.
septic k.
Knemidokoptes

K

NOTES

355

Kniest syndrome
knife
    microtome k.
knife-rest crystal
knight disease
knizocyte
knob
    malarial k.
Knodell histological activity index
knot
Knott technique
Kobelt cyst
Kober test
Köbner phenomenon
Koch
    K. law
    K. old tuberculin
    K. phenomenon
    K. postulate
Kocher-Debré-Semelaigne syndrome
Koch-Weeks bacillus
Koenen tumor
Koenig syndrome
Koerber-Salus-Elschnig syndrome
Kogoj abscess
KOH
    potassium hydroxide
    KOH preparation
    KOH test
Köhler
    K. disease
    K. illumination
Köhlmeier-Degos disease
Kohn one-step staining technique
koilocyte
koilocytosis
koilocytotic
    k. atypia
koilonychia
kokoi venom
Kolmer
    K. test
    K. test with Reiter protein (KRP)
Koongol viruses
Koplik spot
Korean
    K. hemorrhagic fever
    K. hemorrhagic fever virus
Korsakoff syndrome
Koser citrate broth
Koshevnikoff disease
Kossa stain
Kostmann syndrome
Kovats index
Kowarsky test
KP
    keratitic precipitate

KP1
    KP1 antibody
    KP1 immunohistochemical reagent
KP1/CD68 monoclonal antibody
kPa
    kilopascal
KPTT
    kaolin partial thromboplastin time
Krabbe
    K. disease
    K. leukodystrophy
    K. syndrome
kra-kra
K-*ras*
    K-*ras* mutation
    K-*ras* oncogene
kraurosis vulvae
Krause syndrome
Krauss and Neubecker morphologic
    criteria
KRB
    Krebs-Ringer bicarbonate buffer
Krebs
    K. cycle
    K. leukocyte index
Krebs-Henseleit cycle
Krebs-Ringer
    K.-R. bicarbonate buffer (KRB)
    K.-R. phosphate (KRP)
    K.-R. solution
Krishaber disease
Krokiewicz test
Kronecker stain
KRP
    Kolmer test with Reiter protein
    Krebs-Ringer phosphate
Krukenberg tumor
Kruskal-Wallis test
krypton
krypton-85
KS
    ketosteroid
    Klinefelter syndrome
    Kveim-Stilzbach test
KU
    Karmen unit
Kufs disease
Kugelberg-Welander disease
Kühne methylene blue
Kuhnt-Junius disease
Külz cylinder
Kumba virus
Kümmell disease
Kümmell-Verneuil disease
Kunkel
    K. syndrome
    K. test

Kupffer
    K. cell
    K. cell hypertrophy
    K. cell iron deposition
    K. cell sarcoma
kurtosis
kuru
Kurzrok-Ratner test
Kuskokwim syndrome
Kussmaul disease
Kussmaul-Maier disease
KV
    killed vaccine
kV
    kilovolt
kVa
    kilovolt ampere
Kveim
    K. antigen
    K. test
Kveim-Stilzbach
    K.-S. antigen
    K.-S. test (KS)

kvp
    kilovolt peak
KW
    Keith-Wagener
kW
    kilowatt
kwashiorkor
KWB
    Keith-Wagener-Barker
kW-hr
    kilowatt-hour
Kyasanur
    K. Forest disease
    K. Forest disease virus
kyphos
kyphoscoliotic pelvis
kyphosis
    juvenile k.
kyphotic pelvis
Kyrle disease

K

NOTES

λ (*var. of* lambda)
L
    lethal
    light
    liter
        L chain
        L dose
        L layer
        L unit of streptomycin
L_0, Lo
        L. dose
l-
    levorotatory
L-
    sterically related to L-glyceraldehyde
L26 antibody
LA
    latex agglutination
LAA
    leukocyte ascorbic acid
lab
    laboratory
Laband syndrome
Labbé neurocirculatory syndrome
label
    affinity l.
    l. variable
labeling
    cohort l.
    hazardous materials l.
    l. of hazardous materials
    l. index
    in situ DNA nick end l. (TUNEL)
labile
    l. factor
    heat l.
labiomycosis
laboratorian
laboratory (lab)
    clinical l.
    controlled access l.
    l. diagnosis
    face velocity of l. hood
    l. hood
    l. reference (LR)
    restricted access l.
labyrinthica
    otitis l.
labyrinthine
    l. defect (LD)
    l. hydrops
lacerated wound
laceration
Lachesis

Lacis
lac operon
lacrimal calculus
La Crosse virus
lactacidemia
lactacidosis
lactalbumin hydrolysate (LAH)
Lactarius
lactase deficiency
lactate
    l. dehydrogenase (LD, LDH)
    l. dehydrogenase assay
    l. dehydrogenase isoenzyme
    l. dehydrogenase isoenzymes
        determination
    l. dehydrogenase virus
lactated
    l. Ringer solution (LRS)
lactate-pyruvate ratio (L/P)
lactating adenoma
lactational mastitis
lacteal
    l. cyst
    l. fistula
lactenin
lactescence
lactic
    l. acid
    l. acid assay
    l. acid bacteria
    l. acidemia
    l. acidosis
    l. dehydrogenase (LD)
    l. dehydrogenase test
    l. dehydrogenase virus (LDV)
lacticacidemia
Lactobacillaceae
lactobacillary milk
Lactobacillus
    L. acidophilus
    L. brevis
    L. bulgaricus factor (LBF)
    L. bulgaris
    L. casei
    L. catenaformis
    L. fermentum
    L. jensenii
    L. leichmannii
    L. plantarum
lactocele
lactoferrin
lactogen
    human placental l. (hPL)
lactogenic hormone

L

lactoglobulin
  beta l.
  immune l.
β-lactoglobulin (BLG)
lactone dye
lactoperoxidase radioiodination
lactophenol cotton blue
lactose
  l. operon
  l. tolerance test
lactose-litmus broth
lactoside
  ceramide l.
lactosidosis
  ceramide l.
lactosuria
lactosyl ceramide
lacuna
  chondrocyte l.
  Howship l.
lacunar
  l. abscess
  l. cell
  l. resorption
LAD
  leukocyte adhesion deficiency
Ladd
  L. band
  L. syndrome
ladder
  sequence l.
Ladendorff test
LAE
  left atrial enlargement
Laelaps echidninus
Laënnec
  L. cirrhosis
  L. disease
  L. pearl
laesa
  functio l.
Lafora
  L. body
  L. disease
lag
  anaphase l.
  nitrogen l.
  l. phase
  l. time
Lagochilascaris
  L. minor
LAH
  lactalbumin hydrolysate
  left atrial hypertrophy
LAIT
  latex agglutination-inhibition test
LAK
  lymphokine-activated killer cell

lake
  bile l.
laked blood agar
Laki-Lorand factor (LLF)
laky
  l. blood
Lallemand body
LAMB
  lentigines, atrial myxoma, mucocutaneous
    myxomas, and blue nevi
  LAMB syndrome
lambda, λ
  l. chain
lambert
  L. canal
  L. law
Lambert-Eaton syndrome
Lamblia intestinalis
lambliasis
lambo
  lambo l.
lamella, pl. lamellae
  annulate lamellae
  cornoid l.
  elastic lamellae
  external elastic lamellae
  internal elastic lamellae
lamellar
  l. ichthyosis
  l. necrosis
lamina
  basal l.
  glomerular basal l.
  l. propria
laminar
  l. cortical necrosis
  l. cortical sclerosis
  l. flow burner
laminated thrombus
laminin
laminitis
L-amino acid oxidase
LAMP-1
  lysosomal membrane glycoprotein-1
LAMP-2
  lysosomal membrane glycoprotein-2
lamp
  hollow cathode l.
  mercury-vapor l.
  slit l.
  spirit l.
  tungsten arc l.
  tungsten halogen l.
  Wood l.
Lan antigen
Lancefield
  L. classification

L. grouping
L. precipitation test
lanceolate myxoma
Lancereaux-Mathieu disease
lancet fluke
Landouzy-Dejerine progressive muscular dystrophy
Landouzy disease
Landry
L. disease
L. syndrome
Landry-Guillain-Barré (LGB)
L.-G.-B. syndrome
Landschutz tumor
land scurvy
Landsteiner-Donath test
Lane disease
Langdon Down disease
Lange
L. colloidal gold test
L. solution
Langerhans
L. cell
L. cell granulomatosis (LCG)
L. cell histiocytosis
L. granule
islets of L.
langerhansian hormone
Langhans
L. cell
L. giant cell
L. layer
L. type of giant cell reaction
language
algorithm-oriented l. (ALGOL)
artificial l.
assembly l.
high-level l.
low-level l.
machine l.
source l.
Lansing virus
lanthanide
lanthanoid
lanthanum
l. nitrate
lanugo hair
LAP
leucine aminopeptidase
leukocyte alkaline phosphatase
lyophilized anterior pituitary

LAP stain
LAP test
laparomyositis
lapinization
lapinized
Laplace law
Laquer stain for alcoholic hyalin
L-**arabinose dehydrogenase**
L-**arabitol dehydrogenase**
larbish
lardaceous
l. liver
l. spleen
large
l. calorie (C, Cal)
l. cell carcinoma
l. cell lymphoma
l., external transformation-sensitive fibronectin (LETS)
l. granular lymphocyte (LGL)
l. vessel hematocrit (LVH)
large-scale integration
Larrey cleft
Larrey-Weil disease
Larsen
L. disease
L. syndrome
Larsen-Johansson disease
larva, pl. larvae
l. currens
l. fly
fly l.
larva migrans
lepidopterid l.
larval
larvicidal
larvicide
larviparous
larviphagic
laryngeal
l. granuloma
l. lupus
l. nodule
l. papillomatosis
l. polyp
l. tuberculosis
l. web
laryngis
pachyderma l.
laryngitis
laryngomalacia
laryngopharyngitis

NOTES

L

laryngotracheitis
    avian infectious l.
laryngotracheobronchitis (LTB)
Lasègue disease
laser
    l. microprobe
    l. microscope
LaserTweezer
Lash casein hydrolysate-serum medium
Lasiohelea
Lassa
    L. hemorrhagic fever
    L. virus
late
    l. infantile amaurotic familial
      idiocy (LIAFI)
    l. neonatal death
    l. positive component (LPC)
    l. reaction
    l. replicating X chromosome
    l. systolic murmur (LSM)
latency
    distal l.
    l. period (LP)
    terminal l.
latent
    l. allergy
    l. carcinoma
    l. coccidioidomycosis
    l. empyema
    l. heat
    hypermetropia, l. (HL)
    l. infection
    l. iron-binding capacity (LIBC)
    l. membrane protein-1 expression
      (LMP-1)
    l. microbism
    l. period
    l. porphyria
    l. rat virus
    l. stage
late-phase response
lateral
    l. aberrant thyroid carcinoma
    l. vaginal wall smear
latex
    l. agglutination (LA)
    l. agglutination-inhibition test
      (LAIT)
    l. agglutination test
    l. agglutinin
    l. fixation test
    l. flocculation test (LFT)
    l. screen
    l. slide agglutination test
lathyrism
lathyrus protein

Latrodectus
    L. bishopi
    L. geometricus
    L. mactans
LATS
    long-acting thyroid stimulator
    LATS protector
    LATS test
lattice
Lauber disease
Launois-Bensaude syndrome
Launois-Cléret syndrome
Launois syndrome
laurel fever
Laurell technique
Laurence-Biedl syndrome
Laurence-Moon-Bardet-Biedl syndrome
Laurence-Moon-Biedl syndrome
Laurence-Moon syndrome
lauric acid
lauryl sulfate broth
Lauth violet
LAV
    lymphadenopathy-associated virus
lavage
    bronchoalveolar l. (BAL)
    bronchopulmonary l.
    cervicovaginal l.
    gastric l.
    peritoneal l.
Laverania
law
    Ambard l.'s
    Ångstrom l.
    Beer l.
    Behring l.
    Bell-Magendie l.
    Bouguer l.
    Boyle l.
    Charles l.
    Coulomb l.
    Courvoisier l.
    Dalton l.
    Einthoven l.
    Faraday l. of electrolysis
    Farr l.
    Fick l.
    gas l.
    Gay-Lussac l.
    Graham l.
    Halsted l.
    Hamburger l.
    Hardy-Weinberg l.
    Henry l.
    Hooke l.
    ideal gas l.
    inverse-square l.
    Joule l.

Kirchoff l.
Koch l.
Lambert l.
Laplace l.
Marfan l.
l. of mass action
mass action l.
Mendel l.
Newton l. of cooling
Ohm l.
Planck radiation l.
Poiseuille l.
l. of priority
Profeta l.
Raoult l.
right-to-know l.
Snell l.
Starling l.
Stefan-Boltzmann l.
Stokes l.
Virchow l.
Lawford syndrome
Lawless stain
lawn plate
Lawrence-Seip syndrome
layer
cambium l.
depletion l.
germ l.
half-value l. (HVL)
L l.
Langhans l.
plasma l.
sluggish l.
still l.
lazarine leprosy
lazy leukocyte syndrome
LBBB
left bundle-branch block
LBF
Lactobacillus bulgaricus factor
LBI
low serum-bound iron
LBM
lean body mass
LBW
low birth weight
LBWI
low birth weight infant
LC
lethal concentration
lipid cystosome

LCA
leukocyte common antigen
LCA antibody
LCAT
lecithin-cholesterol acyltransferase
LCAT deficiency
LCD
lipochondral degeneration
LCFA
long-chain fatty acid
LCG
Langerhans cell granulomatosis
L-chain
L.-c. disease
L.-c. myeloma
LCIS
lobular carcinoma in situ
LCL
Levinthal-Coles-Lillie (bodies)
lymphocytic leukemia
lymphocytic lymphosarcoma
LCM
left costal margin
lymphatic choriomeningitis
lymphocytic choriomeningitis
LCM virus
LCT
long-chain triglyceride
LD
labyrinthine defect
lactate dehydrogenase
lactic dehydrogenase
Legionnaire's disease
lethal dose
living donor
lymphocyte-defined
L-D
Leishman-Donovan body
LD$_{50}$
median lethal dose
LDH
lactate dehydrogenase
LDH agent
LDL, LDLP
low-density lipoprotein
LDL cholesterol assay
LDL-C
low-density lipoprotein-cholesterol
L-dopa
levodopa
L⁺ dose

NOTES

LDV
  lactic dehydrogenase virus
LE
  leukoerythrogenetic
  lupus erythematosus
    LE body
    LE cell
    LE cell test
    LE factor
    LE phenomenon
    LE test
Le
  Le antigen
Le^a
  Lewis antibody
Le^b
  Lewis antibody
leaching
lead
  l. anemia
  l. apron
  l. assay
  black l.
  l. broth
  l. chromate
  l. citrate
  l. demonstration in tissue
  l. encephalitis
  l. encephalopathy
  l. fixative
  l. gout
  l. hydroxide stain
  l. level
  l. pigmentation
  l. poisoning
  l. stomatitis
leading strand
lead-pipe
  l.-p. colon
  l.-p. rigidity
lean body mass (LBM)
least squares regression
leather-bottle stomach
Leber
  L. disease
  L. optic atrophy
lecithin
lecithinase A
lecithin-cholesterol
  l.-c. acyltransferase (LCAT)
  l.-c. acyltransferase deficiency
lecithin-sphingomyelin
  l.-s. ratio (L/S)
  l.-s. ratio determination
lecithin/sphingomyelin ratio
lectin
lectotype

lectularia
  Acanthia l.
lectularius
  Cimex l.
LED
  lupus erythematosus disseminatus
Lederer anemia
leech
leeching
Lee-White
  L.-W. clotting test
  L.-W. clotting time
  L.-W. clotting time method
  L.-W. method (LW)
left
  l. atrial enlargement (LAE)
  l. atrial hypertrophy (LAH)
  l. bundle-branch block (LBBB)
  l. costal margin (LCM)
  l. frontoanterior position (LFA)
  l. ventricular enlargement (LVE)
  l. ventricular failure (LVF)
  l. ventricular hypertrophy (LVH)
left-sidedness
  bilateral l.
left-to-right ratio (L/R)
leg
  Barbados l.
  elephant l.
  milk l.
  white l.
Legal
  L. disease
  L. test
Legg-Calvé-Perthes disease
Legg disease
Legg-Perthes disease
Legionella
  L. bozemanii
  L. jordanis
  L. longbeachae
  L. pneumophila
  L. pneumophila culture
  L. pneumophila direct fA smear
legionellosis
Legionnaire's
  L. disease (LD)
  L. disease antibody
LEICA
  L. VT1000 E fully automatic
    microtome
  L. VT1000 M semi-automatic
    microtome
Leigh disease
Leiner disease
leiodermia
leiomyoblastoma
leiomyofibroma

leiomyoma
l. cutis
parasitic l.
uterine l.
vascular l.
leiomyomatosis
intravenous l. (IVL)
leiomyosarcoma
pleomorphic l.
Leipzig yellow
Leishman
L. chrome cell
L. stain
Leishman-Donovan body (L-D)
Leishmania
L. braziliensis
L. caninum
L. donovani
L. infantum
L. nilotica
L. peruviana
L. tropica
L. tropica mexicana
leishmaniasis
American l.
l. americana
anergic l.
cutaneous l.
lupoid l.
mucocutaneous l.
naso-oral l.
nasopharyngeal l.
pseudolepromatous l.
l. recidivans
l. serological test
l. tegumentaria diffusa
visceral l.
leishmanicidal
leishmaniosis
leishmanoid
Leitz image analysis system
Leloir disease
lemic
lemniscus, pl. **lemnisci**
lemon yellow
Lendrum
L. inclusion body stain
L. phloxine-tartrazine stain
Lenègre disease
length
focal l.
greatest l. (GL)

Lennert
L. classification
L. lesion
L. lymphoma
Lennox syndrome
lens
achromatic l.
aplanatic l.
electron l.
oil immersion l.
lens-induced uveitis
lenticula
lenticular
l. opacity
l. progressive degeneration
l. protein
lenticulopapular
lentiginosis
periorificial l.
lentigo, pl. **lentigines**
l. maligna
l. maligna melanoma
malignant l.
lentigomelanosis
Lentivirinae
lentivirus
lentogenic
Lenz syndrome
leonina
Toxascaris l.
leonine facies
leontiasis
l. ossea
Leon virus
LEOPARD
lentigines, electrocardiographic
abnormalities, ocular hypertelorism,
pulmonary stenosis, abnormalities of
genitalia, retardation of growth, and
deafness
Lepehne-Pickworth stain
leper
lepidic
Lepidoptera
lepidopterid larva
lepidosis
Lepore thalassemia
Leporipoxvirus
lepori pox virus
lepra
l. cell
l. manchada

L

NOTES

leprechaun facies
leprologist
leprology
leproma
lepromatous
    l. leprosy
lepromin
    l. reaction
    l. skin test
leprosarium
leprose
leprosery
leprostatic
leprosy
    anesthetic l.
    articular l.
    l. bacillus
    borderline l.
    cutaneous l.
    dimorphous l.
    dry l.
    histoid l.
    indeterminate l.
    lazarine l.
    lepromatous l.
    Lucio l.
    macular l.
    Malabar l.
    murine l.
    mutilating l.
    nodular l.
    smooth l.
    trophoneurotic l.
    tuberculoid l.
leprotic
leprous
Leptoconops
leptocyte
leptocytosis
leptokurtic
leptomeningeal
    l. carcinoma
    l. carcinomatosis
    l. cyst
    l. fibrosis
leptomeningitis
    basilar l.
leptomonad
Leptomonas
leptonema
Leptopsylla
    L. segnis
Leptospira
    L. australis
    L. autumnalis
    L. biflexa
    L. canicola
    L. culture

    L. grippotyphosa
    L. hebdomidis
    L. hyos
    L. icterohaemorrhagiae
    L. interrogans
    L. pomona
    L. serodiagnosis
leptospiral jaundice
leptospirosis
    l. icterohemorrhagica
leptospiruria
leptotene
Leptothrix
Leptotrichia
    L. buccalis
Leptotrombidium
    L. akamushi
    L. deliense
Leptus
Leriche syndrome
Leri pleonosteosis
Leri-Weill
    L.-W. disease
    L.-W. syndrome
Lermoyez syndrome
Leroy disease
Lesch-Nyhan syndrome
lesion
    angiocentric immunoproliferative l. (AIL)
    angiocentric lymphoproliferative l.
    Baehr-Lohlein l.
    benign lymphoepithelial l.
    bird's nest l.
    Bracht-Wachter l.
    bull's-eye l.
    central l.
    coin l.
    cold l.
    Councilman l.
    extracapillary l. (ECL)
    fibrohistiocytic l.
    Ghon primary l.
    gross l.
    histocytoid hemangioma-like l. (HHLL)
    histologic l.
    hot l.
    impaction l.
    indiscriminate l.
    initial syphilitic l.
    irritative l.
    Janeway l.
    jet l.
    Kimmelstiel-Wilson l.
    Lennert l.
    Lohlein-Baehr l.
    Mallory-Weiss l.

molecular l.
nonexophytic l.
onion scale l.
organic l.
papulonodular l.
peripheral l.
precancerous l.
precursor l.
primary l.
radial sclerosing l.
ring-wall l.
skip l.
space-occupying l. (SOL, Sol)
spontaneous l. (SPL)
squamous intraepithelial l. (SIL)
structural l.
systemic l.
target l.
trophic l.
verrucopapillary external genital l.
wire-loop l.

LET
leukocyte esterase test
linear energy transfer
lethal (L)
l. coefficient
l. concentration (LC)
l. dose (LD)
l. dwarfism
l. equivalent
l. midline granuloma
l. mutation
synthetic l.
lethargic encephalitis
LETS
large, external transformation-sensitive
fibronectin
Letterer-Siwe disease
Leu
L. 2 antibody
L. 3 antibody
L. 4 antibody
L. 7 antibody
L. 8 antibody
L. 12 antibody
L. 14 antibody
L. 22 antibody
L. 1 antigen
L. M1 antibody
leucin
leucine
l. aminopeptidase (LAP)

l. aminopeptidase test
l. hypoglycemia
leucinosis
leucinuria
Leucocytozoon
leucocytozoonosis
leucofuchsin
leucomethylene blue
leuco patent blue
leucovorin
l. calcium
leucyl
leucyl-RNA synthetase
leukanemia
leukapheresis
leukasmus
leukemia
acute granulocytic l. (AGL)
acute lymphoblastic l. (ALL)
acute lymphocytic l. (ALL)
acute megakaryoblastic l.
acute monoblastic l. (AML, AMoL)
acute monocytic l. (AML, AMoL, MLa)
acute myelocytic l. (AML)
acute myelogenous l.
acute myelomonocytic l. (AMML)
acute nonlymphocytic l. (ANLL)
acute promyelocytic l. (APL)
acute undifferentiated l. (AUL)
adult T-cell l. (ATL)
aleukemic granulocytic l.
aleukemic lymphocytic l.
aleukemic monocytic l.
basophilic l.
basophilocytic l.
blast cell l.
chronic cell l.
chronic granulocytic l. (CGL)
chronic lymphatic l. (CLL)
chronic lymphocytic l. (CLL)
chronic lymphosarcoma l. (CLSL)
chronic monoblastic leukemia (CMoL)
chronic monocytic l. (CMoL)
chronic myelocytic l. (CML)
chronic myelogenous l. (CML)
chronic myelomonocytic l. (MLC)
compound l.
l. cutis
embryonal l.

NOTES

leukemia *(continued)*
    eosinophilic l.
    eosinophilocytic l.
    erythroleukemia
    erythromyeloblastic l.
    feline l.
    l. of fowls
    granulocytic l.
    hairy cell l. (HCL)
    histiocytic l.
    l. immunophenotyping
    leukemic l.
    leukopenic l.
    lymphatic l.
    lymphoblastic l.
    lymphocytic l. (LCL)
    lymphoid l.
    lymphosarcoma cell l.
    mast cell l.
    mature cell l.
    megakaryocytic l.
    meningeal l.
    micromyeloblastic l.
    mixed l.
    mixed cell l.
    monoblastic l.
    monocytic l.
    monomyelocytic l.
    murine l.
    myeloblastic l.
    myelocytic l.
    myelogenic l.
    myelogenous l.
    myeloid l.
    myelomonocytic l.
    Naegeli type of monocytic l.
    neutrophilic l.
    plasma cell l.
    plasmacytic l.
    polymorphocytic l.
    progranulocytic l.
    promyelocytic l.
    Rieder cell l.
    Schilling type of monocytic l.
    smoldering l.
    splenic l.
    stem cell l.
    subacute myelomonocytic l. (MLS)
    subleukemic granulocytic l.
    subleukemic lymphocytic l.
    subleukemic monocytic l.
    thrombocytic l.
    thymic l.
    thymus l. (TL)
leukemic
    l. erythrocytosis
    l. leukemia
    l. myelosis

    l. reticuloendotheliosis
    l. reticulosis
leukemid
leukemogenesis
leukemogenic
leukemoid
    l. reaction
leukin
leukoagglutination
    EDTA-associated l.
leukoagglutinin
leukobilin
leukoblast
    granular l.
leukoblastosis
leukochloroma
leukocidin
leukocytactic
leukocytal
leukocytaxia
leukocyte
    acidophilic l.
    l. acid phosphatase stain
    l. adherence assay test
    l. adhesion deficiency (LAD)
    l. agglutinin
    agranular l.
    l. alkaline phosphatase (LAP)
    alkaline phosphatase activity of
        granular l. (APGL)
    l. alkaline phosphatase method
    l. alloantibodies
    l. antigen
    l. ascorbic acid (LAA)
    l. bactericidal assay test
    basophilic l.
    l. common antigen (LCA)
    l. cream
    cystinotic l.
    l. cytochemistry
    l. differential count
    endothelial l.
    eosinophilic l.
    l. esterase
    l. esterase test (LET)
    filament polymorphonuclear l.
    globular l.
    granular l.
    heterophilic l.
    l. histamine release test
    hyaline l.
    l. inclusion
    l. inhibitory factor
    l. interferon
    lymphoid l.
    mast l.
    motile l.
    multinuclear l.

neutrophilic l.
nonfilament polymorphonuclear l.
nongranular l.
nonmotile l.
oxyphilic l.
polymorphonuclear l. (poly)
polynuclear l.
segmented l.
l. transfusion
transitional l.
Türk irritation l.
leukocyte-poor (LP)
l.-p. red blood cell
leukocythemia
leukocytic
l. crystal
l. hypersegmentation
l. infiltrate
l. margination
l. marrow
l. maturation alteration
l. nuclear hyposegmentation
l. sarcoma
leukocytoblast
leukocytoclasia
leukocytoclasis
leukocytoclastic
l. angiitis
l. vasculitis
leukocytogenesis
leukocytoid
leukocytolysin
leukocytolysis
leukocytolytic
leukocytoma
leukocytometer
leukocytopenia
leukocytoplania
leukocytopoiesis
leukocytosis
absolute l.
agonal l.
basophilic l.
digestive l.
distribution l.
emotional l.
eosinophilic l.
lymphocytic l.
monocytic l.
neutrophilic l.
l. of the newborn
physiologic l.

relative l.
terminal l.
leukocytosis-promoting factor (LPF)
leukocytotactic
leukocytotaxia
leukocytotoxin
Leukocytozoon
leukocytozoonosis
leukocyturia
leukoderma
acquired l.
l. acquisitum centrifugum
leukodystrophy
Alexander l.
globoid l.
Krabbe l.
metachromatic l. (MLD)
metachromatic-type l.
spongy degenerative-type l.
sudanophilic l.
leukoencephalitis
acute epidemic l.
acute hemorrhagic l. (AHLE)
subacute sclerosing l.
leukoencephalopathy
multifocal progressive l.
progressive multifocal l. (PML)
leukoerythroblastic anemia
leukoerythroblastosis
leukoerythrogenetic (LE)
leukogram
leukokeratosis
leukokinetic
leukokinetics
leukokinin
leukokraurosis
leukolymphosarcoma
leukolysin
leukolysis
leukolytic
leukoma
leukomyelopathy
leukon
leukonecrosis
leukonychia
leukoparakeratosis
leukopathia
acquired l.
leukopathy
leukopcdesis
leukopenia
autoimmune l.

L

NOTES

leukopenia *(continued)*
    basophilic l.
    eosinophilic l.
    lymphocytic l.
    monocytic l.
    neutrophilic l.
leukopenic
    l. factor
    l. index
    l. leukemia
    l. myelosis
leukophlegmasia
    l. dolens
leukophoresis
leukoplakia
    l. vulvae
leukoplakic vulvitis
leukopoiesis
leukopoietic
leukopoietin
leukorrhea
leukosarcoma
leukosarcomatosis
leukosis
    avian l.
    enzootic bovine l.
    fowl l.
Leukosporidium
leukostasis
Leukostat stain
leukotactic
    l. assay
leukotaxia
leukotaxine
leukotaxis
leukotic
leukotome
leukotoxin
leukotriene
    l. A, B, C, D
Leukovirus
Leu-M1
    L.-M. antigen
    L.-M. immunoperoxidase stain
Levaditi
    L. method
    L. stain
levamphetamine
levan
levarterenol bitartrate
Levay antigen
Lev disease
level
    antibiotic l.
    barbiturate l.
    Clark l.
    confidence l.
    ethanol l.

    high l.
    isoelectric l.
    lead l.
    low l.
    minimal bactercidal l. (MBL)
    salicylate l.
    signal l.
    significance l.
Levey-Jennings charts
Levine alkaline Congo red stain
Levine-Rosai tumor classification
Levinson test
Levinthal-Coles-Lillie (bodies) (LCL)
Leviviridae
levocardia
    isolated l.
levodopa (L-dopa)
levorotatory (*l-*)
levothyroxine (LT)
levulosemia
levulose tolerance test
levulosuria
Lévy-Roussy syndrome
Lewandowski-Lutz disease
Lewis
    L. acid
    L. antibody (Le^b, Le^a)
    L. base
    L. blood group
Lewy body
Leyden
    L. crystal
    L. disease
Leyden-Möbius syndrome
Leydig
    L. cell adenoma
    L. cell hyperplasia
    L. cell tumor
    interstitial cell of L.
    L. interstitial cell
Leydig-Sertoli cell tumor
LF
    limit flocculation
Lf
    limes flocculation
    Lf dose
LFA
    left frontoanterior position
L-form
LFT
    latex flocculation test
    liver function test
LGB
    Landry-Guillain-Barré
LGL
    large granular lymphocyte
L-glyceric aciduria

LGV
   lymphogranuloma venereum
LH
   luteinizing hormone
L/H cell
Lhermitte-McAlpine syndrome
L-histidine ammonia-lyase
LHPC
   lipomatous hemangiopericytoma
LH-RF
   luteinizing hormone-releasing factor
LH-RH
   luteinizing hormone-releasing hormone
L-hydroxyacyl coenzyme A
LIAFI
   late infantile amaurotic familial idiocy
LIBC
   latent iron-binding capacity
liberator
   histamine l.
Libman-Sacks
   L.-S. disease
   L.-S. endocarditis
   L.-S. syndrome
library
   cDNA l.
   gene l.
LIC
   limiting isorrheic concentration
lice (*pl. of* louse)
lichen
   l. amyloidosis
   l. annularis
   atrophic l. planus
   bullous l. planus
   hypertrophic l. planus
   l. myxedematosus
   l. nitidus
   l. planus
   l. sclerosus et atrophicus
   l. scrofulosorum
   l. simplex chronicus
lichenification
lichenization
lichenoid
   l. dermatitis
   l. eczema
   l. keratosis
   pigmented purpuric l. dermatitis
Lichtheim
   L. disease
   L. syndrome

lidocaine
   l. assay
   l. hydrochloride
Lieberkühn
   crypts of L.
Liebermann-Burchard
   L.-B. reaction
   L.-B. test
lienomedullary
lienomyelogenous
Liesegang ring
life
   average l.
   mean effective l.
   l. table
   technologic l.
   useful l.
Li-Fraumeni cancer syndrome
ligand
   addressing l.
ligandin
ligase
   DNA l.
   polynucleotide l.
light (L)
   black l.
   l. chain
   l. green SF yellowish
   incident l.
   l. microscope
   l. microscopy (LM)
   l. pen
   l. pipe
   polarized l.
   l. reaction (LR)
   stray l.
   strobe l.
   ultraviolet l.
   visible l.
   Wood l.
light-chain disease
light-scattering immunoassay
Lightwood syndrome
Lignac
   L. disease
   L. syndrome
Lignac-Fanconi syndrome
ligneous
   l. struma
   l. thyroiditis
lignoceric acid
ligroin

L

NOTES

Lillie
    L. allochrome connective tissue stain
    L. allochrome method
    L. azure-eosin stain
    L. ferrous iron stain
    L. hematoxylin
    L. sulfuric acid Nile blue stain
limb-girdle muscular dystrophy
limen
    difference l. (DL)
limes
    l. flocculation (Lf)
limit
    assimilation l.
    l. check
    l. dextrin
    l. dextrinosis
    explosive l.
    l. of flocculation
    l. flocculation (LF)
    gas storage l.
    permissible exposure l.
    quantum l.
    l. of resolution
    saturation l.
    storage l.
    within normal l.'s (WNL)
limitations
    container size l.
limiting
    l. isorrheic concentration (LIC)
    l. reactant
Limnatis nilotica
limnemia
limnemic
limnology
limulus
    l. amebocyte lysate assay
    l. lysate test
lincomycin
lindane
Lindau
    L. disease
    L. tumor
Lindau-von Hippel disease
Lindner body
line
    Beau l.
    cell l.
    cement l.
    D l.
    delay l.
    l. of demarcation
    Eberth l.
    emission l.
    equipotential l.
    established cell l.

    l. filter
    grid l.
    Gubler l.
    Head l.
    Hunter-Schreger l.
    M l.
    l. number
    Ohngren l.
    Raji cell l.
    Reid base l. (RBL)
    resonance l.
    l. spectrum
    tender l.
    l. test
    Ullmann l.
    Wegner l.
    Z l.
    Z l.
    l. of Zahn
    Zahn l.
linea, pl. **lineae**
    lineae albicantes
    lineae atrophicae
lineage infidelity
linear
    l. amplifier
    l. attenuation coefficient
    l. energy transfer (LET)
    l. fracture
    l. IgA bullous disease in children
    l. regression
    l. sebaceous nevus syndrome
linearity
    l. check
    photometric l.
line-spread function
Lineweaver-Burk equation
lingua, pl. **linguae**
    anthracosis linguae
lingual goiter
Linguatula
    L. serrata
linguatuliasis
Linguatulidae
linitis
    l. plastica
linkage
    chromosomal l.
    l. disequilibrium
    l. group
    l. map
linnaean system of nomenclature
Linognathus
linoleate
linoleic acid
linolenic acid
Linstowiidae
liotrix

LIP
>lymphocytic interstitial pneumonitis
>lymphoid interstitial pneumonia

lip
>cleft l.
>rhombic l.

liparocele

lipase
>l. assay
>clearing factor l.
>lipoprotein l. (LPL)
>pancreatic l.
>l. 105 stain
>l. 21 stain
>l. test
>triacylglycerol l.

lipedema

lipemia
>absorptive l.
>alimentary l.
>diabetic l.
>postprandial l.
>l. retinalis

lipemic

lipid
>accumulation of complex l.'s
>l. assay
>Ciaccio-positive l.
>l. cystosome (LC)
>l. degeneration
>l. depletion
>l. embolism
>extracellular aggregate alteration l.
>l. histiocytosis
>l. nephrosis
>nuclear aggregate l.
>l. pigment
>l. pneumonia
>l. profile
>l. proteinosis
>l. stain
>l. storage disease
>l. test
>l. transport
>l. transport disorder

lipidemia

lipidized glioma

lipidosis, pl. **lipidoses**
>cerebroside l.
>glycolipid l.
>sphingomyelin l.
>sulfatide l.

lipiduria

lipoarthritis

lipoatrophia
>l. annularis
>l. circumscripta

lipoatrophic diabetes

lipoatrophy
>insulin l.
>partial l.

lipoblastic lipoma

lipoblastoma

lipoblastomatosis

lipocele

lipochondral degeneration (LCD)

lipochondrodystrophy

lipochrome pigmentation

lipocrit

lipocyte

lipodystrophia
>l. intestinalis
>l. progessiva superior

lipodystrophy
>congenital total l.
>inferior l.
>insulin l.
>intestinal l.
>progressive l.

lipoedema

lipofibroma

lipofuscin

lipofuscinosis

lipogenesis

lipogenic

lipogranuloma

lipogranulomatosis
>disseminated l.
>Farber l.

lipogranulomatosis

lipohemia

lipoic acid

lipoid
>l. degeneration
>l. dermatoarthritis
>l. dystrophy
>l. granuloma
>l. nephrosis (LN)
>l. pneumonia
>l. proteinosis

lipoidemia

lipoidosis

lipolipoidosis

lipolysis regulation

L

NOTES

lipolysosome
lipolytic
    l. enzyme
    l. hormone
lipoma
    l. annulare colli
    l. arborescens
    atypical l.
    l. capsulare
    l. cavernosum
    fetal fat cell l.
    l. fibrosum
    infiltrating l.
    lipoblastic l.
    l. myxomatodes
    l. ossificans
    l. petrificans
    pleomorphic l.
    l. sarcomatodes
    l. sarcomatosum
    spindle cell l.
    telangiectatic l.
lipomatoid
lipomatosa
    macrodystrophia l.
lipomatosis, pl. lipomatoses
    encephalocraniocutaneous l.
    mediastinal l.
    multiple symmetric l.
    l. neurotica
lipomatous
    l. hemangiopericytoma (LHPC)
    l. hypertrophy
    l. infiltration
    l. myxoma
    l. polyp
lipomelanic reticulosis
lipomelanin
lipomelanotic reticuloendothelial cell
  hyperplasia
lipomeningocele
lipomucopolysaccharidosis
Liponyssus
lipopeliosis
lipopenia
lipopenic
lipophage
lipophagia
    l. granulomatosis
lipophagic
    l. granuloma
    l. intestinal granulomatosis
lipophagy
lipophilic
lipophyllodes tumor
lipoprotein (LP)
    α-l.
    alpha l.

    l. assay
    beta l.
    l. chylomicron
    l. electrophoresis (LPE)
    l. electrophoresis test
    high-density l. (HDL, HDLP)
    intermediate-density l. (IDL)
    l. lipase (LPL)
    l. lipase deficiency
    low-density l. (LDL, LDLP)
    l. Lp(a)
    l. polymorphism
    pre-β-l.
    very high density l. (VHDL)
    very low density l. (VLDL,
      VLDLP)
lipoprotein-cholesterol
    high-density l.-c. (HDL-C)
    low-density l.-c. (LDL-C)
lipoproteinemia
lipoprotein-X (Lp-X)
liposarcoma
    dedifferentiated l.
    myxoid l.
liposis
liposome
lipotrophic
lipotropic
lipotropin (LPH)
lipotropy
lipovaccine
lipoxenous
lipoxeny
lipping
Lipschütz
    L. cell
    L. disease
    L. ulcer
lipuria
lipuric
liquefacient
liquefaction degeneration
liquefactive
    l. degeneration
    l. necrosis
liquid
    l. chromatography
    combustible l.
    l. crystal
    l. human serum
    l. junction potential
    l. scintillation counter
    l. scintillator
    l. (solution) hybridization
liquid-in-glass thermometer
liquid-liquid
    l.-l. chromatography
    l.-l. junction potential

LIS
  lobular in situ
Lison-Dunn
    L.-D. method
    L.-D. stain
lissamine rhodamine B 200
lissencephalia
lissencephalic
lissencephaly
list
    l. mode
    l. structure
Listerella
Listeria
    L. monocytogenes
listeriosis, listerosis
listing
liter (L)
    millimoles per l. (mM/L, mM/l)
literal
liters per minute (Lpm, lpm)
lithiasis
    l. conjunctivae
    pancreatic l.
lithic acid
lithium
    l. assay
    l. carbonate
    l. carmine
    l. tungstate
lithium-drifted detector
Lithobius
lithocholate
lithocholic acid
lithogenesis
lithogenic
lithogenous
lithogeny
lithoid
lithonephritis
lithopedion
lithotroph
lithuresis
lithureteria
lithuria
litmus
    l. whey
Little disease
littoral cell
littoral-cell angioma
littritis

livedo
    postmortem l.
    l. racemosa
    l. reticularis
    l. reticularis idiopathica
    l. reticularis symptomatica
    l. telangiectatica
    l. vasculitis
livedoid
live oral poliovirus vaccine
liver
    l. battery
    cardiac l.
    l. cell adenoma
    l. cell carcinoma
    fatty l.
    l. flocculation test
    l. fluke
    frosted l.
    l. function test (LFT)
    l. grooves
    hobnail l.
    icing l.
    lardaceous l.
    nutmeg l.
    l. palm
    polycystic l.
    l. profile
    septal fibrosis of l.
    sugar-icing l.
    wandering l.
    waxy l.
lividity
    postmortem l.
living donor (LD)
livor mortis
lixiviation
LJM
    Löwenstein-Jensen medium
L layer
LLF
    Laki-Lorand factor
L-L factor
LLL
    localized leishmania lymphadenitis
LLM
    localized leukocyte mobilization
Lloyd reagent
L-lysine:NAD⁺ oxidoreductase
LM
    light microscopy

NOTES

LMD, LMDX
  low molecular weight dextran
LMP-1
  latent membrane protein-1 expression
LMW
  low molecular weight
LN
  lipoid nephrosis
  lupus nephritis
LN1 antibody
LN2 antibody
LN3 monoclonal antibody
LNPF
  lymph node permeability factor
Lo (*var. of* L$_0$)
Loa
  L. loa
load
  l. factor
loader
loading
  l. dose
  salt l.
lobar
  l. cerebral atrophy
  l. pneumonia
  l. pulmonary atrophy
  l. sclerosis
lobectomy
lobeline
lobitis
Loboa loboi
Lobo disease
loboi
  Loboa l.
lobomycosis
lobopodium
Lobstein
  L. disease
  L. syndrome
lobster claw deformity
lobular
  l. adenocarcinoma
  l. carcinoma
  l. carcinoma in situ (LCIS)
  l. disarray
  l. glomerulonephritis
  infiltrating l. carcinoma (ILC)
  l. neoplasia
  l. pattern
  l. pneumonia
  l. in situ (LIS)
lobulation
  fetal l.
lobule
  peripheral l.
lobulocentric pattern

local
  l. anaphylaxis
  l. anemia
  l. death
  l. exhaust ventilation
  l. glomerulonephritis
  l. immunity
  l. reaction
localization
  eye tumor l.
localized
  l. histiocytosis
  l. inflammation
  l. leishmania lymphadenitis (LLL)
  l. leukocyte mobilization (LLM)
  l. mucinosis
  l. nodular tenosynovitis
  l. osteitis fibrosa
  l. peritonitis
  l. plaque formation (LPF)
  l. scleroderma
locant
location
  storage l.
loci (*pl. of* locus)
Locke-Ringer solution
Locke solution
lock-in amplifier
loculated
  l. architecture
  l. empyema
loculation
loculus, pl. **loculi**
locus, pl. **loci**
  l. ceruleus
  cis-acting l.
  four l.
  histocompatibility l. (HL)
  major histocompatibility l.
LOD score
Loeb deciduoma
Loeffler (*var. of* Löffler)
Loevit
  L. cell
Loewenthal reaction
Löffler, Loeffler
  L. blood culture medium
  L. blood serum
  L. caustic stain
  L. coagulated serum medium
  L. disease
  L. methylene blue
  L. myocarditis
  L. syndrome
logarithm
  common l.
  napierian l.

logarithmic
    l. amplifier
    l. curve
    l. phase
log dilution
logic
    CMOS l.
    complementary metal oxide
      semiconductor l.
    emitter-coupled l. (ECL)
    transistor-transistor l.
    tristate l.
logical record
logit transformation
lognormal distribution
Lohlein-Baehr lesion
loiasis
London force
long
    L. coefficient
    L. formula
    l. incubation hepatitis
    l. terminal repeat sequence (LTR)
long-acting
    l.-a. thyroid stimulating hormone
      test (LATS test)
    l.-a. thyroid stimulator (LATS)
    l.-a. thyroid-stimulator hormone
      assay
long-chain
    l.-c. fatty acid (LCFA)
    l.-c. triglyceride (LCT)
longior
    Tyroglyphus l.
longirostratum
    Exserohilum l.
longispiculata
    Nematodirella l.
loop
    capillary l.
    l. diuretic
    feedback l.
    hairpin l.
    l. of Henle
    hysteresis l.
looping
Looser-Milkman syndrome
loose skin
Lophophora
lophotrichous
Lorain disease
Lorain-Lévi syndrome

lordoscoliosis
lordosis
lordotic
    l. albuminuria
    l. pelvis
Losch nodule
loss
    allele-specific l.
    blood l. (BL)
    eddy-current l.
    estimated blood l. (EBL)
    transepidermal water l. (TWL)
lot
Lou Gehrig disease
Louis-Bar syndrome
louping ill
louping-ill virus
louse, pl. **lice**
    body l.
    chicken l.
    crab l.
    dog l.
    head l.
    pubic l.
    sucking l.
louse-borne typhus
lousiness
lousy
low
    l. birth weight (LBW)
    l. birth weight infant (LBWI)
    l. frequency transduction
    l. grade astrocytoma
    l. level
    l. malignant potential tumor
    l. molecular weight (LMW)
    l. molecular weight dextran (LMD,
      LMDX)
    l. molecular weight kininogen
    l. order
    l. protein (LP)
    l. serum-bound iron (LBI)
low-actinic glass
low-compliance bladder
low-density
    l.-d. lipoprotein (LDL, LDLP)
    l.-d. lipoprotein cholesterol
    l.-d. lipoprotein-cholesterol (LDL-C)
Lowe
    L. disease
    L. syndrome

L

NOTES

low-egg-passage vaccine
Löwenstein-Jensen medium (LJM)
Lowenthal test
lower
    l. nephron nephrosis
    l. respiratory tract smear
Lowe-Terrey-MacLachlan syndrome
low-level language
Lown-Ganong-Levine syndrome
low-pass filter
low-power field (LPF, lpf)
low-voltage
    l.-v. fast (LVF)
    l.-v. foci (LVF)
Loxosceles
    L. laeta
    L. reclusa
Loxotrema ovatum
LP
    latency period
    leukocyte-poor
    lipoprotein
    low protein
    lymphoid plasma
L/P
    lactate-pyruvate ratio
LPC
    late positive component
LPD
    lymphoproliferative disease
LPE
    lipoprotein electrophoresis
LPF
    leukocytosis-promoting factor
    localized plaque formation
    low-power field
    lymphocytosis-promoting factor
lpf
    low-power field
LPH
    lipotropin
L-phase variant
LPHD
    lymphocyte predominance Hodgkin
      disease
LPI
    lysinuric protein intolerance
LPL
    lipoprotein lipase
Lpm, lpm
    liters per minute
Lp-X
    lipoprotein-X
LR
    laboratory reference
    light reaction
L/R
    left-to-right ratio

Lr
    Lr dose
LRS
    lactated Ringer solution
LS, LSA
    lymphosarcoma
LSA/RCS
    lymphosarcoma-reticulum cell sarcoma
LSD
    lysergic acid diethylamide
LSM
    late systolic murmur
L-sulfoiduronate sulfatase
LT
    levothyroxine
    lymphotoxin
LTB
    laryngotracheobronchitis
LTH
    luteotropic hormone
LTR
    long terminal repeat sequence
Lu antigen
Lubarsch
    crystal of L.
    L. crystal
Lucas-Championnière disease
Lucey-Driscoll syndrome
Lucilia
Lucio
    L. leprosy
    L. leprosy phenomenon
Lücke
    L. test
Lucké
    L. adenocarcinoma
    L. carcinoma
    L. virus
lückenschädel
Ludwig angina
lues
luetic
    l. aneurysm
    l. aortitis
Luft
    L. disease
    L. potassium permanganate fixative
Lugol
    L. iodine solution
    L. stain
Lukes-Butler
    L.-B. histologic subclassification
    L.-B. non-Hodgkin lymphoma
      classification
Lukes-Collins classification
lumbago
lumbar
    l. appendicitis

l. puncture
l. spondylosis
lumbrical
lumbricidal
lumbricide
lumbricoid
lumbricosis
lumbricus
lumen, pl. **lumina, lumens**
luminal
luminescence
luminescent
luminophore
luminous
l. flux
l. flux density
l. intensity
Lumi-Phos solution
lumpy
l. jaw
l. skin disease
Luna-Ishak stain
lung
l. abscess
acinic cell tumor of l.
bilobed right l.
bird-breeder's l.
black l.
butterfly l.
cheese worker's l.
collier's l.
cystic disease of l.
diffusing capacity of l.
eosinophilic l.
eosinophilic granuloma of l. (EGL)
farmer's l.
l. fluke
honeycomb l.
human embryo l. (HEL)
hyperlucent l.
malt-worker's l.
mason's l.
miner's l.
mushroom-worker's l.
pseudovascular adenoid squamous
cell carcinoma of the l.
(PASSCL)
rudimentary l.
shock l.
thresher's l.
l. tumor

uremic l.
welder's l.
lunger disease
lungworm
Lunyo virus
lupi
Spirocerca l.
lupiform
lupinine
lupoid
l. hepatitis
l. leishmaniasis
l. ulcer
lupous
lupus
l. band test
chronic discoid l. erythematosus
discoid l. erythematosus (DLE)
disseminated l. erythematosus
(DLE)
l. erythematodes
l. erythematosus (LE)
l. erythematosus cell
l. erythematosus cell test
l. erythematosus disseminatus
(LED)
l. erythematosus inhibitor
l. erythematosus profundus
hydralazine l.
l. hypertrophicus
laryngeal l.
l. livido
l. lymphaticus
l. mutilans
l. nephritis (LN)
l. papillomatosus
l. pernio
l. psoriasis
l. sclerosus
l. sebaceus
l. serpiginosus
l. superficialis
systemic l. erythematosus (SLE)
l. tuberculosus
l. tumidus
l. verrucosus
l. vulgaris
l. vulgaris erythematoides
Luse body
luteal
l. cyst
l. hormone

L

NOTES

lutein
>l. cell

luteinization

luteinized follicular cyst

luteinizing
>l. hormone (LH)
>l. hormone assay
>l. hormone-releasing factor (LH-RF)
>l. hormone-releasing hormone (LH-RH)
>l. principle

luteinoma

Lutembacher syndrome

luteolysis

luteolytic

luteoma
>pregnancy l.

luteotropic hormone (LTH)

luteotropin

lutetium

luteum
>cystic corpus l.

Lutheran
>L. Blood Group
>L. blood group system

lututrin

Lutzomyia

Lutz-Splendore-Almeida disease

lux

luxation

Luxol
>L. fast blue
>L. fast blue stain

luxus heart

Luys body syndrome

LVE
>left ventricular enlargement

LVF
>left ventricular failure
>low-voltage fast
>low-voltage foci

LVH
>large vessel hematocrit
>left ventricular hypertrophy

LW
>Lee-White method

lyase
>argininosuccinate l.
>heparitinsulphate l.

lycopenemia

Lycoperdon

lycoperdonosis

lycophora

lye

Lyell
>L. disease
>L. syndrome

LYG
>lymphomatoid granulomatosis

Lymantria

Lyme
>L. borreliosis
>L. disease
>L. disease serology

Lymnaea

lymph
>aplastic l.
>blood l.
>l. cell
>l. corpuscle
>corpuscular l.
>croupous l.
>dental l.
>l. embolism
>euplastic l.
>fibrinous l.
>germinal center of l. node
>glycerinated l.
>inflammatory l.
>intercellular l.
>intravascular l.
>l. node
>l. node biopsy
>l. node permeability factor (LNPF)
>plastic l.
>l. scrotum
>tissue l.
>vaccine l.
>l. varix

lympha

lymphadenitis
>dermatopathic l.
>Kikuchi l.
>localized leishmania l. (LLL)
>paratuberculous l.
>regional granulomatous l.
>tuberculosis l.
>tuberculous l.

lymphadenoid goiter

lymphadenoma

lymphadenomatosis

lymphadenopathy
>angioimmunoblastic l.
>angioimmunoblastic l. with dysproteinemia (AILD)
>dermatopathic l.
>immunoblastic l.
>silicone l.
>sinus histiocytosis with massive l. (SHML)
>l. syndrome

lymphadenopathy-associated virus (LAV)

lymphadenosis
>benign l.
>malignant l.

lymphadenovarix
lymphangeitis
lymphangiectasia
lymphangiectasis
    cavernous l.
    cystic l.
    intestinal l.
    simple l.
lymphangiectatic
lymphangiectodes
lymphangiitis
lymphangioendothelial sarcoma
lymphangioendothelioma
lymphangioleiomyomatosis
lymphangiology
lymphangioma
    l. capillare varicosum
    l. cavernosum
    l. circumscriptum
    l. cysticum
    l. superficium simplex
    l. tuberosum multiplex
    l. xanthelasmoideum
lymphangiomatosis
lymphangiomatous
lymphangiomycomatosis
lymphangiomyomatosis
lymphangiophlebitis
lymphangiosarcoma
lymphangitis
    l. carcinomatosa
    epizootic l.
    l. epizootica
lymphapheresis
lymphatic
    l. angina
    l. choriomeningitis (LCM)
    l. corpuscle
    l. dissemination theory of
      endometriosis
    l. dyscrasia
    l. edema
    l. leukemia
    l. nevus
    l. sarcoma
lymphatitis
lymphatolysis
lymphatolytic
lymphectasia
lymphedema
    congenital l.
    hereditary l.

    l. praecox
    primary l.
lymphedematous keratoderma
lymphemia
lymphoadenoma
lymphoblast
lymphoblastic
    l. leukemia
    l. lymphoma
    l. lymphosarcoma
lymphoblastoid
lymphoblastoma
    giant follicular l.
lymphoblastosis
lymphocele
lymphocerastism
lymphocyst
lymphocytapheresis
lymphocyte
    activated l.
    l. activation
    atypical l.
    B l.
    l. blastogenic factor
    circulating atypical l.
    cytologic T l. (CTL)
    Downey-type l.
    l. function associated antigen
    helper T l.
    killer l.
    large granular l. (LGL)
    mantle-zone l.
    l. microcytotoxicity assay
    l. mitogenic factor
    nodular poorly differentiated l.
      (NPDL)
    null l.
    plasmacytoid l.
    l. predominance Hodgkin disease
      (LPHD)
    Rieder l.
    l. subset enumeration
    suppressor T l.
    T l.
    l. transfer test
    l. transformation
    l. transformation test
    transformed l.
    tumor-infiltrating l. (TIL, TILS)
lymphocyte-activating factor
lymphocyte-defined (LD)
lymphocyte-mediated cytotoxicity

NOTES

lymphocyte-stimulating hormone
lymphocyte transformation test
lymphocyte-transforming factor
lymphocythemia
lymphocytic
- l. adenohypophysitis
- l. blood cell
- l. choriomeningitis (LCM)
- l. choriomeningitis virus
- l. cuffing
- l. hypophysitis
- l. infiltration of skin
- l. inflammatory infiltrate
- l. interstitial pneumonitis (LIP)
- l. leukemia (LCL)
- l. leukemoid reaction
- l. leukocytosis
- l. leukopenia
- l. lymphoma
- l. lymphosarcoma (LCL)
- l. marrow
- l. series
- l. thymoma
- l. transformation

lymphocytic-histiocytic (L/H cell)
lymphocytoblast
lymphocytolysis
lymphocytoma
- benign l. cutis

lymphocytopenia
lymphocytopoiesis
lymphocytorrhexis
lymphocytosis
- neutrophilic l.

lymphocytosis-promoting factor (LPF)
lymphocytotoxic antibody
lymphocytotoxicity
lymphocytotoxin
lymphoderma
- l. perniciosa

lymphoepithelioma
lymphogenesis
lymphogenic
lymphogenous
- l. embolism
- l. metastasis

lymphogranuloma
- l. benignum
- l. inguinale
- l. malignum
- Schaumann l.
- venereal l.
- l. venereum (LGV)
- l. venereum antigen
- l. venereum titer
- l. venereum virus

lymphogranulomatosis
lymphohematopoiesis

lymphohematopoietic
lymphohistiocytosis
lymphoid
- l. corpuscle
- l. hemoblast of Pappenheim
- l. hyperplasia
- l. hypophysitis
- l. hypoplasia
- l. interstitial pneumonia (LIP)
- l. leukemia
- l. leukocyte
- l. monoclonal antibody
- l. plasma (LP)
- l. polyp
- l. series
- l. stem cell

lymphoid-rich effusion
lymphokine
lymphokine-activated killer cell (LAK)
lympholeukocyte
lymphology
lymphoma
- adult T-cell l. (ATL)
- anaplastic large cell l. (ALCL)
- anaplastic large cell malignant l.
- B-cell l. (BCL)
- benign l.
- benign l. of the rectum
- biphenotypic l.
- Burkitt l. (BL)
- centrocytic l.
- centrocytic/mantle-cell l. (CC/MCL)
- cutaneous l.
- cutaneous T-cell l. (CTCL)
- diffuse histocytic l. (DHL)
- diffuse poorly differentiated l. (DPDL)
- diffuse small cleaved cell l.
- discordant l.
- enteropathy-associated T-cell l. (ETCL)
- extranodal l.
- floral variant of follicular l. (FFL)
- follicular predominantly large cell l.
- follicular predominantly small cleaved cell l.
- giant follicular l.
- histiocytic l. (HL)
- Hodgkin l.
- immunoblastic l.
- l. immunophenotyping
- Ki-1+ l.
- large cell l.
- Lennert l.
- lymphoblastic l.
- lymphocytic l.
- lymphoplasmacytoid l.

lymphosarcoma type malignant l.
macrofollicular l.
malignant l. (ML)
mantle cell l.
marginal zone l.
Mediterranean l.
monocytoid B-cell l.
mucosa-associated lymphoid
   tissue l. (MALToma, MALT
   lymphoma)
nasal T/NK-cell l.
nodular histiocytic l.
non-Hodgkin l.
non-MALT l.
   nonmucosa-associated lymphoid
     tissue lymphoma
nonmucosa-associated lymphoid
   tissue l. (non-MALT lymphoma)
parafollicular B-cell l. (PBCL)
paraimmunoblastic l.
peripheral T-cell l. (PTCL)
plasmacytoid l.
poorly differentiated lymphocytic l.
   (PDLL)
prethymic lymphoblastic l.
pulmonary MALT l.
pyothorax-associated l.
respiratory angiocentric l.
small lymphocytic l. (SLL)
splenic marginal zone l. (SMZL)
stem cell l.
T cell-rich, B-cell l. (TCRBCL)
T/natural killer cell l.
U-cell l.
undifferentiated l. (UL)
Waldeyer ring l.
well-differentiated lymphocytic l.
   (WDLL)
lymphomatoid
   l. granulomatosis (LYG)
   l. papulosis
lymphomatosis
   avian l.
   fowl l.
   ocular l.
   visceral l.
lymphomatous
lymphomyeloma
lymphomyxoma
lymphopathia venereum
lymphopenia

lymphopenic thymic dysplasia
lymphophagocytosis
lymphoplasmacytic
   l. infiltrate
   l. response
lymphoplasmacytoid lymphoma
lymphoplasmapheresis
lymphopoiesis
lymphopoietic
lymphoproliferative
   l. disease (LPD)
   l. disorder
   l. syndrome
lymphoreticular
   l. disease
   l. disorder
   l. system
lymphoreticulosis
   benign inoculation l.
lymphorrhea
lymphorrhoid
lymphosarcoma (LS, LSA)
   l. cell leukemia
   follicular l. (FLSA)
   lymphoblastic l.
   lymphocytic l. (LCL)
   reticulum cell l.
   l. type malignant lymphoma
lymphosarcoma-reticulum cell sarcoma
   (LSA/RCS)
lymphosarcomatosis
lymphosis
lymphostatic verrucosis
lymphotoxicity
lymphotoxin (LT)
lymphuria
Lyon hypothesis
lyonization
lyophilization
lyophilize
lyophilized anterior pituitary (LAP)
Lyponyssus
Lys
   lysine
lysate
lyse
lysemia
lysergic
   l. acid diethylamide (LSD)
   l. acid diethylamide assay

L

NOTES

lysin
    β-l.
    beta l.
lysine (Lys)
    l. dehydrogenase
    l. intolerance
    l. ketoglutarate reductase
lysine-2-oxoglutaryl reductase
lysine-iron agar
lysinemia
lysing agent
lysinogen
lysinogenic
lysinuria
lysinuric protein intolerance (LPI)
lysis
    clot l.
    colloid-osmotic l.
    fibrin plate l.
    follicle l. (Fl)
lysochrome
lysogen
lysogenesis
lysogenic
    l. bacterium
    l. induction
    l. strain
lysogenicity
lysogenization
lysogeny
lysokinase

lysolecithin
lysophosphatidate
lysophosphatide
lysophosphatidyl choline
lysophosphatidylethanolamine
lysophospholipase
lysosomal
    l. membrane glycoprotein-1 (LAMP-1)
    l. membrane glycoprotein-2 (LAMP-2)
    l. protease
    l. storage disease
lysosome
    secondary l.
lysostaphin
lysotype
lysozyme
    l. assay
    egg-white l. (EWL)
    human milk l. (HML)
    l. test
lyssa
Lyssavirus
lysyl
Lyt antigen
lytic
Lytta
lytta
lyze

μ (*var. of* mu)
μμ
    micromicron
μμc
    micromicrocurie
μf, μfd
    microfarad
μL
    microliter
μm
    micrometer
μmm
    micromillimeter
μV
    microvolt
M
    molar
    mucoid
        M antigen
        M band
        M colony
        M component
        M concentration
        M line
        M phase
        M protein
M_1 antigen
MΩ
    megohm
m
    meter
mμ
    millimicron
mμc
    millimicrocurie
mμg
    millimicrogram
mA
    milliampere
MAA
    macroaggregated albumin
MAb, MAB
    monoclonal antibody
        MAb 12C3 monoclonal antibody
MAC
    Mycobacterium avium-intracellulare
Mac387 antibody
Macaca
Macchiavello stain
MacConkey
    M. agar
    M. broth
macerated
    m. fetus
    m. stillbirth

maceration
Machado-Guerreiro test
Mache unit (MU)
machine
    m. error
    Faxitron x-ray m.
    m. language
Machupo virus
MacKenzie
    M. disease
    M. syndrome
Macleod
    M. rheumatism
    M. syndrome
maclurin
MacNeal tetrachrome blood stain
Macracanthorhynchus
    M. hirudinaceus
macrencephaly
macroadenoma
macroaggregate
macroaggregated albumin (MAA)
macroamylase
macroamylasemia
Macrobdella
macrobiote
macroblast
macrocephalic
macrocephaly
macrocheilia, macrochilia
macrochemistry
macrochilia
macrochylomicron
macrocolon
macroconidium, pl. macroconidia
macrocranium
macrocryoglobulin
macrocryoglobulinemia
macrocyst
macrocytase
macrocyte
macrocythemia
    hyperchromatic m.
macrocytic
    m. achylic anemia
    m. anemia of pregnancy
    m. hyperchromia
macrocytosis
macrodystrophia lipomatosa
macroencephalon
macroerythroblast
macroerythrocyte
macrofollicular
    m. adenoma
    m. lymphoma

M

macrogamete
macrogametocyte
macrogamont
macrogamy
macrogastria
macrogenitosomia
    m. praecox
    m. praecox suprarenalis
macroglia
macroglobulin
    α_2-m.
    alpha-2 m.
    m. assay
    α_2-m. inhibitor
macroglobulinemia
    Waldenström m.
macroglobulins
macroglossia
macrogyria
macrohomology
macro-Kjeldahl method
macrolabia
macroleukoblast
macrolide antibiotic
macrolides
macromastia
macromelanosome
macromerozoite
macromethod of Wintrobe
macromolecular
macromolecule
Macromonas
    M. bipunctata
    M. mobilis
macromonocyte
macromyeloblast
macronormoblast
macronormochromoblast
macronucleoli
    eosinophilic m.
macronucleus
macroparasite
macropathology
macrophage
    activated m.
    m. activation factor (MAF)
    m. agglutination factor (MAggF)
    alveolar m.
    armed m.
    associated m.
    m. chemotactic factor (MCF)
    m. colony-stimulating factor
    m. growth factor
    Hansemann m.
    inflammatory m.
    m. inflammatory protein (MIP)
    m. migration inhibition factor
    m. migration inhibition test

    pulmonary alveolar m. (PAM)
    tingible-body m.
macrophage-56
    human alveolar m. (HAM-56)
macrophage-activating factor
macrophage-derived growth factor
macrophage-inhibiting factor (MIF)
macrophagocyte
macropolycyte
macropromyelocyte
macrorchis
    Prosthogonimus m.
macroreticulocyte
macroscopic agglutination
macrosigmoid
macrosis
macrosomia
macrospore
macrostomia
macrothrombocyte
macula, pl. maculae
    m. albida, pl. maculae albidae
    m. atrophica
    m. cerulea
    m. gonorrhoica
    honeycomb m.
    m. lactea
    mongolian m.
    Saenger m.
    m. tendinea
macular
    m. amyloidosis
    m. atrophy
    m. eruption
    m. erythema
    m. leprosy
maculatum
    atrophoderma m.
macule
maculoerythematous
maculopapular eruption
madder
Madelung
    M. disease
    M. neck
mad itch
Madura
    M. boil
    M. foot
Madurella
    M. grisea
    M. mycetomi
maduromycetoma
maduromycosis
maduromycotic mycetoma
maedi
    m. virus

MAF
macrophage activation factor
Maffucci syndrome
magaldrate
magenta
m. I, II, III
acid m.
basic m.
m. O
MAggF
macrophage agglutination factor
maggot
Congo floor m.
rat-tail m.
Magitot disease
magna
Fascioloides m.
magnesium
m. ammonium phosphate
m. assay
m. test
magnesium-activated ATPase
magnet
magnetic
m. core
m. core memory
m. field
m. field strength
m. flux
m. induction
m. moment
m. susceptibility
m. tape
magnetization
magnification (X)
magnitude
signed m.
Maher disease
MAI
Mycobacterium avium-intracellulare
main
m. en griffe
m. en lorgnette
m. frame
maintenance
Majocchi
M. disease
M. granuloma
major
m. agglutinin
m. gene
m. histocompatibility antigen

m. histocompatibility complex
(MHC)
m. histocompatibility locus
m. tranquilizer
MAK6 immunohistochemical reagent
maker
Geometric Data Miniprep slide m.
mal
m. de Cayenne
m. de San Lazaro
Malabar
M. itch
M. leprosy
malabsorption syndrome
malachite
m. green
m. green broth
malacia
malacic
malacoplakia, malakoplakia
m. vesicae
malacosis
malacotic
maladie de Roger
malakoplakia (*var. of* malacoplakia)
malaria
algid m.
benign tertian m.
bilious remittent m.
bovine m.
double tertian m.
falciparum m.
m. film test
gastric algid m.
hemolytic m.
hemorrhagic m.
intermittent m.
malariae m.
malignant tertian m.
ovale m.
pernicious m.
quartan m.
quotidian m.
remittent m.
m. smear
tertian m.
therapeutic m.
vivax m.
malariacidal
malarial
m. cachexia
m. deposition pigment

NOTES

malarial *(continued)*
    m. dysentery
    m. fever
    m. hemoglobinuria
    m. knob
    m. parasite
    m. pigment deposition
    m. pigment stain
    m. rosette
malariology
malarious
Malassez disease
Malassezia
    M. furfur
    M. macfadyani
    M. ovalis
    M. tropica
malate dehydrogenase
malathion
Malayan
    M. filariasis
    M. pit viper venom
Maldonado-San Jose stain
male
    m. castration
    m. hormone
    m. rudimentary uterus
    m. sex chromatin pattern
    m. Turner syndrome
malformation
    Arnold-Chiari m.
    arteriovenous m. (AVM)
    cardiac valvular m.
    cardiovascular m.
    congenital m.
    cutaneous m.
    cystic adenomatoid m.
    Ebstein m.
    m. syndrome
malfunction
Malherbe
    M. calcifying epithelioma
    M. disease
Malibu disease
malic
    m. acid
    m. dehydrogenase (MD)
maligna
    cynanche m.
malignancy
    B-cell m.
malignant
    m. adenoma
    m. anemia
    m. atrophic papulosis
    m. breast tumor
    m. bubo
    m. carbuncle

    m. carcinoid syndrome
    m. catarrhal fever
    m. catarrhal fever virus
    m. catarrh of cattle
    m. dyskeratosis
    m. edema
    m. endocarditis
    m. ependymoma
    m. fibrous histiocytoma (MFH)
    m. giant cell tumor of bone
    m. giant cell tumor of soft parts
    m. glioma
    m. granuloma
    m. hepatoma
    m. histiocytosis
    m. hypertension
    m. jaundice
    m. lentigo
    m. lentigo melanoma
    m. lymphadenosis
    m. lymphoma (ML)
    m. melanoma (MM)
    m. melanoma in situ
    m. melanoma staging
    m. meningioma
    m. mesenchymoma
    m. mesothelioma
    m. mixed mesodermal tumor (MMMT)
    m. mixed müllerian tumor
    m. neoplasm
    m. nephrosclerosis
    m. neurilemoma
    m. pustule
    m. schwannoma
    m. smallpox
    m. synovioma
    m. teratoma (MT)
    m. teratoma intermediate (MTI)
    m. tertian fever
    m. tertian malaria
    m. thymoma
    m. transformation
    m. trophoblastic teratoma (MTT)
Malin syndrome
mallein
    m. test
malleinization
Malleomyces
    M. mallei
    M. malleomyces
    M. pseudomallei
    M. whitmori
mallet finger
Mallophaga
Mallory
    M. aniline blue stain
    M. body

M. collagen stain
M. hyaline
M. iodine stain
M. phloxine stain
M. phosphotungstic acid
  hematoxylin stain
M. stain for actinomyces
M. stain for hemofuchsin
M. trichrome stain
M. triple stain
Mallory-Weiss
  M.-W. lesion
  M.-W. syndrome
  M.-W. tear
Malmejde test
malnourished
  intrauterine fetally m. (IUM)
malnutrition
  protein-calorie m. (PCM)
malocclusion
Maloney leukemia virus
malonic acid
malonyl coenzyme A
malpighii
  stratum m.
malposition
malrotation
  intestinal m.
MALT
  mucosa-associated lymphoid tissue
  MALT lymphoma
malt
  m. agar
  m. extract broth
Malta fever
maltase
MALToma, MALT lymphoma
  mucosa-associated lymphoid tissue
  lymphoma
maltose
maltosuria
malt-worker's lung
malum
  m. articulorum senilis
  m. coxae senile
mammary
  m. calculus
  m. cancer virus of mice
  m. duct ectasia
  m. dysplasia
  m. fistula
  m. Paget disease

m. tumor virus (MTV)
m. tumor virus of mice
mammillitis
  bovine herpes m.
  bovine ulcerative m.
  bovine vaccinia m.
mammitis
mammosomatotropic adenoma
mammotropic hormone (MH)
mammotropin
management
Manan needle
Manchurian hemorrhagic fever
Mancini iodine stain
Mandelin reagent
mandibuloacral dysostosis
mandibulofacial
  m. dysostosis
  m. dysotosis syndrome
  m. dysplasia
mandibulo-oculofacial
  m.-o. dysmorphia
  m.-o. syndrome
maneuver
  Valsalva m.
manganese
  m. assay
  m. poisoning
manganic
manganism
manganous
mange
  sarcoptic m.
manifest hyperopia (Hm)
manifesting heterozygote
Manifold
  Visiprep Solid-Phase Extraction
  Vacuum M.
mannans
mannitol fermentation
Mann methyl blue-eosin stain
mannoheptulosuria
mannose
mannosidosis
Mann-Whitney rank sum statistic
manometer
manometric flame
manometry
MANOVA
  multivariate analysis of variance
Manson disease

NOTES

M

Mansonella
    M. ozzardi
mansonelliasis
mansoni
    Oxyspirura m.
    Schistosoma m.
Mansonia
Mansonoides
Mantel-Cox
    M.-C. method
    M.-C. procedure
mantle
    m. cell lymphoma
    m. sclerosis
    m. zone
mantle-zone lymphocyte
Mantoux
    M. conversion
    M. diameter (MD)
    M. pit
    M. skin test
manuum
MAP
    megaloblastic anemia of pregnancy
    microtubule-associated protein
map
    chromosome m.
    cytogenetic m.
    genetic m.
    linkage m.
    memory m.
    restriction m.
    m. unit
maple
    m. bark strippers' disease
    m. syrup urine
    m. syrup urine disease (MSUD)
maplike skull
mapping
    genetic m.
maprotiline
Maragiliano body
Marañón syndrome
marantic
    m. atrophy
    m. endocarditis
    m. thrombosis
    m. thrombus
marasmic
    m. thrombosis
    m. thrombus
marble
    m. bone
    m. bone disease
Marburg
    M. agent
    M. virus
    M. virus disease

marcescens
    m. marcescens
march
    m. albuminuria
    M. disease
    m. hemoglobinuria
Marchand
    M. adrenals
    M. rest
Marchesani syndrome
Marchi
    M. fixative
    M. reaction
    M. stain
Marchiafava-Bignami disease
Marchiafava-Micheli
    M.-M. anemia
    M.-M. syndrome
marcid
Marcus Gunn syndrome
Marcy agent
Marek
    M. disease (MD)
    M. disease virus
    M. herpesvirus disease (MDHV)
Marfan
    M. disease
    M. law
    M. syndrome
Margaropus
margin
    left costal m. (LCM)
marginal
    m. granulocyte pool (MGP)
    m. insertion of umbilical cord
    m. ulcer
    m. zone lymphoma
marginated chromatin
margination
    leukocytic m.
Margolis syndrome
Marie
    M. disease
    M. syndrome
Marie-Bamberger
    M.-B. disease
    M.-B. syndrome
Marie-Robinson syndrome
Marie-Strümpell disease
Marie-Tooth disease
marijuana, marihuana
marine protein concentrate (MPC)
Marinesco-Garland syndrome
Marinesco-Sjögren syndrome
Marion disease
Marituba virus
Marjolin ulcer

mark
- port-wine m.
- m. sense reader
- strawberry m.
- tape m.
- Unna m.

marker
- allotypic m.
- B-cell m.
- cell m.
- cell surface m.
- m. chromosome
- DNA m.
- endocrine m.
- enzyme m.
- fecal m.
- genetic m.
- HMB-45 m.
- immunohistochemical m.
- myogen m.
- oncofetal m.
- polymorphic genetic m.
- m. rescue
- rhabdomyosarcoma m.
- S-100 m.
- tumor m.
- utrophin m.

Marme reagent

marmoratus
- status m.

marmoset virus

marmot

Maroteaux-Lamy syndrome

Marquis reagent

marrow
- aplastic bone m.
- basophilic m.
- bone m.
- eosinophilic m.
- erythrocytic m.
- leukocytic m.
- lymphocytic m.
- monocytic m.
- neutrophilic m.
- reticulocytic m.

Marseilles fever

Marsh
- M. disease

Marshall
- M. method
- M. syndrome

Marshallagia marshalli

marshalli
- *Marshallagia m.*

Marshall-Marchetti (MM)

marsh fever

Martin
- M. broth
- M. disease

Martin-Lester agar

martius
- m. scarlet blue
- m. yellow

Martorell syndrome

mA-s
- milliampere-second

Masaoka staging criteria

maschaladenitis

maschaloncus

masculinization
- ovarian m.

masculinovoblastoma

mask
- BLB m.
- m. of pregnancy
- tropical m.

masked
- m. message
- m. virus

Mason-Pfizer virus

mason's lung

mass
- m. action law
- atomic m.
- m. attenuation coefficient
- body m. (BM)
- carbon gelatin m.
- m. concentration
- critical m.
- erythrocyte m. (EM)
- exchangeable m.
- fat-free m. (FFM)
- filar m.
- m. fragmentography
- m. infection
- injection m.
- intravascular m. (IVM)
- lean body m. (LBM)
- m. memory
- molecular m.
- m. number (A)
- red blood cell m. (RBCM)
- m. spectrograph
- m. spectrometer

NOTES

mass *(continued)*
    m. spectrometry (MS)
    m. storage
massive
    m. collapse
    m. embolus
    m. hepatic necrosis (MHN)
    m. transfusion
    m. vitreous retraction (MVR)
Masson
    M. argentaffin stain
    M. humid meningioma
    M. pseudoangiosarcoma
    M. trichrome method
    M. trichrome stain
Masson-Fontana ammoniacal silver stain
mast
    m. cell
    m. cell disease
    m. cell hyperplasia
    m. cell leukemia
    m. cell sarcoma
    m. cell staining
    m. cell tumor
    m. leukocyte
mastadenitis
mastadenoma
Mastadenovirus
mastatrophia
mastatrophy
mastauxe
master
    m. file
    M. 2-step test
mastic test
Mastigophora
mastigophorous
mastigote
mastitis
    acute m.
    bovine m.
    chronic cystic m.
    cystic m.
    fibrocystic m.
    gargantuan m.
    glandular m.
    granulomatous m.
    interstitial m.
    lactational m.
    m. neonatorum
    parenchymatous m.
    periductal m.
    phlegmonous m.
    plasma cell m.
    puerperal m.
    retromammary m.
    submammary m.
    suppurative m.

mastocytogenesis
mastocytoma
mastocytosis
mastoid abscess
mastoidea
    otitis m.
mastoiditis
mastoncus
mastopathy
    cystic m.
    fibrocystic m.
Mastophora
mastoplasia
mastoscirrhus
Masugi-type nephrotoxic serum nephritis
material
    Biological Matrix Reference M.'s
    biuret-reactive m. (BRM)
    calibration m.
    control m.
    Cotasil silicone slide coating m.
    cross-reacting m. (CRM)
    explosive m.
    extracellular m. (ECM)
    fluorescent m.
    gonadotropin-inhibitory m. (GIM)
    m. graft
    hazardous m.
    labeling of hazardous m.'s
    Matrix Reference M.'s
    neurosecretory m. (NSM)
    particulate crystalline m.
    primary reference m.
    reactive m.
    reference m.
    m. safety data sheet (MSDS)
    Secondary Reference M.'s
    Simulated Matrix Reference M.'s
    vasodepressor m. (VDM)
    vasoexcitor m. (VEM)
maternal
    m. death
    m. immunity
    m. inheritance
mathematical genetics
Mathieu disease
mating
    assortative m.
    consanguineous m.
    negative assortative m.
    positive assortative m.
    random m.
matrass
matrilineal
matrix
    m. calculus
    myxoid m.
    M. Reference Materials

matter
> interaction of radiation with m.

maturate

maturation
> m. arrest
> m. division
> m. index

mature
> m. abnormal chorion
> m. abnormal chorionic villi
> m. abnormal placenta
> m. bacteriophage
> m. cell leukemia
> m. neutrophil

maturity
> fetal lung m. (FLM)

maturity-onset diabetes

Maunier-Kuhn disease

Maurer
> M. cleft
> M. dots

Mauriac syndrome

MAV
> multinucleated atypia of the vulva

Maxcy disease

maxillitis

maximal
> m. acid output
> m. growth temperature
> m. Histalog test
> m. midflow rate (MMFR)
> m. permissible dose (MPD)
> m. tubular excretory capacity of kidneys (T_m)
> m. tubular reabsorption of glucose (T_{mg})

Maximow stain for bone marrow

maximum
> m. impurities reagent
> m. inhibiting dilution (MID)
> m. permissible concentration (MPC)
> m. temperature
> m. thermometer
> m. urea clearance
> m. urinary concentration (MUC)

maxwell (Mx)

Mayaro virus

Mayer
> M. acid alum hematoxylin stain
> M. hemalum stain
> M. hematoxylin
> M. mucicarmine stain
> M. mucihematein stain

mayer (my)

Mayer-Rokitansky-Küster syndrome

mayfly

May-Grünwald-Giemsa stain

May-Grünwald stain

May-Hegglin
> M.-H. anomaly
> M.-H. body

mazamorra

mazoplasia

Mazzotti test

MB
> methylene blue
> microbiological assay

Mb, MbCO, MbO₂
> myoglobin

mbar
> millibar

MBAS
> methylene blue active substance

MBC
> minimal bactericidal concentration

MbCO (*var. of* Mb)

MBD
> methylene blue dye
> minimal brain damage
> minimal brain dysfunction

MBL
> minimal bactercidal level

MbO₂ (*var. of* Mb)

MBP
> myelin basic protein

MC
> myocarditis

mC
> millicoulomb

MCA
> multichannel analyzer

McArdle disease

McArdle-Schmid-Pearson disease

MCB
> membranous cytoplasmic body

MCBR
> minimum concentration of bilirubin

MCC
> mean corpuscular hemoglobin concentration
> minimum complete-killing concentration

McCallum plaque

McCune-Albright syndrome

NOTES

MCD
> mean cell diameter
> mean of consecutive differences
> mean corpuscular diameter
> medullary cystic disease

MCF
> macrophage chemotactic factor

MCFA
> medium-chain fatty acid

McGadey substrate

MCH
> mean cell hemoglobin
> mean corpuscular hemoglobin

MCHC
> mean cell hemoglobin concentration
> mean corpuscular hemoglobin
>   concentration

mCi
> millicurie

mCi-hr
> millicurie-hour

McLean-Maxwell disease

McLeod phenotype

McMaster technique

McNeer classification

McNemar test

MCP
> mitotic-control protein

MCP-1
> monocyte chemoattractant protein-1

McPhail test

MCR
> metabolic clearance rate

MCT
> mean circulation time
> mean corpuscular thickness

MCTD
> mixed connective-tissue disease

MCV
> mean cell volume
> mean corpuscular volume

MCVr
> reticulocyte mean corpuscular volume

MD
> malic dehydrogenase
> Mantoux diameter
> Marek disease
> Ménétrier disease
> muscular dystrophy
> myocardial damage
> myocardial disease

MDC
> minimum detectable concentration

M-DES stain

MDF
> mean dominant frequency
> myocardial depressant factor

MDHV
> Marek herpesvirus disease

MDNCF
> monocyte-derived neutrophil chemotactic
>   factor

MDR
> multiple drug resistance

MDT
> median detection threshold

MDTR
> mean diameter-thickness ratio

MDUO
> myocardial disease of unknown origin

2 ME
> 2-mercaptoethanol

M/E
> myeloid-erythroid ratio

MEA
> multiple endocrine adenomatosis

meal
> test m.

mean
> m. cell diameter (MCD)
> m. cell hemoglobin (MCH)
> m. cell hemoglobin concentration
>   (MCHC)
> m. cell threshold
> m. cell volume (MCV)
> m. circulation time (MCT)
> m. circulatory hematocrit
> m. of consecutive differences
>   (MCD)
> m. corpuscular diameter (MCD)
> m. corpuscular hemoglobin (MCH)
> m. corpuscular hemoglobin
>   concentration (MCC, MCHC)
> m. corpuscular thickness (MCT)
> m. corpuscular volume (MCV)
> m. deviation
> m. diameter-thickness ratio (MDTR)
> m. dominant frequency (MDF)
> m. dose
> m. dose per unit cumulated
>   activity
> m. effective life
> m. generation time
> m. hemolytic dose (MHD)
> m. square deviation
> m. time between failures

measle

measles
> m. antibody
> atypical m.
> m. convalescent serum
> German m.
> m. immune globulin (human)
> m. immunoglobulin

m., mumps, and rubella vaccine (MMR)
three-day m.
tropical m.
m. virus
m. virus vaccine

measly
measurable
not m. (NM)
measure
measurement
blood volume m.
carbon dioxide combining power m.
end-point m.
kinetic m.
oxygen saturation m.
right anterior m. (RAM)
measuring pipette
meat fiber
mechanical
m. diuretic
m. fragility
m. ileus
m. jaundice
m. styptic
m. vector
mechanism
countercurrent m.
defense m.
Frank-Starling m.
immunological m.
ping-pong m.
mecillinam
Mecistocirrus
Meckel
M. cave
M. diverticulum
M. syndrome
Meckel-Gruber syndrome
Meckel reagent
meconium
m. aspiration
m. ileus
m. peritonitis
m. stain
MED
minimal erythema dose
med
median
media (*pl. of* medium)

medial
m. arteriosclerosis
m. calcification
m. cystic necrosis
m. degeneration
m. necrosis of aorta
median (med)
m. bar of Mercier
m. curative dose (CD_{50})
m. detection threshold (MDT)
m. effective dose (ED_{50})
m. fatal dose (FD_{50})
m. infectious dose (ID_{50})
m. lethal dose (LD_{50})
m. rhomboid glossitis
m. tissue culture dose (TCD_{50})
m. tissue culture infective dose ($TCID_{50}$)
m. unbiased estimate
mediastinal
m. elastofibroma
m. fibrosis
m. lipomatosis
m. pericarditis
mediastinitis
idiopathic fibrous m.
mediastinopericarditis
mediate
m. agglutination
m. contagion
mediation
mediator
chemical m.
pharmacologic m.'s of anaphylaxis
medical
m. bacteriology
m. genetics
m. internal radiation dose (MIRD)
m. laboratory technician
m. mycology
m. pathology
m. record
m. technologist
medicinal scarlet red
medicine
clinical m.
forensic m.
preventive m.
medina infection
Medin disease
medionecrosis
m. of the aorta

NOTES

395

medionecrosis *(continued)*
    m. aortae idiopathica cystica
    cystic m.
Mediterranean
    M. anemia
    familial M. fever (FMF)
    M. fever
    M. lymphoma
Mediterranean-hemoglobin E disease
medium, pl. **media**
    aerotitis media
    aortic tunica media
    Apathy gum syrup m.
    aqueous mounting media
    Bactalert FAN culture m.
    Balamuth culture m.
    bilateral otitis media (BOM)
    Boeck-Drbohlav-Locke egg-
      serum m.
    brain-heart infusion broth m.
    chopped meat m.
    clearing m.
    Columbia m.
    contrast m.
    Cryo-Gel embedding m.
    culture m.
    Czapek-Dox m.
    dermatophyte test m. (DTM)
    dispersive m.
    Eagle basal m.
    Eagle minimum essential m.
    enrichment m.
    Epon tissue embedding media
    Farrant m.
    m. frequency (MF)
    glycerol gelatin m.
    Lash casein hydrolysate-serum m.
    Löffler blood culture m.
    Löffler coagulated serum m.
    Löwenstein-Jensen m. (LJM)
    minimum essential m. (MEM)
    mounting m.
    nonpermissive culture media
    Novy, MacNeal, and Nicolle m.
    nutrient m.
    OF m.
    otitis media (OM)
    oxidation-fermentation m.
    passive m.
    permissive culture media
    Petragnani m.
    PVA lacto-phenol m.
    radiopaque m.
    Rees culture m.
    refracting m.
    secretory otitis media (SOM)
    selective m.
    separating m.

    serous otitis media (SOM)
    sodium chloride (6.5 %)
      culture m.
    support m.
    suppurative chronic otitis media
    tellurite m.
    Thayer-Martin m.
    thioglycollate m.
    tissue culture m. (TCM)
    Tobie, von Brand, and Mehlman
      diphasic m.
    transport m.
    Weinman m.
medium-chain
    m.-c. fatty acid (MCFA)
    m.-c. triglyceride
medium-scale integration
medi virus
medorrhea
medroxyprogesterone
medulla
    adrenal m.
medullary
    m. adenocarcinoma
    m. carcinoma
    m. carcinoma of thyroid
    m. chromaffinoma
    m. cystic disease (MCD)
    m. fibrosarcoma
    m. histiocytic reticulosis
    m. necrosis
    m. sarcoma
    m. sponge kidney
medullization
medulloarthritis
medulloblast
medulloblastoma
    desmoplastic m.
    melanotic m.
medulloepithelioma
    adult m.
medullomyoblastoma
Medusa head
MEG
    megakaryocyte
megabladder
megacaryoblast
megacaryocyte
megacephaly
megacins
megacolon
    aganglionic m.
    chronic idiopathic m.
    congenital m.
    m. congenitum
    idiopathic m.
    toxic m.
megacycle

megacystic syndrome
megacystis
megadolichocolon
megaelectron volt (MeV)
megaesophagus
megagamete
megahertz (MHz)
megakaryoblast
megakaryocyte (MEG)
    basophilic m.
megakaryocytic
    m. aplasia
    m. blood cell
    m. emperipolesis
    m. hyperplasia
    m. hypoplasia
    m. leukemia
    m. myelosis
megakaryocytopoiesis
megalencephaly
megaloblast
megaloblastic
    m. anemia
    m. anemia of pregnancy (MAP)
    m. erythropoiesis
megaloblastoid
megaloblastosis
megalocephaly
megalocystis
megalocyte
megalocythemia
megalocytic anemia
megalocytosis
megaloencephalic
megaloencephalon
megaloencephaly
megaloenteron
megalogastria
megalohcpatia
megalokaryocyte
Megalopyge
megalosplenia
megalospore
megaloureter
megalourethra
megamerozoite
megamitochondria
meganucleus
megarectum
Megaselia
megasigmoid
Megasphaera

megaspore
megathrombocyte
megaureter
megaurethra
megavolt (MV)
megavoltage
meglumine
megohm (MΩ)
megoxycyte
megoxyphil, megoxyphile
megthandrostenolone
meibomian
    m. cyst
    m. stye
meibomitis, meibomianitis
Meige disease
Meigs syndrome
Meinicke
    M. test
    M. turbidity reaction (MTR)
meiocyte
meiosis
meiotic
    m. phase
    m. recombination
Meissel stain
meissnerian differentiation
MEK
    methyl ethyl ketone
melanemia
melaniferous
    m. phagocyte
melanin
    artificial m.
    m. bleaching method
    factitious m.
    m. pigmentation
    m. staining method
    m. test
melanism
melanoameloblastoma
melanoblast
melanoblastoma
melanocarcinoma
    m. of anus
melanocortin
melanocyte
melanocyte-inhibiting hormone
melanocyte-stimulating
    m.-s. hormone (MSH)
    m.-s. hormone-inhibiting factor
    (MIF)

M

NOTES

melanocyte-stimulating *(continued)*
    m.-s. hormone-release-inhibiting hormone
    m.-s. hormone-releasing factor (MRF)
    m.-s. hormone-releasing hormone
melanocytic
    m. nevus
melanocytosis
    pagetoid m. (PM)
melanoderma
    m. cachecticorum
    m. chloasma
    senile m.
melanodermatitis
melanodermic
melanogen
    m. test
melanogenemia
melanogenesis
melanoglossia
melanoid
Melanoides
melanokeratosis
Melanolestes
    M. picipes
melanoleukoderma
melanoma
    acral lentiginous m.
    amelanotic m.
    benign juvenile m.
    Cloudman m.
    cutaneous malignant m. (CMM)
    desmoplastic m.
    epidermotropic metastatic malignant m. (EMMM)
    epithelioid cell m.
    halo m.
    Harding-Passey m.
    juvenile m.
    lentigo maligna m.
    malignant m. (MM)
    malignant lentigo m.
    malignant m. in situ
    minimal deviation m.
    nodular m.
    spindle cell m.
    subungual m.
    superficial spreading m.
melanomatosis
melanonychia
melanopathy
melanophage
melanophore
melanophore-stimulating hormone (MSH)
melanoplakia
melanosarcoma

melanosis
    m. circumscripta precancerosa
    m. coli
    m. corii degenerativa
    neurocutaneous m.
    oculodermal m.
    precancerous m. of Dubreuilh
    Riehl m.
    vagabond's m.
melanosome
    giant m.
melanotic
    m. carcinoma
    m. freckle
    m. medulloblastoma
    m. neuroectodermal tumor
    m. neuroectodermal tumor of infancy
    m. pigment
    m. progonoma
    m. whitlow
melanura
    Culiseta m.
melanuria
melanuric
melasma
    m. universale
melatonin
Melchior syndrome
meleagridis
    Histomonas m.
Meleda disease
melena
Meleney
    M. gangrene
    M. ulcer
melicera
meliceris
melioidosis
melitis
melitose
melituria
    glycosuric m.
    m. inosita
    nondiabetic glycosuric m.
Melkersson-Rosenthal syndrome
Melkersson syndrome
mellitus
    insulin-dependent diabetes m. (IDDM)
    noninsulin-dependent diabetes m. (NIDDM)
Melnick-Needles syndrome
Meloidae
melon seed body
Melophagus
melorheostosis

melting
    m. point (MP)
    m. temperature
MEM
    minimum essential medium
membranacea
    placenta m.
membrane
    acute inflammatory m.
    acute pyogenic m.
    artificial rupture of m.'s (ARM)
    m. attack complex
    basement m.
    Bruch m.
    m. capacitance
    cell m.
    croupous m.
    cytoplasmic m.
    decidual m.
    diphtheritic m.
    epithelial basement m.
    erythrocyte m.
    false m.
    m. filter
    m. filter technique
    glassy m.
    glomerular basement m. (GBM)
    hyaline m.
    Hybond N+ nylon m.
    inflammatory m.
    photoreceptor m. (PRM)
    plasma m.
    m. potential
    premature rupture of (fetal) m.'s
      (PROM)
    prolonged rupture of fetal m.'s
      (PRFM)
    prolonged rupture of (fetal) m.'s
      (PROM)
    prophylactic m.
    m. protein
    pyogenic m.
    rupture of m.'s (ROM)
    semipermeable m.
    m. transport
    undulating m.
    unit m.
membranelle
membranoproliferative glomerulonephritis
  (MPGN)
membranous
    m. acute inflammation

    m. cytoplasmic body (MCB)
    m. glomerulonephritis (MGN)
    m. nephropathy
    m. pharyngitis
membranous-proliferative
  glomerulonephritis
memory
    cache m.
    core m.
    magnetic core m.
    m. map
    mass m.
    scratch-pad m.
MEN
    multiple endocrine neoplasia
    MEN I, II
    MEN syndrome
menadione
menaquinone
mendelevium
mendelian
    m. character
    m. genetics
    m. inheritance
Mendel law
Ménétrier
    M. disease (MD)
    M. syndrome
Mengert shock syndrome
Menghini needle
Mengo
    M. encephalitis
    M. virus
Ménière
    M. disease
    M. syndrome
meningeal
    m. carcinoma
    m. carcinomatosis
    m. hernia
    m. leukemia
    m. sarcoma
    m. sarcomatosis
meningioangiomatosis
meningioma
    angiomatous m.
    clear cell m.
    cutaneous m.
    fibroblastic m.
    malignant m.
    Masson humid m.
    meningothelial m.

M

NOTES

meningioma *(continued)*
    mucinous m.
    psammomatous m.
meningiomatosis
    diffuse m.
meningismus
meningitic streak
meningitis, pl. **meningitides**
    amebic m.
    aseptic m.
    bacterial m.
    basilar m.
    Candida m.
    cerebrospinal m. (CSM)
    cryptococcal m.
    epidemic cerebrospinal m.
    epidural m.
    external m.
    internal m.
    meningococcal m.
    Mollaret m.
    mycotic m.
    neoplastic m.
    occlusive m.
    otitic m.
    pyogenic m.
    serous m.
    subacute m.
    syphilitic m.
    torular m.
    tuberculous m. (TBM)
    viral m.
meningocele
meningocerebral cicatrix
meningocerebritis
meningococcal
    m. meningitis
meningococcemia
meningococcin
meningococcus conjunctivitis
meningocyte
meningoencephalitis
    acute primary hemorrhagic m.
    amebic m.
    biundulant m.
    eosinophilic m.
    herpetic m.
    mumps m.
    m. mumps
    primary amebic m.
    syphilitic m.
meningoencephalocele
meningoencephalomyelitis
meningoencephalopathy
    carcinomatous m.
meningomyelitis
meningomyelocele
meningomyeloradiculitis

meningo-osteophlebitis
meningoradiculitis
meningothelial meningioma
meninguria
menisci (*pl. of* meniscus)
meniscitis
meniscocyte
meniscocytosis
meniscus, pl. **menisci**
    degenerated m.
Menkes syndrome
menometrorrhagia
menopausal
    m. gonadotropin (MG)
    m. syndrome
menopause
    delayed m.
Menopon
menorrhagia
menostasis
menstrual
    m. colic
    m. cycle
    m. sclerosis
    m. stage
Mentha
Menzies method
meperidine
    meperidine hydrochloride
mephenytoin
meprobamate
    m. assay
mEq, meq
    milliequivalent
MER
    methanol-extruded residue
M:E ratio
merbromin
mercaptan
mercapto
mercaptoacetic acid
2-mercaptoethanol (2 ME)
mercaptomerin sodium
mercaptopurine
6-mercaptopurine (6-MP)
mercaptopyrazidopyrimidine (MPP)
mercocresols
mercurialism
mercurial thermometer
mercuric
    m. cyanide
    m. fixative
mercurous
mercury (Hg, Hgb)
    m. assay
    methyl m.
    millimeters of m. (mmHg)
    m. poisoning

mercury-vapor lamp
mercury-wetted relay
merge
merispore
meristematic
meristic variation
Merkel
    M. cell
    M. cell tumor
    M. corpuscle
mermithid
Mermithidae
Mermithoidea
merogenesis
merogenetic
merogony
    diploid m.
    parthenogenetic m.
meromelia
meromicrosomia
meromyarial
meront
merorachischisis
merosporangium
merotomy
merozoite
    m. antigen
merozygote
Merzbacher-Pelizaeus disease
mesangial
    m. nephritis
    m. proliferative glomerulonephritis
mesangiocapillary glomerulonephritis
mesangioproliferative glomerulonephritis
mesangium
    extraglomerular m.
mesaortitis
mesarteritis
mescal
mescaline
mesectic
mesencephalic reticular formation
  (MRF)
mesencephalitis
mesenchymal
    m. cell
    m. differentiation
    m. hamartoma
    m. hyloma
mesenchyme

mesenchymoma
    benign m.
    malignant m.
mesenteric
    m. adenitis
    m. infarction
    m. panniculitis
    m. thrombosis
    m. vascular obstruction
mesenteritis
mesenteron
mesna
mesobacterium
mesoblast
    primitive m.
mesoblastic nephroma
mesocardia
Mesocestoides
    M. variabilis
Mesocestoididae
meso compound
Mesogastropoda
mesogenic
mesolepidoma
mesomelia
mesomelic
    m. dwarfism
mesometanephric carcinoma
mesometritis
meson
mesonephric
    m. adenocarcinoma
    m. cyst
    m. remnant
    m. rest
mesonephroid tumor
mesonephroma
mesoneuritis
    nodular m.
mesophile
mesophilic bacterium
mesophlebitis
mesosigmoiditis
mesosome
mesothelial
    m. cell
    m. cyst
    m. hyloma
    m. sarcoma
mesothelioma
    benign m.
    benign m. of genital tract

M

NOTES

mesothelioma *(continued)*
    fibrous m.
    malignant m.
    sarcomatoid m.
Mesozoa
message
    masked m.
messenger RNA (mRNA)
mesylate
    deferoxamine m.
    ergoloid m.
MET
    metabolic equivalent
Met
metabiosis
metabisulfite test
metabolic
    m. acidosis
    m. alkalosis
    m. antagonism
    m. antagonist
    m. bone disease
    m. clearance rate (MCR)
    m. coma
    m. craniopathy
    m. detoxification
    m. encephalopathy
    m. equivalent (MET)
    m. indican
    m. insufficiency
    m. mucinosis
    m. pathway
    m. pool
metabolism
    aerobic m.
    anaerobic m.
    basal m.
    divalent ion m. (DIM)
    glucose m.
    inborn error of m.
    intermediary m.
    propionate m.
metabolite
metabolizable
metacarpal index
metacentric
metacercaria
metacestode
metachromasia
    α m.
    alpha m.
    β m.
    beta m.
    γ m.
    gamma m.
metachromatic
    m. body
    m. dye

    m. granule
    m. leukodystrophy (MLD)
    m. stain
metachromatic-type leukodystrophy
metachromatism
metachroming
metachromophil, metachromophile
metachronal rhythm
metachronous
metachrosis
metacryptozoite
metagenesis
metagglutinin
metaglobulin
metagonimiasis
Metagonimus
    M. ovatus
    M. yokogawai
metal
    alkali m.
    alkaline earth m.
    heavy m.
    m. oxide semiconductor field effect
        transistor
    m. sol
metal-catalyzed pseudoperoxidation
metaldehyde
metallic
    m. bond
    m. foreign body (MFB)
    m. thermometer
metalloenzyme
metalloflavoprotein
metallophil cell
metallophilia
metalloprotein
metalloscopy
metamere
metameric
metamerism
metamorphosis
    fatty m.
metamyelocyte
    basophilic m.
    eosinophilic m.
    neutrophilic m.
metanephrine
    m. assay
    m. test
metaneutrophil, metaneutrophile
metaniline yellow
metanil yellow
metaphase
    m. cell
    m. chromosome
    m. plate
metaphosphoric acid

metaphysial
- m. dysostosis
- m. dysplasia

metaphysitis

metaplasia
- agnogenic myeloid m.
- apocrine m.
- autoparenchymatous m.
- cartilaginous m.
- chondroid m.
- decidual m.
- endothelial m.
- epidermoid m.
- glandular m.
- Hürthle cell m.
- intestinal m.
- myeloid m. (MM)
- myelosclerosis with myeloid m. (MMM)
- osseous m.
- primary myeloid m.
- secondary myeloid m.
- squamous m.
- squamous m. of amnion
- symptomatic myeloid m.
- tuboendometrioid m.

metaplasis

metaplasm

metaplastic
- m. anemia
- m. carcinoma
- m. columnar epithelium
- m. keratinization
- m. ossification
- m. polyp

metarubricyte
- pernicious anemia type m.

metastable state

metastasis, pl. metastases
- biochemical m.
- calcareous m.
- contralateral axillary m. (CAM)
- hematogenous m.
- lymphogenous m.
- no evidence of distant metastases (MO)
- pulsating m.
- satellite m.

metastasize

metastatic
- m. abscess
- m. calcification

- m. carcinoid syndrome
- m. carcinoma
- m. cascade
- m. mumps
- m. neoplasm
- m. panniculitis
- m. pneumonia
- m. thermometer
- m. tumor

metastrongyle

Metastrongylus
- *M. elongatus*

metatroph

metatrophic

metatropic

metatypical carcinoma

metaxeny (*var. of* metoxeny)

Metazoa

metazoan parasite

metazoonosis

Metchnikoff theory

meteorism

meter (m)
- AccuData Easy glucose m.
- count rate m.
- d'Arsonval m.
- flow m.
- HemoCue glucose m.
- Miles Encore QA glucose m.
- oxygen saturation m. (OSM)
- pH m.
- rate m.
- survey m.

meter-kilogram-second (MKS, mks)
- m.-k.-s. system
- m.-k.-s. unit

methacrylate
- butyl m.
- glycol m.

methacycline

methadone
- m. assay
- m. hydrochloride

methallenestril

methamphetamine
- m. hydrochloride

methanal

methane

Methanobacterium

Methanococcus

methanol
- m. assay

M

NOTES

methanol *(continued)*
> m. fixative
> m. test

methanol-extruded residue (MER)
methaqualone
> m. assay

metHb, MetHb
> methemoglobin

methemalbumin (MHA)
> m. assay

methemalbuminemia
methemalbuminuria
metheme
methemoglobin (metHb, MetHb, MHb)
> m. reductase

methemoglobinemia
> acquired m.
> congenital m.
> enterogenous m.
> hereditary enzymatic-type m.
> primary m.
> secondary m.
> toxic m.

methemoglobinuria
methenamine
> m. hippurate
> m. mandelate
> periodic acid-silver m. (PASM)
> m. silver
> m. silver stain

methenamine-silver
methicillin
methicillin-resistant
> m.-r. coagulase-negative
> *Staphylococcus* (MRCNS)
> m.-r. *Staphylococcus aureus*
> (MRSA)

methicillin-susceptible
> m.-s. coagulase-negative
> *Staphylococcus* (MSCNS)
> m.-s. *Staphylococcus aureus*
> (MSSA)

methine dye
methionine
> *N*-formyl m.
> m. malabsorption syndrome
> m. synthase
> m. test

methionyl
methionyl-RNA synthetase
methisazone
methocycline
method
> Abell-Kendall m.
> acid anhydride m.
> acid-fast staining m.
> acridine orange m.
> agar diffusion m.

alkaline phosphatase m.
Altmann-Gersh m.
AMEX processing and
> embedding m.
analytic m.
antialkaline phosphatase m.
Ashby differential agglutination m.
axon staining m.
Ayoub-Shklar m.
bacterial agar m.
bacterial antigen detection m.
Baker Sudan black m.
Barnett-Bourne acetic alcohol-silver
> nitrate method
Barrnett-Seligman
> dihydroxydinaphthyl disulfide m.
Barrnett-Seligman indoxyl
> esterase m.
Barroso-Moguel and Costero
> silver m.
Baumgartner m.
Beaver direct smear m.
Bengston m.
Bennett sulfhydryl m.
Bennhold Congo red m.
Bensley aniline-acid fuchsin-methyl
> green m.
benzo sky blue m.
Berg chelate removal m.
Bielschowsky m.
Billheimer m.
biotin streptavidin detection m.
black periodic acid m.
Bodian m.
Borchgrevink m.
Brecher-Cronkite m.
Cajal gold sublimate m.
Cajal uranium silver m.
Caldwell-Moloy m.
Camp-Gianturco m.
carbol-fuchsin-methylene blue
> staining m.
cellophane tape m.
cell separation m.
Chang aniline-acid fuchsin m.
Chiffelle and Putt m.
chloranilate m.
chloride m.
cholesterol staining m.
chromate m.
chrome alum hematoxylin-
> phloxine m.
chromolytic m.
Ciaccio m.
clean-catch collection m.
m. of Cleary
cobaltinitrite m.
Coblentz test m.

Colcher-Sussman m.
collagen staining m.
constitutive heterochromatin m.
cooled-knife m.
copper sulfate m.
Craigie tube m.
Credé m.
Crippa lead tetraacetate m.
cysteic acid m.
Dale-Laidlaw clotting time m.
Dane m.
definitive m.
diazo staining m.
Dick m.
Dieterle m.
diffusion m.
digitonin m.
disk sensitivity m.
double antibody m.
Duke m.
dyed starch method
enzymatic digestion m.
enzyme demonstration m.
esterase staining m.
fibrin degradation products m.
fibrinogen m.
field m.
Fite m.
fixed sediment m.
flat substrate m.
Folin and Wu m. (FW)
Fontana-Masson staining m.
Foot reticulin m.
formaldehyde-induced
    fluorescence m.
formalin-ether sedimentation m.
freeze-cleave m.
freeze-etch m.
freeze-fracture-etch m.
frozen section m.
Gallyas m.
glass-bead retention m.
glucose oxidase m.
glycerin m.
Gram m.
Granger m.
Grimelius argyrophil stain m.
Grocott-Gomori methenamine-
    silver m.
Hall m.
Hammerschlag m.
Heublein m.

hexokinase m.
Highman m.
Histofine staining m.
Holmes m.
Holzer m.
H.P. Wright m.
HSU m.
immunofluorescence m.
immunoperoxidase staining m.
indophenol m.
Ivy m.
Jacobsson m.
Jendrassik-Grof m.
Jenner m.
Jones m.
Kaplan-Meier staining m.
Kety-Schmidt m.
Kjeldahl m.
Klump and Bieth m.
Lee-White m. (LW)
Lee-White clotting time m.
leukocyte alkaline phosphatase m.
Levaditi m.
Lillie allochrome m.
Lison-Dunn m.
macro-Kjeldahl m.
Mantel-Cox m.
Marshall m.
Masson trichrome m.
melanin bleaching m.
melanin staining m.
Menzies m.
micro-Kjeldahl m.
Millipore m.
Monte Carlo m.
Movat pentachrome m.
myelin staining m.
myoglobin identification m.
Nichols m.
Nikiforoff m.
Nuclepore m.
Ouchterlony m.
Papanicolaou m.
Penfield m.
periodic acid-Schiff m.
peroxidase staining m.
Pfeiffer-Comberg m.
Pizzolato peroxide-silver m.
plasma thrombin clot m.
Ploton staining m.
polyvinyl alcohol fixative m.
protein separation m.

M

NOTES

method *(continued)*
    Puchtler alkaline Congo red m.
    Puchtler Sirius red m.
    PVA fixative m.
    Quick m.
    Rees-Ecker m.
    reference m.
    Rideal-Walker m.
    RNA-zolB RNA extraction m.
    Sahli m.
    Salzman m.
    Schick m.
    Scotch tape m.
    Shaffer-Hartmann m.
    Somogyi m.
    special reference m.
    Stovall-Black m.
    streptavidin-biotin peroxidase m.
    suction m. (SM)
    Sweet m.
    thermodilution m.
    Thoms m.
    Tietz-Fiereck m.
    two-slide m.
    ultropaque m.
    Van Slyke and Cullen m.
    von Clauss m.
    von Kossa m.
    Warthin-Starry m.
    Welker m.
    Westergren sedimentation rate m.
    Whipple m.
    Wilson m.
    Wintrobe and Landsberg m.
    Wintrobe sedimentation rate m.
    zeta sedimentation ratio m.
    Ziehl-Neelsen m.
    zinc sulfate flotation m.
    ZSR m.
methodology
methotrexate
methoxy
    3-methoxy-4-hydroxymandelic acid
        test
methoxychlor
methoxyhydroxymandelic acid (MOMA)
methyl
    m. acetate
    m. alcohol poisoning
    m. aldehyde
    m. blue
    m. bromide
    m. butyl ketone
    m. chloroform
    m. demeton
    m. ethyl ketone (MEK)
    m. green
    m. green-pyronin stain

    m. isobutyl ketone
    m. mercury
    m. orange
    m. parathion
    m. red (MR)
    m. red test
    m. violet
    m. yellow
N-**methylacetamide**
methylation
methylbenzene
methylene
    m. azure
    m. chloride
    m. dichloride
    m. violet
    m. white
methylene blue (MB)
    m. b. active substance (MBAS)
    m. b. dye (MBD)
    Kühne m. b.
    Löffler m. b.
    new m. b.
    polychrome m. b.
    m. b. stain
    m. b. test
3,4-methylenedioxyamphetamine assays
methylenophil, methylenophile
methylenophilic
methylenophilous
N-**methylformamide**
methylmalonic
    m. acid
    m. acidemia
    m. aciduria
methylmalonyl-CoA decarboxylase
methylmercaptan
methylmorphine
N′-**methylnicotinamide**
methylnitrosourea (MNU)
methylparaben
methylphenylethylhydantoin (MPEH)
5-methylresorcinol
methylrosaniline chloride
methyltransferase
    tetrahydropteroylglutamate m.
methyprylon assay
metMb
    metmyoglobin
metmyoglobin (metMb)
Metopirone test
Metopium
Metorchis
metoxenous
metoxeny, metaxeny
metraterm
metratrophia
metratrophy

metria
metric
    m. data
    m. system
metritis
metrofibroma
metrolymphangitis
metromalacia
metromalacoma
metromalacosis
metronidazole assay
metroperitoneal fistula
metroperitonitis
metrorrhagia
metrosalpingitis
metrotrophic test
Mets
  metastases
metyrapone
    m. stimulation test
    m. test
MeV
  megaelectron volt
mev
  million electron volts
mevalonate
mevinphos
Mexican
    M. hat cell
    M. hat corpuscle
mexiletine
Meyenburg
    M. complex
    M. disease
Meyenburg-Altherr-Uehlinger syndrome
Meyer-Betz syndrome
Meyer disease
Meyer-Schwickerath and Weyers
  syndrome
Meynet node
mezlocillin
MF
  medium frequency
  mycosis fungoides
  myelin figure
mF
  millifarad
mf
  microfilaria
MFB
  metallic foreign body

MFH
  malignant fibrous histiocytoma
MG
  menopausal gonadotropin
  Michaelis-Gutmann body
  myasthenia gravis
    streptococcus MG
mg
  milligram
mg%
  milligrams per deciliter
  milligrams per 100 milliliters
MGAB
  mucous gland adenoma of bronchus
Mg agglutinin
MGH, mgh
  microglandular hyperplasia
  milligram-hour
MGN
  membranous glomerulonephritis
MGP
  marginal granulocyte pool
MH
  mammotropic hormone
mH
  millihenry
MHA
  methemalbumin
  microangiopathic hemolytic anemia
  mixed hemadsorption
MHA-TP
  micro-hemagglutination *Treponema*
    pallidum
    MHA-TP test
MHb
  methemoglobin
MHC
  major histocompatibility complex
    MHC restriction
MHD
  mean hemolytic dose
  minimum hemolytic dose
MHN
  massive hepatic necrosis
MHz
  megahertz
MI
  mitral incompetence
  mitral insufficiency
  myocardial infarction
MIB-1 antigen

NOTES

Mibelli
    M. angiokeratoma
    M. disease
    M. porokeratosis
MIC
  minimal inhibitory concentration
  minimal isorrheic concentration
  minimum inhibitory concentration
MIC2 antibody
mice
    pneumonia virus of m. (PVM)
    SCID m.
    severe combined
      immunodeficient m.
    transgenic m.
micelle
    ferruginous m.
Michaelis-Gutmann body (MG)
Michaelis-Menten equation
miconazole
micrencephalia
micrencephalous
micrencephaly
microabscess
    Munro m.
    Pautrier m.
microadenoma
microaerophile
microaerophilic
    m. streptococcus
microaggregate filter
microalbinuria
microalbuminuria
microaleuriospore
microampere
microanalysis
    energy dispersive x-ray m.
microaneurysm
    retinal m.
microangiopathic hemolytic anemia (MHA)
microangiopathy
    diabetic m.
    thrombotic m.
Microbacterium
Microbank cryopreservative
microbar
microbe
microbial
    m. antagonism
    m. associates
    m. genetics
    m. persistence
    m. variation
    m. vitamin
microbic
    m. dissociation
microbicidal

microbicide
microbid
microbioassay
microbiol.
  microbiological
microbiologic
    m. assay
microbiological (microbiol.)
    m. assay (MB)
microbiologist
microbiology
    m. automation
    m. identification systems
microbiotic
microbism
    latent m.
microblast
microbody
microbroth
microburet
microcell
microcephaly
    encephaloclastic m.
    schizencephalic m.
microchemical balance
microchemistry
microchromosome
Micrococcaceae
Micrococcus
microcolitis
microcolony
microcomputer
microconidium, pl. microconidia
microcoulomb
microcrystalline
microcurie
microcurie-hour
microcyst
microcystic disease of renal medulla
microcyte
microcythemia
microcytic hypochromic anemia
microcytosis
microdensitometer
microdiffusion analysis
microdrepanocytic
    m. anemia
    m. disease
microdrepanocytosis
microdysgenesia
microelectrophoresis
microencephaly
microerythrocyte
microevolution
microfarad (μf, μfd)
microfibril
microfilament
    subplasmalemmal m.

microfilaremia
Microfilaria
    M. bancrofti
    M. streptocerca
microfilaria, pl. **microfilariae (mf)**
microfilariasis
microfilm
microflora
Microflow test
microfollicular
    m. adenoma
    m. goiter
microgamete
microgametocyte
microgamont
microgamy
microglandular
    m. adenosis
    m. hyperplasia (MGH, mgh)
microglioma
microgliomatosis
microgliosis
microglobulin
    β-m.
    $β_2$-m.
    beta m.
    beta-2 m.
microglossia
micrognathia
    m. with peromelia
microgram
micrograph
    electron m.
micrography
microgyria
microhemagglutination assay
micro-hemagglutination-*Treponema pallidum* (MHA-TP)
microhemagglutination-*Treponema pallidum* test
microhematocrit
microhenry
microhistology
microhm
microhomology
microimmunofluorescent test
microincineration
microinfarct
microinjector
microinvasion
microinvasive carcinoma
micro-Kjeldahl method

microleukoblast
microliter (μL)
microlith
microlithiasis
    pulmonary alveolar m. (PAM)
microlymphocytotoxicity assay
micromelia
micromelic dwarfism
micromerozoite
micrometastasis
micrometastatic
    m. disease
micrometer (μm)
micromethod
    buffy coat m.
micrometry
micromicrocurie (μμc)
micromicron (μμ)
micromillimeter (μmm)
micromole
Micromonospora
Micromonosporaceae
micromyeloblast
micromyeloblastic leukemia
micron (mu, μ)
microneme
micronodular
micronodularity
    regenerative m.
micronucleus
microorganism
micropapillary component (MPC)
microparasite
micropathology
microphage
microphagocyte
microphthalmia
micropinocytosis
micropinocytotic vesicle
micropipette, micropipet
microplania
microplethysmography
micropolygyria
micropore
microprecipitation test
micropredation
micropredator
microprobe
    electron m.
    laser m.
microprocessor
microprogram

M

NOTES

micropromyelocyte
microprotein
micropyle
microrefractometer
microroentgen
microscope
> analytical electron m. (AEM)
> BHTU m.
> binocular m.
> color-contrast m.
> comparison m.
> compound m.
> dark-field m.
> dark-ground m.
> electron m. (EM)
> fluorescent m.
> infrared m.
> integrating m.
> interference m.
> JEOL 100 S transmission electron m.
> JEOL 1200 transmission electron m.
> laser m.
> light m.
> Nomarski m.
> Olympus BH2 m.
> phase-contrast m.
> Philips 301 electron m.
> polarizing m.
> reflecting m.
> scanning electron m. (SEM)
> simple m.
> stereoscopic m.
> transmission electron m. (TEM)
> trinocular m.
> ultraviolet m.
> x-ray m.
> Zeiss Axiophot fluorescent m.
> Zeiss Axioplan m.
> Zeiss LSM-10 laser m.
> Zeiss transmission electron m.
microscopic
> m. agglutination
> filter paper m. (FPM)
> m. hematuria
> m. infarct
microscopy
> confocal laser scan m. (CLSM)
> electron m. (EM)
> epifluorescence m.
> fluorescence m.
> immune electron m.
> immunofluorescence m.
> light m. (LM)
> transmission electron m. (TEM)
microsecond

microsomal
> m. enzyme
> m. enzyme system
> m. thyroid antibody
> m. thyroid antibody test
microsome
microspectrophotometry
microspectroscope
microsphere
> aggregated m.
microspherocyte
microspherocytosis
microsplanchnic
microsplenia
Microspora
Microsporasida
microspore
Microsporida
microsporidia
microsporidian
microsporidiasis
microsporidiosis
Microsporon
microsporosis
Microsporum
> *M. audouinii*
> *M. canis*
> *M. canis, var. distortum*
> *M. felineum*
> *M. ferrugineum*
> *M. fulvum*
> *M. furfur*
> *M. gallinae*
> *M. gypseum*
> *M. lanosum*
> *M. nanum*
> *M. persicolor*
> *M. vanbreuseghemi*
microstomia
microsyringe
microtome
> cold m.
> freezing m.
> m. knife
> LEICA VT1000 E fully automatic m.
> LEICA VT1000 M semi-automatic m.
> rocker m.
> rotary m.
> sliding m.
microtonometer
microtoxicity assay
Microtrombidium
microtubule
microtubule-associated protein (MAP)
Microtus
microunit

microvesicle
microvilli
microvillous inclusion disease
Microviridae
microvolt (μV)
microwatt
microwave fixation
microxyphil
microzoon
Micrurus
MID
   maximum inhibiting dilution
   minimal infecting dose
   minimum infective dose
midbody
midbrain
midcarpal
Middlebrook
   M. agar
   M. broth
Middlebrook-Dubos hemagglutination
   test
middle piece of spermatozoon
midge
midline
   m. lethal granuloma
   m. malignant reticulosis granuloma
midzonal necrosis
Mielke bleeding time
Miescher
   M. elastoma
   M. granulomatosis
   M. syndrome
Miescheria
MIF
   macrophage-inhibiting factor
   melanocyte-stimulating hormone-
      inhibiting factor
   migration inhibition factor
   mixed immunofluorescence
migrans
   larva m.
   spiruroid larva m.
   visceral larva m.
migrating
   m. abscess
   m. thrombophlebitis
migration
   m. inhibition factor (MIF)

   m. inhibition test
   m. inhibitory factor test
migration-inhibitory factor
migratory
   m. cell
   m. pneumonia
Mikulicz
   M. cell
   M. disease
   M. syndrome
mild silver protein
Miles Encore QA glucose meter
milia (*pl. of* milium)
miliaria
   apocrine m.
   m. profunda
   m. rubra
miliary
   m. abscess
   m. aneurysm
   m. embolism
   m. fever
   m. granulomatous inflammation
   m. tuberculosis
milium, pl. milia
   colloid m.
   m. cyst
milk
   acidophilus m.
   m. alkali syndrome
   m. anemia
   m. cyst
   m. factor
   lactobacillary m.
   m. leg
   m. spot
milker's
   m. nodes
   m. nodule
   m. nodule virus
Milkman syndrome
milkpox
milky
   m. ascites
   m. urine
Millard-Gubler syndrome
miller's asthma
MILLEX-GS plasma filter

M

NOTES

milliamperage
milliampere (mA)
milliampere-second (mA-s)
millibar (mbar)
millicoulomb (mC)
millicurie (mCi)
millicurie-hour (mCi-hr)
milliequivalent (mEq, meq)
millifarad (mF)
Milligan trichrome stain
milligram (mg)
 m.'s per deciliter (mg%)
 m.'s per 100 milliliters (mg%)
milligram-hour (MGH, mgh)
millihenry (mH)
millilambert (mL)
milliliter (mL)
 milligrams per 100 m.'s (mg%)
millimeter (mm)
 cubic m. (cmm)
 m.'s of mercury (mmHg)
 m.'s partial pressure (mmpp)
millimicrocurie (mμc)
millimicrogram (mμg)
millimicron (mμ)
millimolar (mM)
millimole (mM, mmol)
 m.'s per liter (mM/L, mM/l)
millinormal (mN)
million electron volts (mev)
milliosmole (mOsm)
millipede
Millipore
 M. filter
 M. method
millirad (mrad)
millirem (mrem)
milliroentgen (mR)
millisecond (msec)
millisomolal (mOs)
milliunit (mU)
millivolt (mV, mv)
milliwatt (mW)
Millonig
 M. phosphate buffer
 M. phosphate-buffered formalin
 fixative
Millon-Nasse test
Millon reagent
Mills disease
Milroy disease
Milton disease
Mima
 M. polymorpha
Minamata disease
mince
mineral
 m. foreign body

m. nutrients
m. oil foreign body
m. oil granuloma
mineralization
mineralocorticoid hypertension
miner's
 m. asthma
 m. lung
miniature scarlet fever
minicell
minimal
 m. bactercidal level (MBL)
 m. bactericidal concentration (MBC)
 m. brain damage (MBD)
 m. brain dysfunction (MBD)
 m. deviation melanoma
 m. erythema dose (MED)
 m. growth temperature
 m. infecting dose (MID)
 m. inhibitory concentration (MIC)
 m. isorrheic concentration (MIC)
 m. lethal concentration
 m. lethal dose
 m. morbidostatic dose (MMD)
 m. reacting dose (MRD)
minimal-change
 m.-c. disease
 m.-c. nephrotic syndrome
minimum
 m. bactericidal concentration
 m. complete-killing concentration
 (MCC)
 m. concentration of bilirubin
 (MCBR)
 m. detectable concentration (MDC)
 m. dose causing death or
 malformation of 100% of fetuses
 (T/LD_{100})
 m. essential medium (MEM)
 m. hemolytic dose (MHD)
 m. infective dose (MID)
 m. inhibitory concentration (MIC)
 m. lethal concentration (MLC)
 m. lethal dose (MLD)
 m. mycoplasmacidal concentration
 (MPC)
 m. temperature
 m. thermometer
mink enteritis virus
Minkowski-Chauffard syndrome
minocycline
minor
 m. agglutinin
 M. disease
 m. epilepsy
 m. histocompatibility antigen
 m. histocompatibility complex
 m. tranquilizer

Minot-von Willebrand syndrome
minus strand
minute
> counts per m. (cpm)
> cycles per m. (c/min)
> liters per m. (Lpm, lpm)
> revolutions per m. (rpm)
> m. volume (MV)
mionectic
miostagmin reaction
MIP
> macrophage inflammatory protein
miracidium, pl. **miracidia**
Mirchamp sign
MIRD
> medical internal radiation dose
Mirex
Mirizzi syndrome
mirror-image cell
miscarriage
miscibility
miscible
> infinitely m.
> partially m.
missed abortion
missense mutation
missile wound
mist
mistranslation
Mitchell disease
mite
> grain itch m.
> harvest m.
> kedani m.
> parasitoid m.
> predaceous m.
> red m.
> trombiculid m.
> m. typhus
miticidal
miticide
mitochondria
mitochondrial
> m. antibody
> m. myopathy
mitochondrian
> m. cristae alteration
> m. matrix alteration
> m. membrane alteration
mitochondrion
mitogen
> pokeweed m. (PWM)

mitogenesis
mitogenetic
mitogenic
> m. factor
mitokinetic
mitoplasm
mitosis, pl. **mitoses**
> three-part m.
mitosis-karyorrhexis index (MKI)
mitotic
> m. arrest
> m. cycle
> m. figure
> m. index
> m. poison
mitotic-control protein (MCP)
mitral
> m. atresia
> m. incompetence (MI)
> m. incompetency and stenosis
> m. insufficiency (MI)
> m. stenosis
> m. valve
> m. valve calcification
> m. valve prolapse (MVP)
Mitsuda
> M. antigen
> M. reaction
Mittendorf dots
mixed
> m. acid fermentation
> m. agglutination
> m. agglutination reaction
> m. agglutination test
> m. calculus
> m. cell leukemia
> m. chancre
> m. connective-tissue disease (MCTD)
> m. cryoglobulin syndrome
> m. culture
> m. epithelial-mesenchymal tumor
> m. glioma
> m. hemadsorption (MHA)
> m. hemoglobinopathy
> m. hepatocellular carcinoma
> m. immunofluorescence (MIF)
> m. infection
> m. leukemia
> m. leukocyte culture (MLC)
> m. lymphocyte culture (MLC)
> m. lymphocyte culture reaction

M

NOTES

mixed *(continued)*
m. lymphocyte culture test
m. lymphocyte reaction (MLR)
m. mesodermal tumor
m. squamous cell carcinoma and adenocarcinoma
m. thalassemia
m. thrombus
m. tumor of salivary gland
m. tumor of skin
m. venous (MV)
m. venous blood
m. venous P_{CO_2}
m. venous P_{O_2}
mixing
phenotypic m.
mixoploid
developmental m.
proliferative m.
mixoploidy
mixotrophic
mixture
dextrose solution m. (DSM)
dichloropropene-dichloropropene m.
racemic m.
toxoid-antitoxin m. (TAM)
Miyagawa body
Miyagawanella
Miyasato disease
MK
monkey kidney
MKI
mitosis-karyorrhexis index
MKS, mks
meter-kilogram-second
MKS system
MKS unit
ML
malignant lymphoma
M:L
monocyte-lymphocyte ratio
mL
millilambert
milliliter
MLa
acute monocytic leukemia
MLC
chronic myelomonocytic leukemia
minimum lethal concentration
mixed leukocyte culture
mixed lymphocyte culture
MLC test
MLD
metachromatic leukodystrophy
minimum lethal dose
MLR
mixed lymphocyte reaction

MLS
subacute myelomonocytic leukemia
MLV
Moloney leukemogenic virus
mouse leukemia virus
MM
malignant melanoma
Marshall-Marchetti
multiple myeloma
myeloid metaplasia
MM virus
mM
millimolar
millimole
mm
millimeter
MMD
minimal morbidostatic dose
MMFR
maximal midflow rate
mmHg
millimeters of mercury
mM/L, mM/l
millimoles per liter
MMM
myeloid metaplasia with myelofibrosis
myelosclerosis with myeloid metaplasia
MMMT
malignant mixed mesodermal tumor
M-mode echo
mmol
millimole
mmpp
millimeters partial pressure
MMR
measles, mumps, and rubella vaccine
MMTV
mouse mammary tumor virus
mN
millinormal
mnemonic code
MNS blood group
MNSs antigen
MNU
methylnitrosourea
MO
no evidence of distant metastases
MoAb
monoclonal antibody
mobile
m. gene
m. phase
mobility
electrophoretic m.
mobilization
localized leukocyte m. (LLM)
m. test
Mobiluncus

Möbius
    M. disease
    M. syndrome
modal centromere copy number
mode
    conversational m.
    decay m.
    histogram m.
    list m.
model
    hepatocarcinogenesis m.
modem
moderator band
modification
    racemic m.
modified
    m. amino acid
    m. smallpox
modifier
modifying gene
modular
modulate
modulation
    antigenic m.
    m. transfer function
module
modulus
Moeller-Barlow disease
Mohr pipette
moiety
moist
    m. gangrene
    m. papule
    m. wart
Mokola virus
mol
    mole
molal
molality
molar (M)
    m. absorptivity
    m. concentration
    m. heat capacity
    m. pregnancy
    m. weight
molarity
mold
    CRYO rubber m.
    pink bread m.
mole (mol)
    blood m.
    Breus m.

    carneous m.
    cystic m.
    false m.
    fleshy m.
    m. fraction
    grape m.
    hairy m.
    hydatid m.
    hydatidiform m. (HM)
    invasive m.
    spider m.
    vesicular m.
molecular
    m. anemia
    m. biology
    m. cloning
    m. disease
    m. dispersion
    m. distillation
    m. exclusion chromatography
    m. genetics
    m. lesion
    m. mass
    m. pathology
    m. sieve
    m. sieve chromatography
    m. weight (MW)
molecule
    accessory m.
    adhesion m.
    endothelial-leukocyte adhesion m. (E-LAM)
    intercellular adhesion m.-1 (ICAM-1)
    neural cell adhesion m. (NCAM)
molecule-1
    intercellular adhesion m. (ICAM-1)
Molisch test
Mollarct meningitis
Mollicutes
mollities
mollusc
Mollusca
molluscous
molluscum, pl. mollusca
    m. body
    m. contagiosum
    m. contagiosum virus
    m. corpuscle
    m. fibrosum
    m. fibrosum gravidarum

M

NOTES

molluscum *(continued)*
    m. sebaceum virus
    m. verrucosum
mollusk
Moloney
    M. leukemogenic virus (MLV)
    M. sarcoma virus (MSV)
    M. test
    M. virus
Molten disease
molybdenum
molybdic
molybdous
MOMA
    methoxyhydroxymandelic acid
moment
    dipole m.
    magnetic m.
momentum
monad
Monakow syndrome
monamide
monaminergic
monaminuria
monarthritis
Mönckeberg
    M. arteriosclerosis
    M. degeneration
    M. medial calcification
    M. medial calcific sclerosis
Mondor disease
Monera
moneran
Monge disease
mongol
mongolian
    m. macula
    m. spot
mongolism
mongoloid
Moniezia expansa
monilated
monilethrix
Monilia
Moniliaceae
monilial
    m. esophagitis
moniliasis
    m. pneumonia
moniliform
Moniliformis
    M. moniliformis
moniliid
monitor
    air m.
monitoring
    atmospheric m.

monkey
    m. B virus
    m. kidney (MK)
monkeypox
    m. virus
monoallelic
monoamine
    m. oxidase
    m. oxidase inhibitor
monoaminodicarboxylic acid
monoaminomonocarboxylic acid
monoaminuria
monoamniotic placenta twins
monoassociated
monobasic
    m. acid
    m. potassium phosphate
monoblast
monoblastic leukemia
monocentric
monocephalus
    m. tetrapus dibrachius
    m. tripus dibrachius
monochorionic
    m. diamniotic placenta
    m. diamniotic placenta twin
    m. monoamniotic placenta
monochroic
monochromatic
monochromatism
monochromatophil, monochromatophile
monochromator
monochromic
monochromophil, monochromophile
monoclonal
    m. antibody (MAb, MAB, MoAb)
    m. antiepithelial membrane antigen
    m. band
    m. gammopathy
    m. hypergammaglobulinemia
    m. immunoglobulin
    m. peak
    m. protein
    m. tumor
monocyte
    m. chemoattractant protein-1 (MCP-1)
    m. function test
monocyte-derived neutrophil chemotactic factor (MDNCF)
monocyte-lymphocyte ratio (M:L)
monocytes (monos)
monocytic
    m. angina
    m. blood cell
    m. inflammatory infiltrate
    m. leukemia
    m. leukemoid reaction

m. leukocytosis
m. leukopenia
m. marrow
monocytogenes bacteria
monocytoid
m. B-cell lymphoma
m. cell
monocytopenia
monocytopoiesis
monocytosis
avian m.
monodermal teratoma
monodermoma
Mono-Diff test
monoenoic fatty acid
monoethylglycinexylidide
monogenesis
monogenetic
monogenic character
monogenous
monoglyceride
monohistiocytic series
monohydric alcohol
monohydrochloride
arginine m.
monohydrolase
orthophosphoric ester m.
monoinfection
monoiodotyrosine
monokine
monolayer
monoleptic fever
monomastigote
monomer
fibrin m.
monomeric
monomicrobic
monomorphic adenoma
monomorphism
monomyelocytic leukemia
monomyositis
Mononchus
mononeuritis
m. multiplex
mononeuropathy
mononuclear
m. phagocyte
m. phagocyte system
mononucleate
mononucleosis
infectious m. (IM)
posttransfusion m. (PTM)

mononucleotide
flavin m. (FMN)
monooxygenase
β-m.
beta m.
monopenia
monophasic wave
monophosphate
3',5'-m.
adenosine m. (AMP)
adenosine 3',5'-cyclic m.
cyclic adenosine m.
cyclic guanosine m.
cytidine m.
deoxyadenosine m. (dAMP)
deoxycytidine m.
deoxyguanosine m. (dGMP)
deoxyuridine m. (dUMP)
guanosine m.
hexose m. (HMP)
inosine m.
thymidine m.
uridine m.
xanthosine m.
monophyletic
m. theory
monophyletism
monoplast
monoplastic
monoploid
monopolar
monoptychial
monorecidive
m. chancre
monos
monocytes
monosaccharide
Monoscreen test
monosodium
m. glutamate
m. urate (MSU)
monosome
monosomic cell
monosomy
monospecific
Monosporium apiospermum
Monospot test
Monosticon Dri-Dot test
Monostoma
monostome
monostotic
m. fibrous dysplasia

M

NOTES

monotreme
Monotricha
monotrichate
monotrichous
monounsaturated
monovalent
    m. antiserum
monoxenous
monoxide
    carbon m.
    diffusing capacity for carbon m.
      (D_{CO})
monozoic
monozygotic twins
Monte Carlo method
Montenegro skin test
Montevideo unit (MU)
Moore syndrome
Morand foot
Morax-Axenfeld bacillus
Moraxella
    M. bovis
    M. conjunctivitis
    M. lacunata
    M. nonliquefaciens
    M. osloensis
    M. phenylpyruvica
morbidity
    m. rate
morbility
morbilli
Morbillivirus
morbillivirus
morbus
mordant
    m. solution
mordicans
    calor m.
Morel-Kraepelin disease
Morel syndrome
Morerastrongylus costaricensis
Morgagni
    M. cyst
    M. disease
    M. hernia
    M. nodule
    M. prolapse
    M. sphere
    M. syndrome
Morgagni-Adams-Stokes syndrome
Morgagni-Stewart-Morel syndrome
morgan
Morgan bacillus
Morganella
    M. morganii
moriens
    ultimum m.
morin

Mörner test
morococcus
morphallactic regeneration
morphea
    m. acroterica
    m. alba
    m. guttata
    m. herpetiformis
    m. linearis
    m. pigmentosa
morphine assay
morphodifferentiation
morphogenesis
morphologic
    m. abnormality
morphology
morphometry
Morquio
    M. disease
    M. syndrome
Morquio-Brailsford syndrome
Morquio-Ullrich
    M.-U. disease
    M.-U. syndrome
Morris syndrome
mors, gen. **mortis**
    m. thymica
mortality rate (MR)
mortar kidney
Mortierella
mortification
mortified
mortis (*gen. of* mors)
Morton
    M. disease
    M. syndrome
morula
morular
morule
Morvan
    M. disease
    M. syndrome
mOs
    millisomolal
mosaic
    m. fungus
    m. pattern
    m. wart
mosaicism
Moschcowitz disease
Mosenthal
    M. test
Mosler diabetes
mOsm
    milliosmole
mosquito
mosquitocidal
mosquitocide

Moss classification
Mosse syndrome
mossy foot
mote
    blood m.
mother
    m. cyst
moth patch
motile
    m. leukocyte
    m. serum
motilin
motility test
motion
    brownian m.
    range of m. (ROM)
α-motor neuron
motor neuron disease
Mott cell
mottled enamel
mottling
Motulsky dye reduction test
moulage
mould
Mounier-Kuhn syndrome
mount
    India ink m.
    wet m.
mountant
mounting medium
mouse
    m. cancer
    cancer-free white m. (CFWM)
    m. encephalomyelitis
    m. encephalomyelitis virus
    m. hepatitis
    m. hepatitis virus
    m. leukemia virus (MLV)
    m. mammary tumor virus (MMTV)
    New Zealand m.
    nude m.
    m. parotid tumor virus
    m. poliomyelitis
    m. poliomyelitis virus
    m. thymic virus
    m. unit (m.u., mu, μ)
    m. uterine unit (MUU)
mousepox
    m. virus
mouse-specific lymphocyte antigen
    (MSLA)

mouth
    scabby m.
    sore m.
    tapir m.
    trench m.
movable
    m. heart
    m. testis
Movat
    M. pentachrome method
    M. pentachrome stain
movement
    ameboid m.
    m. artifact
    brownian m.
    euglenoid m.
    streaming m.
moving phase
Mowry colloidal iron stain
MP
    melting point
6-MP
    6-mercaptopurine
MPC
    marine protein concentrate
    maximum permissible concentration
    micropapillary component
    minimum mycoplasmacidal concentration
MPD
    maximal permissible dose
MPEH
    methylphenylethylhydantoin
MPGN
    membranoproliferative
      glomerulonephritis
M phase
MPP
    mercaptopyrazidopyrimidine
MPS
    mucopolysaccharide
MR
    methyl red
    mortality rate
mR
    milliroentgen
mrad
    millirad
MRCNS
    methicillin-resistant coagulase-negative
      Staphylococcus
MRD
    minimal reacting dose

M

NOTES

mrem
   millirem
MRF
   melanocyte-stimulating hormone-
      releasing factor
   mesencephalic reticular formation
mRNA
   messenger RNA
MRSA
   methicillin-resistant *Staphylococcus
      aureus*
MR-VP broth
MS
   mass spectrometry
   mucosubstance
   multiple sclerosis
MSA antibody
MS-1, -2 agent
MSB trichrome stain
MSCNS
   methicillin-susceptible coagulase-
      negative *Staphylococcus*
MSDS
   material safety data sheet
msec
   millisecond
MSH
   melanocyte-stimulating hormone
   melanophore-stimulating hormone
MSLA
   mouse-specific lymphocyte antigen
MSSA
   methicillin-susceptible *Staphylococcus
      aureus*
MSTS
   Musculoskeletal Tumor Society
      MSTS Staging System
MSU
   monosodium urate
MSUD
   maple syrup urine disease
MSV
   Moloney sarcoma virus
   murine sarcoma virus
MT
   antimetallothionein antibody
   malignant teratoma
MTI
   malignant teratoma intermediate
      MTI antibody
MTR
   Meinicke turbidity reaction
MTT
   malignant trophoblastic teratoma
MTV
   mammary tumor virus

MU
   Mache unit
   Montevideo unit
Mu
      M. antigen
mU
   milliunit
m.u.
   mouse unit
mu, μ
   micron
   mouse unit
      mu chain disease
MUC
   maximum urinary concentration
mucase
Mucha disease
Mucha-Habermann
      M.-H. disease
      M.-H. syndrome
mucicarmine
      m. stain
mucigen granules
mucihematein
mucilloid
      psyllium hydrophilic m.
mucin
      m. clot test
      polymorphic epithelial m. (PEM)
**mucin-depleted mucoepidermoid
   carcinoma**
mucinemia
mucinoid degeneration
mucinosa
      alopecia m.
mucinosis
      cutaneous focal m.
      follicular m.
      localized m.
      metabolic m.
      papular m.
      reticular erythematous m. (REM)
      secondary m.
mucinous
      m. adenocarcinoma
      m. atrophy
      m. carcinoma
      m. cyst
      m. cystadenocarcinoma
      m. cystadenoma
      m. degeneration
      m. meningioma
      m. stroma
mucinuria
mucitis
Muckle-Wells syndrome
mucocele
mucoclasis

mucocutaneous
>>   m. leishmaniasis
>>   m. lymph node syndrome
mucoenteritis
mucoepidermoid
>>   m. carcinoma
>>   m. tumor
mucoepithelial dysplasia
mucoid (M)
>>   m. adenocarcinoma
>>   m. colony
>>   m. medial degeneration
Mucolexx
mucolipidosis, pl. **mucolipidoses**
>>   m. I, II, III, IV
mucopeptide
mucopolysaccharidase
mucopolysaccharide (MPS)
>>   acid m. (AMP)
>>   acid m.'s (AMPS)
>>   m. stain
>>   m. staining
>>   m. storage disease
>>   sulfated acid m. (SAM)
>>   m. test
mucopolysaccharidosis,
>>   pl. **mucopolysaccharidoses**
>>   type IS m.
>>   type IVA, B m.
>>   type I–VIII m.
mucopolysacchariduria
>>   abnormal m. (AMPS)
mucoprotein
>>   m. assay
>>   Tamm-Horsfall m.
>>   m. test
mucopurulent
>>   m. exudate
mucopus
Mucor
Mucoraceae
mucormycosis
mucosa
>>   fundic m.
>>   muscularis m.
mucosa-associated
>>   m.-a. lymphoid tissue (MALT)
>>   m.-a. lymphoid tissue lymphoma
>>   (MALToma, MALT lymphoma)
mucosal
>>   m. disease
>>   m. disease virus

>>   m. ischemia
>>   m. neuroma
>>   m. neuroma syndrome
mucosanguineous
mucosanguinolent
mucoserous
mucosubstance (MS)
mucous
>>   m. cast
>>   m. colitis
>>   m. cyst
>>   m. gland adenoma of bronchus
>>   (MGAB)
>>   m. papule
>>   m. patch
>>   m. plaque
>>   m. polyp
>>   m. threads
mucoviscidosis
mucron
Mucuna
mucus
>>   m. extravasation
>>   m. retention
mud fever
Mueller-Hinton
>>   M.-H. agar
>>   M.-H. broth
Muellerius capillaris
Muir-Torre syndrome
mulberry calculus
Mulder test
mule-spinner's cancer
Müller fixative
Muller-Hermelink criteria
müllerian
>>   m. adenosarcoma
>>   m. rest
>>   m. tumor
multicellular
multicentric reticulohistiocytosis
Multiceps
>>   *M. multiceps*
multichannel analyzer (MCA)
multicore disease
multifactorial inheritance
multifocal
>>   m. eosinophilic granuloma
>>   m. fibrosis
>>   m. inflammation
>>   m. osteitis fibrosa
>>   m. progressive leukoencephalopathy

NOTES

multiform
multiformatter
multiforme
glioblastoma m.
multi-infection
multilamellar body
multilobar
multilobated
multilobate placenta
multilobular
multilocular
m. cystic kidney
m. hydatid cyst
multiloculate hydatid cyst
multimeter
multinodular goiter
multinuclear leukocyte
multinucleated
m. atypia of the vulva (MAV)
m. giant cell
multinucleosis
multipapillosa
Parafilaria m.
multipartial
multipartita
placenta m.
multiphasic screening
multiple
m. access
m. adenoma
m. adenomatous polyps
m. allele
m. chemical sensitivity
m. drug resistance (MDR)
m. endocrine adenomatosis (MEA)
m. endocrine neoplasia (MEN)
m. endocrine neoplasia, type 1, 2
m. endocrinoma
m. endocrinopathy
m. epiphysial dysplasia
m. event curve
m. exostosis
m. hamartoma syndrome
m. idiopathic hemorrhagic sarcoma
m. intestinal polyposis
m. lentigines syndrome
m. mucosal neuroma syndrome
m. myeloma (MM)
m. myelomatosis
m. myositis
m. osteochondromas
m. puncture tuberculin test
m. sclerosis (MS)
m. self-healing squamous
epithelioma
m. serositis
m. stage random sample

m. stain
m. symmetric lipomatosis
multiplex
mononeuritis m.
multiplication
vegetative m.
multipolar spindle
Multistix
multitrichous
multivalent
m. vaccine
multivariate analysis of variance
(MANOVA)
multivesicular body
multiwire proportional chamber
mummification
m. necrosis
mumps
m. antibody titer
iodine m.
meningoencephalitis m.
m. meningoencephalitis
metastatic m.
m. sensitivity test
m. serology
m. skin test antigen
m. virus
m. virus culture
m. virus vaccine
Münchausen, Munchausen
M. syndrome
Munchmeyer disease
Munich tumor classification system
Munro
M. abscess
M. microabscess
mural
m. aneurysm
m. endocarditis
m. thrombus
muramic acid
muramidase
Murchison-Sanderson syndrome
murein
Murex *Candida albicans* CA50 test
murexide
muriform
murine
m. hepatitis
m. leprosy
m. leukemia
m. sarcoma virus (MSV)
m. typhus
murmur
ejection m. (EM)
late systolic m. (LSM)
Murphy-Pattee test

Murray
- M. Valley encephalitis
- M. Valley encephalitis virus
- M. Valley rash

murrina

Murutucu virus

Musca
- *M. domestica*

muscarine

muscarinic

muscarinism

Muscidae

muscle
- m. action potential
- m. biopsy
- m. contractile protein
- m. hemoglobin
- m. serum

muscle-specific actin (HHF-35)

musculamine

muscular
- m. atrophy
- m. dystrophy (MD)
- m. rheumatism
- m. rigidity
- m. subaortic stenosis

muscularis
- m. mucosa
- m. propria

musculoaponeurotic fibromatosis

Musculoskeletal
- M. Tumor Society (MSTS)
- M. Tumor Society Staging System

musculotropic

mushroom
- m. poisoning

mushroom-worker's lung

mustard gas

Musto stain

mutagen
- chromosomal m.
- frame-shift m.

mutagenesis

mutagenic

mutagenicity test

mutant
- conditional-lethal m.
- conditionally lethal m.
- m. gene
- Hfr m.
- high-frequency recombination m.

- suppressor-sensitive m.
- temperature-sensitive m.

mutarotation

mutase
- 2,3-diphosphoglycerate m.
- S-methylmalonyl-CoA m.

mutation
- addition-deletion m.
- amber m.
- auxotrophic m.
- clear plaque m.
- cold-sensitive m.
- conditional lethal m.
- constitutive m.
- deletion m.
- feedback inhibition m.
- forward m.
- frame shift m.
- host-range m.
- insertion m.
- K-*ras* m.
- lethal m.
- missense m.
- nonsense m.
- ochre m.
- phage-resistant m.
- pleiotropic m.
- point m.
- rapid-lysis m.
- m. rate
- reading-frame-shift m.
- reverse m.
- semilethal m.
- sex-reversed m.
- silent m.
- somatic m.
- spontaneous m.
- subvital m.
- suppressor m.
- temperature-sensitive m.
- transition m.
- transversion m.
- t-s m.
- ultraviolet light-induced m.

mutilating
- m. keratoderma
- m. leprosy
- m. wound

muton

mutualism

mutualist

NOTES

MUU
    mouse uterine unit
muzzled sperm
MV
    megavolt
    minute volume
    mixed venous
mV, mv
    millivolt
MVE virus
MVP
    mitral valve prolapse
MVR
    massive vitreous retraction
MW
    molecular weight
mW
    milliwatt
Mx
    maxwell
my
    mayer
MY-10 clone stain
Myá disease
myalgia
    epidemic m.
myasis
myasthenia gravis (MG, MyG)
myatrophy
mycelia (*pl. of* mycelium)
mycelial
    m. fungus
    m. pathogen
mycelian
mycelioid
mycelium, pl. **mycelia**
    aerial m.
    nonseptate m.
    septate m.
mycete
mycetism
    m. cerebralis
    m. choliformis
    m. gastrointestinalis
    m. nervosa
    m. sanguinareus
mycetismus
    m. cerebralis
    m. cerebris
    m. choleriformis
    m. gastrointestinalis
    m. nervosus
    m. sanguinarius
mycetogenetic
mycetogenic
mycetogenous
mycetoma
    actinomycotic m.

    Bouffardi black m.
    Bouffardi white m.
    Brumpt white m.
    Carter black m.
    eumycotic m.
    maduromycotic m.
    Nicolle white m.
    Vincent white m.
mycetosis
mycoagglutinin
MycoAKT latex bead agglutination test
mycobacteria (*pl. of* mycobacterium)
    m. culture
Mycobacteriaceae
mycobacterial adjuvant
mycobacteriosis
Mycobacterium
    M. avium
    M. avium-intracellulare (MAC, MAI)
    M. bovis
    M. chelonae
    M. flavescens
    M. fortuitum
    M. gastri
    M. genavense
    M. gordonae
    M. haemophilum
    M. intracellulare
    M. kansasii
    M. leprae
    M. lepraemurium
    M. malmoense
    M. marinum
    M. microti
    M. nonchromogenicum
    M. paratuberculosis
    M. phlei
    M. scrofulaceum
    M. simiae
    M. smegmatis
    M. szulgai
    M. terrae
    M. triviale
    M. tuberculosis
    M. ulcerans
    M. xenopi
mycobacterium, pl. **mycobacteria**
    atypical mycobacteria
    Battey-type m.
    group I-IV mycobacteria
    nonphotochromogenic mycobacteria
    photochromogenic mycobacteria
    scotochromogenic mycobacteria
mycobactin
mycobiotic agar
Mycocandida
mycocide

Mycococcus
mycodermatitis
mycogastritis
mycolic acid
mycologist
mycology
 medical m.
mycomyringitis
mycophage
Mycoplana
 M. bullata
 M. dimorpha
Mycoplasma
 M. buccale
 M. faucium
 M. fermentans
 M. hominis
 M. orale
 M. pneumoniae
 M. salivarium
 M. serology
mycoplasma
 genital m.
 m. pneumonia of pigs
 T-strain m.
mycoplasmal pneumonia
Mycoplasmataceae
Mycoplasmatales
mycopus
mycoside
mycosis, pl. mycoses
 m. cutis chronica
 m. fungoides (MF)
 Gilchrist m.
 m. intestinalis
mycostatic
mycotic
 m. abscess
 m. aneurysm
 m. keratitis
 m. meningitis
mycotica
 otitis m.
mycotoxicosis
mycotoxin
mycovirus
mydriasis
myelapoplexy
myelatelia
myelauxe
myelemia

myelin
 m. basic protein (MBP)
 m. degeneration
 m. figure (MF)
 m. protein
 m. staining method
myelinic degeneration
myelinolysis
 central pontine m.
myelitis
 acute necrotizing m.
 acute transverse m.
 ascending m.
 bulbar m.
 concussion m.
 demyelinated m.
 Foix-Alajouanine m.
 funicular m.
 postinfectious m.
 postvaccinal m.
 subacute necrotizing m.
 systemic m.
 transverse m.
myeloblast
myeloblastemia
myeloblastic
 m. leukemia
 m. protein
myeloblastoma
myeloblastosis
 avian m.
myelocele
myelocyst
myelocystic
myelocystocele
myelocystomeningocele
myelocyte
 m. A, B, C
 basophilic m.
 eosinophilic m.
 neutrophilic m.
myelocythemia
myelocytic
 m. crisis
 m. leukemia
 m. leukemoid reaction
myelocytoma
myelocytomatosis
myelocytosis
myelodiastasis
myelodysplasia
myelodysplastic syndrome

M

NOTES

myelofibrosis
> myeloid metaplasia with m. (MMM)

myelogenic
> m. leukemia
> m. osteopathy
> m. sarcoma

myelogenous
> m. callus
> m. leukemia

myelogone
myelogonium
myeloic
myeloid
> m. cell
> m. depression
> m. hyperplasia
> m. leukemia
> m. metaplasia (MM)
> m. metaplasia with myelofibrosis (MMM)
> m. metaplasia with polycythemia vera (PCV-M)
> m. reticulosis
> m. sarcoma
> m. series
> m. tissue

myeloid-erythroid ratio (M/E)
myeloidosis
myeloleukemia
myelolipoma
myelolymphocyte
myelolysis
myeloma
> Bence Jones m.
> endothelial m.
> giant cell m.
> L-chain m.
> multiple m. (MM)
> m. multiplex
> nonsecretory m.
> plasma cell m.
> plasmacytic m.
> m. protein

myelomalacia
> angiodysgenetic m.

myelomatosis
> multiple m.
> m. multiplex

myelomeningitis
myelomeningocele
myelomonocyte
myelomonocytic leukemia
myelonencephalitis
myelopathic
> m. anemia
> m. polycythemia

myelopathy
> carcinomatous m.
> paracarcinomatous m.
> transverse m.

myeloperoxidase
> m. deficiency
> m. stain
> m. system

myelopetal
myelophthisic
> m. anemia

myelophthisis
myeloplast
myelopoiesis
> extramedullary m.

myelopoietic
myeloproliferative
> m. disease
> m. disorder
> m. syndromes

myeloradiculitis
myeloradiculodysplasia
myeloradiculopolyneuronitis
myelorrhagia
myelorrhaphy
myelosarcoma
myelosarcomatosis
myeloschisis
myelosclerosis
> m. with myeloid metaplasia (MMM)

myelosis
> aleukemic m.
> chronic nonleukemic m.
> erythremic m.
> funicular m.
> leukemic m.
> leukopenic m.
> megakaryocytic m.
> nonleukemic m.
> subleukemic m.

myelosuppression
myelosyringosis
myelotome
myelotomy
myelotoxic
MyG
> myasthenia gravis

myiasis
> cutaneous m.
> facial m.
> gastric m.
> genitourinary m.
> intestinal m.
> nasal m.
> sanguivorous m.

myiosis
myitis

Mylar capacitor
myoatrophy
myoblastoma
    granular cell m.
myoblastomatoid carcinoma
myocardial
    m. anoxia
    m. bridge
    m. damage (MD)
    m. depressant factor (MDF)
    m. disease (MD)
    m. disease of unknown origin
     (MDUO)
    m. infarction (MI)
    m. infarction in dumbbell form
    m. infarction in H-form
    m. ischemia
myocarditis (MC)
    acute isolated m.
    Fiedler m.
    fragmentation m.
    giant cell m.
    indurative m.
    Löffler m.
    rheumatic m.
myocardosis
myocele
myocelialgia
myocelitis
myocellulitis
myocerosis
myoclonic epilepsy
myocyte
    Anitschkow m.
myocytolysis
    m. of heart
myocytoma
MyoD1 regulatory gene
myodegeneration
myodemia
myodiastasis
myoendocarditis
myoepithelial cell
myoepithelioma
myoepithelium
myofascial syndrome
myofascitis
myofibroblast
myofibroblastic
    m. differentiation
    m. mammary stromal tumor
myofibrohistiocytic

myofibroma
myofibromatosis
    infantile m.
myofibrosis
    m. cordis
myofibrositis
myofilament
myogenic paralysis
myogen marker
myoglobin (Mb, MbCO, MbO$_2$)
    m. identification method
    m. test
myoglobinemia
myoglobinuria
    acute paroxysmal m.
myoglobinuric
    m. nephropathy
    m. nephrosis
myoglobulin
myoglobulinuria
myohemoglobin
myoid
myointimal hyperplasia
myoischemia
myokerosis
myokinase
myolipoma
myolysis
    cardiotoxic m.
myoma
myomalacia
myomatous
    m. polyp
myomelanosis
myometritis
myonecrosis
    clostridial m.
myoneme
myoneuroma
myonosus
myopachynsis
myopathic
myopathy
    alcoholic m.
    carcinomatous m.
    centronuclear m.
    congenital m.
    corticosteroid m.
    distal m.
    endocrine m.
    mitochondrial m.
    myotubular m.

M

NOTES

myopathy *(continued)*
    nemaline m.
    rod m.
    thyrotoxic m.
myopericarditis
myoperitonitis
myophosphorylase deficiency glycogenosis
myorrhexis
myosalpingitis
myosarcoma
myosclerosis
myosin
myosis
    endolymphatic stromal m.
myositic
myositis
    acute disseminated m.
    clostridial m.
    epidemic m.
    m. fibrosa
    infectious m.
    interstitial m.
    multiple m.
    m. ossificans
    m. ossificans circumscripta
    m. ossificans progressiva
    ossifying interstitial m.
    proliferative m.
myospherulosis
myotenositis
myotonic dystrophy
myotubular myopathy
Myoviridae
myriapod
Myriapoda
myringitis
    bullous m.
myringomycosis
myristic acid
Myrmecia
myrmecia
myxadenitis
myxadenoma
myxedema
    m. heart
    infantile m.
    pituitary m.
    pretibial m.
myxedematoid

myxedematous
myxemia
myxochondrofibrosarcoma
myxochondroma
Myxococcidium stegomyiae
myxofibroma
myxofibrosarcoma
myxoid
    m. cyst
    m. degeneration
    m. fibroma
    m. liposarcoma
    m. matrix
myxolipoma
myxoliposarcoma
myxoma, pl. **myxomas, myxomata**
    atrial m.
    cardiac m.
    cystic m.
    m. enchondromatosum
    endochondromatous m.
    erectile m.
    m. fibrosum
    infectious m.
    lanceolate m.
    m. lipomatosum
    lipomatous m.
    odontogenic m.
    m. sarcomatosum
    vascular m.
myxomatosis
    cardiac valve m.
    m. virus
myxomatous
    m. degeneration
myxomycete
Myxomycetes
myxoneuroma
myxopapillary ependymoma
myxopapilloma
myxosarcoma
Myxospora
myxospore
Myxosporea
Myxosporidia
myxovirus
Myxozoa
Myzomyia
Myzorhynchus

N
    newton
    normal
n
    normal
NA
    neutralizing antibody
na
    nephrogenic adenoma
NAACLS
    National Accrediting Agency for Clinical
    Laboratory Sciences
nabothian
    n. cyst
    n. follicle
***N*-acetylaspartate acid**
***N*-acetylmuramic acid**
nacreous
    n. ichthyosis
NAD
    nicotinamide adenine dinucleotide
NADH
    nicotinamide adenine dinucleotide
    (reduced form)
    NADH methemoglobin reductase
Nadi reaction
NADP
    nicotinamide adenine dinucleotide
    phosphate
NADPH
    nicotinamide adenine dinucleotide
    phosphate (reduced form)
Naegeli
    N. syndrome
    N. type of monocytic leukemia
Naegleria
NAF
    neutrophil activating factor
Naffziger syndrome
nagana
Nägele pelvis
Nagler reaction
nail
    n. horn
    shell n.
    yellow n.
nail-patella syndrome
Nairobi
    N. sheep disease
    N. sheep disease virus
Nakanishi stain
naked virus

NAME
    nevi, atrial myxoma, myxoid
    neurofibroma, and ephelides
    NAME syndrome
name
    generic n.
NANB hepatitis
nanism
Nannizzia
nanocurie (nCi)
nanofarad (nF)
nanogram (ng)
nanoliter (nL, nl)
nanomelia
nanometer (nm)
nanomole (nmol)
Nanophyetus salmincola
nanosecond (ns, nsec)
nanukayami
NAP
    neutrophil activating protein
nape nevus
naphthol
    α-n.
    alpha n.
    β-n.
    beta n.
    n. poisoning
    n. yellow S
naphthol-ASD chloroacetate esterase
stain
Napier formol-gel test
napierian logarithm
narcosis
    carbon dioxide n.
    nitrogen n.
narcotic
    n. antagonist
    n. blockade
nasal
    n. glioma
    n. myiasis
    n. polyp
    n. smear
    n. T/NK-cell lymphoma
nascent
Nasik vibrio
naso-oral leishmaniasis
nasopharyngeal
    n. culture
    n. leishmaniasis
    n. swab
nasopharyngitis
nasosinusitis

N

National
- N. Accrediting Agency for Clinical Laboratory Sciences (NAACLS)
- N. Cancer Institute (NCI)
- N. Certification Agency for Medical Laboratory Personnel (NCAMLP)
- N. Council of Health Laboratory Services (NCHLS)
- N. Institutes of Health (NIH)
- N. Registry in Clinical Chemistry (NRCC)
- N. Registry of Microbiologists (NRM)

native albumin

natremia, natriemia

natriuresis

natriuretic

natural
- n. antibody
- n. death
- n. dye
- n. focus of infection
- n. hemolysin
- n. immunity
- n. killer (NK)
- n. killer cell
- n. killer cell-stimulating factor (NKSF)
- n. selection

nausea
- epidemic n.

Nauta stain

navicular
- n. arthritis
- n. cell

NB
- neuroblastoma

NBS
- normal blood serum

NBT
- nitroblue tetrazolium
  - NBT dye
  - NBT test

NBTE
- nonbacterial thrombotic endocarditis

NCAM
- neural cell adhesion molecule

NCAMLP
- National Certification Agency for Medical Laboratory Personnel

NCHLS
- National Council of Health Laboratory Services

NCI
- National Cancer Institute

nCi
- nanocurie

NCL-ARm monoclonal antibody
NCL-ARp polyclonal antibody
NCL-ER-LH2 monoclonal antibody
NCL-PCR monoclonal antibody

ND
- neonatal death
- Newcastle disease
- nondisabling
  - ND virus

NDA
- no data available
- no demonstrable antibodies

NDI
- nephrogenic diabetes insipidus

NDP
- net dietary protein

NDV
- Newcastle disease virus

Nebraska calf scours virus

nebulizer
- ultrasonic n. (USN)

nebulous urine

Necator
- *N. americanus*

necatoriasis

neck
- buffalo n.
- bull n.
- Madelung n.
- n. of spermatozoon
- webbed n.

necrobiosis
- n. lipoidica
- n. lipoidica diabeticorum

necrobiotic xanthogranuloma

necrocytosis

necrogenic
- n. wart

necrogenous

necrogranulomatous

necrolysis
- toxic epidermal n. (TEN)

necroparasite

necropathy

necrophagocytosis

necrophilic

necropsy

necroscopy

necrose

necrosis
- acidophilic n.
- acute inflammatory n.
- acute tubular n. (ATN)
- aseptic n.
- avascular n.
- bridging hepatic n.
- caseation n.
- caseous n.

central n.
central hemorrhagic n. (CHN)
centrilobular n.
coagulation n.
coagulative n.
colliquative n.
cortical n.
cystic medial n. (CMN)
cytodegenerative n.
cytotoxic n.
diffuse n.
ductular piecemeal n.
epiphysial aseptic n.
fat n.
fibrinoid n.
focal n.
gangrenous n.
hyaline n.
inflammatory n.
ischemic n.
lamellar n.
laminar cortical n.
liquefactive n.
massive hepatic n. (MHN)
medial cystic n.
medullary n.
midzonal n.
mummification n.
papillary n.
peripheral n.
periportal n.
piecemeal n.
postpartum pituitary n.
progressive emphysematous n.
radiation n.
radium n.
renal cortical n.
renal medullary n.
renal papillary n.
sclerosing hyaline n.
septic n.
simple n.
spotty lobular n.
subcutaneous fat n. of newborn
suppurative n.
total n.
tumor n.
n. tumor
Zenker n.
zonal n.
necrospermia
necrosteon

necrosteosis
necrotic
    n. cirrhosis
    n. cyst
    n. inflammation
necrotizing
    n. angiitis
    n. arteriolitis
    n. bronchopneumonia
    n. encephalitis
    n. encephalomyelopathy
    n. enterocolitis
    n. factor
    n. fasciitis
    n. glomerulonephritis
    n. granulomatous inflammation
    n. lobar pneumonia
    n. pancreatitis
    n. papillitis
    n. sialometaplasia
    n. ulcerative gingivitis (NUG)
    n. ulcerative gingivostomatitis
    n. vasculitis
NED
    no evidence of disease
needle
    n. aspiration cytology
    Bard n.
    Becton-Dickinson n.
    Crown n.
    n. culture
    Manan n.
    Menghini n.
Neer shoulder fracture I, II, III
Neethling virus
Neftel disease
neg
    negative
negative (neg)
    n. anergy
    n. assortative mating
    n. base excess
    n. catalyst
    n. control enzyme induction
    n. control repression
    n. cytotaxis
    false n.
    n. neutrotaxis
    n. phase
    Rh n.
    Rhesus factor n. (Rh neg)
    n. stain

N

NOTES

negative *(continued)*
n. strand virus
n. variation (NV)
Negishi virus
Negri
N. body
N. corpuscle
Neisser
diplococcus of N.
N. stain
Neisseria
N. *flavescens*
N. *gonorrhoeae*
N. *gonorrhoeae* culture
N. *gonorrhoeae* smear
N. *lactamica*
N. *meningitidis*
N. *mucosa*
N. *sicca*
N. *subflava*
neisseria
anaerobic n.
Neisseriaceae
Nelson
N. syndrome
N. tumor
nemaline myopathy
nemathelminth
Nemathelminthes
nematicidal
nematicide
nematization
nematoblast
nematocide
Nematoda
nematode
nematodiasis
Nematodirella longispiculata
Nematodirus
nematoid
nematologist
nematology
Nematomorpha
nematosis
nematospermia
neoantigens
Neoascaris vitulorum
neocytosis
neoformation
neogenesis
neomembrane
neonatal
n. anemia
n. bilirubin
n. calf diarrhea virus
n. death (ND, NND)
n. hepatitis
n. herpes

n. hypoglycemia
n. isoerythrolysis
n. necrotizing enterocolitis
n. screening
neonatorum
anemia n.
anoxia n.
atelectasis n.
blennorrhea n.
conjunctivitis n.
ophthalmia n.
pemphigus n.
neopathy
neoplasia
cervical intraepithelial n. (CIN)
intratubular germ cell n.
lobular n.
multiple endocrine n. (MEN)
multiple endocrine n., type 1, 2
prostatic intraepithelial n. (PIN)
trophoblastic n.
vulvar intraepithelial n. (VIN)
neoplasm
adipocytic n.
adnexal n.
adrenal n.
benign n.
epithelial n.
epithelioid soft-tissue n. (ESTN)
histoid n.
interdigitating papillary n.
malignant n.
metastatic n.
oncocytic papillary n.
pancreatic endocrine n. (PEN)
synchronous n.
neoplastic
n. arachnoiditis
n. meningitis
neoprecipitin test (NPT)
neopterin
Neorickettsia helmintheca
Neospora canium
neoteny
Neotestudina rosati
neotype
neovascularization
nephelometer
nephelometric inhibition assay (NIA)
nephelometry
nephradenoma
nephrectasia
nephrectasis
nephredema
nephrelcosis
nephridium
nephritic
n. calculus

n. factor
n. syndrome
nephritis, pl. **nephritides**
   acute n.
   acute interstitial n. (AIN)
   analgesic n.
   anti-basement membrane n.
   anti-kidney serum n.
   bacterial n.
   chronic n.
   chronic interstitial n. (CIN)
   Ellis types 1 and 2 n.
   focal n.
   glomerular n.
   n. gravidarum
   hemorrhagic n.
   hereditary n. (HN)
   immune complex n.
   interstitial n.
   lupus n. (LN)
   Masugi-type nephrotoxic serum n.
   mesangial n.
   nephrotoxic n. (NTN)
   scarlatinal n.
   serum n.
   subacute n.
   suppurative n.
   syphilitic n.
   transfusion n.
   tuberculous n.
   tubular interstitial n.
   tubulointerstitial n.
   uranium n.
nephritogenic
nephroblastoma
nephrocalcinosis
nephrocystosis
nephrogenic
   n. adenoma (na)
   n. diabetes insipidus (NDI)
   n. rest
nephrohydrosis
nephrolith
nephrolithiasis
nephrolysin
nephrolysis
nephrolytic
nephroma
   embryonal n.
   mesoblastic n.
nephromalacia
nephromegaly

nephropathia epidemica
nephropathic
nephropathy
   acute uric acid n.
   analgesic n.
   Balkan n.
   Danubian endemic familial n.
   diabetic n.
   gouty n.
   hemoglobinuric n.
   hypokalemic n.
   IgA n.
   IgM n.
   immune complex n.
   membranous n.
   myoglobinuric n.
   sickle cell n.
   tubulointerstitial n. (TIN)
nephrophthisis
   familial juvenile n. (FJN)
nephroptosia
nephroptosis
nephropyelitis
nephrosclerosis
   arterial n.
   arteriolar n.
   benign n. (BNS)
   hyaline n.
   hyperplastic n.
   intercapillary n.
   malignant n.
   senile n.
nephrosclerotic
nephrosis, pl. **nephroses**
   acute n.
   amyloid n.
   bile n.
   cholemic n.
   familial n.
   hemoglobinuric n.
   hypokalemic n.
   hypoxic n.
   lipid n.
   lipoid n. (LN)
   lower nephron n.
   myoglobinuric n.
   osmotic n.
   toxic n.
   tubular n.
   vacuolar n.
nephrospasia
nephrospasis

N

NOTES

nephrotic
    n. syndrome (NS)
nephrotoxic
    n. antibody (NTAB)
    n. nephritis (NTN)
    n. serum
nephrotoxin
nephrotuberculosis
Nernst equation
nerve
    n. growth factor (NGF)
    n. growth factor antiserum
nervosa
    anorexia n.
nesidioblastoma
nesidioblastosis
nesslerization
nesslerize
Nessler reaction
nest
    Brunn epithelial n.
    cell n.
    epithelial n.
net
    Chiari n.
    chromidial n.
    n. dietary protein (NDP)
    n. protein ratio (NPR)
    n. protein utilization (NPU)
Netherton syndrome
network
    chromatin n.
Neufeld
    N. capsular swelling
    N. reaction
Neumann disease
neu-oncogene
neural
    n. cell adhesion molecule (NCAM)
    n. cyst
    n. tube defect
neuralgic amyotrophy
neuraminic acid
neuraminidase
    n. digestion
neuraminoglycoprotein
    alpha-2 n.
α_2-**neuraminoglycoprotein**
neuridine
neurilemmitis
neurilemoma
    acoustic n.
    ameloblastic n.
    Antoni type A n.
    Antoni type B n.
    malignant n.
neurilemosarcoma
neurility

neurimotility
neurimotor
neurinoma
    acoustic n.
neuritic
    n. atrophy
    n. plaque
neuriticum
    atrophoderma n.
neuritis
    adventitial n.
    allergic n.
    branchial n. (BN)
    experimental allergic n. (EAN)
    paralytic brachial n. (PBN)
neuroallergy
neuroarthropathy
neuroastrocytoma
neuroblast
neuroblastic
neuroblastoma (NB)
    olfactory n.
neuroborreliosis
neurochitin
neurochoroiditis
neurocristic hamartoma
neurocristopathy
neurocutaneous
    n. melanosis
    n. phacomatosis syndrome
neurocytolysis
neurocytoma
    central n.
neurodermatitis
neuroectodermal tumor
neuroencephalomyelopathy
neuroendocrine
    n. cell
    n. differentiation
neuroepithelioma
neuroepithelium
neurofibril
neurofibrillary degeneration
neurofibroma
    plexiform n.
    storiform n.
neurofibromatosis (NF)
    abortive n.
    central type n.
    incomplete n.
neurofibrosarcoma
neurofilament
    n. protein
    n. triplet polypeptide (NFP)
neurogenic
    n. arthropathy
    n. bladder
    n. muscular atrophy (NMA)

n. sarcoma
n. shock
neurogliomatosis
neurohypophyseal hormone
neurohypophysis
neurokeratin
neuroleptic malignant syndrome
neuroleukin
neurolymphomatosis
n. gallinarum
neurolysin
neuroma
acoustic n.
amputation n.
n. cutis
false n.
fibrillary n.
mucosal n.
pancinian n.
plexiform n.
n. telangiectodes
traumatic n.
Verneuil n.
neuromalacia
neuromatosis
neuromelanin
neuromelaninogenesis
neuromuscular choristoma
neuromyelitis
neuromyopathy
carcinomatous n.
neuromyositis
neuron
alpha motor n.
bipolar n.
α-motor n.
neuronal
n. hyperplasia
n. intestinal dysplasia
neuron-associated class III β-tubulin
neuronevus
neuronophage
neuronophagia
neuron-specific enolase (NSA, NSE)
neuro-oncology
neuropathic
n. albuminuria
n. arthritis
neuropathology (NP)
neuropathy
amblyopia n.
amyloid n.

diabetic n.
entrapment n.
hereditary sensory radicular n.
hypertrophic interstitial n.
peripheral n. (PN)
retrobulbar n.
subacute myelo-optical n. (SMON)
vincristine n.
neuroplexus
neuroretinitis
neuroretinopathy
neurosarcocleisis
neurosarcoidosis
neurosarcoma
neuroschwannoma
neurosclerosis
neurosecretory
n. granules
n. material (NSM)
Neurospora
neurosyphilis
neurothekeoma
neurotome
neurotoxin
neurotrophic atrophy
neurotropic virus
neurovaccine
neurovascular hamartoma
neurovirus
Neusser granule
neutral
n. buffered formalin fixative
n. lipid storage disease
n. red
n. stain
neutralization
n. test (NT)
viral n.
neutralizing (NT)
n. antibody (NA)
neutral protamine Hagedorn (insulin) (NPH)
neutral red
neutron
slow n.
thermal n.
neutropenia
cyclic n.
periodic n.
neutropenic angina
neutrophil, neutrophile
n. activating factor (NAF)

NOTES

N

neutrophil *(continued)*
    n. activating protein (NAP)
    band n.
    n. chemotactant factor
    filamented n.
    giant n.
    n. granule
    granules of developing n.'s
    hypersegmented n.
    immature n.
    juvenile n.
    mature n.
    polymorphonuclear n. (PMN)
    rod n.
    segmented n.
    stab n.
neutrophilia
    giant n.
neutrophilic
    n. chemotactic factor
    n. hyperplasia
    n. infiltrate
    n. leukemia
    n. leukocyte
    n. leukocytosis
    n. leukopenia
    n. lymphocytosis
    n. marrow
    n. metamyelocyte
    n. myelocyte
    n. promyelocyte
neutrophilopenia
neutrophilous
neutrotaxis
    indifferent n.
    negative n.
nevi (*pl. of* nevus)
nevocarcinoma
nevocyte
nevocytic nevus
nevoid
    n. elephantiasis
    n. hypertrichosis
nevolipoma
nevose
nevous
nevoxanthoendothelioma
nevus, pl. **nevi**
    acquired n.
    n. anemicus
    n. angiomatodes
    apocrine n.
    n. arachnoideus
    n. araneus
    nevi, atrial myxoma, myxoid
      neurofibroma, and ephelides
      (NAME)
    balloon cell n.

    basal cell n.
    bathing trunk n.
    Becker n.
    blue rubber-bleb nevi
    capillary n.
    n. cavernosus
    n. cell
    cellular blue n.
    comedo n.
    n. comedonicus
    compound n.
    congenital n.
    connective tissue n.
    dermal n.
    dermal-epidermal n.
    dysplastic n.
    n. elasticus of Lewandowski
    epidermic-dermic n.
    epithelioid cell n.
    faun tail n.
    flame n.
    n. flammeus
    n. follicularis keratosis
    giant blue n.
    giant pigmented n.
    halo n.
    intradermal n.
    Ito n.
    Jadassohn n.
    Jadassohn-Tièche n.
    junction n.
    junctional n.
    n. lipomatodes, n. lipomatosus
    lymphatic n.
    n. lymphaticus
    melanocytic n.
    nape n.
    nevocytic n.
    nodal n.
    organoid n.
    Ota n.
    pigmented hair epidermal n.
    n. pigmentosus
    n. pilosus
    sebaceous n.
    n. sebaceus
    spider n.
    spindle cell n.
    Spitz n.
    spongy n.
    strawberry n.
    Sutton n.
    n. syringocystadenomatosus
      papilliferus
    systematized n.
    n. unius lateris
    vascular n.

n. venosus
verrucous n.

new

n. fuchsin
n. growth
n. methylene blue
N. World hookworm
N. Zealand mice

newborn

n. crossmatch
hemolytic disease of n. (HDN)
n. hemolytic disease
n. hemorrhagic disease
icterus gravis of n.
n. respiratory syndrome
n. screen

Newcastle

N. disease (ND)
N. disease virus (NDV)
N. virus disease (NVD)

Newcastle-Manchester bacillus
Newcomer fixative
newton (N)

N. law of cooling

Nezelof

N. syndrome
N. type of thymic alymphoplasia

NF

neurofibromatosis

nF

nanofarad

N_5-formyl FH$_4$
N-formyl methionine
NFP

neurofilament triplet polypeptide

ng

nanogram

NGF

nerve growth factor
NGF antiserum

NGU

nongonococcal urethritis

NHA

nonspecific hepatocellular abnormality

NHC

nonhistone chromosomal
NHC protein

NHS

normal horse serum
normal human serum

NIA

nephelometric inhibition assay

niacin test
niche

ecologic n.

Nichols

N. method
N. reagent

nick
nickel

Raney n.

Nickerson-Kveim

N.-K. test
N.-K. test reaction

Nicklès test
Nicolas-Favre disease
Nicolle

N. stain for capsules
N. white mycetoma

Nicol prism
Nicotiana
nicotinamide

n. adenine dinucleotide (NAD)
n. adenine dinucleotide phosphate (NADP)
n. adenine dinucleotide phosphate (reduced form) (NADPH)
n. adenine dinucleotide (reduced form) (NADH)

nidal
NIDDM

noninsulin-dependent diabetes mellitus

Nidoko disease
nidus, pl. nidi
Nieden disease
Niemann disease
Niemann-Pick

N.-P. cell
N.-P. disease (NPD)
N.-P. type of histiocyte

nigra

substantia n.

nigricans

pseudoacanthosis n.

nigrities
nigrosin, nigrosine
Nigrospora
NIH

National Institutes of Health

Nikiforoff method
Nikolsky sign
Nikon microprocessor-controlled camera
nil disease

NOTES

Nile blue
    N. b. A
    N. b. fat stain
nilotica
    Limnatis n.
ninhydrin-Schiff
    n.-S. reaction
    n.-S. stain for proteins
nipple discharge cytology
Nippostrongylus
Nissl
    N. body
    N. stain
    N. substance alteration
nit
nitrate
    n. agar
    n. broth
    lanthanum n.
    peroxyacetal n. (PAN)
    n. reduction test
    silver n.
    n. utilization test
nitrifying bacterium
nitrite
nitritoid reaction
nitrituria
nitroanilene poisoning
Nitrobacter
Nitrobacteraceae
nitroblue
    n. tetrazolium (NBT)
    n. tetrazolium dye
    n. tetrazolium stain
    n. tetrazolium test
Nitrocystis
nitro dye
nitrogen
    alkali-soluble n. (ASN)
    amino acid n. (AAN)
    n. balance
    blood urea n. (BUN)
    n. dilution
    n. distribution
    n. equivalent
    n. lag
    n. narcosis
    nonprotein n.
    n. partition
    serum urea n. (SUN)
    undetermined n.
    urea n. (UN)
    urinary n.
    urine urea n. (UUN)
***p*-nitrophenylic acid**
nitropropiol test

nitroprusside
    sodium n.
    n. test
nitroso dye
nitroso-indole-nitrate test
nitrosourea agent
***p*-nitrosulfathiazole**
nitrous acid
NIXIE tube
njovera
NK
    natural killer
NK cell
NKH
    nonketotic hyperosmotic
NKSF
    natural killer cell-stimulating factor
Nl
    normal
nL, nl
    nanoliter
NLT
    normal lymphocyte transfer test
NM
    not measurable
nm
    nanometer
NMA
    neurogenic muscular atrophy
nmol
    nanomole
NND
    neonatal death
NNN
    Novy, MacNeal, and Nicolle
no
    n. data available (NDA)
    n. demonstrable antibodies (NDA)
    n. evidence of disease (NED)
    n. evidence of distant metastases (MO)
    n. evidence of primary tumor (TO)
    n. reflow phenomenon
    n. serious abnormality (NSA)
    n. significant abnormality (NSA)
    n. significant defect (NSD)
    n. significant deviation (NSD)
    n. significant difference (NSD)
    n. significant disease (NSD)
Noack syndrome
Noble stain
Nocard bacillus
Nocardia
    N. asteroides
    N. brasiliensis
    N. caviae
    N. culture
    N. dacryolith

N. farcinica
N. leishmanii
N. lutea
N. madurae
Nocardiaceae
nocardiasis
nocardiosis
noctalbuminuria
nodal nevus
node
    Babès n.
    Bouchard n.
    delphian n.
    Dürck n.
    Haygarth n.
    Heberden n.
    Hensen n.
    hilar n. (HN)
    lymph n.
    Meynet n.
    milker's n.'s
    Osler n.
    Ranvier n.
    SA n.
    sentinel n.
    signal n.
    singer's n.
    Troisier n.
    Virchow n.
nodosa
    arteritis nodosa
    arthritis nodosa
    periarteritis nodosa (PAN, PN)
    polyarteritis n. (PAN, PN)
    salpingitis isthmica nodosa
    trichorrhexis n.
    vasitis n.
nodose
    n. ganglion
    n. rheumatism
nodositas
nodosity
nodous
nodular
    n. amyloidosis
    n. arteriosclerosis
    n. body
    n. calcific aortic stenosis
    n. colloid goiter
    n. embryo
    n. fasciitis
    n. glomerulosclerosis

    n. hidradenoma
    n. histiocytic lymphoma
    n. hyperplasia of prostate
    n. hyperplastic goiter
    n. leprosy
    n. melanoma
    n. mesoneuritis
    n. mesothelial hyperplasia
    n. nonsuppurative panniculitis
    n. non-X histiocytosis
    n. panencephalitis
    n. paragranuloma (NP)
    n. poorly differentiated lymphocyte (NPDL)
    n. regenerative hyperplasia
    n. sclerosing Hodgkin disease (NSIID)
    n. sclerosis
    n. subepidermal fibrosis
    n. syphilid
    n. transformation of the liver
    n. tuberculid
    n. vasculitis
nodularis
    prurigo n.
nodulate
nodulated
nodulation
nodule
    apple jelly n.
    Aschoff n.
    Caplan n.
    cold n.
    Dalen-Fuchs n.
    fibrocalcific n.
    fibrosiderotic n.
    fibrous n.
    Gamna-Gandy n.
    Hoboken n.
    hot n.
    Jeanselme n.
    juxta-articular n.
    laryngeal n.
    Losch n.
    milker's n.
    Morgagni n.
    parenchymal n.
    rheumatic n.
    rheumatoid n.
    Schmorl n.
    siderotic n.

NOTES

nodule *(continued)*
    Sister Joseph n.
    subcutaneous n.
nodulous
Noguchia
    N. granulosus
Nomarski microscope
nomenclature
    binary n.
    binomial n.
    chromosome n.
nomogram
    acid-base n.
    blood volume n.
    cartesian n.
    Radford n.
    Siggaard-Andersen alignment n.
nomograph
non-A
    non-A hepatitis
    n.-A, non-B hepatitis
    n.-A, non-B hepatitis virus
non-A,
nonagglutinating vibrio
nonbacterial
    n. gastroenteritis virus
    n. thrombotic endocarditis (NBTE)
    n. verrucous endocarditis
non-B hepatitis
nonbirefringent
nonbursate
noncaseating granuloma
noncellular
nonchromaffin paraganglioma
noncommunicating hydrocephalus
nonconjugative plasmid
nonconsanguinous
nondiabetic glycosuric melituria
nondisabling (ND)
    nonsymptomatic, n. (NSND)
nondisease
nondisjunction
nonelectrolyte
nonesterified fatty acid
nonexophytic lesion
**nonfilament polymorphonuclear
    leukocyte**
nongonococcal urethritis (NGU)
nongranular leukocyte
nonhemolytic
    n. jaundice
    n. streptococcus
nonhistone
    n. chromosomal (NHC)
    n. chromosomal protein
non-Hodgkin lymphoma
nonideal solution

nonimmune
    n. agglutination
    n. fetal hydrops
    n. serum
nonimmunity
noninfectious
noninfiltrating lobular carcinoma
noninflammatory edema
noninsulin-dependent
    n.-d. diabetes mellitus (NIDDM)
nonionic detergent
nonisolated proteinuria
nonketotic
    n. hyperglycemia
    n. hyperglycinemia
    n. hyperosmotic (NKH)
nonleukemic myelosis
nonlipid histiocytosis
non-MALT lymphoma
nonmelanosomal
nonmotile
    n. leukocyte
    n. organism (*O*)
**nonmucosa-associated lymphoid tissue
    lymphoma (non-MALT lymphoma)**
non-necrotizing
    n.-n. granuloma
    n.-n. granulomatous inflammation
Nonne-Milroy disease
Nonne-Milroy-Meige syndrome
nonneoplastic
nonobstructive jaundice
nonoccluded virus
nonossifying fibroma
nonparametric
nonpathogenic
nonpermissive culture media
nonphotochromogenic mycobacteria
nonprecipitable antibody
nonprecipitating antibody
nonprotein
    n. nitrogen
    n. nitrogen test
nonradioisotopic immunoassay
nonreactive (NR)
    n. pattern
nonrenal
    n. azotemia
    n. death (NRD)
nonrespiratory alkalosis
nonresponder tolerance
nonrotation
    n. of intestine
    n. of kidney
nonsecretor
nonsecretory myeloma

nonsense
 n. mutation
 n. triplet
nonseptate mycelium
nonsister chromatid
non-small-cell carcinoma (NSCLC)
nonspecific (NS)
 n. anergy
 n. hepatocellular abnormality
 (NHA)
 n. protein
 n. therapy
 n. urethritis (NSU)
nonstructural gene
nonsuppressible
 n. insulin-like activity (NSILA)
nonsymptomatic (NS)
nonsymptomatic, nondisabling (NSND)
nontoxic goiter (NTG)
nontransmural myocardial infarction
nontropical sprue
nontypable (NT)
nonunion
 n. fracture
nonvascular
nonviable
Noonan syndrome
Nordau disease
normal (N, n, Nl, NR)
 n. animal
 n. antibody
 n. antithrombin
 n. antitoxin
 n. blood serum (NBS)
 n. body temperature
 n. cholesteremic xanthomatosis
 diphtheria toxin n. (DTN)
 n. horse serum (NHS)
 n. human plasma
 n. human serum (NHS)
 n. human serum albumin
 n. lymphocyte transfer test (NLT)
 n. opsonin
 n. plasma (NP)
 n. rabbit serum (NRS)
 n. reference serum (NRS)
 n. serum
 n. single dose (NSD)
 n. toxin
 upper limits of n. (ULN)
 n. value

normoblast
 acidophilic n.
 basophilic n.
 intermediate n.
 orthochromatic n.
 orthochromatophilic n.
 polychromatic n.
 polychromatophilic n.
normoblastic
normoblastosis
normocalcemia
normochromia
normochromic
 n. anemia
normocyte
normocytic anemia
normocytosis
normoerythrocyte
normoglycemia
normoglycemic
 n. glycosuria
normokalemia, normokaliemia
normolipemic xanthoma planum
normoplasia
normovolemia
Norris corpuscle
North American blastomycosis
Northern
 N. blot analysis
 N. blot technique
 N. blot test
Norwalk
 N. agent
 N. disease
 N. virus
NOS
 not otherwise specified
nose
 cleft n.
 dog n.
Nosema
Nosematidae
nosocomial
 n. anemia
 n. infection
nosomycosis
nosophyte
Nosopsyllus
 N. fasciatus
nosotoxic
nosotoxin

N

NOTES

not
n. measurable (NM)
n. otherwise specified (NOS)
n. recorded (NR)
n. resolved (NR)
n. significant (NS)
n. statistically significant (NSS)
n. sufficient (NS)
n. sufficient quantity (NSQ)
notanencephalia
notation
scientific n.
notencephalocele
notencephalus
notochord
Notoedres cati
NOVA Celltrak 12 hematology analyzer
Novelli stain
Novy, MacNeal, and Nicolle (NNN)
N. M. a. N. medium
Novy rat disease
NP
neuropathology
nodular paragranuloma
normal plasma
nucleoplasmic index
NPD
Niemann-Pick disease
NPDL
nodular poorly differentiated lymphocyte
NPH
neutral protamine Hagedorn (insulin)
NPR
net protein ratio
NPT
neoprecipitin test
NPU
net protein utilization
NR
nonreactive
normal
not recorded
not resolved
NRBC
nucleated red blood cell
NRCC
National Registry in Clinical Chemistry
NRD
nonrenal death
NREM sleep
NRM
National Registry of Microbiologists
NRS
normal rabbit serum
normal reference serum
NS
nephrotic syndrome
nonspecific

nonsymptomatic
not significant
not sufficient
ns, nsec
nanosecond
NSA
neuron-specific enolase
no serious abnormality
no significant abnormality
NSCLC
non-small-cell carcinoma
NSD
normal single dose
no significant defect
no significant deviation
no significant difference
no significant disease
NSE
neuron-specific enolase
NSE stain
nsec (*var. of* ns)
nanosecond
NSHD
nodular sclerosing Hodgkin disease
NSILA
nonsuppressible insulin-like activity
NSM
neurosecretory material
NSND
nonsymptomatic, nondisabling
NSQ
not sufficient quantity
NSS
not statistically significant
NSU
nonspecific urethritis
NT
neutralization test
neutralizing
nontypable
NTAB
nephrotoxic antibody
Ntaya virus
n-**tetracosanoic acid**
NTG
nontoxic goiter
NTN
nephrotoxic nephritis
nubecula
nuchal
n. fibroma
n. hemangioma
n. rigidity
nuclear
n. aggregate lipid
n. aplasia
n. chain
n. crystalline aggregate

n. dust
n. envelope
n. fast red stain
n. hyperchromasia
n. inclusion body
n. isomerism
n. lipid aggregate
n. magnetic resonance spectroscopy
n. membrane alteration
n. pore alteration
n. pseudoinclusion
n. sap alteration
n. shape alteration
n. size alteration
n. stain
n. vacuolization
nuclear-cytoplasmic
n.-c. ratio
n.-c. ratio alteration
nucleated
n. red blood cell (NRBC)
nucleation
heterogeneous n.
nuclei (*pl. of* nucleus)
nucleic acid
infectious n. a.
nucleic acid probe
nucleocapsid
nucleoid
nucleolar-associated chromatin
nucleolar-nuclear ratio
nucleoli
nucleolonema
nucleolus
Nucleophaga
nucleophagocytosis
nucleophile
nucleoplasmic index (NP)
nucleoprotein
nucleosidase
nucleosome
nucleotidase
5′ nucleotidase
nucleotide
cyclic n.
diphosphopyridine n. (DPN, DPNH)
pyridine n.
nucleotidylexotransferase
DNA n.
nucleotidyltransferase
DNA n.
RNA n.

nucleotoxin
Nuclepore
N. filter
N. method
nucleus, pl. nuclei
dentate n.
droplet nuclei
hyperchromatic nuclei
Klein-Gumprecht shadow nuclei
shadow n.
stripped n.
trophic n.
vesicular n.
wrinkled n.
nude mouse
NUG
necrotizing ulcerative gingivitis
null
n. cell
n. lymphocyte
null-cell adenoma
null-point potentiometer
number
acid n.
atomic n.
Avogadro n.
CI n.
color index n.
complex n.
CT n.
dibucaine n. (DN)
diploid n.
fluoride n.
haploid n.
imaginary n.
iodine n.
line n.
mass n. (A)
modal centromere copy n.
oxidation n.
random n.
real n.
Reynold n.
turnover n.
wave n.
numbering
stereospecific n.
numerical
n. aperture
n. hypertrophy
n. karyotype
n. taxonomy

NOTES

nummiform
nummular
    n. dermatitis
    n. eczema
    n. sputum
nummulation
nutmeg liver
nutrient
    n. agar
    n. broth
    n. medium
    mineral n.'s
nutritional
    n. anemia
    n. cirrhosis

Nuttallia
NV
    negative variation
NVD
    Newcastle virus disease
Nyctotherus
nymph
nymphal
nymphitis
nympholabial
nymphoncus
Nyssorhynchus
nystagmus
    periodic alternating n. (PAN)
    positional alcohol n. (PAN)

O
O agglutination
O agglutinin
O antigen
O colony

O
nonmotile organism

OA
osteoarthritis

OAAD
ovarian ascorbic acid depletion

OAD
obstructive airway disease

OAF
osteoclast activating factor

OAP
osteoarthropathy

oasthouse urine disease
oat
o. cell
o. cell carcinoma

oatmeal-tomato paste agar
OAV
oculoauriculovertebral
OAV dysplasia
OAV syndrome

OB
osteoblastoma

O&B
opium and belladonna

Obermayer test
Obermeier spirillum
Obermüller test
obesity
object
o. code
o. program

objective
achromatic o.
aplanatic o.
apochromatic o.
dry o.
flat-field o.
fluorite o.
immersion o.
semiapochromatic o.
o. synonym

obligate
o. aerobe
o. anaerobe
o. autotroph
o. parasite

oblique fracture
obliterans
thromboangiitis o. (TAO)

obliterating
o. arteritis
o. endarteritis

obliteration
fibrous o.

obliterative
o. arachnoiditis
o. bronchitis
o. inflammation
o. pericarditis
o. pleuritis

obnubilation
OBS
organic brain syndrome

observation
censored o.

Obstetrics
International Federation of
Gynecology and O. (FIGO)

obstipation
obstructed testis
obstruction
ball-valve o.
biliary o.
bladder neck o. (BNO)
chronic airway o. (CAO)
closed-loop o.
complete o.
extrahepatic o. (EHO)
intestinal o. (IO)
mesenteric vascular o.
partial o.
ureteropelvic o.
ureterovesical o.
urethral o.
urinary o.

obstructive
o. airway disease (OAD)
o. appendicitis
o. atelectasis
o. cirrhosis
o. diverticulitis
o. emphysema
o. hyperbilirubinuria
o. jaundice

obstruent
obturating embolism
obturation
occlude
occluded virus
occludens
zonula o.

occlusion
internal carotid artery o. (ICAO)

O

occlusion *(continued)*
    thrombotic o.
    o. time (OT)
occlusive meningitis
occult
    o. bleeding
    o. blood
    o. blood test
    o. carcinoma
occulta
    spina bifida o.
occupational
    o. lung disease
    O. Safety and Health
      Administration (OSHA)
ocellus
OCG
    oral cholecystogram
ochratoxin
ochre mutation
Ochromyia
    O. anthropophaga
ochronosis
ochronotic
    o. arthritis
OCT
    ornithine carbamoyltransferase
    oxytocin challenge test
octal
octane
octanoic acid
Octomitidae
Octomitus hominis
Octomyces
    O. etiennei
octulosonic acid
ocular
    o. cytology
    o. hypertelorism
    o. lymphomatosis
    o. muscle dystrophy (OMD)
ocular-mucous membrane syndrome
oculoauriculovertebral (OAV)
    oculoauriculovertebral dysplasia
oculobuccogenital syndrome
oculocerebrorenal syndrome
oculodentodigital (ODD)
    o. dysplasia
    o. syndrome
oculodermal melanosis
oculoencephalic angiomatosis
oculoglandular tularemia
oculomandibulodyscephaly
oculomycosis
oculovertebral
    o. dysplasia
    o. syndrome

OD
    optical density
    outside diameter
ODD
    oculodentodigital
      ODD dysplasia
      ODD syndrome
odditis
odontoameloblastoma
odontoblast
Odontobutis
odontogenic
    o. cyst
    o. fibroma
    o. fibrosarcoma
    o. myxoma
odontoma
    ameloblastic o.
    complex o.
    compound o.
    fibroameloblastic o.
odoratism
Oe
    oersted
oersted (Oe)
oesophagostomiasis
Oesophagostomum
    O. apiostomum
    O. bifurcum
    O. stephanostomum
Oestridae
oestrids
oestrosis
Oestrus
    O. hominis
    O. ovis
OF
    Ovenstone factor
    oxidation-fermentation
      OF medium
OFD syndrome
off-line
Ogilvie syndrome
O'Grady prognostic indices
OGTT
    oral glucose tolerance test
Oguchi disease
Ohara disease
ohm
Ohm law
ohmmeter
ohne Hauch
Ohngren line
OHP
    oxygen under high pressure
17-OHP
    17-hydroxyprogesterone
***o*-hydroxyphenylacetic acid**

oidia
Oidiomycetes
oidiomycin
oidiomycosis
oidium
OIF
    oil immersion field
oil
    anise o.
    bergamot o.
    cedar o.
    chenopodium o.
    clove o.
    croton o.
    o. cyst
    distilled o.
    o. embolism
    essential o.
    eucalyptus o.
    fatty o.
    fixed o.
    flaxseed o.
    o. immersion
    o. immersion field (OIF)
    o. immersion lens
    origanum o.
    red o.
    o. red O stain
    safflower o.
    sandalwood o.
    santal o.
    sesame o.
    o. tumor
    turpentine o.
    o. vaccine
    volatile o.
    water in o. (W/O)
    o. in water (O/W)
oil-water ratio (O/W)
oily granuloma
Okazaki segment
OKT
    Ortho-Kung T
    OKT cell
olatile alkali
old
    o. infarct
    o. myocardial infarction (OMI)
    o. thrombus
    o. tuberculin (OT)
    O. World hookworm
oleaginous

oleandomycin
oleate
olecranarthropathy
olefin
oleic
    o. acid
    o. acid I 125
    o. acid uptake test
oleogranuloma
oleoma
oleoresin
    aspidium o.
olfactory
    o. cell
    o. esthesioneuroblastoma
    o. neuroblastoma
OLGC
    osteoclast-like giant cell
OLH
    ovine lactogenic hormone
Oligella urethralis
oligemia
oligemic
olighemia
oligoclonal
    o. band
    o. banding
oligocystic
oligocythemia
oligodactyly
oligodendroblastoma
oligodendrocyte
oligodendroglia
    o. stain
    o. staining
oligodendroglioma
    anaplastic o.
    pleomorphic o.
oligodynamic
oligo-1,6-glucosidase
oligohydramnios
oligomeganephronia
oligomenorrhea
oligomer
oligomeric plasmid
oligonucleotide
    allele-specific o. (ASO)
    o. probe
oligopeptide
oligophrenia
oligosaccharide
oligospermatism

O

NOTES

oligospermia
oligotrophic
oligozoospermatism
oligozoospermia
oliguria
olivocerebellar atrophy
olivopontocerebellar atrophy
Ollier disease
Olmer disease
olympian forehead
Olympus BH2 microscope
OM
    otitis media
OMD
    ocular muscle dystrophy
omega
Omenn syndrome
omentitis
omentovolvulus
OMI
    old myocardial infarction
omicron
omitis
OMM
    ophthalmomandibulomelic
        OMM dysplasia
        OMM syndrome
omnibus hypothesis
OMPA
    otitis media, purulent, acute
omphalelcosis
omphalitis
omphalocele
omphalophlebitis
Omsk
    O. hemorrhagic fever
    O. hemorrhagic fever virus
Onchocerca
    O. caecutiens
    O. cervicalis
    O. lienalis
    O. volvulus
onchocerciasis
onchocercid
Onchocercidae
onchocercosis
Oncocerca
oncocyte
oncocytic
    o. adenoma
    o. hepatocellular tumor
    o. papillary cystadenoma
    o. papillary neoplasm
oncocytoma
    renal o.
oncofetal
    o. antigen
    o. marker

oncogene
    bcl-2 o.
    c-fos o.
    cyclin D1 o.
    HER-2/neu o.
    Ki-67 o.
    K-*ras* o.
    retroviral o.
oncogenesis
oncogenic
    o. virus
oncogenous
oncoides
oncologist
oncology
oncolysis
oncolytic
oncoma
Oncomelania
oncoplastic carcinoma
oncoprotein antigen
Oncorhynchus
oncornavirus
oncosis
oncosphere
oncotic
    o. pressure
oncotropic
Oncovirinae
oncovirus
on-demand system
one-side alternative
one-tailed test
onion
    o. body
    o. scale lesion
onionskin changes
o-nitrophenyl-β-galactosidase (ONPG)
onocytoma
ONPG
    o-nitrophenyl-β-galactosidase
    ONPG test
Onthophagus
ontogeny
onychatrophia
onychia
onychitis
onychoheterotopia
onycholysis
onychoma
onychomycosis
onycho-osteodysplasia
onychophosis
onychorrhexis
o'nyong-nyong
    o.-n. fever
    o.-n. fever virus
onyxitis

oocyst
oocyte
oogenesis
oogonium
ookinete
oolemma
oomycosis
oophoritic cyst
oophoritis
oophorocystosis
oophoroma
oophorosalpingitis
oophorous
    cumulus o.
oosome
Oospora
oosporangium
oospore
ootid
ootype
OP
    osmotic pressure
    OP code
O&P, O & P
    ova and parasites
    O&P test
opacification
opacity
    corneal o. (CO)
    lenticular o.
opalescent
opalgia
Opalski cell
opaque
OPD4 antibody
open
    o. angle glaucoma
    o. circuit
    o. tuberculosis
opera-glass hand
operating
    o. cycle
    o. system
    o. time
operation
    o. code
    comparison o.
    parallel o.
    serial o.
    symmetry o.
    unattended laboratory o.

operational amplifier
operative
operator
    o. gene
operculated
operculum
operon
    arabinose o.
    lac o.
    lactose o.
    tra o.
    transfer o.
ophryogenes
    ulerythema o.
Ophryoscolecidae
ophthalmia
    gonococcal o.
    gonorrheal o.
    o. neonatorum
    spring o.
    sympathetic o.
ophthalmitis
    sympathetic o.
ophthalmomandibulomelic (OMM)
    ophthalmomandibulomelic dysplasia
ophthalmomycosis
ophthalmomyiasis
ophthalmopathy
    infiltrative o.
ophthalmoplegia
ophthalmoplegic-type progressive
    muscular dystrophy
ophthalmosteresis
ophthalmovascular choke
opiate assay
opioid
opisthomastigote
opisthorchiasis
opisthorchid
Opisthorchiidae
Opisthorchioidea
Opisthorchis
    O. felineus
    O. noverca
    O. viverrini
opisthorchosis
opisthotonos
Opitz disease
opium
    belladonna and o. (B&O)
    o. and belladonna (O&B)

O

NOTES

Oppenheim
    O. disease
    O. syndrome
Oppenheim-Urbach disease
opportunistic
    o. infection
    o. pathogen
opsin
opsinogen
opsogen
opsonic
    o. action
    o. index
opsonin
    bacterial o.
    common o.
    immune o.
    normal o.
    specific o.
    thermolabile o.
    thermostable o.
opsonization
opsonocytophagic
opsonometry
opsonophilia
opsonophilic
optic
    o. atrophy
    geometric o.'s
    o. nerve glioma
    o. papillitis
    physical o.'s
optical
    o. activity
    o. density (OD)
    o. glass
    o. isomer
    o. isomerism
    o. path
    o. purity
    o. rotary dispersion (ORD)
    o. rotation
optimal growth temperature
OptiMax immunostaining system
optimizing compiler
optimum temperature
Optochin susceptibility test
OPV
    oral poliovirus vaccine
OR
    OR circuit
    OR gate
oral
    o. antibiotic
    o. cavity cytology
    o. cholecystogram (OCG)
    o. flora
    o. glucose tolerance test (OGTT)
    o. lactose tolerance test
    o. pathology
    o. poliovirus vaccine (OPV)
    o. smear
oral-facial-digital
orange
    acridine o. (AO)
    ethyl o.
    methyl o.
    orange G
    victoria o.
OraSure HIV-1 Oral Specimen Collection Device
orbital
    o. abscess
    hybrid o.
Orbivirus
orcein
    acetic o.
    acid o.
    o. stain
orchella
orchiatrophy
orchidic hormone
orchiditis
orchidoblastoma
orchidoptosis
orchiepididymitis
orchil
orchioblastoma
orchiocele
orchioncus
orchitic
orchitis
    autoimmune o.
    granulomatous o.
orcin
orcinol
    o. test
ORD
    optical rotary dispersion
order
    low o.
ordinal variable
ordinate
orf
    o. virus
organ
    accessory o.
    o. culture
    floating o.
    o. perfusion
    ptotic o.
    supernumerary o.
    target o.
    o. tolerance dose (OTD)
    wandering o.
organelle

organic
    o. acid
    o. brain syndrome (OBS)
    o. chemistry
    o. contracture
    o. disease
    o. lesion
    o. phosphate
    o. radical (R)
organification defect
organism
    Arizona o.
    calculated mean o. (CMO)
    hypothetical mean o. (HMO)
    indicator o.
    nonmotile o. (*O*)
    photosynthetic o.
    pleuropneumonia-like o. (PPLO)
    Rickett o.
    Vincent o.
organization
organized
    o. hematoma
    o. pneumonia
    o. thrombus
organizer
    procentriole o.
organizing inflammation
organochlorine insecticides
organo-chloro pesticide
organogenesis
organoid
    o. nevus
    o. tumor
organoma
organometallic compound
organophosphate
    o. compound
    o. insecticides
organotaxis
organothiophosphate compound assay
organotroph
organotropic
    o. bacterium
organotropism
organotropy
organ-specific
    o.-s. antigen
Oriboca virus
oriental
    O. blood fluke
    o. hemoptysis
    O. lung fluke
    O. lung fluke disease
    O. ringworm
    o. sore
orifice
    golf-hole ureteral o.
origanum oil
origin
    amyloid of immunoglobulin o. (AIO)
    amyloid of unknown o. (AUO)
    anomalous o.
    fever of undetermined o. (FUO)
    fever of unknown o. (FUO)
    myocardial disease of unknown o. (MDUO)
    pyrexia of unknown o. (PUO)
original tuberculin (TO)
oris
    pachyderma o.
Ormond disease
ornate
ornithine
    o. aminotransferase
    o. carbamoyltransferase (OCT)
    o. carbamoyl transferase assay
    o. carbamoyltransferase deficiency
    o. decarboxylase
    o. transcarbamoylase
    o. transcarbamylase deficiency
ornithinemia
ornithine-oxo-acid aminotransferase
ornithinuria
Ornithobilharzia
Ornithodoros
    O. coriaceus
Ornithonyssus
ornithosis
    o. virus
orodigitofacial dysostosis
orofaciodigital syndrome (OFD syndrome)
Oropouche virus
orosomucoid
orotate phosphoribosyltransferase
orotic
    o. acid
    o. aciduria
orotidine-5′-phosphate decarboxylase
orotidylate decarboxylase
Oroya fever

O

NOTES

orphan
    enterocytopathogenic dog o.
    respiratory enteric o. (REO)
    o. virus
orseillin BB
Ortalidae
Orth
    O. fixative
    O. fluid
    O. solution
    O. stain
orthochromatic
    o. normoblast
orthochromatophilic normoblast
orthochromophil, orthochromophile
orthocytosis
orthoiodohippurate
orthokeratosis
Ortho-Kung T (OKT)
Orthomyxoviridae
orthomyxovirus
orthophosphoric
    o. acid
    o. ester monohydrolase
Orthopodomyia
Orthopoxvirus
orthopoxvirus
Orthoptera
orthoptic transplantation
Orthorrhapha
orthostatic
    o. albuminuria
    o. hypertension
    o. hypotension
    o. proteinuria
orthotolidine
osazone test
OSBT
    ovarian serous borderline tumor
oscheitis
oschelephantiasis
oscheohydrocele
oscillation
oscillator
oscilloscope
    storage o.
Osgood-Schlatter disease
OSHA
    Occupational Safety and Health
    Administration
Osler
    O. disease
    O. erythema
    O. node
Osler-Vaquez disease
Osler-Weber-Rendu disease
OSM
    oxygen saturation meter

Osm
    osmole
osmic
    o. acid
    o. acid fixative
osmic acid
osmicate
osmication
osmification
osmiophilic
osmiophobic
osmium
    o. tetroxide
    o. tetroxide stain
osmolal clearance
osmolality
    calculated serum o.
osmolar
    o. gap
osmolarity
osmole (Osm)
osmolute
osmometer
    freezing point depression o.
    vapor pressure depression o.
osmometry
osmophil
osmosis
osmotic
    o. coefficient
    o. diuretic
    o. fragility
    o. fragility test
    o. hemolysis
    o. nephrosis
    o. pressure (OP)
    o. shock
osseous
    o. ankylosis
    o. hydatid
    o. hydatid cyst
    o. metaplasia
    o. polyp
ossificans
    pelvospondylitis o.
ossification
    abnormal endochondral o.
    metaplastic o.
ossifying
    o. fibroma
    o. inflammation
    o. interstitial myositis
ostealgia
osteitic
osteitis
    caseous o.
    central o.
    o. condensans

condensing o.
cortical o.
o. deformans
o. fibrosa circumscripta
o. fibrosa cystica
o. fibrosa disseminata
hematogenous o.
localized o. fibrosa
multifocal o. fibrosa
sclerosing o.
o. tuberculosa multiplex cystica

ostemia
ostempycsis
osteoarthritis (OA)
hyperplastic o.
osteoarthropathy (OAP)
hypertrophic pulmonary o.
idiopathic hypertrophic o. (IHO)
pneumogenic o.
pulmonary o.
secondary hypertrophic o. (SHO)
osteoblast
osteoblastoma (OB)
osteocalcin
osteocarcinoma
osteocartilaginous exostosis
osteochondral
osteochondritis
o. deformans juvenilis
o. deformans juvenilis dorsi
o. dissecans
syphilitic o.
osteochondrodystrophia deformans
osteochondrodystrophy
osteochondroma
multiple o.'s
osteochondromatosis
synovial o.
osteochondrosarcoma
osteochondrosis
osteoclasia
osteoclasis
osteoclast activating factor (OAF)
osteoclastic resorption
osteoclast-like giant cell (OLGC)
osteoclastoma
osteocystoma
osteocyte
osteodermatopoikilosis
osteodermatous
osteodermia
osteodiastasis

osteodysplasty
osteodystrophia
osteodystrophy
Albright hereditary o.
renal o.
osteoectasia
osteofibroma
osteofibrosis
osteofibrous dysplasia of Campanacci
osteogenesis
o. imperfecta
o. imperfecta congenita
o. imperfecta tarda
osteogenic sarcoma
osteohalisteresis
osteohypertrophy
osteoid osteoma
osteolathyrism
osteolipochondroma
osteolysis
osteolytic
osteoma
o. cutis
fibrous o.
giant osteoid o.
o. medullare
osteoid o.
parosteal o.
o. spongiosum
osteomalacia
senile o.
osteomalacic
o. pelvis
osteomatoid
osteomyelitis
Garré sclerosing o.
pyogenic o.
tuberculous o.
osteomyelodysplasia
osteomyelofibrotic syndrome
osteomyelosclerosis
osteon
osteoncus
osteonecrosis
osteo-onychodysplasia
hereditary o. (HOOD)
osteopathia
o. condensans
o. striata
osteopathy
alimentary o.

O

NOTES

osteopathy *(continued)*
    disseminated condensing o.
    myelogenic o.
osteopenia
osteoperiostitis
osteopetrosis
    o. acro-osteolytica
    o. gallinarum
osteopetrotic
osteophlebitis
osteophyma
osteophyte
osteopoikilosis
osteoporosis
    o. circumscripta
    o. circumscripta cranii
    juvenile o.
    posttraumatic o.
osteoporotic
osteopulmonary arthropathy
osteoradionecrosis
osteosarcoma
    parosteal o.
    periosteal o.
osteosclerosis
    o. congenita
osteosclerotic
    o. anemia
osteosis
    o. cutis
    o. eburnisans monomelica
    parathyroid o.
osteospongioma
osteosteatoma
osteothrombosis
Ostertag
    streptococcus of O.
Ostertagia
ostitic
ostitis
ostosis
ostraceous
Ostrum-Furst syndrome
Ostwald viscosimeter
OT
    occlusion time
    old tuberculin
Ota nevus
Ot antigen
OTD
    organ tolerance dose
otic abscess
otitic
    o. meningitis
otitis
    o. desquamativa
    o. diphtheritica
    o. externa

    o. labyrinthica
    o. mastoidea
    o. media (OM)
    o. media, purulent, acute (OMPA)
    o. mycotica
    o. sclerotica
otoacariasis
otobiosis
Otobius
otocerebritis
otocyst
Otodectes
otodectic
otoencephalitis
otolith
otomandibular
    o. dysostosis
    o. syndrome
Otomyces
    O. hageni
    O. purpureus
otomycosis
    o. aspergillina
otorrhagia
otorrhea
otosclerosis
ototoxic drug
OTR
    Ovarian Tumor Registry
Otto
    O. disease
    O. pelvis
Ouchterlony
    O. immunodiffusion
    O. method
    O. technique
    O. test
Oudin immunodiffusion
ounce (oz)
outer dense fibers of spermatozoon
outlier
output
    basal acid o. (BAO)
    o. capacitor
    carbon dioxide o. ($\overset{\circ}{V}_{CO_2}$)
    CO_2 o.
    o. impedance
    maximal acid o.
    peak acid o. (PAO)
outside diameter (OD)
ova (*pl. of* ovum)
ovalbumin
ovale
    anatomically patent foramen o.
    o. malaria
    prematurely closed foramen o.
ovalocyte
ovalocytic anemia

ovalocytosis
ovarian
>   o. ascorbic acid depletion (OAAD)
>   o. ascorbic acid depletion test
>   o. cyst
>   o. granulosa cell tumor
>   o. hormone
>   o. masculinization
>   o. pregnancy
>   o. serous borderline tumor (OSBT)
>   o. tubular adenoma
>   O. Tumor Registry (OTR)
>   o. varicocele

ovarii
>   *Pseudomyxoma o.*

ovarioncus
ovariosalpingitis
ovaritis
ovary
>   polycystic o.

ovatum
>   *Loxotrema o.*

oven
Ovenstone factor (OF)
overdominance
overflow
overlap
>   spectral o.

overlapping inversion
overload
>   circulatory o.

overwintering
ovine
>   o. lactogenic hormone (OLH)
>   o. progressive pneumonia

ovinia
oviposit
oviposition
ovipositor
ovogonium
ovolarviparous
ovotestis
OvuKIT
ovulational sclerosis
ovum, pl. **ova**
>   blighted o.
>   ova and parasites (O&P, O & P)

OvuQUICK
O/W
>   oil in water
>   oil-water ratio

Owren disease

oxacillin sodium
oxalate
>   ammonium o.
>   calcium o.
>   o. calculus
>   double o.

oxalemia
oxalic
>   o. acid
>   o. acid assay
>   o. acid stain

oxalism
oxaloacetate decarboxylase
oxaloacetic acid
oxalosis
oxaluria
oxazin
>   o. dye

oxazine dye
Oxford unit
oxidant
>   total o.

oxidase
>   aldehyde o.
>   D-amino acid o.
>   L-amino acid o.
>   coproporphyrinogen o.
>   glucose o.
>   homogentisate o.
>   p-hydroxyphenylpyruvate o.
>   hydroxyproline o.
>   monoamine o.
>   proline o.
>   protoporphyrinogen o.
>   o. reaction
>   sulfite o.
>   o. test

oxidation
>   fatty acid o.
>   o. number
>   o. state

oxidation-fermentation (OF)
>   o.-f. medium
>   o.-f. test

oxidation-reducing potential
oxidation-reduction
>   o.-r. indicator
>   o.-r. reaction

oxidative
>   o. phosphorylation
>   o. phosphorylation inhibitor
>   o. phosphorylation uncouplers

NOTES

oxide
    aluminum o.
    ethylene o.
    vitamin K_1 o.
oxidize
oxidizer
oxidizing
    o. agent
    o. gas
oxidoreductase
    L-lysine:NAD^+ o.
oximeter
    cuvet o.
oximetry
oxo acid
3-oxobutyric acid
oxoglutarate dehydrogenase
2-oxoglutaric acid
2-oxoisovalerate dehydrogenase
oxolinic acid
oxonium ion
5-oxoproline
4-oxoproline reductase
oxoprolinuria
5-oxoprolinuria
oxyacoia
oxyaphia
oxybiotin
oxycephalia
oxycephalic
oxycephaly
oxychromatic
oxychromatin
oxygen
    o. acceptor
    o. affinity anoxia
    o. affinity hypoxia
    o. analyzer
    o. capacity of blood
    cerebral metabolic rate of o.
      (CMRO)
    o. consumption
    o. content of blood
    o. effect
    forced inspiratory o. (FI_{O2}, FIO_2)
    fraction of inspired o. (FI_{O2}, FIO_2)
    o. half-saturation pressure of
      hemoglobin
    o. poisoning
    o. quotient (QO_2, qO_2)

    o. saturation
    o. saturation measurement
    o. saturation meter (OSM)
    o. tension
    o. under high pressure (OHP)
    o. uptake
    o. utilization coefficient
oxygenase
oxygenated hemoglobin
oxygenation
oxygenator
oxygen-hemoglobin dissociation curve
oxyhemoglobin (HbO_2)
oxyhemogram
oxyhemograph
oxyntic cell
oxyphil, oxyphile
    o. adenoma
    o. cell
    o. chromatin
    o. granule
    o. inclusion body
oxyphilic
    o. endometrioid adenocarcinoma
    o. leukocyte
    o. papillary carcinoma
oxypolygelatin
oxypurinol
Oxyspirura mansoni
oxytalan
    o. fiber
    o. fiber stain
oxytetracycline
oxytocin challenge test (OCT)
Oxytrema
Oxyurata
oxyuriasis
oxyuricide
oxyurid
Oxyuridae
Oxyuris
    O. incognita
    O. vermicularis
Oxyuroidea
oz
    ounce
ozone
ozonization
ozonolysis
Ozzards filaria

Ψ (*var. of* upsilon)
P

  plasma
  pressure
  probability
    P antigen
    P blood group
    P and P test
    P value
P₁
  parental generation
p24 antigen
p53 gene
P$_{CO_2}$ electrode
P$_{Na}$
  plasma sodium
PA

  pathology
  pernicious anemia
  phakic-aphakic
  pregnancy-associated
  primary anemia
Pa
  pascal
Paas disease
PAB, PABA
  p-aminobenzoic acid
pacchionian granulation
pacemaker
  wandering p.
Pacheco parrot disease virus
pachyacria
pachycephalia
pachycephalic
pachycephalous
pachycephaly
pachychromatic
pachydactylia
pachydactylous
pachydactyly
pachyderma
  p. laryngis
  p. lymphangiectatica
  p. oris
  p. verrucosa
  p. vesicae
pachydermatocele
pachydermatosis
pachydermatous
pachydermia
pachydermic
pachydermoperiostosis
pachygyria
pachyhymenia
pachyhymenic

pachyleptomeningitis
pachylosis
pachymenia
pachymenic
pachymeningitis
  adhesive chronic p.
  chronic adhesive p.
  p. externa
  fibrous hypertrophic p.
  hemorrhagic p.
  hypertrophic cervical p.
  p. interna
  pyogenic p.
pachymeningopathy
pachynema
pachynsis
pachyntic
pachyonychia
  p. congenita
pachyperiostitis
pachyperitonitis
pachypleuritis
pachysalpingitis
pachysalpingo-ovaritis
pachysomia
pachytene
pachyvaginalitis
pachyvaginitis
  p. cystica
pacinitis
pack
package
  dual-in-line p.
packed
  p. cell volume (PCV)
  p. human blood cells
  p. red blood cells
  p. red cells (PRC)
packet
packing ratio
paclitaxel
PACONA
  periodic acid-concanavalin A
  PACONA technique
Padykula-Herman
  P.-H. stain for myosin ATPase
Paecilomyces
paecilomycosis
Paederus
PAF
  platelet-activating factor
  platelet-aggregating factor
  pulmonary arteriovenous fistula
PAGE
  polyacrylamide gel electrophoresis

P

Paget
    P. cell
    P. disease
    P. disease of bone
    P. disease of breast
    P. test
Paget-Eccleston stain
pagetic
pagetoid
    p. melanocytosis (PM)
    p. reticulosis
PAGMK
    primary African green monkey kidney
PAH
    p-aminohippuric acid
PAH
    postatrophic hyperplasia
    pulmonary artery hypertension
PAHA
    p-aminohippuric acid
painful-bruising syndrome
painless jaundice
pair
    base p. (bp)
    conjugate redox p.
    electron p.
    ion p.
    kilobase p. (kbp)
    p. production
pairing
    base p.
    exchange p.
    p. segment
    somatic p.
pajaroello
Palaemonetes
palate
    cleft p.
palatitis
pale
    p. infarct
    p. thrombus
paleopathology
palindrome
palindromia
palindromic encephalopathy
palisade
palisading granuloma
palladium (Pd)
    p. chloride
palm
    liver p.
palmar
    p. crease
    p. erythema
    p. fibromatosis
palmellin
Palmgren silver impregnation stain

palmitate
palmitic acid
palmitoleate
palmitoleic acid
palmoplantar keratoderma
palsy
    cerebral p. (CP)
    progressive bulbar p.
    progressive supranuclear p. (PSP)
    pseudobulbar p.
paludal
    p. fever
Paludina
paludism
PAM
    pulmonary alveolar macrophage
    pulmonary alveolar microlithiasis
***p*-aminobenzoic acid (PAB, PABA)**
***p*-aminohippuric acid (PAH, PAHA)**
pampinocele
PAN
    periarteritis nodosa
    periodic alternating nystagmus
    peroxyacetal nitrate
    polyarteritis nodosa
    positional alcohol nystagmus
panacinar emphysema
panagglutinable
panagglutination
panagglutinins
panangiitis
panarteritis
panarthritis
panatrophy
panbronchiolitis
    diffuse p. (DFB)
pancake kidney
pancarditis
pancervical smear
pancinian neuroma
Pancoast
    P. syndrome
    P. tumor
pancreas, pl. pancreata
    aberrant p.
    accessory p.
    amount of insulin extractable
      from p. (AIEP)
    annular p.
    p. antigen retrieval
    Baggenstoss change in p.
    cystic fibrosis of p. (CFP)
    fibrocystic disease of the p.
pancreatemphraxis
pancreatic
    p. amylase
    p. calculus
    p. cholera

p. colic
p. colipase
p. encephalopathy
p. endocrine neoplasm (PEN)
p. islet cell antibody test
p. islet stain
p. juice
p. lipase
p. lithiasis
p. polypeptide
ribonuclease (p.)
p. RNase
p. tumor
pancreatitis
acute hemorrhagic p.
calcifying p.
chronic p.
chronic fibrosing p.
hemorrhagic p.
necrotizing p.
relapsing p.
pancreatoblastoma
pancreatolith
pancreatolithiasis
pancreatomegaly
pancreolith
pancreoprivic
pancreozymin (PZ)
pancreozymin-cholecystokinin (PZ-CCK)
pancreozymin-secretin test
pancytopenia
autoimmune p.
congenital p.
Fanconi p.
pandemic
pandemicity
Pandy
P. reaction
P. test
panel
panencephalitis
nodular p.
subacute sclerosing p. (SSPE)
Paneth
P. cell
P. cell-like change (PCLC)
Pangonia
panhyperemia
panhypopituitarism
postpuberal p.
postpubertal p.
prepubertal p.

panimmunity
pankeratin
panleukopenia
p. virus (PLV)
p. virus of cats
panlobular emphysema
panmixis
panmyelophthisis
panmyelosis
Panner disease
panniculitis
cytophagic histiocytic p.
mesenteric p.
metastatic p.
nodular nonsuppurative p.
relapsing febrile nodular p.
panophthalmitis
panoptic
p. stain
pansclerosis
panspermia
pansporoblast
pansporoblastic
Panstrongylus
PANTA antimicrobial agent
pantachromatic
pantaloon embolism
pantanencephaly
pantatrophia
pantatrophy
pantetheine
pantomorphia
pantomorphic
pantothenic
p. acid
p. acid assay
p. acid unit
pantoyl-β-alanine
pantoyl beta alanine
pantropic virus
panzerherz
panzootic
PAO
peak acid output
PAOD
peripheral arterial occlusive disease
peripheral arteriosclerotic occlusive
disease
PAP
peroxidase-antiperoxidase
primary atypical pneumonia
pulmonary alveolar proteinosis

NOTES

P

PAP *(continued)*
    PAP complex
    PAP immunoperoxidase stain
    PAP technique
Pap
   Papanicolaou
    P. smear
    P. stain
    P. test
papain
Papanicolaou (Pap)
    P. examination
    P. method
    P. smear
    P. smear test
    P. stain
Papaver
paper
    alkannin p.
    azolitmin p.
    p. capacitor
    p. chromatography
    Congo red p.
    p. mill worker's disease
    probability p.
    p. radioimmunosorbent test
papilla
    exophytic p.
papillar villous hyperplasia
papillary
    p. adenocarcinoma
    p. adenoma of large intestine
    p. adenomatous polyp
    p. cystadenoma
    p. cystadenoma lymphomatosum
    p. cystic adenoma
    p. ectasia
    p. ependymoma
    p. hidradenoma
    p. hyperplasia
    p. infolding
    p. muscle dysfunction
    p. muscle syndrome
    p. necrosis
    p. serous cystadenocarcinoma
    p. syringadenoma
    p. transitional cell carcinoma
    p. tumor
papillary, marginal, attached (gingivitis) (PMA)
papillary/verrucous architecture
papilledema
papillitis
    anal p.
    chronic lingual p.
    necrotizing p.
    optic p.
papilloadenocystoma

papillocarcinoma
papilloma
    p. acuminatum
    basal cell p.
    p. canaliculum
    canine oral p.
    choroid plexus p.
    p. diffusum
    duct p.
    p. durum
    fibroepithelial p.
    hard p.
    hyperkeratotic p.
    infectious p. of cattle
    p. inguinale tropicum
    intracystic p.
    intraductal p.
    inverted p.
    keratotic p.
    p. molle
    rabbit p.
    Shope p.
    soft p.
    squamous cell p.
    transitional cell p.
    p. venereum
    verrucous p.
    villous p.
    p. virus
papillomatosis
    p. of breast
    confluent and reticulate p.
    florid oral p.
    intraductal p.
    juvenile p.
    laryngeal p.
    subareolar duct p.
papillomatous
Papillomavirus
papillomavirus
Papillon-Léage and Psaume syndrome
Papillon-Lefèvre syndrome
PAPI stain
Papovaviridae
papovavirus
pappataci
    p. fever
    p. fever virus
Pappenheimer
    P. body
Pappenheim stain
papula, pl. papulae
papular
    p. mucinosis
    p. scrofuloderma
    p. stomatitis virus of cattle
    p. tuberculid

papule
    moist p.
    mucous p.
    prurigo p.
papuliferous
papuloerythematous
papulonecrotic tuberculid
papulonodular lesion
papulonodule
papulosis
    bowenoid p.
    lymphomatoid p.
    malignant atrophic p.
papulosquamous
papulovesicular
PAPVC
    partial anomalous pulmonary venous
      connection
papyraceous scar
para-aminobenzoic acid
para-aminodimethylaniline
para-aminohippurate
    p.-a. clearance
para-aminohippuric acid
para-appendicitis
parabiosis
parabiotic
parabola
Parabuthus
paracanthoma
paracanthosis
paracarcinomatous
    p. encephalomyelopathy
    p. myelopathy
paracarmine
    p. stain
paracasein
paracentesis
paracholera vibrio
Parachordodes
parachromatopsia
parachute reflex
paracoagulants
paracoagulation test
paracoccidioidal granuloma
Paracoccidioides brasiliensis
paracoccidioidin
paracoccidioidomycosis
paracolitis
Paracolobactrum
    P. aerogenoides
    P. arizonae

    P. coliforme
    P. intermedium
paracolon bacillus
paracolpitis
paracrine
    p. stimulation
paracystitis
paracytic
paradenitis
paradidymis
paradoxical
    p. embolism
    p. embolus
Par. aff.
   part affected
paraffin
    bismuth iodoform p. (BIP)
    p. block
    p. cancer
    p. immunoperoxidase (PIP)
    p. tumor
paraffin-embedded
    p.-e. tissue (PET)
    p.-e. tissue section
paraffinoma
Parafilaria multipapillosa
paraflagella
paraflagellate
paraflagellum
parafollicular
    p. B-cell lymphoma (PBCL)
    p. cell
paraformaldehyde
Parafossarulus
parafrenal abscess
parafuchsin
paraganglioma
    chromaffin p.
    nonchromaffin p.
Paragon blue stain
paragonimiasis
Paragonimus
    P. africanus
    P. caliensis
    P. heterotremus
    P. kellicotti
    P. mexicanus
    P. westermani
Paragordius
    P. cintus
    P. tricuspidatus
    P. varius

NOTES

P

paragranuloma
    nodular p. (NP)
parahemophilia
parahormone
parahypophysis
paraimmunoblast cell
paraimmunoblastic lymphoma
parainfluenza
    p. antibody test
    p. viral serology
    p. virus
    p. virus antigen
    p. virus culture
    p. virus, types 1, 2, 3, 4
parakeratosis
    p. pustulosa
    p. scutularis
    p. variegata
parakeratotic tiering
paralbuminemia
paraldehyde
    p. assay
    p. poisoning
paraleprosis
parallel
    p. circuit
    p. grid
    p. operation
parallergic
paralysis, pl. paralyses
    acute atrophic p.
    fowl p.
    immune p.
    immunological p.
    infectious bulbar p.
    myogenic p.
    tick p.
    vasomotor p.
paralyssa
paralytic
    p. brachial neuritis (PBN)
    p. ileus
paralyzable detector
paramagnetic resonance of electrons
paramastigote
Paramax reagent
Paramecium
    P. coli
paramecium, pl. paramecia
paramesonephric rest
parameter
paramethasone
parametric abscess
parametritic
    p. abscess
parametritis
parametrium
Paramoeba

paramorphia
paramorphic
Paramphistomatidae
paramphistomiasis
Paramphistomum
paramyloid
paramyloidosis
paramyotonia
    p. congenita
Paramyxoviridae
Paramyxovirus
paramyxovirus
paraneoplasia
paraneoplastic
    p. acrokeratosis
    p. encephalomyelopathy
    p. pemphigus
    p. syndrome
paranephric abscess
paraneuron
parapedesis
paraphimosis
paraphysial, paraphyseal
    p. cyst
paraplast
Paraponera
Parapoxvirus
parapox virus
paraproctitis
paraprostatitis
paraprotein
paraproteinemia
parapsoriasis
    p. en plaque
    p. guttata
    p. lichenoides
    p. lichenoides et varioliformis acuta
    p. varioliformis
paraquat assay
pararama
pararosanilin
pararosaniline
Parasa
Parasaccharomyces
    P. ashfordi
parasalpingitis
Parascaris equorum
parascarlatina
parasite
    accidental p.
    extracellular p.
    facultative p.
    intermittent p.
    intracellular p.
    malarial p.
    metazoan p.
    obligate p.
    ova and p.'s (O&P, O & P)

periodic p.
permanent p.
protozoan p.
spurious p.
temporary p.
parasitemia
parasite screen
parasitic
p. castration
p. chylocele
p. cyst
p. ectopic pregnancy
p. embolus
p. fetus
p. granuloma
p. hemoptysis
p. leiomyoma
p. thyroiditis
p. twin
parasiticidal
parasiticide
parasitism
parasitize
parasitocenose
parasitogenesis
parasitogenic
parasitoid
p. mite
Parasitoidea
parasitologist
parasitology
parasitome
parasitosis
parasitotropic
parasitotropism
parasitotropy
paraspadias
Parastrongylus
parastruma
parasympathomimetic
parasynovitis
parasyphilis
paratcnesis
paratenic host
parathion
methyl p.
parathormone (PTH)
parathyrin
parathyroid
p. chief cell
p. cyst
p. extract (PTE)

p. hormone (PTH)
p. hormone secretion (rate) (PTHS)
p. osteosis
p. oxyphil cell
p. transitional cell
p. tumor
p. wasserhelle cell
parathyroidin
paratope
paratrophic
paratuberculous
p. lymphadenitis
p. pneumonia
paratyphlitis
paratyphoid
p. fever (types A, B, and C)
p. immunization
paravaccinia
p. virus
paravaginitis
paravirus
Parazoa
parazoon
parchment
p. heart
p. skin
parectasia
parectasis
parencephalia
parencephalocele
parencephalous
parenchyma
parenchymal nodule
parenchymatitis
parenchymatous
p. degeneration
p. goiter
p. keratitis
p. mastitis
parent
p. cyst
parentage
parental generation (P_1)
parenteral
paresis
general p. (GP)
parietal
p. cell
p. cell antibody
p. fistula
p. thrombus
Parietti broth

NOTES

P

463

Parinaud oculoglandular syndrome
Paris
    P. classification
    P. green
    P. yellow
parity
    p. bit
    p. check
Park aneurysm
Parkinson
    P. disease (PD)
    P. facies
parkinsonian syndrome
parkinsonism
Park-Williams
    P.-W. bacillus
    P.-W. fixative
paromomycin
paromphalocele
paronychia
    herpetic p.
paroophoritic cyst
paroophoritis
parorchidium
parosteal
    p. fasciitis
    p. osteoma
    p. osteosarcoma
parosteitis
parosteosis, parostosis
parostitis
parotid abscess
parotiditis
    epidemic p.
    postoperative p.
    punctate p.
parotitis
    p. syndrome
    p. virus epidemic
parovaritis
paroxysm
paroxysmal
    p. aciduria
    p. cold hemoglobinuria (PCH)
    p. hypertension
    p. nocturnal hemoglobinuria (PNH)
parrot
    P. disease
    p. fever
    p. virus
Parry disease
Parry-Romberg syndrome
pars compacta
Parson disease
part affected (Par. aff.)
parthenogenesis
parthenogenetic merogony

partial
    p. agglutinin
    p. anomalous pulmonary venous connection (PAPVC)
    p. antigen
    p. identity pattern
    p. lipoatrophy
    p. obstruction
    p. reaction of degeneration (PRD)
    p. remission (PR)
    p. thromboplastin time (PTT)
    p. thromboplastin time test
    p. trisomy
partially miscible
partial pressure
    p. p. of carbon dioxide
    p. p. of nitrogen
    p. p. of oxygen
    p. p. of water vapor
partial-thickness burn
particle
    α-p.
    alpha p.
    β-p.
    beta p.
    charged p.
    chromatin p.
    Dane p.
    defective interfering p.
    DI p.
    elementary p.
    p. transport time (PTT)
    Zimmermann elementary p.
α-particle detector
particulate
    p. crystalline material
    p. crystalline material deposition
    settled p.
    suspended p.
partition
    p. coefficient
    nitrogen p.
parvilocular cyst
Parvobacteriaceae
Parvoviridae
Parvovirus
    P. B 19
parvovirus
parvum
    Chrysosporium p.
Paryphostomum
    P. sufrartyfex
PAS
    periodic acid-Schiff
    pulmonary artery stenosis
    PAS reaction

PAS stain
PAS test
pascal (Pa)
PASCC
    pseudovascular adenoid squamous cell
      carcinoma
Paschen body
PASH
    pseudoangiomatous stromal hyperplasia
PASM
    periodic acid-silver methenamine
passage
    blind p.
    serial p.
Passalurus ambiguus
PASSCL
    pseudovascular adenoid squamous cell
      carcinoma of the lung
passé
    coma dé p.
passive
    p. agglutination
    p. Arthus reaction
    p. congestion
    p. cutaneous anaphylactic reaction
    p. cutaneous anaphylaxis (PCA)
    p. cutaneous anaphylaxis test
    p. hemagglutination (PHA)
    p. hemagglutination test
    p. hemolysis
    p. immunity
    p. immunization
    p. medium
    p. prophylaxis
    p. sensitization
    p. transfer
    p. transference
    p. transport
Passovoy factor
Pasteur
    P. effect
    P. pipette
    P. vaccine
Pasteurella
    P. enterocolitica
    P. haemolytica
    P. multocida
    P. pestis
    P. pneumotropica
    P. pseudotuberculosis
    P. septica

    P. tularensis
    P. ureae
pasteurellosis
pasteurization
Patau syndrome
patch
    gray p.
    herald p.
    moth p.
    mucous p.
    Peyer p.
    salmon p.
    shagreen p.
    soldier's p.
    p. test
    white p.
Patein albumin
Patella disease
patent
    p. blue V dye
    p. foramen ovale
paternity testing
Paterson-Brown-Kelly syndrome
Paterson-Kelly syndrome
Paterson syndrome
path
    pathology
      optical path
pathergy
pathoanatomic background
pathobiology
pathoclisis
pathogen
    mycelial p.
    opportunistic p.
pathogenesis
pathogen-free
    specific p.-f. (SPF)
pathogenic
pathogenicity
    bacterial p.
pathognomonic
pathography
pathologic
    p. anatomy
    p. calcification
    p. cell
    p. diagnosis
    p. dislocation
    p. fracture
    p. glycosuria
    p. histology

NOTES

P

pathologist
pathology (PA, path)
 anatomic p.
 anatomical p.
 cellular p.
 clinical p.
 comparative p.
 dental p.
 experimental p.
 functional p.
 general p.
 geographic p.
 humoral p.
 internal p.
 medical p.
 molecular p.
 oral p.
 solidistic p.
 special p.
 surgical p.
pathometric
pathometry
pathomorphism
pathonomia
pathonomy
pathophysiologic
pathophysiology
pathotype
pathovar
pathway
 alternative complement p.
 amphibolic p.
 biosynthetic p.
 classical complement p.
 coagulation p.
 Embden-Meyerhof p.
 Entner-Doudoroff p.
 extrinsic p.
 hexose monophosphate p. (HMP)
 intrinsic p.
 metabolic p.
 pentose phosphate p. (PPP)
 phosphogluconate oxidative p.
 reentrant p.
Patois virus
pattern
 angiocentric p.
 angiodestructive p.
 arborizing p.
 gel electrophoresis p.
 identity p.
 indeterminate p.
 lobular p.
 lobulocentric p.
 male sex chromatin p.
 mosaic p.
 nonreactive p.
 partial identity p.

 polyclonal p.
 storiform p.
 trabecular p.
 vesicular chromatin p.
 XX/XY sex chromosome p.
 zellballen p.
patulous
paucicellular
 p. area
Paul
 P. reaction
 P. test
Paul-Bunnell-Barrett test
Paul-Bunnell test
Pautrier
 P. abscess
 P. microabscess
Pauwel femoral neck fracture
Pauzat disease
Pavy disease
Payr disease
PB
 protein binding
PBC
 primary biliary cirrhosis
PBCL
 parafollicular B-cell lymphoma
PBD
 proliferative breast disease
PBG
 porphobilinogen
P-50 blood gas
PBN
 paralytic brachial neuritis
PBS
 phosphate buffered saline
PC
 platelet count
pc
 picocurie
PCA
 passive cutaneous anaphylaxis
PCB
 polychlorinated biphenyl
PCD
 polycystic disease
 posterior corneal deposit
PCH
 paroxysmal cold hemoglobinuria
pCi
 picocurie
PCLC
 Paneth cell-like change
PCM
 protein-calorie malnutrition
PCNA
 proliferating cell nuclear antigen

PCO$_2$, pCO$_2$
  carbon dioxide pressure
PCP
  pentachlorophenol
PCR
  plasma clearance rate
  polymerase chain reaction
    allele-specific PCR (A-PCR)
PCT
  plasmacrit
  porphyria cutanea tarda
  prothrombin consumption time
PCV
  packed cell volume
  polycythemia vera
PCV-M
  myeloid metaplasia with polycythemia
    vera
PD
  Parkinson disease
  plasma defect
  pulmonary disease
Pd
  palladium
PDGF
  platelet-derived growth factor
PDLL
  poorly differentiated lymphocytic
    lymphoma
PE
  pulmonary edema
  pulmonary embolism
peak
    absorption p.
    p. acid output (PAO)
    p. amplitude
    p. area
    biclonal p.
    p. broadening
    coincidence sum p.
    p. height
    iodine escape p.
    kilovolt p. (kvp)
    p. kilovoltage (pkV)
    monoclonal p.
    p. secretory flow rate (PSFR)
    p. transmittance
peak-to-peak amplitude
pearl
    epithelial p.
    keratin p.
    Laënnec p.

    squamous p.
    p. tumor
pearl-worker's disease
peau d'orange
pectenitis
pectenosis
pectin
pectinate
    p. body
Pectinibranchiata
Pectobacterium
    P. carotovorum
pectoris
    angina p. (AP)
pectus
    p. carinatum
    p. excavatum
    p. gallinatum
    p. recurvatum
pederin
pedes (*pl. of* pes)
Pedi-BacT
pedicellate
pedicellation
pedicle
pedicular
pediculate
pediculation
pediculi
pediculicide
Pediculoides ventricosus
pediculosis
pediculous
Pediculus
    P. humanus
    P. humanus capitis
    P. humanus corporis
    P. inguinalis
    P. pubis
pediculus
pedigree chart
pedis
pedogenesis
peduncle
pedunculate
pedunculated polyp
peeling
peenash
peg
    rete p.
PEI
    phosphate excretion index

NOTES

P

Pel-Ebstein
    P.-E. disease
    P.-E. fever
Pelecypoda
Pelger-Huët nuclear anomaly
peliosis
    p. hepatis
    p. hepatitis
Pelizaeus-Merzbacher disease
pellagra
    p. preventive (PP)
Pellegrini disease
Pellegrini-Stieda disease
pellicle
pellicular
pelliculous
Pellizzi syndrome
pellucid
pelta
peltation
pelves (*pl. of* pelvis)
pelvic
    p. abscess
    p. cellulitis
    p. inflammatory disease (PID)
    p. kidney
pelvirectal achalasia
pelvis, pl. **pelves**
    beaked p.
    caoutchouc p.
    frozen p.
    hardened p.
    kyphoscoliotic p.
    kyphotic p.
    lordotic p.
    Nägele p.
    p. obtecta
    osteomalacic p.
    Otto p.
    Prague p.
    pseudo-osteomalacic p.
    rachitic p.
    Rokitansky p.
    rostrate p.
    rubber p.
    scoliotic p.
    spider p.
    split p.
    spondylolisthetic p.
pelvospondylitis ossificans
PEM
    polymorphic epithelial mucin
pemphigoid
    benign mucosal p.
    bullous p.
    cicatricial p.
pemphigus
    p. antibodies

    benign mucous membrane p.
    p. crouposus
    p. erythematosus
    familial benign p.
    p. foliaceus
    p. gangrenosus
    p. leprosus
    p. neonatorum
    paraneoplastic p.
    p. vegetans
    p. vulgaris
PEN
    pancreatic endocrine neoplasm
pen
    light p.
pencil dosimeter
Pendred syndrome
pendulous heart
penetrability
penetrance
    complete p.
    incomplete p.
penetrans
    Sarcopsylla p.
    Tunga p.
penetrating
    p. radiation
    p. ulcer
    p. wound
penetrometer
Penfield method
penicillamine
penicilli (*pl. of* penicillus)
penicillin
    p. G
    p. V
penicillinase
    p. test
penicillin-fast
penicillinosis
penicillin, streptomycin, and tetracycline (PST)
Penicillium
    P. barbae
    P. bouffardi
    P. minimum
    P. montoyai
    P. notatum
    P. patulum
    P. spinulosum
penicillus, pl. **penicilli**
penile fibromatosis
penitis
pentachlorophenol (PCP)
pentaene
pentaerythritol tetranitrate
pentagastrin test
pentamer

pentamethyl violet
pentamidine
Pentastoma
    P. constrictum
    P. denticulatum
    P. taenioides
pentastomiasis
Pentastomida
Pentatrichomonas
    P. ardin delteili
pentatrichomoniasis
pentavalent gas gangrene antitoxin
penta-X chromosomal aberration
pentene
penton
    p. antigen
pentose
    p. assay
    p. phosphate pathway (PPP)
    p. shunt
pentoside
pentosuria
    alimentary p.
    essential p.
    idiopathic p.
    primary p.
peplomer
peplos
Pepper syndrome
pepsin (PPS)
    p. A
pepsinogen assay
pepsinuria
peptic
    p. cell
    p. esophagitis
    p. ulcer (PU)
peptidase
peptide
    anionic neutrophil activating p.
      (ANAP)
    p. bond
    C p.
    calcitonin gene-related p. (CGRP)
    p. group
    p. hormone
    phenylthiocarbamoyl p.
    PTC p.
    trefoil p.
    vasoactive intestinal p. (VIP)
peptidoglycan
Peptococcaceae

Peptococcus
    P. anaerobius
    P. asaccharolyticus
    P. constellatus
    P. magnus
    P. prevotii
peptone shock
peptone-starch-dextrose (PSD)
Peptostreptococcus
    P. anaerobius
    P. intermedius
    P. lanceolatus
    P. micros
    P. prevotii
    P. productus
PER
    protein efficiency ratio
per
    p. contiguum
    p. continuum
    p. second (ps)
peracetic
    p. acid
    p. acid-Schiff reaction
peracid
perambulating ulcer
percent
5 percent dextrose in water (D5W, D5
    & W, D_5W)
percentile
perchlorate
    p. discharge test
    potassium p.
perchloric acid
perchloroethylene
percolate
percolation
percreta
    placenta p.
percutaneous
    p. radiofrequency gangliolysis
    p. renal puncture
perencephaly
perester
perfect
    p. fungus
    p. stage
    p. state
    p. yeast
perforated
    p. diverticulitis
    p. gastric ulcer

NOTES

P

perforating
    p. abscess
    p. fibers of Sharpey
    p. ulcer
    p. wound
perforation
    inflammatory p.
perforin
performic
    p. acid
    p. acid reaction
    p. acid-Schiff reaction (PFAS)
performin
perfusate
perfuse
perfusion
    organ p.
    p. pressure
    pulmonary p.
periadenitis
periangiocholitis
periangitis
periaortitis
periapical
    p. abscess
    p. granuloma
periappendiceal abscess
periappendicitis
    p. decidualis
periarteritis
    p. gummosa
    p. nodosa (PAN, PN)
    syphilitic p.
periarticular abscess
peribiliary gland hamartoma
peribronchiolitis
peribronchitis
pericanalicular fibroadenoma
pericardia (*pl. of* pericardium)
pericardial
    p. cyst
    p. fluid examination
    p. friction rub
    p. serum
    p. tuberculosis
pericardii
    concretio p.
pericarditic
pericarditis
    adherent p.
    adhesive p.
    bacterial p.
    carcinomatous p.
    chronic constrictive p.
    constrictive p.
    fibrinous p.
    fungal p.
    hemorrhagic p.

    idiopathic p.
    internal adhesive p.
    mediastinal p.
    p. obliterans
    obliterative p.
    postmyocardial infarction p.
    postpericardiotomy p.
    posttraumatic p.
    purulent p.
    rheumatic p.
    serofibrinous p.
    p. sicca
    suppurative p.
    tuberculous p.
    uremic p.
    p. villosa
    viral p.
pericardium, pl. pericardia
    adherent p.
    bread-and-butter p.
    p. fibrosum
    p. serosum
    shaggy p.
pericentral fibrosis
pericholangitis
perichondritis
    relapsing p.
pericolitis
    p. dextra
    p. sinistra
pericolonitis
pericolpitis
pericranitis
pericryptal fibroblast
pericrypt eosinophilic enterocolitis
pericystitis
pericystium
pericyte
    Rouget p.
    p. of Zimmermann
peridesmitis
perididymitis
peridium
peridiverticulitis
periductal mastitis
periduodenitis
periencephalitis
perienteritis
periesophagitis
perifocal
perifollicular
perifolliculitis
perigastritis
periglandulitis
perihepatitis
perijejunitis
perilymphangitis
perimeningitis

perimetritis
perimuscular fibrosis
perimyelitis
perimyoendocarditis
perimyositis
perimysiitis
perimysitis
perinatal
    p. death
    p. mortality rate (PMR)
perinea (*pl. of* perineum)
perineovaginal fistula
perinephric abscess
perinephritis
perineum, pl. **perinea**
    watering-can p.
perineural
    p. fibroblastoma
    p. invasion
perineurial cell
perineurioma
perineuronal satellite cell
perinuclear
    p. cisterna
    p. space
period
    eclipse p.
    effective refractory p. (ERP)
    incubation p. (IP)
    induction p.
    latency p. (LP)
    latent p.
    prepatent p.
    refractory p. (RP)
    relative refractory p. (RRP)
periodate-lysing-paraformaldehyde
  fixative
periodate-Schiff procedure
periodic
    p. acid
    p. acid-concanavalin A (PACONA)
    p. acid-Schiff (PAS)
    p. acid-Schiff method
    p. acid-Schiff reaction
    p. acid-Schiff technique
    p. acid-Schiff test
    p. acid-silver methenamine (PASM)
    p. alternating nystagmus (PAN)
    p. disease
    p. edema
    p. neutropenia
    p. parasite

    p. peritonitis
    p. polyserositis
    p. syndrome (PS)
    p. wave
periodicity
periodontal
    p. cyst
    p. disease
periodontitis
perioophoritis
perioophorosalpingitis
periorchitis
    p. hemorrhagica
periorificial lentiginosis
periosteal
    p. chondroma
    p. fibroma
    p. fibrosarcoma
    p. ganglion
    p. implantation
    p. osteosarcoma
    p. sarcoma
periosteitis
    p. fibrosa
periosteoma
periosteomedullitis
periosteomyelitis
periosteophyte
periosteosis
periostitis
periostoma
periostosis, pl. **periostoses**
periostosteitis
periovaritis
peripachymeningitis
peripancreatitis
peripheral
    p. aneurysm
    p. arterial occlusive disease
    (PAOD)
    p. arteriosclerotic occlusive disease
    (PAOD)
    p. blood
    p. blood preparation
    p. blood smear
    p. blood stem cell infusion
    p. chemoreceptor
    p. circulatory failure
    p. dysostosis
    p. edema
    p. lesion
    p. lobule

NOTES

P

peripheral (*continued*)
    p. necrosis
    p. neuroectodermal tumor (PNET)
    p. neuropathy (PN)
    p. odontogenic fibroma
    p. protein
    p. resistance (PR)
    p. resistance unit (PRU)
    p. T-cell lymphoma (PTCL)
    p. total resistance (PTR)
    p. vascular disease (PVD)
    p. vein plasma (PVP)
periphlebitic
periphlebitis
Periplaneta
periplasm
periplast
peripolesis
periporitis
periportal
    p. cardiomyopathy
    p. fibrosis
    p. necrosis
periproctitis
periprostatitis
peripylephlebitis
perirectal abscess
perirectitis
perirenal insufflation
perisalpingo-ovaritis
perisigmoiditis
perispermatitis
    p. serosa
perisplanchnitis
perisplenitis
    hyaline p.
perispondylitis
peristalsis disorder
peristasis
peristatic hyperemia
peristoma
peristome
periston
peristrumous
perisynovial
peritendinitis
    p. calcarea
    p. serosa
peritenontitis
perithecium
perithelioma
perithyroiditis
peritoneal
    p. cancer
    p. dialysis
    p. fluid examination
    p. hemodialysis

    p. hernia
    p. lavage
peritonei
    pseudomyxoma p.
peritoneopathy
peritonitis
    acute diffuse p.
    adhesive p.
    benign paroxysmal p.
    bile p.
    chemical p.
    chyle p.
    circumscribed p.
    p. deformans
    diaphragmatic p.
    diffuse p.
    p. encapsulans
    feline infectious p.
    fibrinous p.
    fibrocaseous p.
    gas p.
    general p.
    gonococcal p.
    localized p.
    meconium p.
    periodic p.
    productive p.
    septic p.
    tuberculous p.
peritonsillar abscess
Peritrichida
peritrichous
periungual fibroma
periureteral abscess
periureteritis
    p. plastica
periurethral abscess
periurethritis
perivaginitis
perivascular cuff
perivasculitis
perivenular cell
perivisceritis
Perkin-Elmer/Cetus DNA Thermal Cycler
perlèche
Perls
    P. Prussian blue stain
    P. reaction
    P. test
permanent parasite
permanganate
    potassium p.
permeability
    p. quotient (PQ)
    p. of vacuum
permeable
permease

permeation
permissible exposure limit
permissive culture media
permittivity of vacuum
Permount slide fixative
permutation
Permutit
perniciosiform
pernicious
    p. anemia (PA)
    p. anemia type metarubricyte
    p. anemia type prorubricyte
    p. anemia type rubriblast
    p. malaria
perniosis
peroneal muscular atrophy
perosseous
peroxidase
    benzidine method for myoglobin p.
    DAKO Envision System P.
    endogenous p.
    glutathione p.
    hepatocatalase p. (HCP)
    horseradish p.
    p. reaction
    s-ABC p.
    p. stain
    p. staining method
peroxidase-antiperoxidase (PAP)
    p.-a. complex
    p.-a. technique
peroxidase-conjugated lotus tetragonolobus
peroxidation
peroxide
    acyl p.
    alkyl p.
    hydrogen p.
peroxisome
peroxyacetal nitrate (PAN)
peroxyacylnitrate
peroxysulfide
    ammonium p.
Perrin-Ferraton disease
Persian Gulf syndrome
persistence
    microbial p.
persistent
    p. chronic hepatitis
    p. filaria
    p. tolerant infection (PTI)
    p. truncus arteriosus (PTA)

persister
perstans
    acrodermatitis p.
    erythema dyschromicum p.
PERT
    program evaluation and review technique
Perthes disease
Pertik diverticulum
Pertofrane
pertussis
    p. immune globulin
    p. immunoglobulin
    p. serology
    p. vaccine
pes, pl. pedes
    p. febricitans
pessary
    p. cell
    p. corpuscle
pest
    fowl p.
    swine p.
pesticemia
pesticide
    chlorinated hydrocarbon p.
    cyclodiene hydrocarbon p.
    organo-chloro p.
pestiferous
pestilence
pestilential
Pestivirus
PET
    paraffin-embedded tissue
    preeclamptic toxemia
peta
petechia, pl. petechiae
    Tardieu petechiae
petechial
    p. angioma
    p. hemorrhage
petechiasis
petit mal epilepsy
Petragnani medium
Petri
    P. dish
    P. test
petriellidiosis
Petriellidium
    P. boydii
petrifaction
petroleum ether
petrositis

NOTES

P

petrous
petrousitis
Pette-Döring disease
Peutz-Jeghers
    P.-J. polyp
    P.-J. syndrome
Peutz syndrome
pexis
Peyer patch
peyote
Peyronie disease
PF
    platelet factor
pF
    picofarad
PFAS
    performic acid-Schiff reaction
Pfaundler-Hurler syndrome
PFC
    plaque-forming cell
Pfeiffer
    P. bacillus
    P. blood agar
    P. disease
    P. phenomenon
    P. syndrome
Pfeiffer-Comberg method
PFP
    platelet-free plasma
PFU
    plaque-forming unit
PG
    prostaglandin
    pyoderma gangrenosum
pg
    picogram
PGDR
    plasma-glucose disappearance rate
PGH
    pituitary growth hormone
PGI
    potassium, glucose, and insulin
PGP
    postgamma proteinuria
    protein gene product
PgR
    progesterone receptor
PGTR
    plasma glucose tolerance rate
PH
    prostatic hypertrophy
    pulmonary hypertension
Ph
    Philadelphia chromosome
        Ph chromosome
Ph$_1$
    Philadelphia chromosome

pH
    hydrogen ion concentration
        pH alteration
        pH electrode
        pH indicator
        pH meter
PHA
    passive hemagglutination
    phytohemagglutinin
    plasminogen activator inhibitor assay
    pulse height analyzer
phacoanaphylactic uveitis
phacoanaphylaxis
phacoma
phacomalacia
phacomatosis
phacosclerosis
PHA-E
    Phaseolus vulgaris erythroglutinin
Phaenicia sericata
phaeohyphomycosis
phaeomycotic cyst
phaeosporotrichosis
phage
    β-p.
    beta p.
    defective p.
    p. genetics
    temperate p.
phagedena
    p. gangrenosa
    p. nosocomialis
phagedenic
    p. ulcer
phage-resistant mutation
phagocyte
    alveolar p.
    p. dysfunction
    endothelial p.
    globuliferous p.
    melaniferous p.
    mononuclear p.
    sessile p.
phagocytic
    p. cell immunocompetence profile
    p. dysfunction disorders
      immunodeficiency
    p. histiocyte
    p. index
phagocytin
phagocytize
phagocytoblast
phagocytolysis
phagocytolytic
phagocytose
phagocytosis
    induced p.

spontaneous p.
vacuole alteration p.
phagolysis
phagolysosome
phagolytic
phagosome
phagotype
phakic-aphakic (PA)
phako-anaphylactic-endophthalmitis
phakoma
phakomatosis
phalanx, pl. **phalanges**
tufted p.
phallitis
phalloidin
phallolysin
phalloncus
phaneroplasm
phanerosis
phanerozoite
phantom
p. corpuscle
Hine-Duley p.
p. tumor
pharmacodynamics
pharmacogenetics
pharmacokinetics
pharmacologic mediators of anaphylaxis
PharmChek seat patch drug detection test
pharyngeal
p. calculus
p. pouch syndrome
pharyngitic
pharyngitis
atrophic p.
croupous p.
follicular p.
gangrenous p.
glandular p.
granular p.
p. herpetica
p. hypertrophica lateralis
membranous p.
p. sicca
Pharyngobdellida
pharyngoconjunctival
p. fever
p. fever virus
pharyngoesophageal diverticulum
pharyngokeratosis

pharyngolaryngitis
pharyngolith
pharyngomycosis
pharyngorhinitis
pharyngoscleroma
pharyngotonsillitis
phase
continuous p.
disperse p.
eclipse p.
exponential p.
G_0 p.
G_1 p.
G_2 p.
inductive p.
p. lag
lag p.
logarithmic p.
M p.
meiotic p.
mobile p.
moving p.
negative p.
positive p.
radial growth p.
S p.
stationary p.
vertical growth p.
phase-contrast microscope
Phaseolus vulgaris **erythroglutinin (PHA-E)**
phasmid
Phasmidia
phenacetin breath test
phenacetolin
phenaceturic acid
phenanthrene
phenazopyridine hydrochloride
phencyclidine
p. assay
phene
phenobarbital
p. assay
phenocopy
phenodeviant
phenogenetics
phenol
p. assay
p. coefficient
p. sulfatase
phenolemia

NOTES

P

phenolphthalein
p. test
phenolsulfonphthalein (PSP)
p. test
phenoluria
phenom
phenomenon, pl. phenomena
adhesion p.
anarchic p.
Arias-Stella p.
Arthus p.
atavistic p.
Bordet-Gengou p.
Danysz p.
Debré p.
Denys-Leclef p.
d'Herelle p.
Donath-Landsteiner p.
Ehrlich p.
erythrocyte adherence p.
Felton p.
generalized Shwartzman p.
Gengou p.
Hamburger p.
Houssay p.
Huebener-Thomsen-Friedenreich p.
immune adherence p.
Jod-Basedow p.
Kanagawa p.
Köbner p.
Koch p.
LE p.
Lucio leprosy p.
no reflow p.
Pfeiffer p.
prozone p.
quellung p.
Raynaud p.
red cell adherence p.
Sanarelli p.
Sanarelli-Shwartzman p. (SSP)
Schultz-Charlton p.
second-set p.
Splendore-Hoeppli p.
Theobald Smith p.
Twort p.
Twort-d'Herelle p.
phenon
phenothiazine
p. tranquilizer
p. tranquilizers assays
phenothiazines
phenotype
Bombay p.
McLeod p.
secretor p.
phenotypic
p. adaptation

p. mixing
p. variance
phenotyping
alpha-1 antitrypsin p.
α_1-antitrypsin p.
phenoxypenicillin
phentolamine test
phenylacetic acid
phenylacetylglutamine
phenylalanine
p. agar
p. assay
p. hydroxylase
p. test
p. tolerance index
phenylalanine-4-monooxygenase
phenylalanyl
phenylamine
phenylbutazone assay
phenylcarbinol
phenylethyl alcohol blood agar
phenylhydrazine
phenylketonuria (PKU)
p. test
phenyllactic acid
phenylpyruvic
p. acid
p. acid test
p. amentia
phenylpyruvicaciduria
phenylthiocarbamide
phenylthiocarbamoyl (PTC)
p. peptide
phenylthiourea
phenytoin
p. assay
pheochrome
p. cell
pheochromoblastoma
pheochromocyte
pheochromocytoma
pheomelanin
pheresis
pheromone
phialide
phialoconidium
Phialophora
P. compactum
P. dermatitidis
P. gougerotii
P. jeanselmei
P. mutabilis
P. parasitica
P. repens
P. richardsia
P. spinifera
P. verrucosa
phialophore

Phialophore-type conidiophore
phialospore
Philadelphia
    P. chromosome (Ph, Ph$_1$)
Philip gland
Philips 301 electron microscope
Philopia casei
phimosis
PHLA
    postheparin lipolytic activity
phlebarteriectasia
phlebectasia
phlebectopia
phlebectopy
phlebemphraxis
phlebeurysm
phlebismus
phlebitic
phlebitis
    adhesive p.
    p. nodularis necrotisans
    puerperal p.
    septic p.
    sinus p.
phlebography
phlebolite
phlebolith
phlebolithiasis
phlebometritis
phlebomyomatosis
phlebosclerosis
phlebostenosis
phlebothrombosis
Phlebotominae
phlebotomine
phlebotomist
Phlebotomus
    P. argentipes
    P. chinensis
    P. intermedius
    P. macedonicum
    P. noguchi
    P. papatasii
    P. sergenti
    P. verrucarum
    P. vexator
phlebotomus
    p. fever
    p. fever virus
Phlebovirus
phlegm

phlegmasia
    p. alba dolens
    cellulitic p.
    p. cerulea dolens
    p. malabarica
    thrombotic p.
phlegmon
    diffuse p.
    emphysematous p.
    gas p.
phlegmonous
    p. abscess
    p. adenitis
    p. cellulitis
    p. enteritis
    p. gastritis
    p. mastitis
    p. ulcer
phlogocyte
phlogocytosis
phlogogenic
phlogogenous
phlogosin
phlogotherapy
phloridzin, phlorhizin
    p. diabetes
    p. glycosuria
phloroglucin
phloroglucinol
phloroglucol
phloxine
phloxine-tartrazine stain
phlyctenular
    p. conjunctivitis
    p. keratoconjuctivitis
phlyctenule
phlyctenulosis
Phobetron
Phocas disease
phocomelia
phocomelic dwarfism
Phoma
    P. hibernica
phorate
phoresis
phoresy
Phoridae
Phormia regina
phorocytosis
phorozoon

NOTES

P

phos
        alk p.
            alkaline phosphatase
phosgene
        p. (choking gas) (CG)
phosphatase
        acid p.
        alkaline p. (alk phos, alk phos)
        bisphosphoglycerate p.
        cupric ion-inhibited acid p.
        diphosphoglycerate p.
        leukocyte alkaline p. (LAP)
        placental alkaline p. (PLAP)
        polyclonal anti-placental alkaline p.
          (PLAP)
        prostatic acid p.
        serum p.
        serum alkaline p. (SAP)
        tartrate-inhibited acid p.
        tartrate resistant acid p. (TRACP)
        p. test
        total serum prostatic acid p.
          (TSPAP)
        p. unit
phosphate
        acid p.
        ammonium magnesium p.
        p. assay
        p. buffer
        p. buffered formalin
        p. buffered saline (PBS)
        calcium p.
        carbamyl p.
        creatine p.
        deoxyguanosine p.
        deoxyuridine p.
        dibasic potassium p.
        dihydroxyacetone p.
        dolichol p.
        p. excretion index (PEI)
        p. group transfer potential
        guanosine 3':5'-cyclic p.
        high-energy p.
        inorganic p.
        Krebs-Ringer p. (KRP)
        magnesium ammonium p.
        monobasic potassium p.
        nicotinamide adenine dinucleotide p.
          (NADP)
        organic p.
        potassium p.
        primaquine p.
        tribasic potassium p.
        tricresyl p.
        tri-o-cresyl p.
        triple p.
3-phosphate
4-phosphate

5-phosphate
6-phosphate
phosphatemia
phosphatidalcholine
phosphatidalethanolamine
phosphatidate
phosphatid histiocytosis
phosphatidic acid
phosphatid-type histiocytosis
phosphatidylcholine
phosphatidylcholine-cholesterol
    acyltransferase
phosphatidylethanolamine
phosphatidylglycerol
phosphatidylinositide
phosphatidylinositol
phosphatidylserine (PS)
phosphaturia
phosphide
        zinc p.
phosphine
phosphoadenosine diphosphosulfate
3'-phosphoadenosine-5'-phosphosulfate
phosphocholine
phosphocreatine
phosphodiesterase
        sphingomyelin p.
phosphoenolpyruvate
phosphoethanolamine
phosphofluoridate
        diisopropyl p.
6-phosphofructokinase
phosphofructokinase deficiency
phosphoglucomutase
phosphogluconate
        p. dehydrogenase
        6-p. dehydrogenase assay
        p. oxidative pathway
6-phospho-D-gluconate
6-phosphogluconic acid
6-phospho-D-gluconolactone
3-phosphoglyceraldehyde
2-phospho-D-glycerate
3-phospho-D-glycerate
phosphoglycerate kinase
phosphoglycerides
phosphoglyceromutase
phosphoguanidine
phosphohexokinase
phosphohexose isomerase deficiency
phosphokinase
        creatine p.
        serum creatine p. (SCPK)
phospholipase
        p. A$_2$, B, C
phospholipid
        p. assay
        p. staining

p. test
p. type anticoagulant
p. vesicle
5-phosphomevalonic acid
phosphomolybdic
p. acid
p. acid stain
phosphomonoesterase
phosphonoacetic acid
4′-phosphopantetheine
phosphoprotein
phosphopyridoxal
phosphor
phosphorescence
phosphorescent
phosphoribomutase (PRM)
5-phosphoribosyl-1-amine
phosphoribosyltransferase
hypoxanthine guanine p.
orotate p.
phosphoric
p. acid
p. acid test
p. monoester hydrolase
phosphoruria
phosphorus
p. assay
phosphorus-32
phosphorylase
p. deficiency
glycogen p.
inosine p.
p. kinase
purine nucleoside p.
phosphorylated thiamin
phosphorylation
oxidative p.
substrate level p.
tyrosine p.
phosphorylation-dependent/independent
neurofilament epitope
phosphorylation-independent NF-H/M
epitope
3-phosphoserine
phosphotransferase
phosphotungstic
p. acid (PTA)
p. acid hematoxylin (PTAH)
p. acid stain
phosphotungstic acid (PTA)
phosphuria
phot

photoallergic sensitivity
photoallergy
photoautotroph
photoautotrophic
photocatalysis
photocatalyst
photocell
photochemical
p. reaction
p. smog
photochemistry
photochromogen
photochromogenic
p. mycobacteria
photochromogenicity
photocoagulation
photoconductive cell
photocontact dermatitis
photodecomposition
photodermatitis
photodetector
photodiode
photodissociation
photodistribution
photodynamic sensitization
photoelectric effect
photoelectrometer
photoelectron
photogenesis
photogenic
photographic effect
photoheterotroph
photoheterotrophic
photolithotroph
photolithotrophic
photoluminescence
photoluminescent
photolysis
photolytic
photometer
double-beam p.
filter p.
flame p.
photometric
p. accuracy
p. linearity
p. reproducibility
photometry
flame p.
photomicrograph
photomicrography
photomicroscope

NOTES

P

photomicroscopy
photomultiplier tube
photomyoclonic response
photon counting
photoorganotroph
photoorganotrophic
photo-patch test
photopeak detection efficiency
photophoresis
    extracorporeal p.
photophthalmia
photoreaction
photoreactivation
photoreceptor membrane (PRM)
photoresistor
photoretinitis
photosensitive
    p. porphyria
photosensitivity
photosensitization
photostable
photosynthesis
photosynthetic organism
phototaxis
phototoxic
    p. contact dermatitis
    p. sensitivity
phototoxicity
phototransistor
phototrophic
phototropism
phototube
photovoltaic cell
photuria
PHP
    primary hyperparathyroidism
    pseudohypoparathyroidism
    pyridoxylated hemoglobin-
      polyoxyethylene
phrenoptosia
phrenosin
phrygian cap
pH-stat
phthalein test
phthalic acid
phthalocyanine dye
phthalylsulfathiazole
phthinoid
phthiriasis
Phthirus
    P. pubis
phthisic, phthisical
phthisis
Phycomycetes
phycomycetosis
phycomycosis
p-hydroxybenzoic acid
p-hydroxyphenyllactic acid

p-hydroxyphenylpyruvic acid
phyla (*pl. of* phylum)
phylacagogic
phylactic
phylaxis
phyllodes
    cystosarcoma p. (CP)
    p. tumor
phylloquinone
phylogeny
phylum, pl. phyla
phyma
phymatoid
phymatorrhysin
phymatosis
Physa
physaliferous
physaliform
physaliformis
    ecchordosis p.
physaliphore
physaliphorous
    p. cell
physalis
Physaloptera
    P. caucasica
    P. mordens
physalopteriasis
Physalopteridae
physical
    p. adsorption
    p. allergy
    p. chemistry
    p. diagnosis
    p. half-life
    p. optics
    p. record
Physick pouch
physicochemical
physics
    health p.
physiochemical
physiologic
    p. albuminuria
    p. anemia
    p. chemistry
    p. equilibrium
    p. hypertrophy
    p. hypogammaglobulinemia
    p. incompatibility
    p. leukocytosis
    p. saline solution
    p. sclerosis
    p. unit
physiological saline solution (PSS)
physisorption
Physocephalus sexalatus
physocephaly

Physopsis
physostigmine salicylate
phytanic acid
phytic acid
phytin
phytoagglutinin
Phytobdella
phytobezoar
Phytoflagellata
phytohemagglutinin (PHA)
    p. assay
phytoid
phytol
phytolectin
Phytomastigina
Phytomastigophora
Phytomastigophorasida
Phytomastigophorea
phytomitogen
phytophotodermatitis
phytopneumoconiosis
phytotoxic
phytotoxin
PI
    proliferative index
    protamine insulin
    protease inhibitor
    pulmonary incompetence
    pulmonary infarction
pi
    p. bond
PIA
    plasma insulin activity
pia-arachnitis
pian
Piazza test
pica
Picchini syndrome
Pichia
    P. membranaefaciens
Pick
    P. atrophy
    P. body
    P. cell
    P. disease
    P. syndrome
    P. tubular adenoma
picket cell
pickwickian
    p. disease
    p. syndrome

picloram
picocurie (pc, pCi)
picofarad (pF)
picogram (pg)
picometer (pm)
picopicogram (ppg)
Picornaviridae
picornavirus
picosecond (ps)
picramic acid
picrate test
picric
    p. acid
    p. acid fixative
    p. stain
picrocarmine
    p. stain
picroformol
    p. fixative
picro-Mallory trichrome stain
picronigrosin
    p. stain
picrotoxin
PID
    pelvic inflammatory disease
    plasma iron disappearance
PIDT
    plasma-iron disappearance time
PIE
    pulmonary infiltration and eosinophilia
    pulmonary interstitial emphysema
    PIE syndrome
piebald skin
piece
    Fab p.
    Fc p.
piecemeal necrosis
piedra
    black p.
    p. nostras
    white p.
Piedraia
    P. hortae
Pierre Robin syndrome
piezoelectric effect
piezogenic
PIF
    prolactin-inhibiting factor
    proliferation inhibitory factor
pigeon
    p. breast

NOTES

P

pigeon *(continued)*
- p. breast deformity
- p. breeder disease

pigment
- accumulation of p.
- anthracotic p.
- bile p.
- bilharzial deposition p.
- calculous p.
- p. calculus
- ceroid p.
- cirrhosis p.
- endogenous p.'s and deposits
- epithelial p.
- exogenous p.'s and deposits
- formalin p.
- p. granule
- hematogenous p.
- hepatogenous p.
- p. induration of the lung
- lipid p.
- malarial deposition p.
- melanotic p.
- pseudomelanosis p.
- respiratory p.
- wear-and-tear p.

pigmentary
- p. cirrhosis
- p. degeneration
- p. dermatosis

pigmentation
- arsenic p.
- bismuth p.
- exogenous p.
- hematin p.
- hematoidin p.
- hemofuscin p.
- hemoglobin p.
- lead p.
- lipochrome p.
- melanin p.
- porphyrin p.
- wear-and-tear p.

pigmented
- p. ameloblastoma
- p. dermatofibrosarcoma protuberans
- p. epulis
- p. hair epidermal nevus
- p. pilocytic astrocytoma
- p. purpuric lichenoid dermatitis
- p. villonodular synovitis (PVNS)
- p. villonodular tenosynovitis

pigmentolysin
pigmentosa
- retinitis p.

pig skin
PII
- plasma inorganic iodine

Pike streptococcal broth
Pila
pilar
- p. cyst
- p. sheath acanthoma
- p. tumor of scalp

pilaris
- p. keratosis
- pityriasis rubra p. (PRP)

pile
- sentinel p.

piles
pili
Pilidae
piliferous cyst
pilimiction
pilin
pilocystic
pilocytic astrocytoma
piloid
- p. astrocytoma

pilomatrixoma
pilonidal
- p. cyst
- p. fistula
- p. sinus

pilus
- F p.
- I p.
- R p.
- sex p.

PIN
- prostatic intraepithelial neoplasia

pinacyanol
Pindborg tumor
pineal
- p. cyst
- p. germinoma
- p. secretory rate

pinealocyte
pinealoma
- ectopic p.
- extrapineal p.

pinealopathy
pineoblastoma
pineocytoma
ping-pong
- p.-p. bone
- p.-p. mechanism

pink
- p. bread mold
- p. puffer (emphysema) (PP)

pinkeye
Pinkus disease
pinocyte
pinocytosis

pinocytotic
  p. vesicle
  p. vessel
pinosome
pinta
pinworm
  p. preparation
pioepithelium
pion
Piophila casei
PIP
  paraffin immunoperoxidase
pipe
  light p.
piperacillin
piperazine
pipe-smoker's cancer
pipestem
  p. artery
  p. cirrhosis
  p. fibrosis
pipette, pipet
  blowout p.
  graduated p.
  measuring p.
  Mohr p.
  Pasteur p.
  serologic p.
  TC p.
  TD p.
  transfer p.
  volumetric p.
  washout p.
Pirenella
piriform
Piroplasma
Piroplasmida
piroplasmosis
Pirquet
  P. cutaneous tuberculin test
  P. reaction
Pisces
Pistol
  Cameco Syringe P.
PIT
  plasma iron turnover
pit
  Mantoux p.
  tubular p.
pitch wart
pitch-worker's cancer

PITR
  plasma iron turnover rate
pitting edema
Pittsburgh pneumonia agent
pituicyte
pituicytoma
pituitary
  p. adamantinoma
  p. adenoma
  p. ameloblastoma
  p. basophilia
  p. basophilism
  p. dwarf
  p. dwarfism
  p. endocrine disorder
  p. function test
  p. gonadotropic failure
  p. gonadotropin
  p. growth hormone (PGH)
  p. hormone
  lyophilized anterior p. (LAP)
  p. myxedema
  p. stalk section
  p. tumor
pituitary-like
  anterior p. (APL)
pityriasic
pityriasis
  p. alba
  p. capitis
  p. lichenoides et varioliformis acuta
  (PLEVA)
  p. nigra
  p. rosea
  p. rubra
  p. rubra pilaris (PRP)
  p. versicolor
Pityrosporon
  P. orbiculare
  P. ovale
  P. versicolor
Pityrosporum
  P. furfur
  P. orbiculare
  P. ovale
PIVKA
  protein induced by vitamin K antagonism
Pizzolato peroxide-silver method
PK, P-K
  Prausnitz-Küstner
  PK reaction

NOTES

P

483

PKU
  phenylketonuria
    PKU test
pkV
  peak kilovoltage
PL
  placebo
  placental lactogen
placebo (PL)
placenta
    p. accreta
    battledore p.
    bilobate p.
    p. circummarginata
    circumvallate p.
    dichorionic diamniotic p.
    duplex p.
    p. fenestrata
    p. increta
    mature abnormal p.
    p. membranacea
    monochorionic diamniotic p.
    monochorionic monoamniotic p.
    multilobate p.
    p. multipartita
    p. percreta
    premature abnormal p.
    prematurely separated p.
    premature separation of p.
    p. previa
    p. spuria
    p. succenturiata
    p. triloba
    trilobate p.
    p. tripartita
    twin p.
    p. twin
placentae
  ablatio p.
placental
    p. alkaline phosphatase (PLAP)
    p. and fetoplacental function tests
    p. hormone
    p. polyp
    p. residual blood volume (PRBV)
    p. site trophoblastic tumor
    p. steroid sulfatase deficiency
    p. thrombosis
    p. transmogrification
placental lactogen (PL)
placentation bleeding
placentitis
placentoma
plagiocephaly
Plagiorchiidae
Plagiorchioidea
Plagiorchis

plague
    p. bacillus
    black p.
    bubonic p.
    cattle p.
    cellulocutaneous p.
    duck p.
    fowl p.
    hemorrhagic p.
    pneumonic p.
    rabbit p.
    septicemic p.
    p. serum
    sylvatic p.
    urban p.
    p. vaccine
plakins
plakoglobin
Planck
    P. constant
    P. radiation law
plane
    focal p.
    symmetry p.
    p. wart
planimetry
plankter
plankton
planktonic
Planorbarius
planorbid
Planorbidae
Planorbis
plant
    p. agglutinin
    p. antitoxin
    p. indican
    p. protease test (PPT)
    p. toxin
    p. virus
Plantago
plantar
    p. fibromatosis
    p. wart
planuria
planus
    atrophic lichen p.
    bullous lichen p.
PLAP
  placental alkaline phosphatase
  polyclonal anti-placental alkaline
    phosphatase
plaque
    atheromatous p.
    attachment p.
    bacterial p.
    dental p.
    Hollenhorst p.

McCallum p.
mucous p.
neuritic p.
pleural p.
senile p.
p. technique
plaque-forming
 p.-f. cell (PFC)
 p.-f. cell assay
 p.-f. unit (PFU)
plasm
plasma (P)
 p. accelerator globulin
 p. activation
 adsorbed p.
 antihemophilic p.
 antihemophilic p. human
 antilymphocyte p. (ALP)
 anti-*Pseudomonas* human p.
  (APHP)
 p. bicarbonate
 blood p.
 p. blood cell
 p. cell dyscrasia
 p. cell granuloma
 p. cell hepatitis
 p. cell hyperplasia
 p. cell infiltrate
 p. cell leukemia
 p. cell mastitis
 p. cell myeloma
 p. cell pneumonia
 p. clearance
 p. clearance rate (PCR)
 p. clotting factor
 p. clotting time
 p. defect (PD)
 p. depletion
 p. exchange
 p. expander
 p. factor X
 p. fibronectin
 fresh frozen p. (FFP)
 frozen p. (FP)
 p. glucose tolerance rate (PGTR)
 p. hemoglobin test
 p. inorganic iodine (PII)
 p. insulin activity (PIA)
 p. iodoprotein disorder
 p. iron disappearance (PID)
 p. iron turnover (PIT)
 p. iron turnover rate (PITR)

p. labile factor
p. layer
lymphoid p. (LP)
p. marinum
p. membrane
normal p. (NP)
normal human p.
p. oncotic pressure (POP)
peripheral vein p. (PVP)
platelet-free p. (PFP)
platelet-poor p. (PPP)
platelet-rich p. (PRP)
p. protein
p. protein fraction (PPF)
p. renin activity (PRA)
salted p.
p. sodium (P_{Na})
p. stain
p. substitute
p. therapy
p. thrombin clot method
p. thromboplastin antecedent (PTA)
p. thromboplastin antecedent
 deficiency
p. thromboplastin component (PTC)
p. thromboplastin factor (PTF)
p. thromboplastin factor B
p. triglyceride
p. volume (PV)
p. volume expander
plasmablast
plasmacrit (PCT)
 p. test
plasmacyte
plasmacytic
 p. blood cell
 p. leukemia
 p. myeloma
plasmacytoid
 p. lymphocyte
 p. lymphoma
plasmacytoma
 extramedullary solitary p. (EMP)
plasmacytosis
plasma expander
plasmagene
plasma-glucose disappearance rate
 (PGDR)
plasma-iron disappearance time (PIDT)
plasmalemma
plasmalogen
plasmal reaction

NOTES

P

plasmapheresis
plasmarrhexis
plasmatic
  p. stain
plasmic
  p. stain
plasmid
  bacteriocinogenic p.
  conjugative p.
  F p.
  infectious p.
  p. integration
  nonconjugative p.
  oligomeric p.
  R p.
  resistance p.
  rough p.
  p. transfer
  transmissible p.
plasmin
  p. coagulation
  p. prothrombins conversion factor
    (PPCF)
plasminogen
  p. activator
  p. activator inhibitor
  p. activator inhibitor assay (PHA)
  p. assay
plasminokinase
plasminoplastin
plasmocrine vacuole
plasmocyte
plasmocytic leukemoid reaction
plasmodial
Plasmodiidae
Plasmodium
  P. falciparum
  P. malariae
  P. ovale
  P. pleurodyniae
  P. vivax
  P. vivax minuta
plasmodium
  p. embolism
  exoerythrocytic p.
Plasmodromata
plasmoid humor
plasmokinin
plasmolysis
plasmolytic
plasmolyze
plasmon
plasmoptysis
plasmorrhexis
plasmoschisis
plasmotomy
plasmotropic
plasmotropism

plasmotype
plasmozyme
plastic
  p. bronchitis
  p. corpuscle
  p. induration
  p. lymph
  p. pleurisy
  p. section stain
plasticizer
plastid
  blood p.
plate
  Abbé test p.
  blood p.
  blood agar p. (BAP)
  cough p.
  counting p.
  Covalink MicroElisa culture p.
  p. culture
  epiphyseal p.
  equatorial p.
  flood p.
  Hospidex microtiter p.
  lawn p.
  pour p.
  spread p.
  streak p.
  theoretical p.
  p. thrombosis
platelet
  p. actomyosin
  p. adhesion test
  p. adhesiveness test
  p. agglutination
  p. agglutinin
  p. aggregation
  p. aggregation test
  p. antibody
  p. autoantibody
  p. cofactor
  p. cofactor I, II, V
  p. concentrate
  p. count (PC)
  p. defect (PLD)
  p. factor (PF)
  p. factor 1, 2, 3, 4
  p. GPIIb/IIIa
  p. isoantibody
  p. membrane glycoprotein
  p. retention test
  p. sizing
  p. survival test
  p. thrombosis
  p. thrombus
  p. tissue factor
  p. transfusion
  in vivo adhesive p. (IVAP)

platelet-activating
 p.-a. factor (PAF)
platelet-aggregating factor (PAF)
platelet-derived growth factor (PDGF)
platelet-free plasma (PFP)
plateletpheresis
platelet-poor
 p.-p. blood (PPB)
 p.-p. plasma (PPP)
platelet-rich plasma (PRP)
platelike
plating
platinosis
platinum group
platybasia
platycyte
platyhelminth
Platyhelminthes
platykurtic
PLD
 platelet defect
pleated sheet
plebeius
 Vaginulus p.
plectonemic coil
plciotropic mutation
pleiotropy
Pleistophora
pleochroic
pleochroism
pleochromatic
pleochromatism
pleocytosis
pleokaryocyte
pleomorphic
 p. adcnoma
 p. carcinoma
 p. leiomyosarcoma
 p. lipoma
 p. oligodendroglioma
 p. rhabdomyosarcoma
 p. xanthoastrocytoma (PXA)
pleomorphism
pleonosteosis
 Leri p.
Pleospora
plerocercoid
plerocercus
Plesiomonas
plcural
 p. calculus
 p. fibrin ball

 p. fibroma
 p. fluid
 p. fluid examination
 p. friction rub
 p. plaque
 p. tuberculosis
pleurisy
 adhesive p.
 benign dry p.
 costal p.
 diaphragmatic p.
 dry p.
 encysted p.
 epidemic benign dry p.
 epidemic diaphragmatic p.
 fibrinous p.
 hemorrhagic p.
 interlobular p.
 plastic p.
 productive p.
 proliferating p.
 pulmonary p.
 purulent p.
 sacculated p.
 serofibrinous p.
 serous p.
 suppurative p.
 visceral p.
 wet p.
 p. with effusion
pleuritic
pleuritis
 acute fibrinous p.
 fibrinous p.
 obliterative p.
 rcactive eosinophilic p. (REP)
pleuritogenous
Pleuroceridae
pleurodesis
pleurodynia
 epidemic p.
pleurogenous
pleurohcpatitis
pleurolith
pleuropericarditis
pleuropneumonia
pleuropneumonia-like organism (PFLO)
pleuropulmonary blastoma
pleurorrhea
PLEVA
 pityriasis lichenoides et varioliformis
 acuta

NOTES

P

plexiform
> p. neurofibroma
> p. neuroma
> p. schwannoma

Plexiglas

plexitis

plexogenic pulmonary arteriopathy

plexosarcoma

PLH
> pulmonary lymphoid hyperplasia

plica, pl. **plicae**

Plimmer body

ploidy
> DNA p.

plot
> Scatchard p.

Ploton staining method

plotter

PLS
> prostaglandin-like substance

PLT
> psittacosis-lymphogranuloma venereum-trachoma (group)

plug
> Dittrich p.
> Traube p.

plumbism

Plummer disease

Plummer-Vinson syndrome

plump cell

pluricentric blastoma

pluriglandular adenomatosis

pluripotent
> p. myeloid stem cell

pluripotential stem cell

pluriresistant

plus strand

plutonium

PLV
> panleukopenia virus

PM
> pagetoid melanocytosis
> polymorph
> postmortem

pm
> picometer

PMA
> papillary, marginal, attached (gingivitis)
> progressive muscular atrophy

PMB
> polymorphonuclear basophil

PMC
> pseudomembranous colitis

PMD
> primary myocardial disease
> progressive muscular dystrophy

PME
> polymorphonuclear eosinophil

p-methoxyamphetamine assay

PMF
> progressive massive fibrosis

PML
> progressive multifocal leukoencephalopathy

PMN
> polymorphonuclear neutrophil

PMR
> perinatal mortality rate
> proportionate morbidity ratio
> proportionate mortality ratio

PMS
> postmitochondrial supernatant
> pregnant mare serum

PMSG
> pregnant mare serum gonadotropin

PMT
> pseudosarcomatous myofibroblastic tumor

PN
> periarteritis nodosa
> peripheral neuropathy
> pneumonia
> polyarteritis nodosa
> pyelonephritis

PNEC
> pulmonary neuroendocrine cell

PNET
> peripheral neuroectodermal tumor
> primitive neuroectodermal tumor

pneumarthrosis

pneumatic

pneumatinuria

pneumatocele

pneumatoides
> cystitis p.

pneumatosis
> p. cystoides intestinalis
> p. intestinalis cystica

pneumaturia

pneumobacillus
> Friedländer p.

pneumococcal
> p. pneumonia
> p. polysaccharide
> p. vaccine

pneumococcemia

pneumococci (*pl. of* pneumococcus)

pneumococcidal

pneumococcolysis

pneumococcosuria

pneumococcus, pl. **pneumococci**

pneumoconiosis, pl. **pneumoconioses**
> coal workers' p. (CWP)

pneumocystiasis

Pneumocystis
> P. carinii

    P. carinii pneumonia
    P. fluorescence
    P. pneumoniae
pneumocystosis
pneumocyte
    granular p.
pneumoderma
pneumogenic osteoarthropathy
pneumohemopericardium
pneumohemothorax
pneumohydroperitoneum
pneumohydrothorax
pneumohypoderma
pneumolith
pneumolithiasis
pneumomalacia
pneumomediastinum
pneumomycosis
pneumonia (PN)
    acute gelatinous p.
    aspiration p.
    atypical primary p.
    bronchial p.
    bronchiolitis obliterans with
      organizing p. (BOOP)
    caseous p.
    central p.
    chemical p.
    confluent p.
    core p.
    desquamative interstitial p. (DIP)
    diffuse interstitial p.
    p. dissecans
    double p.
    Eaton agent p.
    eosinophilic p.
    focal p.
    Friedländer p.
    fungal p.
    gangrenous p.
    giant cell p.
    giant cell interstitial p. (GIP)
    Hecht p.
    hemorrhagic p.
    hypostatic p.
    inhalation p.
    p. interlobularis purulenta
    interstitial giant cell p.
    interstitial plasma cell p.
    Klebsiella p.
    lipid p.
    lipoid p.

    lobar p.
    lobular p.
    lymphoid interstitial p. (LIP)
    metastatic p.
    migratory p.
    moniliasis p.
    mycoplasmal p.
    mycoplasma p. of pigs
    necrotizing lobar p.
    organized p.
    ovine progressive p.
    paratuberculous p.
    plasma cell p.
    pneumococcal p.
    Pneumocystis carinii p.
    primary atypical p. (PAP)
    primary influenza virus p.
    rheumatic p.
    septic p.
    staphylococcal p.
    streptococcal p.
    suppurative p.
    p. tularemia
    unresolved lobar p.
    uremic p.
    viral p.
    p. virus of mice (PVM)
    virus p. of pigs
    wandering p.
pneumoniae
    Chlamydia p.
    Pneumocystis p.
pneumonic
    p. plague
pneumonitis
    aspiration p.
    chemical p.
    desquamative interstitial p. (DIP)
    hypersensitivity p.
    interstitial p.
    lymphocytic interstitial p. (LIP)
    pulmonary p.
    rheumatic p.
    uremic p.
    usual interstitial p. (UIP)
    p. virus
pneumonoconiosis
pneumonocyte
pneumonomoniliasis
pneumonomycosis
Pneumonyssus simicola
pneumoperitoneum

NOTES

P

pneumoperitonitis
pneumopleuritis
pneumoretroperitoneum
pneumoserothorax
pneumothorax (PT, Px)
    spontaneous p.
    therapeutic p.
Pneumovirus
pneumovirus
PNH
    paroxysmal nocturnal hemoglobinuria
PNU
    protein nitrogen unit
pocket
    p. dosimeter
pocketed calculus
poculum
podarthritis
podedema
poditis
podocyte
podophyllin resin
Podoviridae
POEMS
    polyneuropathy, organomegaly,
    endocrinopathy, monoclonal
    gammopathy, and skin changes
      POEMS syndrome
POES growth promoting enrichment
poetin
Pogonomyrmex
pOH
    hydroxyl concentration
poik
    poikilocyte
poikiloblast
poikilocyte (poik)
    tail p.
poikilocythemia
poikilocytosis
poikiloderma
    p. atrophicans and cataract
    p. atrophicans vasculare
    p. of Civatte
    p. congenitale
poikilodermatomyositis
poikilothrombocyte
point
    boiling p. (bp)
    end p.
    equivalence p.
    p. estimate
    freezing p. (FP)
    growing p.
    ice p.
    ignition p.
    p. of inflection
    isoelectric p.

    isosbestic p.
    melting p. (MP)
    p. mutation
    radix p.
    set p.
    thermal death p.
    triple p.
pointed
    p. condyloma
    p. wart
pointer variable
point-of-care testing
poise
Poiseuille
    P. law
    P. space
poison
    P. Control Center
    industrial p.
    mitotic p.
poisoning
    antimony p.
    arsenic p.
    blood p.
    carbon disulfide p.
    carbon monoxide p.
    carbon tetrachloride p.
    chloroform p.
    cyanide p.
    desquamative interstitial p.
    ethyl alcohol p.
    food p.
    heavy-metal p.
    lead p.
    manganese p.
    mercury p.
    methyl alcohol p.
    mushroom p.
    naphthol p.
    nitroanilene p.
    oxygen p.
    paraldehyde p.
    salmonella p.
    scombroid p.
    systemic p.
    tetrachlorethane p.
    thallium p.
Poisson distribution
Poisson-Pearson formula
poker spine
pokeweed mitogen (PWM)
Poland syndrome
polar
    p. anemia
    p. body
    p. compound
    p. coordinates
polarimeter

polarimetry
polarity
polarizability
polarization
polarize
polarized light
polarizer
polarizing microscope
polarogram
polarography
Polhemus-Schafer-Ivemark syndrome
policeman
     rubber p.
polio
   poliomyelitis
polioclastic
poliodystrophia
     p. cerebri progressiva infantilis
poliodystrophy
     progressive cerebral p.
polioencephalitis
     p. infectiva
poliomyelitis (polio)
     acute anterior p.
     acute bulbar p.
     anterior acute p.
     chronic anterior p.
     p. I, II, III titer
     p. immune globulin (human)
     immunization reaction p.
     p. immunoglobulin
     mouse p.
     p. vaccine
     virus p.
     p. virus
poliovaccine
     inactivated p. (IPV)
poliovirus
     p. hominis
     p. vaccine
Polistes
polka fever
pollen
     p. antigen
     p. extract
Pollenia
pollenosis
pollinosis
polonium
poly
   polymorphonuclear leukocyte

polyacrylamide
     p. gel
     p. gel electrophoresis (PAGE)
polyadenitis
polyadenopathy
polyadenosis
polyadenylate tail
polyadenylation
polyadenylic acid
polyagglutination
polyamide
polyamine
polyamine-methylene resin
polyangiitis
polyanion
polyarteritis
     p. nodosa (PAN, PN)
polyarthritis
     p. chronica
     p. chronica villosa
     epidemic p.
     p. rheumatica acuta
     vertebral p.
polyA tail
polybasic acid
polyblast
polychlorinated
     p. biphenyl (PCB)
     p. biphenyl assay
polychondritis
     chronic atrophic p.
     relapsing p.
polychromasia
polychromatia
polychromatic
     p. cell
     p. normoblast
polychromatocyte
polychromatocytosis
polychromatophil, polychromatophile
     p. cell
polychromatophilia
polychromatophilic
     p. normoblast
     p. rubricyte
polychromatosis
polychrome
     p. methylene blue
     p. methylene blue stain
polychromemia
polychromia
polychromophil

NOTES

P

polychromophilia
polyclave
polyclonal
   p. activator
   p. antibody
   p. anti-carcinoembryonic antigen
   p. anti-placental alkaline
      phosphatase (PLAP)
   p. anti-S-100 protein
   p. gammopathy
   p. hypergammaglobulinemia
   p. pattern
   p. tumor
polycystic
   p. change
   p. disease (PCD)
   p. disease of kidneys
   p. kidney
   p. liver
   p. liver disease
   p. ovary
   p. ovary disease
   p. ovary syndrome
   p. renal disease
polycythaemica
   polyemia p.
polycythemia
   compensatory p.
   p. hypertonica
   myelopathic p.
   relative p.
   p. rubra
   p. rubra vera
   splenomegalic p.
   p. vera (PCV, PV)
polycytokeratin
polycytosis
polydactyly
polydeoxyribonucleotide synthetase
Polydesmus
polydysplasia
polydystrophia
polydystrophic
   p. dwarfism
polydystrophy
polyelectrolyte
polyembryony
polyemia
   p. aquosa
   p. hyperalbuminosa
   p. polycythaemica
   p. serosa
polyendocrine
   p. adenomatosis
   p. autoimmune disease
polyene antibiotic
polyenoic acid
polyester

polyethylene
   p. glycol
   p. glycol precipitation assay
polygenic inheritance
polygon
   frequency p.
polygyny
polygyria
polyhedral
   p. body
   p. cell
polyhelminthism
polyhydramnios
polyhydric alcohol
polykaryocyte
   Warthin-Finkeldey type p.
polykaryon
polyleptic fever
polymastia
polymastigote
polymer
   addition p.
   condensation p.
   poly-(methyl methacrylate) p.
   vinyl p.'s
polymerase
   p. chain reaction (PCR)
   DNA p.
   RNA p.
polymerization
polymerize
polymetaphosphate
polymethine dye
poly-(methyl methacrylate) polymer
polymicrobial
polymicrolipomatosis
polymitus
polymorph (PM)
polymorphic
   p. epithelial mucin (PEM)
   p. genetic marker
   p. light eruption
   p. reticulosis
polymorphism
   balanced p.
   lipoprotein p.
   restriction fragment length p.
      (RFLP)
polymorphocyte
polymorphocytic leukemia
polymorphonuclear
   p. basophil (PMB)
   p. eosinophil (PME)
   p. leukocyte (poly)
   p. leukocytic infiltrate
   p. neutrophil (PMN)
   p. neutrophil chemotactic factor

polymorphous
    p. eruption
    p. lymphoid infiltrate
polymyalgia
    p. arteritica
    p. rheumatica
polymyositis
polymyxin
    p. B sulfate
    p. E
polynesic
polyneuritic-type hypertrophic muscular atrophy
polyneuritiformis
    heredopathia atactia p. (HAP)
polyneuritis
    acute idiopathic p.
    infectious p.
polyneuropathy
polyneuropathy, organomegaly, endocrinopathy, monoclonal gammopathy, and skin changes (POEMS)
polynuclear leukocyte
polynucleate
polynucleolar
polynucleosis
polynucleotide
    p. ligase
polyol dehydrogenase
polyolefin
Polyomavirus
polyoma virus
polyoncosis, polyonchosis
    cutaneomandibular p.
polyostotic
    p. fibrous dysplasia
polyp
    adenomatous p.
    aural p.
    bleeding p.
    bronchial p.
    cardiac p.
    cellular p.
    cervical p.
    choanal p.
    cholesterol p.
    cloacogenic p.
    cockscomb p.
    colorectal p.
    cystic p.
    endometrial p.

    familial juvenile p. (FJP)
    fibrinous p.
    fibroepithelial p.
    fibrous p.
    fleshy p.
    gastric p.
    gelatinous p.
    granulomatous p.
    hamartomatous p.
    hydatid p.
    hyperplastic p.
    inflammatory p.
    juvenile p.
    laryngeal p.
    lipomatous p.
    lymphoid p.
    metaplastic p.
    mucous p.
    multiple adenomatous p.'s
    myomatous p.
    nasal p.
    osseous p.
    papillary adenomatous p.
    pedunculated p.
    Peutz-Jeghers p.
    placental p.
    regenerative p.
    retention p.
    sessile p.
    small intestine p.
    umbilical p.
    vascular p.
    villous p.
polyparasitism
polypeptide
    adrenocorticotropic p. (ACTP)
    gastric inhibitory p. (GIP)
    neurofilament triplet p. (NFP)
    pancreatic p.
    vasoactive intestinal p. (VIP)
polyphaga
    Acanthamoeba p.
polyphase
polyphasic wave
polyphenism
polyphenotypia
polypheny
polyphosphoric acid
polyphyletic
    p. theory
polyphyletism
polypi (*pl. of* polypus)

NOTES

P

polypiform
polyplasmia
Polyplax
Polyplis
polyploid
polyploidy
polypnea
polypoid
      p. adenoma
      p. hyperplasia
polyposis
      p. coli
      familial intestinal p.
      multiple intestinal p.
polypous
      p. endocarditis
      p. gastritis
polypropylene
polypus, pl. **polypi**
polypyrrylmethane
polyradiculoneuritis
polyradiculoneuropathy
polyradiculopathy
polyribosome
polysaccharide
      cryptococcal p.
      pneumococcal p.
      specific soluble p.
polyserositis
      familial paroxysmal p.
      familial recurrent p.
      periodic p.
polysialic acid
polysinusitis
polysomaty
polysome
polysomic
polysomy
polysorbate
polyspermy
polysplenia syndrome
polystyrene
polytendinitis
polytene chromosome
polyteny
polytetrafluoroethylene
poly(U)
polyunsaturated fatty acid (PUFA)
polyunsaturated-to-saturated fatty acids
  ratio (P/S)
polyuridylic acid
polyvalent
      p. allergy
      p. antiserum
      p. serum
      p. vaccine
polyvinyl
      p. alcohol (PVA)

      p. alcohol fixative method
      p. chloride
polyvinylpyrrolidone
polyzoic
Pomatiopsis
Pompe disease
ponceau D xylidine
Poncet disease
Ponfick shadow
ponos
Pontamine sky blue stain
Pontiac fever
pontine angle tumor
pool
      circulating granulocyte p. (CGP)
      gene p.
      marginal granulocyte p. (MGP)
      metabolic p.
      rapidly miscible p. (RMP)
      total blood granulocyte p. (TBGP)
      vaginal p.
pooled
      p. blood serum
      p. estimate
poorly
      p. compliant bladder
      p. differentiated lymphocytic
        lymphoma (PDLL)
POP
   plasma oncotic pressure
popcorn cell
popliteal aneurysm
pop-off technique
population
      p. biology
      p. cytogenetics
      disomic p.
      p. genetics
      p. sample (PS)
P:O ratio
porcine
      p. adenovirus
      p. hemagglutinating
        encephalomyelitis virus
      p. transmissible gastroenteritis
porcupine skin
pore
      alveolar p.
porencephalia
porencephalic
porencephalitis
porencephalous
porencephaly
Porges-Meier test
Porges-Salomon test
Porifera
pork tapeworm
porocele

porocephaliasis
Porocephalidae
porocephalosis
Porocephalus
    P. armillatus
    P. clavatus
    P. constrictus
    P. denticulatus
poroconidium
porokeratosis
    actinic p.
    disseminated superficial actinic p. (DSAP)
    Mibelli p.
poroma
    eccrine p.
porosis, pl. poroses
    cerebral p.
porosity
porospore
porotic
porphin
porphobilinogen (PBG)
    p. deaminase
    p. synthase
    p. synthase assay
porphyria
    acute intermittent p. (AIP)
    congenital p.
    congenital crythropoietic p. (CEP)
    p. cutanea tarda (PCT)
    erythrohcpatic p.
    erythropoietic p.
    hepatic p.
    hereditary coproporphyria (HCP)
    latent p.
    photosensitive p.
    protoporphyria
    South African type p.
    symptomatic p.
    variegate p.
porphyrin
    p. assay
    p. pigmentation
    p. test
porphyrinuria
porphyruria
porrigo
    p. favosa
    p. furfurans
    p. lupinosa
    p. scutulata

port
portal
    p. cirrhosis
    p. hypertension
    p. pyemia
    p. system
    p. triad
    p. vein thrombosis (PVT)
portal-systemic encephalopathy (PSE)
Porter-Silber (PS)
    P.-S. chromogen (PSC)
    P.-S. chromogens test
    P.-S. reaction
Porteus maze test
Porthetria
Portmann classification
portocaval shunt
port-wine
    p.-w. mark
    p.-w. stain
Posada disease
Posada-Wernicke disease
position
    p. isomerism
    left frontoanterior p. (LFA)
positional alcohol nystagmus (PAN)
positive
    p. anergy
    p. assortative mating
    p. control enzyme induction
    p. control repression
    false p.
    p. neutrolaxis
    p. phase
    positive cytotaxis
    p. pressure
    Rh p.
    Rhesus factor p.
    p. stain
    wcakly p. (WP)
    p. whiff test
positron
    p. annihilation
    p. bcta decay
post
    postmortem
postabsorptive state
postatrophic hyperplasia (PAH)
postchromation
postchroming
postdiction
postductal coarctation of aorta

NOTES

P

posterior
    p. corneal deposit (PCD)
    p. pituitary hormone
    p. spinal sclerosis
    p. subcapsular cataract (PSC)
    p. urethritis
    p. wall infarct (PWI)
postgamma proteinuria (PGP)
posthemorrhagic anemia
postheparin lipolytic activity (PHLA)
posthepatic cirrhosis
posthepatitic cirrhosis
posthitis
postholith
postinfectious
    p. allergic encephalitis
    p. encephalomyelitis
    p. glomerulonephritis
    p. myelitis
postmaturity
postmenopausal
    p. atrophy
    p. syndrome
postmitochondrial supernatant (PMS)
postmordant
postmordanting
postmortem (PM, post)
    p. clot
    p. examination
    p. hypostasis
    p. livedo
    p. lividity
    p. pustule
    p. suggillation
    p. thrombus
    p. tubercle
    p. wart
postmyocardial infarction pericarditis
postnecrotic
    p. cirrhosis
postoperative
    p. parotiditis
    p. repair
postpartum (PP)
    p. hemorrhage (PPH)
    p. pituitary necrosis
postpericardiotomy pericarditis
postprandial (PP)
    p. blood sugar (PPBS)
    p. glucose
    p. lipemia
postprimary tuberculosis
postpuberal panhypopituitarism
postpubertal
    p. hyperpituitarism
    p. panhypopituitarism
postpump syndrome (PPS)

postpyknotic
postradiation dysplasia (PRDX)
postrema
    area p.
postrenal
    p. albuminuria
    p. azotemia
postrubella syndrome
poststenotic dilatation
poststreptococcal
    p. glomerulonephritis (PSGN)
posttransfusion
    p. hepatitis (PTH)
    p. mononucleosis (PTM)
posttransplant
    p. lymphoproliferative disease (PTLD)
    p. lymphoproliferative disorder (PTLPD)
posttraumatic
    p. epilepsy
    p. leptomeningeal cyst
    p. osteoporosis
    p. pericarditis
postulate
    Ehrlich p.
    Koch p.
postural
    p. albuminuria
    p. proteinuria
postvaccinal
    p. encephalitis
    p. myelitis
postvaccination allergic encephalitis
potable
Potamidae
Potamon
potassium
    p. acidosis
    p. alkalosis
    p. *p*-aminosalicylate
    p. assay
    p. chlorate
    p. cyanide
    p. dichromate
    p. ferrocyanide
    glucose, insulin, and p. (GIK)
    p. hydroxide (KOH)
    p. hydroxide test
    p. hydroxide test
    p. metabisulfate stain
    p. perchlorate
    p. permanganate
    p. permanganate stain
    p. phosphate
    p. thiocyanate
    total body p. (TBK)
    total exchangeable p. measurement

potassium-42
potassium, glucose, and insulin (PGI)
potato
    p. dextrose agar
    p. tumor of neck
potency
    homeopathic symbol for decimal
      scale of p.'s (X)
potential
    atypical polypoid adenomyofibroma
      of low malignant p. (APA-LMP)
    cervical somatosensory evoked p.
    decomposition p.
    diffusion p.
    Donnan p.
    electric p.
    electrode p.
    p. energy
    half-wave p.
    junction p.
    liquid-liquid junction p.
    membrane p.
    muscle action p.
    oxidation-reducing p.
    phosphate group transfer p.
    redox p.
    reduction p.
    resting membrane p.
    standard electrode p.
    standard reduction p.
    visual evoked p. (venostasis)
    zeta p.
    zoonotic p.
potentiometer
    direct-reading p.
    null-point p.
    slide-wire p.
potentiometric titration
potentiometry
Pott
    P. abscess
    P. aneurysm
    P. disease
Potter
    P. disease
    P. facies
    P. syndrome
Potter-Bucky grid
potters' asthma
pouch
    Physick p.
pouchitis

Poulet disease
poultry handler's disease
pounds per square inch (p.s.i.)
pour plate
povidone
povidone-iodine
Powassan
    P. encephalitis
    P. virus
power
    p. amplifier
    apparent p.
    carbon dioxide combining p.
    p. resistor
    resolving p.
    p. supply
pox
    Kaffir p.
    p. virus
Poxviridae
poxvirus
    p. officinalis
PP
    pellagra preventive
    pink puffer (emphysema)
    postpartum
    postprandial
    prothrombin-proconvertin
    protoporphyrin
PPB
    platelet-poor blood
PPBS
    postprandial blood sugar
PPCA
    proserum prothrombin conversion
      accelerator
PPCF
    plasmin prothrombins conversion factor
PPD
    purified protein derivative
      PPD skin test
PPD-S
    purified protein derivative-standard
PPF
    plasma protein fraction
ppg
    picopicogram
PPH
    postpartum hemorrhage
    primary pulmonary hypertension
PPHP
    pseudo-pseudohypoparathyroidism

NOTES

P

PPLO
pleuropneumonia-like organism
PPP
pentose phosphate pathway
platelet-poor plasma
PPR
Price precipitation reaction
PPS
pepsin
postpump syndrome
PPT
plant protease test
Ppt, ppt
precipitate
prepared
PQ
permeability quotient
PR
partial remission
peripheral resistance
progesterone receptor
protein
Pr
prism
PRA
plasma renin activity
progesterone assay
Prader bead standard
Prader-Willi syndrome
P-radiolabeled DNA probe fragment
Prague pelvis
prairie itch
pralidoxime chloride
praseodymium
Prausnitz-Küstner (PK, P-K)
P. antibody
P. reaction
P. test
prazosin hydrochloride
PRBV
placental residual blood volume
PRC
packed red cells
PRCA
pure red cell agenesis
pure red cell aplasia
PRD
partial reaction of degeneration
PRDX
postradiation dysplasia
preadaptation
preadenomatous
prealbumin
thyroxine-binding p. (TBPA)
preamplifier
pre-B cell
prebetalipoprotein
precancer

precancerous
p. dysplasia
p. lesion
p. melanosis of Dubreuilh
prechroming
precipitant
precipitate (Ppt, ppt)
keratitic p. (KP)
keratotic p.
precipitating antibody
precipitation
double antibody p.
immune p.
p. test
tuberculin p. (TP)
precipitin
p. curve
p. reaction
p. test
tube p. (TP)
precipitinogen
precipitinogenoid
precipitogen
precipitoid
precipitophore
precision
P. QI-D handheld blood glucose test
p. resistor
Precision-G handheld blood glucose test
precocious
p. adrenarche
p. pseudopuberty
p. puberty
precocity
precursor lesion
predaceous mite
predecidual
p. alteration
predeposit autologous transfusion
prediabetes
predictive
p. value
p. value of negative test
p. value of positive test
predispose
predisposing cause
predisposition
prednisone
bleomycin, p.
cyclophosphamide, doxorubicin hydrochloride, vincristine (Oncovin), p. (CHOP)
cyclophosphamide, THP-doxorubicin, vincristine, p. (THPCOP)
daunorubicin, cytarabine, 6-mercaptopurine, p. (DCMP)
preductal coarctation of aorta

preeclampsia
preeclamptic toxemia (PET)
preeruptive
prefibrinolysin
pregnancy
    aborted ectopic p.
    corpus luteum of p.
    p. cycle
    ectopic p. (EP)
    extrauterine p.
    p. luteoma
    megaloblastic anemia of p. (MAP)
    molar p.
    ovarian p.
    parasitic ectopic p.
    ruptured ectopic p.
    p. test
    toxemia of p.
    tubal p.
    p. urine (PU)
    voluntary interruption of p. (VIP)
pregnancy-associated (PA)
pregnanediol assay
pregnanetriol
pregnant
    p. mare serum (PMS)
    p. mare serum gonadotropin
      (PMSG)
pregnenolone
prehepatic hypoproteinemia
preictal
preinvasive
Preiser disease
Preisz-Nocard bacillus
prekallikrein
preleukemia
prelytic sphere
premalignant
premammary abscess
premature
    p. abnormal placenta
    p. infant
    p. rupture
    p. rupture of (fetal) membranes
      (PROM)
    p. senility syndrome
    p. separation of placenta
prematurely
    p. closed foramen ovale
    p. separated placenta
prematurity
premonocyte

premorbid
premunition
premunitive
premyeloblast
premyelocyte
prenatal
    p. diagnosis
    p. screening
preneoplastic
prenyl group
preovulatory
preparation
    allergenic protein p.'s
    biomechanical p.
    broken cell p.
    cell block p.
    corrosion p.
    cytologic filter p.
    heart-lung p.
    impression p.
    ThinPrep cytologic p.
    Trichomonas p.
preparative immunofiltration
prepared (Ppt, ppt)
prepatent period
preproprotein
prepubertal
    p. hyperpituitarism
    p. panhypopituitarism
preputial
    p. calculus
preputii
    smegma p.
prepyloric atresia
prerenal
    p. albuminuria
    p. azotemia
presacral insufflation
presbycardia
presbyopia
presenile spontaneous gangrene
presentation
    antigen p.
    compound p.
preservative
PreservCyt fixative
prespermatogonia
pressor
    p. amine
    p. base
    p. substance
pressure (P)

NOTES

P

pressure *(continued)*
    arterial p.
    p. atrophy
    barometric p.
    carbon dioxide p. (PCO_2, pCO_2)
    central venous p.
    cerebrospinal fluid p.
    colloidal osmotic p. (COP)
    continuous distending p. (CDP)
    end-systolic p. (ESP)
    millimeters partial p. (mmpp)
    oncotic p.
    osmotic p. (OP)
    oxygen under high p. (OHP)
    partial p.
    plasma oncotic p. (POP)
    positive p.
    pulmonary p.
    pulse p.
    screen filtration p. (SFP)
    selection p.
    standard temperature and p.
    standard temperature and p., dry
      (STPD)
    systemic arterial p. (SAP)
    p. urticaria
    vapor p.
    venous p.
pressure-volume curve
presumptive heterophil test
presuppurative
prethymic lymphoblastic lymphoma
pretibial myxedema
prevalence rate
prevention
preventive
    p. medicine
    pellagra p. (PP)
    p. treatment
previa
    placenta p.
previous value check
prezone
PRFM
    prolonged rupture of fetal membranes
PRH
    prolactin-releasing hormone
priapism
priapitis
Price-Jones curve
Price precipitation reaction (PPR)
primaquine
    p. phosphate
    p. sensitivity
primaquine-sensitive anemia
primary
    p. active transport
    p. adrenal insufficiency

p. African green monkey kidney
    (PAGMK)
p. agammaglobulinemia
p. amebic meningoencephalitis
p. amenorrhea
p. amyloidosis
p. anemia (PA)
p. atelectasis
p. atypical pneumonia (PAP)
p. biliary cirrhosis (PBC)
p. bubo
p. carcinoma
p. cardiomyopathy
p. coccidioidomycosis
p. coil
p. colors
p. complex
p. constriction
p. culture
p. endocardial sclerosis
p. erythroblastic anemia
p. fibrinolysis
p. fibromyalgia syndrome
p. glaucoma
p. granule
p. herpetic stomatitis
p. hyperaldosteronism
p. hyperparathyroidism (PHP)
p. hyperplasia
p. hypoadrenocorticism
p. hypogammaglobulinemia
p. immune response
p. influenza virus pneumonia
p. irritant
p. Ki-1 lymphoma of brain
p. lesion
p. lymphedema
p. methemoglobinemia
p. myeloid metaplasia
p. myocardial disease (PMD)
p. pentosuria
p. pulmonary hypertension (PPH)
p. pyoderma
p. reaction
p. reference material
p. refractory anemia
p. rejection
p. renal calculus
p. renal tubular acidosis
p. repair
p. sclerosing cholangitis
p. sequestrum
p. sex character
p. standard
p. structure
p. thrombocythemia
p. transcript
p. trisomy

p. tuberculosis
p. union
primed lymphocyte typing
primer
primerite
primidone
p. assay
primite
primitive
p. erythroblast
p. mesoblast
p. neuroblastic cell
p. neuroectodermal tumor (PNET)
primordial
p. dwarf
p. germ cell
p. sex cell
primordium, pl. **primordia**
primulin
principal
p. cell
p. focus
p. piece of spermatozoon
principle
antianemic p.
Fick p.
follicle-stimulating p.
hematinic p.
immediate p.
luteinizing p.
prothrombin-converting p.
proximate p.
ultimate p.
uncertainty p.
Pringle disease
printed circuit
Prinzmetal angina
prion
Prionurus
prism (Pr)
adamantine p.
Nicol p.
prismatic
pristanic acid
private antigen
privileged site
PRL
prolactin
PRM
phosphoribomutase
photoreceptor membrane

pro
prothrombin
proaccelerin
proactivator
C3 p.
C3 p. convertase
probabilistic
probability (P)
conditional p.
p. distribution
p. paper
significance p.
probable error
probacteriophage
defective p.
proband
probe
allele-specific oligonucleotide p.
ASO p.
centromere enumeration p. (CEP)
DNA p.
fluorescent p.
nucleic acid p.
oligonucleotide p.
p. patent foramen ovale
radioactive p.
viral p.
probiosis
probiotic
probit transformation
Probstymayria vivipara
procainamide
p. assay
procaine hydrochloride
procapsid
Procarbazine
Procaryotae
procaryote (*var. of* prokaryote)
procaryotic
procedure
Cherry-Crandall p.
concentration p.
Cryptosporidium diagnostic p.
evacuation p.
helminth identification p.
hypophysis staining p.
Jatlow-Nadim p.
Mantel-Cox p.
periodate-Schiff p.
procentriole organizer
procercoid

NOTES

P

501

process
p. control
filiform p.
foot p.
iterative p.
styloid p.
ThinPrep slide p.
processing
antigen p.
automatic tissue p.
interactive p.
RNA p.
tissue p.
processor
front-end p.
procidentia
procoagulant
procollagen
proconvertin
proctatresia
proctectasia
proctencleisis, proctenclisis
proctitis
chronic ulcerative p.
idiopathic p.
proctocele
proctocolitis
proctodeal
proctodeum
proctopolypus
proctoptosis
proctosigmoiditis
proctostenosis
prodigiosin
prodromal stage
product
cleavage p.
contact activation p.
cross p.
decay p.
dot p.
end p.
fibrin breakdown p.
fibrin degradation p. (FDP)
fibrin/fibrinogen degradation p.
(FDP)
fibrinogen breakdown p. (FBE)
fibrinogen split p. (FSP)
fibrinolytic split p. (FSP)
fibrin-split p.
fission p.
gene p.
protein gene p. (PGP)
scalar p.
solubility p.
spallation p.
substitution p.

vector p.
waste p.
production
carbon dioxide p.
CO_2 p.
excessive heat p. (EHP)
pair p.
production-defect anemia
productive
p. inflammation
p. peritonitis
p. pleurisy
proenzyme
proerythroblast
proerythrocyte
Professional Standards Review
Organization (PSRO)
Profeta law
profibrinolysin
Profichet
P. disease
P. syndrome
proficiency survey
profile
biochemical p.
cell volume p. (CVP)
fatty acid p.
kidney p.
liver p.
phagocytic cell
immunocompetence p.
test p.
profunda
miliaria p.
progenitor cell
progeny
progeria
p. with cataract
p. with microphthalmia
progeroid
progestational
p. agent
p. hormone
progesteroid
progesterone
p. assay (PRA)
p. receptor (PgR, PR)
p. receptor assay
p. unit
progestin
progestogen
proglottid
proglottis
prognathism
prognosis
prognostic factor

progonoma
    p. of jaw
    melanotic p.
program
    p. evaluation and review technique (PERT)
    object p.
    safety p.
    source p.
    survey p.
programming
    temperature p.
progranulocyte
progranulocytic leukemia
progravid
progressive
    p. bacterial synergistic gangrene
    p. bulbar palsy
    p. cerebellar dyssynergia
    p. cerebral poliodystrophy
    p. cleavage
    p. emphysematous necrosis
    p. hypocythemia
    p. lipodystrophy
    p. massive fibrosis (PMF)
    p. multifocal leukoencephalopathy (PML)
    p. muscular atrophy (PMA)
    p. muscular dystrophy (PMD)
    p. pigmentary dermatosis
    p. pneumonia virus
    p. spinal muscular atrophy
    p. staining
    p. subcortical encephalopathy
    p. supranuclear palsy (PSP)
    p. systemic sclerosis (PSS)
    p. transformation of germinal centers (PTGC)
    p. vaccinia
prohormone
proinsulin
projection
    Fischer p.
    transmandibular p.
Prokaryotae
prokaryote, procaryote
prokaryotic
prolactin (PRL)
    chorionic growth hormone p. (CGP)
    p. release-inhibiting hormone

    p. test
    p. unit
prolactin-inhibiting factor (PIF)
prolactinoma
prolactin-producing adenoma
prolactin-releasing
    p.-r. factor
    p.-r. hormone (PRH)
prolapse
    mitral valve p. (MVP)
    Morgagni p.
prolapsed umbilical cord
proleukocyte
proliferans
    retinitis p.
proliferating
    p. cell nuclear antigen (PCNA)
    p. endarteritis
    p. pleurisy
    p. systematized angioendotheliomatosis
    p. tricholemmal cyst
proliferation
    cell p.
    cholangiolar p.
    p. cyst
    diffuse mesangial p.
    p. inhibitory factor (PIF)
    T-cell p.
proliferative
    acute p. (AP)
    p. breast disease (PBD)
    p. bronchiolitis
    p. chronic arthritis
    p. cyst
    p. fasciitis
    p. glomerulonephritis
    p. glomerulopathy
    p. index (PI)
    p. inflammation
    p. intimitis
    p. mixoploid
    p. myositis
    p. stage
    p. synovitis
proliferous cyst
proline
    p. dehydrogenase
    p. hydroxylase
    p. oxidase
proline,2-oxoglutarate dioxygenase
prolinemia

NOTES

P

prolinuria
prolonged
    p. bleeding time
    p. coagulation time
    p. rupture of fetal membranes
      (PRFM)
    p. rupture of (fetal) membranes
      (PROM)
prolyl
prolymphocyte
    p. cell
PROM
    premature rupture of (fetal) membranes
    prolonged rupture of (fetal) membranes
Promace-MOPP
promastigote
promegakaryoblast
promegakaryocyte
promegaloblast
prometaphase banding
promethium
promoblast
promonocyte
promoter
    cancer p.
    eosinophil stimulation p. (ESP)
    tumor p.
promoting agent
promotion
promyelocyte
    basophilic p.
    eosinophilic p.
    neutrophilic p.
promyelocytic leukemia
pronormoblast
pronucleus
proof
    constructive p.
    existence p.
propagating thrombosis
propagation
propagule
propanenitrile
propanoic acid
1-propanol
2-propanol
proparathyroid hormone
propenal
propepsin
properdin
    p. assay
    p. factor A, B, D, E
    p. system
prophage
    defective p.
prophase
prophlogistic

prophylactic
    p. membrane
    p. serum
    p. treatment
prophylaxis
    active p.
    chemical p.
    passive p.
propidium iodide solution
propionate
    p. carboxylase
    p. metabolism
Propionibacteriaceae
Propionibacterium
    P. acnes
    P. avidum
    P. granulosum
    P. lymphophilum
propionic
    p. acid
    p. acidemia
    p. aciduria
propionicacidemia
propionitrile
propionyl-CoA carboxylase
proplasia
proplasmacyte
proportional
    p. count
    p. counter
proportionate
    p. morbidity ratio (PMR)
    p. mortality ratio (PMR)
propositus, pl. **propositi**
propoxur
propoxyphene
    p. assay
propranolol
    p. assay
propria
    muscularis p.
proprotein
propyl alcohol
propylene
    p. glycol
prorubricyte
    pernicious anemia type p.
proscolex
prosection
prosector
    p. tubercle
    p. wart
proserum prothrombin conversion
  accelerator (PPCA)
prosodemic
p-**rosolic acid**
prosopalgia
prosopectasia

prosoplasia
prososstomate trematode
prospective study
prostacyclin
prostaglandin (PG)
- p. A
- p. B
- p. D_2
- p. E_2
- p. E_1
- p. endoperoxide
- p. $F_2\alpha$
- p. $F_1\alpha$
- p. F_1 alpha
- p. F_2 alpha
- p. G_2
- p. H_2
- p. I_2
- p. test

prostaglandin-like substance (PLS)
prostanoic acid
prostatectomy
- transurethral p. (TURP)

prostate specific antigen
prostate-specific antigen (PSA)
prostatic
- p. acid phosphatase
- p. adenoma
- p. calculus
- p. hypertrophy (PH)
- p. intraepithelial neoplasia (PIN)
- p. tumor

prostatitic
prostatitis
prostatocystitis
prostatolith
prostatomegaly
prostatovesiculitis
prosthetic group
Prosthogonimus macrorchis
prot
- protein

protactinium
Protac venom
protamine
- p. insulin (PI)
- p. sulfate
- p. sulfate test
- p. titration test
- p. zinc insulin (PZI)

protanomaly
protanopia

Protargol stain
protean
protease
- p. inhibitor (PI)
- lysosomal p.
- slow-moving p. (SMP)

α_1-protease inhibitor (α_1PI)
protection
- radiation p.
- p. test

protective protein
protector
- LATS p.

protein (PR, prot)
- accumulation of p.
- acute phase p.
- acyl carrier p.
- anti-S-100 p.
- antiviral p.
- p. assay
- *bcl*-2 p.
- Bence Jones p. (BJP)
- p. binding (PB)
- p. breakdown
- p. buffer
- p. C
- carrier p.
- catabolite activator p.
- conjugated p.
- copper storage p.
- corticosteroid-binding p.
- C-reactive p. (CRP)
- p. deficiency anemia
- p. denaturation
- derived p.
- dietary p.
- p. efficiency ratio (PER)
- p. electrolyte
- p. electrophoresis
- p. fever
- fibrinolytic p.
- fibrous p.
- foreign p.
- G. p.
- p. gene product (PGP)
- glial fibrillary acidic p. (GFAP)
- globular p.
- heat-shock p.
- HER-2 p.
- HER-2/neu p.
- heterologous p.
- high p. (HP)

NOTES

protein *(continued)*
    p. hydrolysate
    immune p.
    p. induced by vitamin K antagonism (PIVKA)
    integral p.
    intermediate filament p.
    iron-sulfide p.
    Kolmer test with Reiter p. (KRP)
    lenticular p.
    low p. (LP)
    M p.
    macrophage inflammatory p. (MIP)
    membrane p.
    microtubule-associated p. (MAP)
    mild silver p.
    mitotic-control p. (MCP)
    monoclonal p.
    monocyte chemoattractant p.-1 (MCP-1)
    muscle contractile p.
    myelin p.
    myelin basic p. (MBP)
    myeloblastic p.
    myeloma p.
    net dietary p. (NDP)
    neurofilament p.
    neutrophil activating p. (NAP)
    NHC p.
    p. nitrogen unit (PNU)
    nonhistone chromosomal p.
    nonspecific p.
    peripheral p.
    plasma p.
    polyclonal anti-S-100 p.
    protective p.
    p. quotient
    reactive p. (RP)
    respiratory p.
    retinol-binding p. (RBP)
    p. S
    S-100 p.
    p. separation method
    p. shock
    p. shock therapy
    simple p.
    sterol carrier p.
    stress p.
    structural p.
    p. synthesis
    Tamm-Horsfall p.
    p. test
    thyroxine-binding p. (TBP)
    total p. (TP)
    total serum p. (TSP)
    unwinding p.
proteinase
    Bothrops atrox serine p.

    p. K
    Staphylococcus aureus neutral p.
protein-binding
    competitive p. (CPB)
protein-bound
    p.-b. iodine
    p.-b. iodine assay
    p.-b. iodine test
    p.-b. iodine-131 test
protein-calorie malnutrition (PCM)
proteinemia
protein-losing enteropathy
proteinosis
    alveolar p.
    lipid p.
    lipoid p.
    pulmonary alveolar p. (PAP)
proteinuria
    Bence Jones p.
    gestational p.
    isolated p.
    nonisolated p.
    orthostatic p.
    postgamma p. (PGP)
    postural p.
proteoglycan
proteolipid
proteolysis
proteolytic enzyme
Proteomyces
Proteomyxidia
proteose
proteosuria
Proteus
    P. inconstans
    P. mirabilis
    P. morganii
    P. OX-19
    P. rettgeri
    P. stuartii
    P. vulgaris
proteus group
prothoracicotropic hormone
prothrombase
prothrombin (pro)
    p. accelerator
    p. complex
    p. consumption test
    p. consumption time (PCT)
    p. deficiency
    p. and proconvertin test
    p. time (PT)
    p. time test
prothrombinase
prothrombin-converting principle
prothrombinogen
prothrombinopenia
prothrombin-proconvertin (PP)

prothrombokinase
    p. factor
proticity
protic solvent
protime
protirelin
protist
Protista
protistologist
protistology
protium
Protobacterieae
protobe
protobiology
protocol
protocoproporphyria
    p. hereditaria
Protoctista
Protocult test
protodiastolic
protoerythrocyte
protofilament
protogonoplasm
protoleukocyte
protomerite
protometrocyte
proton
    p. acceptor
    p. acid
    p. donor
    p. tautomer
protonephridium
proton-motive hypothesis
proto-oncogene
    bcl-2 p.
protoplasm
protoplasmic
    p. astrocyte
    p. astrocytoma
protoplasmolysis
protoplast fusion
protoporphyria
    erythropoietic p. (EPP)
protoporphyrin (PP)
    p. assay
    erythrocyte p. (EP)
    p. test
protoporphyrinogen oxidase
protoporthyrinuria
protospore
Protostrongylus rufescens

Prototheca
    P. ciferrii
    P. filamenta
    P. segbwema
    P. wickerhamii
    P. zopfii
protothecosis
prototrophic
prototype
Protozoa
protozoa (*pl. of* protozoon)
protozoal
    p. dysentery
protozoan
    p. parasite
protozoiasis
protozoicide
protozoologist
protozoology
protozoon, pl. **protozoa**
protozoophage
protransglutaminase
protriptyline assay
protrude
protrusio acetabuli
protrusion
protuberance
protuberans
    dermatofibrosarcoma p. (DFSP)
    fibrous dysplasia p.
proud flesh
proventriculus
Providencia
    P. alcalifaciens
    P. providenciae
    P. stuartii
provirus
provisional callus
provitamin
provocation typhoid
provocative
    p. chelation test
    p. diagnosis
    p. Wassermann test
Prowazek-Greeff body
Prowazekia
Prower factor
Prower-Stuart factor
proximate
    p. cause
    p. principle

NOTES

P

prozone
  p. phenomenon
  p. reaction
PRP
  pityriasis rubra pilaris
  platelet-rich plasma
PRU
  peripheral resistance unit
prune
  p. belly
  p. belly syndrome
prune-juice
  p.-j. expectoration
  p.-j. sputum
prurigo
  p. nodularis
  p. papule
Prussian
  P. blue
  P. blue stain
prussiate
prussic acid
PS
  periodic syndrome
  phosphatidylserine
  population sample
  Porter-Silber
  pulmonary stenosis
  pyloric stenosis
P/S
  polyunsaturated-to-saturated fatty acids
    ratio
pS2
ps
  per second
  picosecond
PSA
  prostate-specific antigen
psammocarcinoma
Psammolestes
psammoma
  p. body
  Virchow p.
psammomatous
  p. meningioma
psammous
PSC
  Porter-Silber chromogen
  posterior subcapsular cataract
PSD
  peptone-starch-dextrose
PSE
  portal-systemic encephalopathy
psec
Pselaphephilia
pseudacromegaly
pseudalbuminuria
Pseudallescheria boydii

pseudallescheriasis
Pseudamphistomum
  P. truncatum
pseudarthrosis
pseudelminth
pseudinoma
pseudoacanthosis nigricans
pseudoachondroplasia
pseudoachondroplastic spondyloepiphysial
  dysplasia
pseudoacini
pseudoagglutination
pseudo-ainhum
pseudoalbuminuria
pseudoaldosteronism
pseudoallele
pseudoanaphylactic
  p. shock
pseudoanaphylaxis
pseudoanemia
pseudoaneurysm
pseudoangiomatous stromal hyperplasia
  (PASH)
pseudoangiosarcoma
  Masson p.
pseudoarthrosis
pseudobacillus
pseudobacterium
pseudobulbar palsy
pseudocarcinomatous
  p. change
  p. hyperplasia
pseudocartilaginous
pseudocast
pseudocelom
pseudocholesteatoma
pseudocholinesterase
  p. deficiency
pseudochromhidrosis
pseudochylous ascites
pseudocirrhosis
pseudocolloid
  p. of lips
pseudocowpox
  p. virus
pseudocoxalgia
pseudocyesis
pseudocylindroid
pseudocyst
pseudodecidual
pseudodiphtheria
pseudodiploid
pseudodiverticulum
pseudodysentery
pseudoepitheliomatous hyperplasia
pseudoerysipelas
pseudoexfoliation
pseudofollicular proliferation center

pseudo-Gaucher cell
pseudoglanders
pseudoglomerulus
pseudoglucosazone
Pseudogordius
pseudogout
pseudogynecomastia
Pseudohazis
pseudohematuria
pseudohermaphrodism
pseudohermaphroditism
pseudohernia
pseudoheterotopia
pseudohydrocephaly
pseudohydronephrosis
pseudohyperkalemia
pseudohyperparathyroidism
pseudohyperplasia
pseudohypertrophic
pseudohypertrophy
pseudohypha
pseudohyponatremia
pseudohypoparathyroidism (PHP)
pseudoinclusion
    nuclear p.
pseudointraligamentous
pseudoisochromatic
pseudolepromatous leishmaniasis
pseudolipoma
pseudolithiasis
pseudolobule
pseudolymphocyte
pseudolymphocytic choriomeningitis virus
pseudolymphoma
    Spiegler-Fendt p.
    p. of Spiegler-Fendt
pseudolysogenic
    p. strain
pseudolysogeny
pseudomalignancy
pseudomamma
pseudomelanosis
    p. coli
    p. pigment
pseudomembrane
pseudomembranous
    p. acute inflammation
    p. bronchitis
    p. colitis (PMC)
    p. enterocolitis
    p. gastritis
pseudomonad

Pseudomonadaceae
Pseudomonadales
Pseudomonadineae
Pseudomonas
    P. acidovorans
    P. aeruginosa
    P. alcaligenes
    P. cepacia
    P. diminuta
    P. eisenbergii
    P. fluorescens
    P. fragi
    P. kingii
    P. mallei
    P. maltophilia
    P. multivorans
    P. nonliquefaciens
    P. paucimobilis
    P. pseudoalcaligenes
    P. pseudomallei
    P. putida
    P. putrefaciens
    P. pyocyanea
    P. stutzeri
    P. syncyanea
    P. testosteroni
    P. viscosa
Pseudomonilia
pseudomucinous
    p. cyst
    p. cystadenocarcinoma
    p. cystadenoma
    p. degeneration
pseudomycelium
pseudomyiasis
Pseudomyxoma
    P. ovarii
pseudomyxoma
    p. peritonei
pseudoneoplasm
pseudoneuroma
pseudo-osteomalacia
pseudo-osteomalacic
    p. pelvis
pseudoparakeratosis
pseudoparasite
pseudoparenchyma
pseudoperiodic
pseudoperoxidation
    metal-catalyzed p.
pseudophlegmon
    Hamilton p.

NOTES

P

pseudophyllid
Pseudophyllidea
pseudophyllidean
pseudoplatelet
pseudopod
pseudopodium, pl. pseudopodia
pseudopolycythemia
pseudopolydystrophy
pseudopolyp
pseudopolyposis
pseudo-pseudohypoparathyroidism
   (PPHP)
pseudopuberty
   precocious p.
pseudorabies
   p. virus
pseudoreaction
pseudoreplica
pseudorheumatism
pseudorosette
pseudorubella
pseudosarcoma
pseudosarcomatous
   p. fasciitis
   p. myofibroblastic tumor (PMT)
pseudosclerosis
   Jakob-Creutzfeldt p.
   Westphal-Strümpell p.
pseudosmallpox
Pseudostertagia bullosa
pseudostoma, pl. pseudostomas,
   pseudostomata
pseudostratified
pseudothalidomide syndrome
Pseudothelphusa
pseudothrombocytopenia
   EDTA-dependent p.
pseudotrichiniasis
pseudotrichinosis
pseudotruncus arteriosus
pseudotubercle
pseudotuberculosis bacillus
pseudotubular degeneration
pseudotumor
   inflammatory p.
pseudo-Turner syndrome
pseudouridine excretion
pseudovacuole
pseudovariola
pseudovascular
   p. adenoid squamous cell
     carcinoma (PASCC)
   p. adenoid squamous cell
     carcinoma of the lung (PASSCL)
pseudoventricle
pseudoxanthoma
   p. cell
   p. elasticum (PXE)

pseudoxanthomatous transformation
PSFR
   peak secretory flow rate
     PSFR assay
PSGN
   poststreptococcal glomerulonephritis
p.s.i.
   pounds per square inch
psilocin
Psilocybe
psilocybin
psittacosis
   p. inclusion body
   p. titer
   p. virus
psittacosis-lymphogranuloma venereum-
   trachoma (group) (PLT)
psoas abscess
psorelcosis
psorenteritis
Psorergates
psoriasiform dermatitis
psoriasis
   p. arthropica
   exfoliative p.
   generalized pustular p. of
     Zambusch
   pustular p.
   p. vulgaris
psoriatic arthritis
Psorophora
Psoroptes
PSP
   phenolsulfonphthalein
   progressive supranuclear palsy
PSRO
   Professional Standards Review
     Organization
PSS
   physiological saline solution
   progressive systemic sclerosis
PST
   penicillin, streptomycin, and tetracycline
Psychodidae
psychogenic purpura
psychomotor epilepsy
psychosine
psychrophile
psychrophilic bacterium
psyllium hydrophilic mucilloid
PT
   pneumothorax
   prothrombin time
PTA
   persistent truncus arteriosus
   phosphotungstic acid
   plasma thromboplastin antecedent

PTA deficiency
PTA stain
PTAH
phosphotungstic acid hematoxylin
PTAH stain
PTC
phenylthiocarbamoyl
plasma thromboplastin component
PTC deficiency
PTC peptide
PTCL
peripheral T-cell lymphoma
PTE
parathyroid extract
pulmonary thromboembolism
PTED
pulmonary thromboembolic disease
pteridine
pterin
pteroic acid
pteronyssinus
Dermatophagoides p.
pteroylglutamic acid
pteroylpolyglutamate
pterygium
congenital p.
p. syndrome
pterygoid chest
Pterygota
PTF
plasma thromboplastin factor
PTGC
progressive transformation of germinal
centers
PTH
parathormone
parathyroid hormone
posttransfusion hepatitis
PTH assay
pthiriasis
Pthirus
PTHS
parathyroid hormone secretion (rate)
PTI
persistent tolerant infection
PTLD
posttransplant lymphoproliferative
disease
PTLPD
posttransplant lymphoproliferative
disorder

PTM
posttransfusion mononucleosis
ptomaine
ptomainemia
ptomatine
ptosed
ptosis, pl. **ptoses**
ptotic
p. organ
PTR
peripheral total resistance
PTT
partial thromboplastin time
particle transport time
ptyalocele
PU
peptic ulcer
pregnancy urine
puberty
delayed p.
precocious p.
pubic
p. louse
p. tuberosity
public
p. antigen
p. health bacteriology
Puchtler
P. alkaline Congo red method
P. Sirius red method
Puchtler-Sweat
P.-S. stain
P.-S. stain for basement
membranes
P.-S. stain for hemoglobin and
hemosiderin
PUE
pyrexia of unknown etiology
puerperal
p. eclampsia
p. fever
p. mastitis
p. phlebitis
p. septicemia
p. thrombosis
puerperium
PUFA
polyunsaturated fatty acid
puffball
Pulex
P. irritans
pulicicide

NOTES

Pulicidae
Pullularia
    P. pullulans
pullulate
pullulation
pulmolith
pulmonale
    cor p.
pulmonary
    p. adenomatosis
    p. alveolar macrophage (PAM)
    p. alveolar microlithiasis (PAM)
    p. alveolar proteinosis (PAP)
    p. alveolus
    p. angiomyolipoma
    p. arteriovenous fistula (PAF)
    p. artery hypertension (PAH)
    p. artery stenosis (PAS)
    p. aspergillosis
    p. atresia
    p. blastoma
    p. blood flow
    p. bulla
    p. capillary blood volume
    p. congestion
    p. disease (PD)
    p. distomiasis
    p. docimasia
    p. dysmaturity syndrome
    p. edema (PE)
    p. embolism (PE)
    p. emphysema
    p. eosinophilia
    p. fibrosis
    p. fistula
    p. function test
    p. glomangiosis
    p. hamartoma
    p. hemosiderosis
    p. hypertension (PH)
    p. hypostasis
    p. incompetence (PI)
    p. infarct
    p. infarction (PI)
    p. infiltration and eosinophilia (PIE)
    p. insufficiency
    p. interstitial emphysema (PIE)
    p. lymphoid hyperplasia (PLH)
    p. MALT lymphoma
    p. neuroendocrine cell (PNEC)
    p. osteoarthropathy
    p. perfusion
    p. perfusion scan
    p. pleurisy
    p. pneumonitis
    p. pressure
    p. sarcoidosis

    p. stenosis (PS)
    p. surfactant
    p. thromboembolic disease (PTED)
    p. thromboembolism (PTE)
    p. tuberculosis
    p. venous congestion (PVC)
    p. ventilation scan
pulmonitis
pulp
    putrescent p.
pulpar cell
pulpefaction
pulpiform
pulpitis
    putrescent p.
pulsating
    p. empyema
    p. metastasis
pulse
    p. height analyzer (PHA)
    p. pressure
pulsed-field
    p.-f. gel electrophoresis
pulseless disease
pulsellum
pulsion
    p. diverticulum
pultaceous
pump
punch
    p. biopsy
punctate
    p. basophilia
    p. keratoderma
    p. parotiditis
punctiform
punctum
    p. vasculosum
puncture
    femoral p.
    lumbar p.
    percutaneous renal p.
Puntius
PUO
    pyrexia of unknown origin
pupa
pupil
    Adie p.
    Argyll Robertson p.
pupiparous
pure
    p. antiandrogen
    chemically p. (CP)
    p. culture
    p. red cell agenesis (PRCA)
    p. red cell anemia
    p. red cell aplasia (PRCA)

purified
 p. protein derivative (PPD)
 p. protein derivative-standard (PPD-S)
 p. protein derivative of tuberculin
puriform
purine
 p. bodies test
 p. nucleoside phosphorylase
 p. and pyrimidine bases
purinemia
purity
 optical p.
 radiochemical p.
 radionuclidic p.
Purkinje cell
puromucous
purple
 bromcresol p.
 bromocresol p.
purpura
 allergic p.
 anaphylactoid p.
 p. angioneurotica
 p. annularis telangiectodes
 autoimmune thrombocytopenic p.
 fibrinolytic p.
 p. fulminans
 p. hemorrhagica
 Henoch p.
 Henoch-Schönlein p.
 hyperglobulinemic p.
 idiopathic thrombocytopenic p. (ITP)
 immune thrombocytopenic p.
 psychogenic p.
 Schönlein p.
 thrombocytopenic p. (TP)
 thrombotic thrombocytopenic p. (TTP)
 Waldenström p.
purpurea
 Claviceps p.
purpureus
 Rhinoestrus p.
purpuric
purpuriferous
purpurigenous
purpurin
purpurinuria
purpuriparous
Purtscher disease

purulence
purulency
purulent
 p. encephalitis
 p. inflammation
 p. pericarditis
 p. pleurisy
 p. synovitis
purulenta
 thromboarteritis p.
puruloid
pus
 blue p.
 p. cell
 cheesy p.
 p. corpuscle
 curdy p.
 green p.
 ichorous p.
 sanious p.
push-pull amplifier
pustular
 p. bacterid
 p. inflammation
 p. psoriasis
pustule
 malignant p.
 postmortem p.
 spongiform p. of Kogoj
pustulosis
 p. vacciniformis acuta
Putnam-Dana syndrome
putrefaction
putrescent
 p. pulp
 p. pulpitis
putrescentiae
 Tyrophagus p.
putrescine
putrid throat
putty kidney
puzzles
 blood p.
PV
 plasma volume
 polycythemia vera
PVA
 polyvinyl alcohol
 PVA fixative method
 PVA lacto-phenol medium
PVC
 pulmonary venous congestion

NOTES

P

513

PVD
peripheral vascular disease
PVM
pneumonia virus of mice
PVM virus
PVNS
pigmented villonodular synovitis
PVP
peripheral vein plasma
PVT
portal vein thrombosis
PWI
posterior wall infarct
PWM
pokeweed mitogen
Px
pneumothorax
PXA
pleomorphic xanthoastrocytoma
PXE
pseudoxanthoma elasticum
pyarthrosis
pycnomitosis
pyelectasia
pyelectasis
pyelitic
pyelitis
p. cystica
p. glandularis
pyelocaliectasis
pyelocystitis
pyelonephritic kidney
pyelonephritis (PN)
acute p.
ascending p.
chronic p. (CPN)
xanthogranulomatous p.
pyeloureterectasis
pyemia
cryptogenic p.
portal p.
pyemic
p. abscess
p. embolism
Pyemotes tritici
Pyemotidae
pyencephalus
pyesis
pygomelus
pygopagus
pyknodysostosis
pyknomorphous
pyknosis
pyknotic
p. index
Pyle disease
pylemphraxis
pylephlebectasia

pylephlebectasis
pylephlebitis
pylethrombophlebitis
pylethrombosis
pyloric stenosis (PS)
pyloristenosis
pyloritis
pyloroduodenitis
pyloroptosia
pyloroptosis
pylorostenosis
Pym fever
pyocele
pyocelia
pyocephalus
circumscribed p.
external p.
internal p.
pyocin
pyocolpos
pyocyanic
pyocyanin
pyocyanogenic
pyocyanolysin
pyocyst
pyocyte
pyoderma
chancriform p.
p. gangrenosum (PG)
primary p.
secondary p.
p. vegetans
pyodermatitis
pyodermatosis
pyogen
pyogenesis
pyogenetic
pyogenic
p. bacterium
p. fever
p. granuloma
p. infection
p. membrane
p. meningitis
p. osteomyelitis
p. pachymeningitis
p. salpingitis
pyogenous
pyohemia
pyoid
pyometra
pyometritis
pyomyositis
pyonephritis
pyonephrolithiasis
pyonephrosis
pyopericarditis
pyopericardium

pyoperitoneum
pyoperitonitis
pyopoiesis
pyopoietic
pyopyelectasis
pyorrhea
pyosalpinx
pyosemia
pyosepticemia
pyosis
pyospermia
pyostatic
pyothorax
pyothorax-associated lymphoma
pyoureter
pyoverdin
pyoxanthin
pyoxanthose
pyramidal disease
pyran
pyranose
pyranoside
pyrazinamide
Pyrazus
pyrenemia
Pyrenochaeta romeroi
pyrenoid
pyrethrin
pyrethrum
Pyrex
pyrexia
    p. of unknown etiology (PUE)
    p. of unknown origin (PUO)
pyridine
   alum-precipitated p. (APP)
   p. nucleotide
pyridoxal-5'-phosphate
pyridoxamine
4-pyridoxic acid
pyridoxilated stroma-free hemoglobin
  solution
pyridoxine
pyridoxylated hemoglobin-polyoxyethylene
  (PHP)
pyriform
pyriformis
    Tetrahymena p.
pyrimethamine assay
pyrimidine base
pyrogallol
pyrogallolphthalein

pyrogen
pyrogenic
pyroglobulin
pyroglobulinemia
pyroglobulins
pyroglutamase
pyroglutamate hydroxylase
pyroglutamicaciduria
pyrolysis
pyronin
    p. B
    p. G
    p. Y
pyroninophilia
pyrophosphatase
   inorganic p.
pyrophosphate
   inorganic p.
pyrophosphohydrolase
   ATP p.
pyrophosphoric acid
pyroracemic acid
pyrotoxin
pyrrol
    p. blue
    p. blue stain
    p. cell
pyrrole
pyrrolidone carboxylate
pyrroline
   p.-5-carboxylate reductase
   1-p.-5-carboxylate dehydrogenase
pyruvate
   p. carboxylase
   p. kinase
   p. kinase assay
   p. kinase deficiency
pyruvic
   p. acid
   p. acid assay
Pythium insidiosum
pythogenesis
pythogenic
pythogenous
pyuria
PZ
   pancreozymin
PZ-CCK
   pancreozymin-cholecystokinin
PZI
   protamine zinc insulin

NOTES

P

Q

Q
   coulomb
     Q fever
     Q fever titer

Q_{10}
   temperature coefficient

Q_B
   total body clearance

Q-banding stain

QC
   quality control

Q-enzyme

QF
   quality factor

QI
   quality improvement

QNS
   quantity not sufficient

QO_2, qO_2
   oxygen quotient

QP
   quanti-Pirquet reaction

QRZ
   wheal reaction time

quadrant
quadrigeminal
quadriplegia
quadripolar
quadriradial
quadrivalent
quail bronchitis virus
qualitative
   q. analysis
quality
   q. control (QC)
   q. control chart
   q. factor (QF)
   q. improvement (QI)
quanta (*pl. of* quantum)
quantasome
quantile
quantimeter
quanti-Pirquet reaction (QP)
quantitation test
quantitative
   q. analysis
   q. hypertrophy
   q. inheritance
quantity
   not sufficient q. (NSQ)
   q. not sufficient (QNS)
quantotrope
quantum, pl. quanta
   q. limit
   q. yield

Quaranfil virus
quarantine
quark
quartan
   q. fever
   q. malaria
quartile
quartz
quasicontinuous inheritance
quasidiploid
quasidominance
quasidominant inheritance
quaternary
   q. structure
   q. syphilis
Queckenstedt test
quellung
   q. phenomenon
   q. reaction
   q. test
quenching
   fluorescence q.
queue
Quick
   Q. method
   Q. test
QuickVue Chlamydia test
quiet hip disease
quinacrine
   q. banding
   q. chromosome banding stain
   q. hydrochloride
quinaldine red
Quincke
   Q. disease
   Q. edema
quinhydrone
   q. electrode
quinidine assay
quinine
   q. assay
   q. carbacrylic resin
   q. carbacrylic resin test
Quinlan test
quinoline dye
quinolinic acid
quinone
quinovose
Quinquaud disease
quinquevalent
quinsy
quintana
   Bartonella q.

quotidian
> q. fever
> q. malaria

quotient
> albumin q.
> blood q.
> caloric q.
> cerebral glucose oxygen q.
>   (CG/OQ)

circadian q. (CQ)
oxygen q. (QO_2, qO_2)
permeability q. (PQ)
protein q.
rachidean q.
reaction q.
respiratory q.

R

Behnken unit
organic radical
Rankine (scale)
Réaumur scale
regression coefficient
Rinne test
rough
R antigen
R colony
R determinant
R factor
R pilus
R plasmid

2R

chromotrope 2R

R-250

Coomassie brilliant blue R-250

RA

rheumatoid arthritis
RA cell
RA latex fixation test

rabbit

r. antidog-thymus serum (RADTS)
r. antimouse-thymocyte (RAMT)
r. antimouse-thymocyte serum
r. antirat-lymphocyte serum
(RARLS)
r. aorta-contracting substance
r. blood agar
r. fibroma
r. fibroma virus
r. kidney (RK)
r. myxoma virus
r. papilloma
r. plague
r. test

rabbitpox

r. virus

rabid
rabies

r. immune globulin
r. immunoglobulin
r. vaccine
r. vaccine, Flury strain egg-passage
r. virus
r. virus, Flury strain
r. virus, Kelev strain

race
racemase
racemate
racemic

r. mixture
r. modification

racemization

racemose

r. aneurysm
r. hemangioma

rachidean quotient
rachischisis
rachitic

r. pelvis
r. rosary

rachitis

r. fetalis
r. fetalis annularis
r. fetalis micromelica
r. intrauterina
r. uterina

racial
racquet hypha
RAD

right axis deviation

rad

radiation absorbed dose

Radford nomogram
radial

r. aplasia-thrombocytopenia
syndrome
r. growth phase
r. immunodiffusion (RID)
r. scar
r. sclerosing lesion
r. styloid tendovaginitis
r. symmetry

radian
radiant energy
radiation

r. absorbed dose (rad)
r. anemia
β r.
braking r.
r. chimera
r. colitis
r. counter
r. damage
r. dermatitis
r. dermatosis
r. dose
r. effects
electromagnetic r.
general r.
r. hazard
r. injury
ionizing r.
r. measuring unit
r. necrosis
penetrating r.
r. protection

R

radiation *(continued)*
    r. sickness
    ultraviolet r.
radiative capture
radical
    free r.
    organic r. (R)
    r. scavenger
radicular cyst
radiculitis
radiculoganglionitis
radiculomeningomyelitis
radiculomyelopathy
radiculoneuropathy
radiculopathy
radioactive
    r. concentration
    r. constant
    r. decay
    r. drug
    r. equilibrium
    r. iodide uptake test
    r. iodinated human serum albumin (RIHSA)
    r. iodinated serum albumin (RISA)
    r. iodine (^{131}I, RAI)
    r. iodine uptake (RAIU, RIU)
    r. iodine uptake test
    r. probe
    r. waste
radioactivity
radioallergosorbent
    r. assay test (RAST)
    r. test (RAST)
radioassay
    C1q r.
radioautography
radiobiology
radiochemical purity
radiochromatogram
radiodense
radiodensity
radiodermatitis
radioenzymatic assay (REA)
radiography
    body-section r.
    breast specimen r.
    stereoscopic r.
radioimmunoassay (RIA)
    r. automation
    solid-phase r.
radioimmunodiffusion
radioimmunoelectrophoresis
radioimmunoprecipitation
    r. assay
radioimmunosorbent test (RIST)

radioiodinated
    r. fatty acid (RIFA)
    r. serum albumin
radioiodination
    lactoperoxidase r.
radioisotope
radioisotopic
    r. culture
    r. immunoassay
radiolabeled
radioligand assay
radiolysis
radiometer
radionecrosis
radionuclide
radionuclidic purity
radiopaque medium
radiopharmaceutical
radioreceptor assay (RRA)
radioresistant
radioresponsiveness
radiosensitivity test (RST)
radium necrosis
radius
    r. of resolution
    thrombocytopenia with absence of r. (TAR)
    r. of view
radix point
radon
RADTS
    rabbit antidog-thymus serum
RAE
    right atrial enlargement
Raeder paratrigeminal syndrome
RAF
    rheumatoid arthritis factor
raffinose
ragocyte
RAH
    right atrial hypertrophy
RAI
    radioactive iodine
    RAI test
Raillietina
    R. celebensis
    R. demerariensis
raillietiniasis
raised colony
RAIU
    radioactive iodine uptake
Raji
    R. cell
    R. cell line
    R. cell radioimmune assay
RAM
    right anterior measurement
Raman spectroscopy

Rambourg
    R. chromic acid-phosphotungstic
    acid stain
    R. periodic acid-chromic
    methenamine-silver stain
ramex
Ramon flocculation
Ramsay Hunt syndrome
Ramsden eyepiece
RAMT
    rabbit antimouse-thymocyte
rancid
rancidification
rancidity
random
    r. coil
    r. error
    r. genetic drift
    r. mating
    r. number
    r. number generator
    r. plasma glucose test
    r. urine specimen
    r. variable
randomization
random sample
    multiple stage r. s.
    simple r. s.
    stratified r. s.
Rancy nickel
range
    r. of motion (ROM)
    semiinterquartile r.
Ranikhet disease
ranine tumor
rank
    r. correlation coefficient
    r. sum test
ranked data
Ranke formula
Rankine
    R. (scale) (R)
    R. temperature scale
    R. thermometer
Ranson pyridine silver stain
RANTES
    regulated on activation, normal T
    expressed and secreted
    RANTES cycle
ranula
    r. pancreatica
ranular cyst

Ranvier node
Raoult law
rape
rapid
    R. ANA II test
    r. grower
    r. plasma reagin (RPR)
    r. plasma reagin test
    r. recompression -- high pressure
    oxygen (RR-HPO)
rapidly
    r. miscible pool (RMP)
    r. progressive glomerulonephritis
    (RPGN)
rapid-lysis mutation
RapiTex Hp test
Rapoport test
Rappaport classification
rare
    r. base cutters
    R. Donor File
    r. earth element
RARLS
    rabbit antirat-lymphocyte serum
RAS
    renal artery stenosis
rash
    antitoxin r.
    astacoid r.
    black currant r.
    hydatid r.
    Murray Valley r.
    serum r.
Rasmussen aneurysm
RAST
    radioallergosorbent assay test
    radioallergosorbent test
rat
    r. ovarian hyperemia (ROH)
    r. ovarian hyperemia test
    r. tapeworm
    r. thymus antiserum (RATHAS)
    r. unit (RU)
    r. virus (RV)
    Wistar r.
rat-bite
    r.-b. disease
    r.-b. fever
rate
    acid-secretion r.
    adjusted r.
    age-adjusted r.

R

NOTES

rate *(continued)*
- age-specific r.
- aldosterone excretion r. (AER)
- aldosterone secretion r. (ASR)
- aldosterone secretory r. (ASR)
- amebic prevalence r. (APR)
- attack r.
- basal metabolic r. (BMR)
- basal secretory flow r. (BSFR)
- bone formation r. (BFR)
- case fatality r.
- cause-specific death r.
- cerebral cortex perfusion r. (CPR)
- cerebral metabolic r. (CMR)
- circulation r.
- r. constant
- corrected sedimentation r. (CSR)
- cortisol production r. (CPR)
- cortisol secretion r. (CSR)
- count r.
- crude r.
- decay r.
- dose r.
- error r.
- erythrocyte sedimentation r. (ESR)
- failure r.
- flotation r.
- flow r. (FR)
- glomerular filtration r. (GFR)
- incidence r.
- infant mortality r. (IMR)
- intrauterine growth r. (IUGR)
- maximal midflow r. (MMFR)
- metabolic clearance r. (MCR)
- r. meter
- morbidity r.
- mortality r. (MR)
- mutation r.
- peak secretory flow r. (PSFR)
- perinatal mortality r. (PMR)
- pineal secretory r.
- plasma clearance r. (PCR)
- plasma-glucose disappearance r. (PGDR)
- plasma glucose tolerance r. (PGTR)
- plasma iron turnover r. (PITR)
- prevalence r.
- reaction r.
- red cell iron turnover r.
- renin-release r. (RRR)
- Rourke-Ernstein sedimentation r.
- secondary attack r.
- secretion r. (SR)
- sedimentation r. (SR)
- ζ sedimentation r. (ZSR)
- somnolent metabolic r. (SMR)
- specific r.
- standardized r.

- testosterone production r. (TPR)
- Westergren sedimentation r.
- Wintrobe sedimentation r.
- work metabolic r. (WMR)

rate-controlling step

ratellina
- *Grisonella r.*

RATHAS
- rat thymus antiserum

Rathke
- R. cleft cyst
- R. pouch tumor

ratings
- reactivity hazard r.

ratio
- acid-base r. (A/B)
- activity r.
- ADP/ATP r.
- A/G r.
- ALT:AST ratio
- amniotic fluid
  - lecithin/sphingomyelin r.
- amylase-creatinine clearance r.
- AT/GC r.
- base r.
- body hematocrit-venous
  - hematocrit r. (BH/VH)
- bound-free r. (B/F)
- branching r.
- BUN/creatinine r.
- cholesterol-phospholipid r. (C/P)
- common mode rejection r. (CMRR)
- conversion r.
- crude mortality r. (CMR)
- cumulated activity r.
- De Ritis r.
- dextrose-nitrogen r. (DN)
- free T_4 r.
- glucose nitrogen r. (GN)
- granulocyte-erythroid r. (G/E)
- grid r.
- IgG r.'s
- International Normalized R. (INR)
- IRI/G r.
- ketogenic-antiketogenic r.
- lactate-pyruvate r. (L/P)
- lecithin-sphingomyelin r. (L/S)
- lecithin/sphingomyelin r.
- left-to-right r. (L/R)
- L/S
  - lecithin-sphingomyelin ratio
- M:E r.
- mean diameter-thickness r. (MDTR)
- monocyte-lymphocyte r. (M:L)
- myeloid-erythroid r. (M/E)
- net protein r. (NPR)
- nuclear-cytoplasmic r.
- nucleolar-nuclear r.

oil-water r. (O/W)
packing r.
P:O r.
polyunsaturated-to-saturated fatty acids r. (P/S)
proportionate morbidity r. (PMR)
proportionate mortality r. (PMR)
protein efficiency r. (PER)
resin-uptake r. (RUR)
reversed albumin-globulin r.
r. scale
ζ sedimentation r. (ZSR)
selectivity r.
standard morbidity r.
standard mortality r. (SMR)
therapeutic r.
thyroid-to-serum r. (TSR)
T_4:TBG R.
urine-plasma r. (U/P)
rat-tail maggot
Rattus
Rauscher leukemia virus
RAV
Rous-associated virus
ray
β r.
beta r.
cathode r.
corresponding r.
δ r.
delta r.
γ r.
gamma r.
grenz r.
Rayer disease
Raymond-Cestan syndrome
Raynaud
R. disease (RD)
R. phenomenon
RBA
rose bengal antigen
R-banding stain
rbc, RBC
red blood cell
red blood count
RBC/hpf
red blood cells per high power field
RBCM
red blood cell mass
RBCV
red blood cell volume

RBE
relative biological effectiveness
RBL
Reid base line
RBP
retinol-binding protein
RC
red cell
red cell cast
RC circuit
RCBV
regional cerebral blood volume
RCC
red cell count
renal cell carcinoma
RCF
red cell folate
relative centrifugal force
RCM
red cell mass
RCS
reticulum cell sarcoma
RCV
red cell volume
RD
Raynaud disease
reaction of (to) degeneration
resistance determinant
rd
rutherford
RDE
receptor-destroying enzyme
RDI
rupture-delivery interval
rDNA
recombinant DNA
ribosomal DNA
RDS
respiratory distress syndrome
RDW
red cell diameter width
reticulocyte distribution width
RE
regional enteritis
REA
radioenzymatic assay
reabsorb
reabsorption
react
reactance
capacitive r.
inductive r.

R

NOTES

reactant
acute phase r.
limiting r.
reaction
accelerated r.
acid r.
acrosome r.
acute hemolytic transfusion r.
acute phase r.
addition r.
alkaline r.
allergic r.
allergic transfusion r.
alloxan-Schiff r.
amphoteric r.
anamnestic r.
anaphylactic r.
anaphylactic transfusion r.
anaphylactoid r.
anoxia r.
antigen-antibody r.
antigen-antiglobulin r. (AAR)
argentaffin r.
Arias-Stella r.
Arthus r.
Ascoli r.
associative r.
autoimmune r.
azo coupling r.
bacterial transfusion r.
Bauer r.
Bence Jones r.
Berthelot r.
biuret r.
Bloch r.
blocking antibody r.
Bordet and Gengou r.
Burchard-Liebermann r.
capsular precipitation r.
Carr-Price r.
cell-mediated r.
chain r.
Chantemesse r.
chemical r.
cholera-red r.
CHR r.
Christeller r.
chromaffin r.
clot r.
cocarde r.
colloidal gold r.
complement-fixation r.
constitutional r.
contrast media r.
cross r.
cutaneous r.
cytotoxic r.
DAB r.

Dale r.
dark r.
decidual r.
r. of degeneration (DeR, DR)
delayed hemolytic transfusion r.
delayed hypersensitivity r.
depot r.
dermotuberculin r.
diaminobenzidine r.
diazo r.
digitonin r.
Dold r.
dopa r.
early r.
Edman r.
Ehrlich benzaldehyde r.
Ehrlich diazo r.
elimination r.
endergonic r.
endogenous antigen-cell-bound
  antibody r.
endogenous antigen-circulating
  antibody r.
endogenous antigen-transferred
  antibody r.
endogenous antigen-transferred cell-
  bound antibody r.
enthalpy of r.
exergonic r.
false-negative r.
false-positive r.
febrile nonhemolytic transfusion r.
Felix-Weil r. (FWR)
Fernandez r.
ferric chloride r. of epinephrine
Feulgen r.
first-order r.
fixation r.
flocculation r. (FR)
focal r.
foreign body r.
Forssman antigen-antibody r.
Frei-Hoffmann r.
fuchsinophil r.
Fujiwara r.
furfurol r.
gel diffusion r.
Gell and Coombs r.
generalized Sanarelli-Shwartzman r.
  (GSSR)
generalized Shwartzman r. (GSR)
Gerhardt r.
giant cell r.
glycine-arginine r.
graft-versus-host r. (GVHR)
graft-versus-host disease r.
Grimelius argyrophil r.
group r.

Gruber-Widal r.
GVH r.
hemoclastic r.
hemolytic transfusion r.
Henle r.
Herxheimer r.
heterophil antigen r.
hypersensitivity r.
id r.
r. of identity
immediate hypersensitivity r.
immune r.
incompatible blood transfusion r.
inflammatory r.
r. intermediate
intracutaneous r.
intradermal r. (IDR)
iodate r. of epinephrine
iodine r. of epinephrine
irreversible r.
Jaffe r.
Jarisch-Herxheimer r.
Jones-Mote r.
Langhans type of giant cell r.
late r.
lepromin r.
leukemoid r.
Liebermann-Burchard r.
light r. (LR)
local r.
Loewenthal r.
lymphocytic leukemoid r.
Marchi r.
Meinicke turbidity r. (MTR)
miostagmin r.
Mitsuda r.
mixed agglutination r.
mixed lymphocyte r. (MLR)
mixed lymphocyte culture r.
monocytic leukemoid r.
myelocytic leukemoid r.
Nadi r.
Nagler r.
Nessler r.
Neufeld r.
Nickerson-Kveim test r.
ninhydrin-Schiff r.
nitritoid r.
r. of nonidentity
oxidase r.
oxidation-reduction r.
Pandy r.

r. of partial identity
PAS r.
passive Arthus r.
passive cutaneous anaphylactic r.
Paul r.
peracetic acid-Schiff r.
performic acid r.
performic acid-Schiff r. (PFAS)
periodic acid-Schiff r.
Perls r.
peroxidase r.
photochemical r.
Pirquet r.
PK r.
plasmal r.
plasmocytic leukemoid r.
polymerase chain r. (PCR)
Porter-Silber r.
Prausnitz-Küstner r.
precipitin r.
Price precipitation r. (PPR)
primary r.
prozone r.
quanti-Pirquet r. (QP)
quellung r.
r. quotient
r. rate
reagin r.
redox r.
reversed Prausnitz-Küstner r.
reverse transcriptase-polymerase
   chain r. (RT-PCR)
rheumatoid factor r.
Sakaguchi r.
Schmorl r.
Schultz r.
Schultz-Charlton r.
Schultz-Dale r.
second-order r.
serum r.
Shwartzman r.
sigma r. (SR)
skin r.
specific r.
streptococcal toxin immunization r.
substitution r.
symptomatic r.
Szent-Györgyi r.
tetanus toxin immunization r.
thermoprecipitin r.
r. time (RT)
r. of (to) degeneration (RD)

R

NOTES

reaction *(continued)*
    transferred antigen-cell-bound
      antibody r.
    transferred antigen-transferred
      antibody r.
    transfusion r.
    Treponema pallidum
      immobilization r.
    triketohydrindene r.
    tuberculin r.
    tuberculin-type r.
    type III hypersensitivity r.
    typhoid immunization r.
    vaccinoid r.
    Voges-Proskauer r.
    VP r.
    Wassermann r. (WR, Wr)
    Weidel r.
    Weil-Felix r. (WFR)
    Weinberg r.
    wheal-and-erythema r.
    wheal-and-flare r.
    Widal r.
    Yorke autolytic r.
    zero-order r.
    Zimmermann r.
reactivate
reactivation
    dark r.
reactive
    r. astrocyte
    r. cell
    r. eosinophilic pleuritis (REP)
    r. follicular hyperplasia
    r. hyperemia (RH)
    r. hyperemia blood flow (RHBF)
    r. material
    r. protein (RP)
    weakly r. (WR, Wr)
reactivity
    r. hazard ratings
reactone red test
reactor
    biologic false-positive r. (BFR)
readability
reader
    mark sense r.
reading frame
reading-frame-shift mutation
readout
readthrough
reagent
    Bazolyze r.
    Benedict-Hopkins-Cole r.
    Bial r.
    chlorous acid r.
    Cleland r.
    Coleman-Schiff r.

    diazo r.
    Drabkin r.
    Edlefsen r.
    Ehrlich diazo r.
    Eosinofix r.
    Esbach r.
    Folin-Ciocalteu r.
    Fouchet r.
    FPN r.
    Frohn r.
    furfural r.
    Girard r.
    gold chloride r.
    r. grade
    Gram-Sure r.
    Günzberg r.
    Hahn oxine r.
    Hammarsten r.
    Hanker-Yates r.
    HORM collagen r.
    Ilosvay r.
    Kasten fluorescent Schiff r.
    KP1 immunohistochemical r.
    Lloyd r.
    MAK6 immunohistochemical r.
    Mandelin r.
    Marme r.
    Marquis r.
    maximum impurities r.
    Mecke r.
    Millon r.
    Nichols r.
    Paramax r.
    Rosenthaler-Turk r.
    Sanger r.
    Schaer r.
    Scheibler r.
    Schiff r.
    Selivanoff r.
    Sickledex r.
    Stravigen immunohistochemical r.
    r. strip
    Sulkowitch r.
    Vectabond r.
    Vecta-Stain immunohistochemical r.
reagin
    atopic r.
    automated r.
    rapid plasma r. (RPR)
    r. reaction
reaginic
    r. antibody
real
    r. number
    r.-time
real-time clock
reanneal

rearrangement
    bcl-1/PRAD1 gene r.
    breakpoint cluster region r.
    immunoglobulin gene r.
reassociation
    r. of DNA
    DNA r.
Réaumur
    R. scale (R)
    R. thermometer
Rebuck skin window technique
recalcification time
receiver operating characteristic
recent
    r. embolus
    r. infarct
    r. thrombus
receptoma
receptor
    α-adrenergic r.
    β-adrenergic r.
    alpha adrenergic r.
    androgen r.
    antiestrogen r.
    antiprogesterone r.
    B cell antigen r.
    beta adrenergic r.
    cell surface r.
    epidermal growth factor r. (EGFR)
    estradiol r.
    estrogen r. (ER)
    Fc r.
    folic acid r.
    hormone r.
    J r.
    juxtapulmonary-capillary r.
    progesterone r. (PgR, PR)
    r. site
    soluble interleukin-2 r.
    somatostatin r.
    T-cell r. (TCR)
    T cell antigen r.
    X-linked human androgen r.
      (HUMARA)
receptor-destroying enzyme (RDE)
recessive
    r. character
    r. gene
    r. inheritance
recipient

reciprocal
    r. transfusion
    r. translocation
Recklinghausen
    R. disease
    R. disease of bone
    R. disease type I
    R. tumor
Recklinghausen-Applebaum syndrome
Reclus disease
recognition
    antigen r.
    r. factor
recombinant
    r. DNA (rDNA)
    r. strain
    r. vector
recombination
    r. frequency
    genetic r.
    high-frequency r. (Hfr)
    meiotic r.
RecombiPlasTin thromboplastin
recon
record
    logical r.
    medical r.
    physical r.
recorded
    not r. (NR)
recorder
recording
    r. electrode
    r. thermometer
recovery time
recrudescent
    r. typhus
    r. typhus fever
recticulum
    endoplasmic r.
rectification
rectifier
    bridge r.
    full-wave r.
    half-wave r.
    silicon-controlled r.
rectitis
rectocele
rectocolitis
rectolabial fistula
rectostenosis
rectourethral fistula

NOTES

rectovaginal fistula
rectovesical fistula
rectovestibular fistula
rectovulvar fistula
recurrence risk
recurrent
    r. albuminuria
    r. carcinoma
    r. encephalopathy
    r. inflammation
    r. upper respiratory tract infection
    (RURTI)
recurring digital fibromas of childhood
recursion
recursive
    r. definition
    r. subroutine
recurvatum
    pectus r.
red
    alizarin r.
    amidonaphthol r.
    r. atrophy
    Biebrich scarlet r.
    r. blood cell (rbc, RBC)
    r. blood cell cast
    r. blood cell count
    r. blood cell enzyme deficiency
    r. blood cell mass (RBCM)
    r. blood cell morphology
    r. blood cells per high power
    field (RBC/hpf)
    r. blood cell survival
    r. blood cell urinary cast
    r. blood cell volume (RBCV,
    VRBC)
    r. blood count (rbc, RBC)
    brilliant vital r.
    calcium r.
    r. cell (RC)
    r. cell adherence phenomenon
    r. cell adherence test
    r. cell aplasia
    r. cell cast (RC)
    r. cell count (RCC)
    r. cell diameter width (RDW)
    r. cell distribution width
    r. cell folate (RCF)
    r. cell fragility
    r. cell fragmentation syndrome
    r. cell indices
    r. cell iron turnover rate
    r. cell mass (RCM)
    r. cell survival test
    r. cell volume (RCV)
    chlorophenol r.
    chlorphenol r.
    chrome r.

    Congo r.
    r. corpuscle
    cresol r.
    Darrow r.
    r. degeneration
    r. half-moon
    r. hepatization
    r. induration
    r. infarct
    medicinal scarlet r.
    methyl r. (MR)
    r. mite
    neutral r.
    r. oil
    quinaldine r.
    ruthenium r.
    scarlet r.
    scharlach r.
    Sirius r.
    r. squill
    r. thrombus
    toluylene r.
    trypan r.
    turkey r.
    r. venous blood (RVB)
    vital r.
redia
redox
    r. couple
    r. indicator
    r. potential
    r. reaction
reduce
reduced
    r. glutathione (GSH)
    r. hematin
    r. hemoglobin
    r. nicotinamide-adenine dinucleotide
reducing
    r. agent
    r. substances in urine
    r. sugar
reductant
reductase
    acetoacetyl-CoA r.
    cytochrome b_5 r.
    dihydrofolate r. (DHFR)
    dihydropteridine r.
    folate r.
    glutathione r.
    lysine ketoglutarate r.
    lysine-2-oxoglutaryl r.
    methemoglobin r.
    NADH methemoglobin r.
    4-oxoproline r.
    pyrroline-5-carboxylate r.
    L-xylulose r.

reduction
  r. division
  r. potential
  tetrazolium r. (TR)
reduplication
reduvid, reduviid
Reduviidae
Reduvius
redwater disease
Reed-Hodgkin disease
reed relay
Reed-Sternberg cell (RS)
reentrant pathway
Rees culture medium
Rees-Ecker
  R.-E. fluid
  R.-E. method
REF
  renal erythropoietic factor
refect
reference
  common r.
  r. distribution
  r. electrode
  laboratory r. (LR)
  r. material
  r. method
  r. strain
  r. value
Refetoff syndrome
reflecting microscope
reflection
  angle of r.
  diffuse r.
  specular r.
  total internal r.
reflex
  esophagosalivary r.
  parachute r.
  Roger r.
  viscerotrophic r.
reflux
  r. esophagitis
  hepatojugular r.
  vesicoureteral r.
refract
refracting medium
refraction
  angle of r.
  double r.
  index of r.
refractive index (RI)

refractometer
refractory
  r. period (RP)
  r. sideroblastic anemia
Refsum disease
Regan isoenzyme
Regaud fixative
regeneration
  atypical r.
  compensatory r.
  epimorphic r.
  morphallactic r.
regenerative
  r. blood shift
  r. endometrium
  r. micronodularity
  r. polyp
regia
  aqua r.
regina
  Phormia r.
region
  antigen-binding r.
  C r.
    constant region
  complementarity determining r.
  constant r. (C region)
  critical r.
  hinge r.
  homogeneously staining r.
  hypervariable r.
  I r.
  variable r.
regional
  r. cerebral blood volume (RCBV)
  r. colitis
  r. enteritis (RE)
  r. enterocolitis
  r. granulomatous lymphadenitis
  r. ilcitis (RI)
register
  index r.
  shift r.
registry
  tumor r.
Regitine
regressing atypical histiocytosis
regression
  r. coefficient (R)
  r. curve
  least squares r.
  linear r.

NOTES

regressive staining
regulated
    r. area
    r. on activation, normal T
      expressed and secreted (RANTES)
regulation
    genetic r.
    lipolysis r.
regulator
    current r.
    r. gene
    voltage r.
regulatory
    r. albuminuria
    r. gene
    r. sequence
regurgitation
    cardiac valvular r.
    r. jaundice
rehydration
Reichmann
    R. disease
    R. syndrome
Reid
    R. base line (RBL)
    R. index
Reifenstein syndrome
reinfection
    r. tuberculosis
Reinke
    R. crystal
reinnervation
reinoculation
Reinsch test
Reiter
    R. disease
    R. protein complement-fixation
      (RPCF)
    R. protein complement-fixation test
      (RPCFT)
    R. syndrome
    R. test
Reitland-Franklin (unit) (RF)
rejected
    total graft area r. (TGAR)
rejection
    accelerated r.
    acute cellular r.
    allograft r.
    chronic allograft r.
    first-set r.
    first-set graft r.
    graft r.
    homograft r.
    hyperacute r.
    primary r.
    second set r.
    second-set graft r.

rejuvenescence
relapse
relapsing
    r. febrile nodular panniculitis
    r. fever
    r. pancreatitis
    r. perichondritis
    r. polychondritis
relation
    Duane-Hunt r.
    equivalence r.
relationship
    host-parasite r.
relative
    r. biological effectiveness (RBE)
    r. centrifugal force (RCF)
    r. erythrocytosis
    r. fluorescence (RF)
    r. hepatic dullness (RHD)
    r. immunity
    r. leukocytosis
    r. polycythemia
    r. refractory period (RRP)
    r. retention time
    r. sagittal depth (RSD)
    r. sensitivity
    r. specific activity (RSA)
    r. specificity
    r. standard deviation (RSD)
    r. value index (RVI)
relaxin
relay
    mercury-wetted r.
    reed r.
release
    renin r. (RR)
releasing
    r. factor (RF)
    r. hormone (RH)
REM
    reticular erythematous mucinosis
    REM syndrome
remission
    partial r. (PR)
remittent
    r. malaria
    r. malarial fever
remnant
    Cloquet canal r.
    mesonephric r.
    sinus venosus r.
renal
    r. adenocarcinoma
    r. agenesis
    r. amyloidosis
    r. artery stenosis (RAS)
    r. azotemia
    r. blockade

r. calculus
r. carbuncle
r. carcinosarcoma
r. cast
r. cell carcinoma (RCC)
r. colic
r. cortical adenoma
r. cortical necrosis
r. cyst
r. cystic disease
r. diabetes
r. erythropoietic factor (REF)
r. function study (RFS)
r. function test
r. glycosuria
r. hematuria
r. hemorrhage
r. hypertension
r. hypoplasia
r. infarction
r. insufficiency
r. medullary necrosis
r. oncocytoma
r. osteodystrophy
r. papillary necrosis
r. plasma flow (RPF)
r. pressor substance (RPS)
r. threshold
r. threshold for glucose
r. tubular acidosis (RTA)
r. tumor
r. vascular resistance (RVR)
r. vein renin activity (RVRA)
r. vein renin concentration (RVRC)
r. vein thrombosis (RVT)
r. venous renin assay (RVRA)
renaturation
DNA r.
Renaut body
Rendu-Osler-Weber syndrome
Rendu-Weber-Osler disease
renin
r. assay
r. release (RR)
renin-aldosterone axis
renin-angiotensin-aldosterone system
renin-release rate (RRR)
rennin
renomegaly
renovascular hypertension
Renpenning syndrome
Renshaw cell

REO
respiratory enteric orphan
REO virus
Reoviridae
Reovirus
reovirus-like agent
reovirus, types 1, 2, 3
REP
reactive eosinophilic pleuritis
repair
density-dependent r.
DNA r.
fibrous r.
postoperative r.
primary r.
secondary r.
reparative
r. giant cell granuloma
repeat
interspersed r.'s
inverted r.
variable number tandem r.'s (VNTRs)
repeatability
wavelength r.
repeated DNA sequences
reperfusion
repetitive stimulation
replacement
aortic valve r. (AVR)
r. fibrosis
replenisher
replica
r. grating
replicase
replicate
replication
r. cycle
r. fork
r. and transfer (RTF)
replicative form
replicator
replicon
repolarization
repression
catabolite r.
end-product r.
enzyme r.
negative control r.
positive control r.
repressor gene

NOTES

reproducibility
　　photometric r.
reproduction
　　asexual r.
　　sexual r.
reptilase
　　r. fibrin
reptilase-R time
Reptilia
repullulation
repulsion
RES
　　reticuloendothelial system
resazurin
rescue
　　marker r.
resection
　　transurethral r. (TUR)
reserve
　　r. cell
　　r. cell carcinoma
　　r. cell hyperplasia
reservoir
　　chromatin r.
　　r. host
　　r. of infection
　　r. of virus
reset
residual
　　r. abscess
　　r. body
　　r. carcinoma
　　r. urine
residue
　　methanol-extruded r. (MER)
　　spill r.
resin
　　anion-exchange r.
　　cation-exchange r.
　　cholestyramine r.
　　Epon-Araldite r.
　　epoxy r.
　　Harleco synthetic r.
　　ion-exchange r.
　　podophyllin r.
　　polyamine-methylene r.
　　quinine carbacrylic r.
resin-uptake ratio (RUR)
resistance
　　bacteriophage r.
　　cerebrovascular r. (CVR)
　　r. determinant (RD)
　　r. factor
　　insulin r.
　　internal r. (IR)
　　multiple drug r. (MDR)
　　peripheral r. (PR)
　　peripheral total r. (PTR)

　　r. plasmid
　　renal vascular r. (RVR)
　　systemic r. (SR)
　　systemic vascular r. (SVR)
　　r. thermometer
　　total r. (TR)
　　total peripheral r. (TPR)
　　total pulmonary r.
　　total pulmonary vascular r. (TPVR)
　　r. transfer factor (RTF)
　　r. unit (RU)
　　vascular r. (VR)
　　r. to venous return (RVR)
resistance-inducing factor (RIF)
resistance-transferring episome
resistivity
resistor
　　carbon r.
　　carbon-film r.
　　r. color code
　　composition r.
　　power r.
　　precision r.
　　trimming r.
　　variable r.
　　wire-wound r.
resolution
　　energy r.
　　limit of r.
　　radius of r.
　　spectral r.
resolve
resolved
　　not r. (NR)
resolvent
resolving
　　r. power
　　r. time
resonance
　　electron paramagnetic r.
　　electron spin r. (ESR, esr)
　　r. fluorescence
　　r. line
resorcin
resorcin-fuchsin
resorcinol
　　r. phthalic anhydride
　　r. test
resorcinolphthalein
　　r. sodium
resorption
　　bone r.
　　lacunar r.
　　osteoclastic r.
Resource Conservation and Recovery Act
respirator brain

respiratory
- r. acidosis
- r. alkalosis
- r. angiocentric lymphoma
- r. burst
- r. chain
- r. distress syndrome (RDS)
- r. distress syndrome of the newborn
- r. enteric orphan (REO)
- r. enteric orphan virus
- r. exanthematous virus
- r. illness (RI)
- r. infection virus
- r. insufficiency
- r. pigment
- r. protein
- r. quotient
- r. scleroma
- r. syncytial virus (RSV)
- r. syncytial virus antibody test
- r. syncytial virus antigen
- r. syncytial virus antigen test
- r. syncytial virus culture
- r. syncytial virus serology
- r. tract fluid (RTF)
- r. viral disease

respiratory failure
- acute r. f. (ARF)
- chronic r. f.

response
- anamnestic r.
- biphasic r.
- booster r.
- early-phase r.
- galvanic skin r. (GSR)
- R. GM granulocyte count
- host r.
- immune r. (Ir)
- isomorphic r.
- late-phase r.
- lymphoplasmacytic r.
- photomyoclonic r.
- primary immune r.
- reticulocyte r.
- secondary immune r.
- sensitization r. (SR)
- spectral r.
- stringent r.
- total r. (TR)

responsibility
- safety r.

rest
- aberrant r.
- adrenal r.
- cartilaginous r.
- congenital r.
- embryonal r.
- epithelial r.
- Erdheim r.
- Marchand r.
- mesonephric r.
- müllerian r.
- nephrogenic r.
- paramesonephric r.
- Walthard cell r.
- wolffian r.

restiform

resting
- r. cell
- r. membrane potential

restitope

restricted access laboratory

restriction
- r. endonuclease
- r. enzyme
- r. fragment length polymorphism (RFLP)
- r. map
- MHC r.

restrictive

retained
- r. foreign body (RFB)
- r. placental fragment
- r. products of conception
- r. testis

retardation
- growth r.

rete
- r. cell tumor
- r. cyst of ovary
- r. peg
- r. ridges
- r. testis

retention
- r. cyst
- r. index
- r. jaundice
- mucus r.
- r. polyp
- r. time
- r. volume

retic
- reticulocyte

NOTES

reticular
    r. cell
    r. degeneration
    r. erythematous mucinosis (REM)
    r. keratitis
    r. substance
reticulated corpuscle
reticulating colliquation
reticulation
reticulatum
    atrophoderma r.
reticulin
    r. fiber
    r. stain
    r. staining
reticulocyte (retic)
    r. count
    r. distribution width (RDW)
    hemoglobin content of r.'s (HCr)
    r. hemoglobin distribution width (HDW)
    r. mean corpuscular volume (MCVr)
    r. response
    shift r.
    stress r.
reticulocytic
    r. marrow
    r. production index (RPI)
reticulocytopenia
reticulocytosis
reticuloendothelial
    r. cell hyperplasia
    r. sarcoma
    r. system (RES)
reticuloendothelioma
reticuloendotheliosis
    avian r.
    leukemic r.
    systemic r.
reticuloendothelium
reticulohistiocytic granuloma
reticulohistiocytoma
reticulohistiocytosis
    multicentric r.
reticuloid
    actinic r.
reticulopenia
reticulosis
    benign inoculation r.
    histiocytic medullary r.
    leukemic r.
    lipomelanic r.
    medullary histiocytic r.
    midline malignant reticulosis r.
    myeloid r.
    pagetoid r.
    polymorphic r.

reticulotomy
reticulum
    agranular endoplasmic r.
    r. cell
    r. cell hyperplasia
    r. cell lymphosarcoma
    r. cell sarcoma (RCS, RSA)
    granular endoplasmic r.
    sarcoplasmic r.
    r. stain
retinae
    ablatio r.
retinal
    r. anlage tumor
    r. aplasia
    r. detachment
    r. embolism
    r. microaneurysm
retinitis
    r. pigmentosa
    r. proliferans
retinoblastoma
retinoic acid
retinol
retinol-binding protein (RBP)
retinopathy
    circinate r.
    diabetic r. (DR)
retoperithelium
retort
Retortamonas
    R. intestinalis
retothelioma
retractile testis
retraction
    clot r.
    massive vitreous r. (MVR)
retrieval
    information r.
    pancreas antigen r.
retrobulbar
    r. abscess
    r. neuropathy
retrocecal abscess
retrocolic hernia
retroflexion
retrograde
    r. chromatolysis
    r. degeneration
    r. embolism
    r. intussusception
retrolental fibroplasia (RLF)
retromammary mastitis
retroperitoneal
    r. fibromatosis
    r. fibrosis
    r. gas insufflation
retroperitoneum

retroperitonitis
 idiopathic fibrous r.
retropharyngeal abscess
retroplasia
retrospective study
retrosternal hernia
retroversion
retroviral oncogene
Retroviridae
retrovirus
 AKT8 r.
Rettgerella rettgeri
Rett syndrome
return
 resistance to venous r. (RVR)
Reuss
 R. formula
 R. test
revaccination
reverse
 r. agglutination
 r. banding
 r. bias
 r. genetics
 r. grouping
 r. immunoelectrophoresis
 r. mutation
 r. passive hemagglutination
 r. T_3
 r. transcriptase
 r. transcriptase-polymerase chain
  reaction (RT-PCR)
 r. transcription
 r. triiodothyronine (rT_3)
reversed
 r. albumin-globulin ratio
 r. passive anaphylaxis
 r. Prausnitz-Küstner reaction
reversible calcinosis
reversion
revertant
revision
 fusiform skin r. (FSR)
revivescence
revolutions per minute (rpm)
Reye syndrome
Reynold number
RF
 Reitland-Franklin (unit)
 relative fluorescence
 releasing factor

 rheumatic fever
 rheumatoid factor
RFB
 retained foreign body
RFLA
 rheumatoid factor-like activity
RFLP
 restriction fragment length polymorphism
RFS
 renal function study
RH
 reactive hyperemia
 releasing hormone
Rh
 Rhesus factor
 Rh agglutinin
 Rh antigen
 Rh blocking test
 Rh blood group
 Rh factor
 Rh incompatibility
 Rh isoimmunization syndrome
 Rh negative
 Rh null syndrome
 Rh pos
 Rh positive
 Rh type
 Rh typing
rh
 rheumatic
Rhabdiasoidea
Rhabditida
rhabditiform
Rhabditis
 R. hominis
rhabdocyte
rhabdoid
Rhabdomonas
rhabdomyoblast
rhabdomyoblastic
 r. differentiation
rhabdomyolysis
 acute recurrent r.
 familial paroxysmal r.
 idiopathic paroxysmal r.
rhabdomyoma
rhabdomyosarcoma
 alveolar r.
 botryoid r.
 embryonal r.
 r. marker
 pleomorphic r.

R

NOTES

rhabdosarcoma
Rhabdoviridae
rhabdovirus
rhagades
rhagadiform
rhagiocrine vacuole
RHBF
    reactive hyperemia blood flow
RHD
    relative hepatic dullness
    rheumatic heart disease
Rh$_o$(D)
    R. immune globulin
    R. immunoglobulin
    R. typing
rheobase
rheostat
rheostosis
rheotaxis
rheotropism
rhestocythemia
rhesus
    R. factor (Rh)
    R. factor negative (Rh neg)
    R. factor positive
    r. monkey kidney (RMK)
rheum
    rheumatic
rheumatic (rh, rheum)
    r. arteritis
    r. arthralgia
    r. carditis
    r. disease
    r. endocarditis
    r. fever (RF)
    r. heart disease (RHD)
    r. myocarditis
    r. nodule
    r. pericarditis
    r. pneumonia
    r. pneumonitis
    r. valvulitis
rheumatid
rheumatism
    articular r.
    chronic r.
    gonorrheal r.
    inflammatory r.
    Macleod r.
    muscular r.
    nodose r.
    tuberculous r.
rheumatismal
rheumatoid
    r. agglutinator
    r. ankylosing spondylitis
    r. aortitis
    r. arteritis

    r. arthritis (RA)
    r. arthritis factor (RAF)
    r. episcleritis
    r. factor (RF)
    r. factor-like activity (RFLA)
    r. factor reaction
    r. factor test
    r. heart disease
    r. nodule
rhinitis
    acute r.
    allergic .r.
    atrophic r.
    atrophic r. of swine
    fetid r.
    r. nervosa
    vasomotor r. (VMR)
rhinoantritis
Rhinocladiella
Rhinocladium
rhinocleisis
rhinoentomophthoromycosis
rhinoestrosis
Rhinoestrus purpureus
rhinolaryngitis
rhinomucormycosis
rhinomycosis
rhinonasopharyngitis
rhinonecrosis
rhinopharyngitis
    r. mutilans
rhinophycomycosis
rhinophyma
rhinopneumonitis
    equine r. (ERP)
rhinoscleroma
    r. bacillus
rhinosporidiosis
Rhinosporidium seeberi
rhinotracheitis
    feline viral r.
    infectious bovine r. (IBR)
Rhinovirus
rhinovirus
    bovine r.
    equine r.
Rhipicentor
Rhipicephalus
    R. sanguineus
Rhizobiaceae
Rhizobium
Rhizoglyphus
    R. parasiticus
rhizoid
rhizomelia
rhizoplast
Rhizopoda
Rhizopodasida

Rhizopodea
Rhizopus
    R. *arrhizus*
    R. *equinus*
    R. *niger*
    R. *nigricans*
    R. *prolixus*
    R. *rhizopodoformis*
Rh neg
    Rhesus factor negative
rhodamine
    r. B
    r. stain
rhodanate
rhodanic acid
rhodanile blue
rhodanine stain
Rhodesian trypanosomiasis
Rhodnius
Rhodococcus equi
Rhodophyllus sinuatus
Rhodotorula
    R. *mucilaginosa*
    R. *rubra*
rhodotorulosis
rho factor
RhoGAM vaccine
rhombic lip
rhombocele
rhomboidal sinus
Rhombomys
rhopheocytosis
rhoptry
Rhus
    R. toxicodendron antigen
    R. venenata antigen
rhypophagy
rhysodes
    Acanthamoeba r.
rhythm
    circadian r.
    isochronal r.
    metachronal r.
rhytidosis
RI
    refractive index
    regional ileitis
    respiratory illness
RIA
    radioimmunoassay
Ribas-Torres disease
ribavirin

Ribbert theory
riboflavin
    r. assay
    r. loading test
    r. unit
riboflavin-5′-phosphate
ribonuclease (RNase, RNAse)
    r. (pancreatic)
    r. solution
ribonucleic acid (RNA)
ribonucleoprotein (RNP)
    r. complex
    small nuclear r.'s (SNRPs)
ribonucleoside
ribonucleoside-5′-phosphate
    thymine r.
ribonucleotide
riboprobe
    digoxigenin-labeled r.
    EBER1 r.
    U6 r.
ribose
ribose-1-phosphate
ribose-5-phosphate
ribosomal
    r. DNA (rDNA)
    r. RNA (rRNA)
ribosome
ribosome-lamella complex
ribosuria
ribothymidylic acid
ribovirus
ribulose
ribulose-5-phosphate
rice body
rice-flour breath test
rice-Tween agar
Richards-Rundle syndrome
Richet aneurysm
Richter
    R. hernia
    R. syndrome
ricin
ricinoleic acid
rickets
    acute r.
    celiac r.
    hemorrhagic r.
Rickett organism
Rickettsia
    R. *akamushi*
    R. *akari*

R

NOTES

Rickettsia (continued)
  R. *australis*
  R. *burnetii*
  R. *canada*
  R. *conorii*
  R. *diaporica*
  R. *mooseri*
  R. *muricola*
  R. *nipponica*
  R. *orientalis*
  R. *pavlovskii*
  R. *pediculi*
  R. *prowazekii*
  R. *quintana*
  R. *rickettsii*
  R. *sibirica*
  R. *tsutsugamushi*
  R. *typhi*
  R. *wolhynica*
Rickettsiaceae
rickettsiae
rickettsial
rickettsialpox
rickettsia vaccine, attenuated
rickettsiosis
rickettsiostatic
RID
  radial immunodiffusion
Rida virus
Rideal-Walker
  R.-W. coefficient
  R.-W. method
ridge
  interpapillary r.
  rete r.'s
riding embolism
Riechert-Mundiger stereotactic device
Riedel
  R. disease
  R. struma
  R. thyroiditis
Rieder
  R. cell
  R. cell leukemia
  R. lymphocyte
Rieger syndrome
Riehl melanosis
RIF
  resistance-inducing factor
RIFA
  radioiodinated fatty acid
rifamide
rifampicin
rifampin
rifamycin, rifomycin
Rift
  R. Valley fever
  R. Valley fever virus

Riga-Fede disease
Rigg disease
right
  r. anterior measurement (RAM)
  r. atrial enlargement (RAE)
  r. atrial hypertrophy (RAH)
  r. axis deviation (RAD)
  r. ovarian vein syndrome
  r. ventricular enlargement (RVE)
  r. ventricular hypertrophy (RVH)
  r. ventricular hypoplasia
right-handed
  r.-h. alpha helix
  r.-h. α-helix
right-to-know law
rigidity
  decerebrate r.
  lead-pipe r.
  muscular r.
  nuchal r.
rigor
  r. mortis
rigorous
RIHSA
  radioactive iodinated human serum
  albumin
Riley-Day syndrome
Riley-Smith syndrome
Rimini test
rinderpest
  r. virus
Rindfleisch cell
ring
  aromatic r.
  Balbiani r.
  Bandl r.
  Biondi r.
  r. chromosome
  contractile r.
  corrin r.
  r. counter
  Kayser-Fleischer r.
  Liesegang r.
  r. precipitin test
  Schatzki r.
  signet r.
  vascular r.
  Waldeyer r.
ring-chain tautomer
Ringer
  R. lactate solution (RLS)
  R. solution
ring-wall lesion
ringworm
  r. of beard
  black-dot r.
  r. of body
  crusted r.

r. of foot
r. of genitocrural region
gray-patch r.
honeycomb r.
r. of nails
Oriental r.
r. of scalp
scaly r.
Tokelau r.
Rinne test (R)
Rio-rad protein assay
ripening
ripple
r. counter
r. factor
r. voltage
RISA
radioactive iodinated serum albumin
RISA test
risk
r. factor
recurrence r.
RIST
radioimmunosorbent test
ristocetin cofactor
Ritter disease
Ritter-Oleson (RO)
R. technique
RIU
radioactive iodine uptake
riziform
RK
rabbit kidney
RLF
retrolental fibroplasia
RLS
Ringer lactate solution
RMK
rhesus monkey kidney
RMP
rapidly miscible pool
RMSF
Rocky Mountain spotted fever
RNA
ribonucleic acid
chromosomal RNA (cRNA)
heterogeneous nuclear RNA (hnRNA)
RNA nucleotidyltransferase
RNA polymerase
RNA processing
ribosomal RNA (rRNA)

transfer RNA (tRNA)
translation control RNA (tcRNA)
RNA tumor virus
RNAase
RNA-driven hybridization
RNA-RNA hybridization
RNase, RNAse
ribonuclease
RNase A
alkaline RNase
RNase I
pancreatic RNase
RNA-zolB RNA extraction method
RNP
ribonucleoproptcin
RNP complex
RO
Ritter-Oleson
Roaf syndrome
robertsonian translocation
Roberts syndrome
Robinow syndrome
Robinson disease
Robin syndrome
Roble disease
Robson
R. stage I, II renal carcinoma
robust
robustness
ROC
roccellin
Rochalimaea
R. henselae
R. quintana
Roche Septi-Chek blood culture system
rocker microtome
rocket immunoelectrophoresis
Rocky
R. Mountain spotted fever (RMSF)
R. Mountain spotted fever antibody test
R. Mountain spotted fever serology
R. Mountain spotted fever vaccine
rod
Auer r.
r. myopathy
r. neutrophil
rodenticide
rodent ulcer
Rodrigues aneurysm
rod-shaped
roentgen

NOTES

roetheln
Roger
>R. disease
>maladie de R.
>R. reflex
>R. syndrome

ROH
>rat ovarian hyperemia

Rokitansky
>R. disease
>R. pelvis

Rokitansky-Aschoff sinus
Rokitansky-Küster-Hauser syndrome
rolandic epilepsy
roll
>iliac r.
>r. tube

Rollet stroma
roll-tube technique
ROM
>range of motion
>rupture of membranes

Romaña sign
Romano-Ward syndrome
Romanowsky blood stain
Romberg
>R. disease
>R. syndrome
>R. trophoneurosis

romeroi
>*Pyrenochaeta r.*

Römer test
ronds
>corps r.

ronnel
room
>cold r.
>r. temperature

root-mean-square
ropalocytosis
Ropes test
rosacea
>acne r.

rosacea-like tuberculid
Rosai-Dorfman disease
rosanilin
>r. dye

rosaniline
rosary
>rachitic r.

rosati
>*Neotestudina r.*

rose
>r. bengal
>r. bengal antigen (RBA)
>r. bengal radioactive (^{131}I) test
>r. bengal sodium

>r. cold
>R. test

rosea
>pityriasis r.

Rose-Bradford kidney
Rosenbach
>R. disease
>R. syndrome
>R. test

Rosenbach-Gmelin test
Rosenow veal-brain broth
Rosenthal
>R. fiber
>R. syndrome

Rosenthaler-Turk reagent
Rosenthal-Kloepfer syndrome
roseola
>epidemic r.
>r. infantilis
>r. infantum virus
>r. vaccination

rosette
>E r.
>EAC r.
>erythrocyte r.
>Homer-Wright r.
>malarial r.
>r. test

rosette-forming cell
Rose-Waaler test
Rosewater syndrome
p-rosolic acid
Ross
>R. River fever
>R. River virus

Rossbach disease
Ross-Jones test
rostellum
rostrate pelvis
rotamer
rotary microtome
rotation
>axis of r.
>optical r.
>specific r.

rotavirus
>r. serology

Rotazyme test
röteln
rotenone
Roth
>R. disease
>R. syndrome

Roth-Bernhardt
>R.-B. disease
>R.-B. syndrome

Rothera nitroprusside test
Rothmann-Makai syndrome

R

Rothmund syndrome
Rothmund-Thomson syndrome
Rotor syndrome
Rotter
    R. syndrome
    R. test
rot value
Rouget
    R. cell
    R. pericyte
rough (R)
    r. bacterium
    r. colony
    r. determinant
    r. factor
    r. plasmid
rough-smooth variation
Roughton-Scholander
    R.-S. apparatus
    R.-S. syringe
Rougnon-Heberden disease
rouleau, pl. **rouleaux**
    rouleaux formation
round
    r. atelectasis
    r. cell sarcoma
rounding
roundworm
Rourke-Ernstein sedimentation rate
Rous
    R. sarcoma
    R. sarcoma virus (RSV)
    R. test
    R. tumor
Rous-associated virus (RAV)
Roussy-Dejerine syndrome
Roussy-Lévy
    R.-L. disease
    R.-L. syndrome
routine
    r. test dilution (RTD)
    trace r.
Roux
    R. bottle
    R. spatula
    R. stain
Rovsing syndrome
Rowntree and Geraghty test
RP
    reactive protein
    refractory period

RPCF
    Reiter protein complement-fixation
RPCFT
    Reiter protein complement-fixation test
RPF
    renal plasma flow
RPGN
    rapidly progressive glomerulonephritis
RPI
    reticulocytic production index
rpm
    revolutions per minute
RPR
    rapid plasma reagin
        RPR test
RPS
    renal pressor substance
RR
    renin release
RRA
    radioreceptor assay
RR-HPO
    rapid recompression -- high pressure
      oxygen
rRNA
    ribosomal RNA
RRP
    relative refractory period
RRR
    renin-release rate
RS
    Reed-Sternberg cell
RSA
    relative specific activity
    reticulum cell sarcoma
RSD
    relative sagittal depth
    relative standard deviation
RST
    radiosensitivity test
RSV
    respiratory syncytial virus
    Rous sarcoma virus
        RSV culture
R-S variation
Rs virus
RT
    reaction time
rT$_3$
    reverse triiodothyronine
RTA
    renal tubular acidosis

NOTES

RTD
    routine test dilution
RTF
    replication and transfer
    resistance transfer factor
    respiratory tract fluid
RT-PCR
    reverse transcriptase-polymerase chain
      reaction
RU
    rat unit
    resistance unit
rub
    pericardial friction r.
    pleural friction r.
Rubarth
    R. disease
    R. disease virus
rubber
    r. pelvis
    r. policeman
rubeanic acid
rubella
    r. antibody test
    congenital r. syndrome
    r. HI test
    r. serology
    r. virus (RV)
    r. virus culture
    r. virus vaccine, live
rubeola
    r. serology
    r. virus
rubescent
rubidomycin
rubidus
    Hyostrongylus r.
rubine
rubin S
Rubinstein syndrome
Rubinstein-Taybi syndrome
Rubin test
Rubivirus
rubivirus
Rubner test
rubor
rubra
    miliaria r.
    trichomycosis r.
rubratoxin
rubredoxin
rubriblast
    pernicious anemia type r.
rubricyte
    polychromatophilic r.
rubrum
    r. Congo
    r. scarlatinum

ruby spot
rudimentary
    r. finger
    r. lung
    r. structure
    r. testis syndrome
Rud syndrome
rufescens
    Protostrongylus r.
Ruge solution
rule
    Clark r.
    Goriaew r.
ruminantium
    Cowdria r.
Rummo disease
rump
    crown r. (CR)
Rumpel-Leede test
Rundles-Falls syndrome
Runeberg formula
runt disease
runting syndrome
Runyon classification
rupture
    inflammatory r.
    r. of membranes (ROM)
    premature r.
ruptured
    r. aneurysm
    r. ectopic pregnancy
    r. myocardial infarct
    r. umbilical cord
rupture-delivery interval (RDI)
RUR
    resin-uptake ratio
RURTI
    recurrent upper respiratory tract infection
Rushton body
Russell
    R. body
    R. syndrome
    R. unit
    R. viper
    R. viper venom
    R. viper venom clotting time
Russell-Crooke cell
Russian
    R. autumn encephalitis
    R. autumn encephalitis virus
    R. spring-summer encephalitis
      (Eastern subtype)
    R. spring-summer encephalitis virus
    R. spring-summer encephalitis
      (Western subtype)
    R. tick-borne encephalitis
Russula emetica

Rust
    R. disease
    R. syndrome
rusts
rusty sputum
ruthenium red
rutherford (rd)
Rutherford scattering
rutidosis
Ruysch disease
RV
    rat virus
    rubella virus
      RV time
RVB
    red venous blood
RVE
    right ventricular enlargement

RVH
    right ventricular hypertrophy
RVI
    relative value index
RVR
    renal vascular resistance
    resistance to venous return
RVRA
    renal vein renin activity
    renal venous renin assay
RVRC
    renal vein renin concentration
RVT
    renal vein thrombosis
Rye classification

R

NOTES

S
serum
smooth
soluble
sulfur
supravergence
Svedberg unit
Svedberg unit of sedimentation
  coefficient
    S antigen
    S colony
    S phase
    S unit of streptomycin
S-100
    S. antibody
    S. marker
    S. protein
    S. protein antigen
s
second
SA
sarcoma
secondary amenorrhea
secondary anemia
serum albumin
Stokes-Adams
    SA node
SAB
significant asymptomatic bacteriuria
s-ABC peroxidase
saber
    s. shin
    s. tibia
Sabethes
Sabhi agar
Sabin-Feldman
    S.-F. dye test
    S.-F. syndrome
Sabin vaccine
sabot
    coeur en s.
Sabouraud dextrose and brain heart
  infusion agar
sabulous
sac
    aneurysmal s.
sacbrood
saccaromyces
    Busse s.
saccharase
saccharephidrosis
saccharic acid
saccharin
saccharoid
saccharometer

Saccharomonospora viridis
Saccharomyces
    S. albicans
    S. anginae
    S. apiculatus
    S. cantliei
    S. capillitii
    S. carlsbergensis
    S. cerevisiae
    S. coprogenus
    S. epidermica
    S. galacticolus
    S. glutinis
    S. hominis
    S. lemonnieri
    S. mellis
    S. mycoderma
    S. neoformans
    S. pastorianus
Saccharomycetaceae
Saccharomycetales
saccharomycosis
L-saccharopine
saccharopine dehydrogenase
saccharopinuria
Saccharopolyspora rectivirgula
saccharorrhea
saccharosuria
Saccomanno fixative
saccular
    s. aneurysm
    s. bronchiectasis
sacculated
    s. aneurysm
    s. pleurisy
SACD
    subacute combined degeneration
Sachs disease
Sachs-Georgi (S-G)
    S. test
saddle embolism
Saenger macula
Saethre-Chotzen syndrome
safety
    s. glasses
    s. program
    s. responsibility
    s. shower
safflower oil
safranin O
safranophil, safranophile
SAG
    Swiss-type agammaglobulinemia
sagitta
    Dipus s.

S

sago spleen
SAH
    subarachnoid hemorrhage
Sahli method
sailor's skin
Saint Anthony fire
Sakaguchi reaction
Sakamoto poorly differentiated
  carcinoma
Saksenaea
salicylamide
salicylate
    s. assay
    s. level
    physostigmine s.
salicylic
    s. acid
    s. acid test
salicylism
salicylsalicylic acid
salicylsulfonic acid
salicyluric acid
salimeter
saline
    s. agglutination test
    s. agglutinin
    phosphate buffered s. (PBS)
    s. solution
    s. technique
salinometer
Salisbury common cold virus
saliva
salivary
    s. amylase
    s. calculus
    s. corpuscle
    s. gland anlage tumor (SGAT)
    s. gland tumor
    s. gland virus (SGV)
    s. gland virus disease
    s. virus
Salk vaccine
salmincola
    Nanophyetus s.
    Troglotrema s.
Salmonella
    S. arizonae
    S. cholerae-suis
    S. derby
    S. enteritidis
    S. enteritidis serotype *agona*
    S. enteritidis serotype *heidelberg*
    S. enteritidis serotype *hirschfeldii*
    S. enteritidis serotype *infantis*
    S. enteritidis serotype *montevideo*
    S. enteritidis serotype *newport*
    S. enteritidis serotype *paratyphi A*
    S. enteritidis serotype *schottmülleri*

    S. enteritidis serotype *typhimurium*
    S. gallinarum
    S. hirschfeldii
    S. indiana
    S. infantis
    S. minnesota
    S. montevideo
    S. muenchen
    S. newington
    S. oranienburg
    S. paratyphi
    S. schottülleri
    S. sendai
    S. thompson
    S. titer
    S. typhi
    S. typhimurium
    S. typhisuis
    S. typhosa
    S. virginia
salmonella, pl. salmonellae
    s. agglutinin
    s. group
    s. poisoning
Salmonella-Shigella (SS)
Salmonella-Shigella agar
salmonellosis
salmon patch
salpingioma
salpingitis
    chronic interstitial s.
    follicular s.
    foreign body s.
    gonorrheal s.
    s. isthmica nodosa
    pyogenic s.
salpingo-oophoritis
salpingoperitonitis
salsalate
salt
    s. agglutination
    s. antagonism
    bile s.'s
    s. bridge
    diazonium s.
    s. dye
    hexazonium s.'s
    s. loading
    s. sensitivity
    tetrazonium s.
saltation
Saltatoria
saltatory
    s. conduction
salted
    s. plasma
    s. serum
salting-in

salting-out
salt-losing crisis
saluresis
saluretic
salvage therapy
salvarsanized serum
Salvia
    S. horminium
    S. sclarea
Salzman method
SAM
    sulfated acid mucopolysaccharide
samarium
sample
    s. distribution
    s. interaction
    population s. (PS)
    random s.
    s. steady state
sampler
sampling
    chorionic villus s. (CVS)
San
    S. Joaquin fever
    S. Joaquin Valley fever
    S. Miguel sea lion virus
Sanarelli phenomenon
Sanarelli-Shwartzman phenomenon (SSP)
Sanchez Salorio syndrome
sand
    s. body
    brain s.
    s. granule
    intestinal s.
    s. tumor
    urinary s.
sandal foot
sandalwood oil
Sanders disease
sandfly
    s. fever
    s. fever virus
Sandhoff disease
sandpaper gallbladder
sandworm
Sanfilippo syndrome
Sanford test
Sanger reagent
sanguifacient
sanguiferous
sanguification

sanguinarius
    mycetismus s.
sanguineous
    s. cyst
    s. infiltration
sanguinolent
sanguinopurulent
sanguis
Sanguisuga
sanguivorous
    s. myiasis
sanies
saniopurulent
sanioserous
sanious
    s. pus
sanitary bacteriology
sanitization
santal oil
santonin
SAP
    scrum alkaline phosphatase
    systemic arterial pressure
sap
    cell s.
saponifiable fraction
saponification
saponin
    hemolysin s.
    steroid s.
    triterpenoid s.
Sappinea
    S. diploidea
sapremia
saprobe
saprobic
saprogen
saprogenic
sapronosis
saprophilous
saprophyte
saprophytic
Saprospira
saprozoic
saprozoonosis
saramycetin
Sarcina
sarcina
sarcocele
sarcocyst
sarcocystin
Sarcocystis

NOTES

sarcocystosis
sarcocyte
sarcode
Sarcodina
sarcogenic cell
sarcoid
    Boeck s.
    s. granuloma
    granuloma s.
    Spiegler-Fendt s.
sarcoidal granuloma
sarcoidosis
    hypercalcemic s.
    pulmonary s.
sarcolemma
sarcoma (SA)
    alveolar soft part s.
    ameloblastic s.
    angiolithic s.
    avian s.
    botryoid s.
    s. botryoides
    cerebellar s.
    clear cell s.
    endometrial stromal s. (ESS)
    endothelial s.
    epithelioid s.
    Ewing s. (ES)
    fascicular s.
    follicular dendritic cell s.
    giant cell s.
    giant cell monstrocellular s. of
      Zülch
    granulocytic s.
    hemangioendothelial s.
    Hodgkin s.
    immunoblastic s.
    Jensen s.
    juxtacortical osteogenic s.
    Kaposi s.
    Kupffer cell s.
    leukocytic s.
    lymphangioendothelial s.
    lymphatic s.
    lymphosarcoma-reticulum cell s.
      (LSA/RCS)
    mast cell s.
    medullary s.
    meningeal s.
    mesothelial s.
    multiple idiopathic hemorrhagic s.
    myelogenic s.
    myeloid s.
    neurogenic s.
    osteogenic s.
    periosteal s.
    reticuloendothelial s.
    reticulum cell s. (RCS, RSA)

    round cell s.
    Rous s.
    small cell s.
    spindle cell s.
    stromal s.
    synovial s.
    telangiectatic osteogenic s.
    undifferentiated s.
Sarcomastigophora
sarcomata, pl. sarcomas, sarcomata
sarcomatoid
    s. carcinoma
    s. mesothelioma
sarcomatosis
    meningeal s.
sarcomatous
sarcomere
sarcomeric actin
sarconeme
Sarcophaga
    S. carnaria
    S. dux
    S. fuscicauda
    S. haemorrhoidalis
    S. nificornis
    S. rubicornis
Sarcophagidae
sarcoplasm
sarcoplasmic reticulum
Sarcopsylla penetrans
Sarcopsyllidae
Sarcoptes scabiei
sarcoptic
    s. mange
sarcoptid
Sarcoptidae
sarcoptidosis
sarcosine dehydrogenase
sarcosinemia
sarcosis
Sarcosporidia
sarcosporidiosis
sarcostosis
sarcotic
SART
    standard acid reflux test
SAS
    supravalvular aortic stenosis
sat
    saturated
satellite
    s. abscess
    s. colony
    s. metastasis
satellitosis
saturated (sat)
    ambient temperature and
      pressure, s. (ATPS)

body temperature, ambient
pressure, s. (BTPS)
s. fatty acid
s. hydrocarbon
s. solution (SS)
s. solution of potasium iodide
(SSKI)
saturation
s. analysis
s. current
s. hybridization
s. index (SI)
s. limit
oxygen s.
transferrin s.
saturnina
arthralgia s.
saturnine
s. encephalopathy
s. gout
Saundby test
Saunders disease
sauriasis
sauriderma
sauriosis
sauroderma
sausage finger
Savill disease
sawtooth wave
saxitoxin
SB
serum bilirubin
SBE
subacute bacterial endocarditis
SBF
splanchnic blood flow
SBTI
soybean trypsin inhibitor
SC
sickle cell
subcutaneous
scabby mouth
scabiei
Sarcoptes s.
scabies
scalar product
scalded skin syndrome (SSS)
scale
absolute temperature s.
Baumé s. (B)
Benoist s. (B)
Celsius temperature s. (C)

centigrade s.
centigrade temperature s. (C)
customary temperature s.
Fahrenheit temperature s. (F)
full s.
Gaffky s.
gray s.
Hamilton Rating S. (HRS)
hydrometer s.
interval s.
Kelvin temperature s.
Rankine temperature s.
ratio s.
Réaumur s. (R)
scalene node biopsy (SNB)
scalenus anticus syndrome
scaler
scaler-timer
scalloping
scalp contusion
scaly ringworm
scan
bone marrow s.
dot s.
fluorescence-activated cell sorter s.
(FACscan)
gallium s.
s. information density
pulmonary perfusion s.
pulmonary ventilation s.
scandium
scanner
scanning
s. electron microscope (SEM)
s. sequence
scaphohydrocephalus
scaphoid facies
scar
s. cancer
s. carcinoma
cigarette-paper s.
hypertrophic s.
papyraceous s.
radial s.
scarabiasis
**Scarff-Bloom-Richardson tumor grading
system**
scarification test
scarlatina
anginose s.
s. hemorrhagica
s. latens

S

NOTES

549

scarlatina *(continued)*
  s. maligna
  s. rheumatica
  s. simplex
scarlatinal
  s. nephritis
scarlatinella
scarlatiniform
scarlatinoid
scarlatinum
  rubrum s.
scarlet
  Biebrich s.
  s. fever (SF)
  s. fever antitoxin
  s. fever erythrogenic toxin
  s. red
  s. red stain
  s. red sulfonate
  water-soluble s.
SCAT
  sheep cell agglutination test
Scatchard
  S. equation
  S. plot
scatemia
scatologic
scatology
scatoma
scatophagy
scatoscopy
scatter diagram
scattergram
scattering
  elastic s.
  inelastic s.
  Rutherford s.
scatterplot
Scaurus
scavenger
  s. cell
  radical s.
SCC
  squamous cell carcinoma
S-CCK-Pz test
SCD
  subacute combined degeneration (of
    spinal cord)
  sudden cardiac death
  sudden coronary death
Scedosporium apiospermum
SCG
  serum chemistry graft
Schaedler blood agar
Schaeffer-Fulton stain
Schaer reagent
Schafer syndrome
Schaffer test

**Schales and Schales method for
  chloride**
Schallibaum solution
Schamberg
  S. dermatitis
  S. disease
Schanz
  S. disease
  S. syndrome
scharlach red
Schatzki ring
Schaudinn fixative
Schaumann
  S. body
  S. disease
  S. lymphogranuloma
  S. syndrome
Scheibler reagent
Scheie syndrome
Scheloribates
schematic
scheme
  decay s.
  Facklam classification s.
Schenck disease
Scheuermann disease
Schick
  S. method
  S. test
  S. test toxin
Schiff
  S. base
  S. reagent
  S. stain
Schilder disease
Schiller test
Schilling
  S. blood count
  S. index
  S. test
  S. type of monocytic leukemia
Schimmelbusch disease
Schirmer
  S. syndrome
  S. test
schistocelia
schistocystis
schistocyte
schistocytosis
schistorrhachis
Schistosoma
  S. haematobium
  S. intercalatum
  S. japonicum
  S. mansoni
Schistosomatidae
Schistosomatoidea

schistosome
    s. granuloma
schistosomiasis
    s. serological test
schistosomicidal
schistosomicide
schistosomulum
schizencephalic microcephaly
schizencephaly
Schizoblastosporion
schizocyte
schizocytosis
schizogenesis
schizogony
schizogyria
schizomycete
Schizomycetes
schizont
schizonticide
Schizophora
Schizophyllum commune
Schizosaccharomyces
schizotonia
Schizotrypanum cruzi
schizozoite
Schlatter disease
Schlatter-Osgood disease
Schmid-Fraccaro syndrome
Schmidt syndrome
Schmitz bacillus
Schmorl
    S. bacillus
    S. disease
    S. ferric-ferricyanide reduction stain
    S. nodule
    S. picrothionin stain
    S. reaction
Schneider carmine
schneideri
    Elaeophora s.
Scholz disease
Schönbein test
Schönlein
    S. disease
    S. purpura
Schönlein-Henoch disease
Schottmüller disease
Schridde
    S. cancer hairs
    S. syndrome

Schroeder
    S. disease
    S. syndrome
Schüffner
    S. dots
    S. granule
Schüller
    S. disease
    S. syndrome
Schüller-Christian
    S.-C. disease
    S.-C. syndrome
Schultz
    S. disease
    S. reaction
    S. stain
    S. syndrome
Schultz-Charlton
    S.-C. phenomenon
    S.-C. reaction
Schultz-Dale
    S.-D. reaction
    S.-D. test
Schumm test
Schwann cell
schwannian
schwannoma
    acoustic s.
    cellular s.
    malignant s.
    plexiform s.
schwannosis
Schwartz
    S. syndrome
Schwarz test
Schweninger-Buzzi
    S.-B. anetoderma
    S.-B. disease
Schweninger-Buzzi disease
sciatica
SCID
    severe combined immunodeficiency
    SCID mice
scientific notation
scimitar sign
scintillation
    s. camera
    s. count
    s. counter
    s. crystal
    s. technique

S

NOTES

scintillator
    liquid s.
scirrhosity
scirrhous
    s. carcinoma
scirrhus
SCIS
    surface carcinoma in situ
scissiparity
SCK
    serum creatine kinase
SCLC
    small cell lung carcinoma
scleradenitis
scleratogenous
scleredema
    s. adultorum
sclerema
    s. adiposum
    s. neonatorum
sclerencephaly
scleriasis
scleroatrophy
sclerodactyly
scleroderma
    localized s.
scleroderma antibody
sclerodermatitis
sclerodermatous
sclerogenic
sclerogenous
scleroid
scleroma
    respiratory s.
scleromalacia
scleromyxedema
sclero-oophoritis
sclerosal
sclerose
sclerosing
    s. adenosis
    s. cholangitis
    s. hemangioma
    s. hyaline necrosis
    s. inflammation
    s. keratitis
    s. osteitis
    s. sinusitis
sclerosis, pl. scleroses
    Alzheimer s.
    amyotrophic lateral s. (ALS)
    arterial s.
    arteriocapillary s.
    arteriolar s.
    bone s.
    Canavan s.
    cardiac s.
    combined s.

    s. corii
    s. cutanea
    diffuse infantile familial s.
    disseminated s.
    endocardial s.
    glomerular s.
    hippocampal s.
    hyaline s.
    idiopathic hypercalcemic s. of infants
    insular s.
    laminar cortical s.
    lobar s.
    mantle s.
    menstrual s.
    Mönckeberg medial calcific s.
    multiple s. (MS)
    nodular s.
    ovulational s.
    physiologic s.
    posterior spinal s.
    primary endocardial s.
    progressive systemic s. (PSS)
    subacute combined s.
    systemic s.
    tuberous s.
    unicellular s.
    vascular s.
    s. of white matter
sclerostenosis
Sclerostoma
sclerotic
    s. body
    s. gastritis
    s. kidney
    s. stomach
sclerotica
    otitis s.
sclerotium
sclerotylosis
sclerous
scoleces (*pl. of* scolex)
scoleciasis
scoleciform
scolecoid
scolecology
scolex, pl. scoleces
scoliotic pelvis
Scolopendra
scombroid poisoning
scop
    scopolamine
scopolamine (scop)
scopometer
Scopulariopsis
    S. americana
    S. aureus
    S. blochi

S. brevicaulis
S. cinereus
S. koningi
S. minimus
scopulariopsosis
scorbutic
    s. dysentery
    s. gingivitis
score
    Gleason s.
    initial prognostic s. (IPS)
    LOD s.
    standard s.
    Z s.
Scorpiones
Scorpionida
Scotch tape method
scotochromogen
scotochromogenic
    s. mycobacteria
scotoma, pl. **scotomata**
scotopic
Scott tap water substitute
SCPK
    serum creatine phosphokinase
scrape
scraper
    cervical s.
scrapie
scratch-pad memory
scratch test
screen
    amino acid s.
    s. burn
    s. filtration pressure (SFP)
screening
    automated multiphasic s. (AMS)
    cytologic s.
    genetic s.
    multiphasic s.
    neonatal s.
    prenatal s.
    s. test
screw-worm
scrobiculate
scrofula
scrofuloderma
    s. gummosa
    papular s.
    tuberculous s.
    ulcerative s.
    verrucous s.

scrofulotuberculosis
scrofulous
scroll ear
scrotitis
scrotum, pl. **scrota, scrotums**
    lymph s.
    watering-can s.
scrub typhus
SCT
    sex chromatin test
    staphylococcal clumping test
scum
scurvy
    land s.
scuta (*pl. of* scutum)
Scutigera
scutula (*pl. of* scutulum)
scutular
scutularis
    parakeratosis s.
scutulum, pl. **scutula**
scutum, pl. **scuta**
SD
    septal defect
    serologically defined
    serum defect
    spontaneous delivery
    standard deviation
    streptodornase
        SD antigen
SDS
    sudden death syndrome
SDS-gel
    S.-g. electrophoresis
    S.-g. filtration chromatography
SDS-PAGE
    sodium dodecyl sulfate-polyacrylamide
    gel electrophoresis
SE
    standard error
sea-blue
    s.-b. histiocyte
    s.-b. histiocyte disease
seal
    hermetic s.
sealed envelope technique
sealing
    impulse s.
search
Seattle classification
seatworm
sea urchin granuloma

S

NOTES

sebaceous
s. adenocarcinoma
s. adenoma
s. carcinoma
s. cyst
s. epithelioma
s. horn
s. nevus
s. tubercle
sebolith
seborrhea
seborrheic
s. dermatitis
s. keratosis
s. verruca
s. wart
seborrheica
acanthoma verrucosa s.
Sebright bantam syndrome
sebum
Secernentasida
Secernentia
Seckel syndrome
secobarbital
second (s)
cycles per s. (cps)
s. degree
s. degree burn
s. degree frostbite
s. degree heart block
s. degree radiation injury
s. filial generation (F_2)
kilocycles per s. (kcps)
per s. (ps)
s. set rejection
vibration s. (v.s.)
secondary
s. active transport
s. agammaglobulinemia
s. amenorrhea (SA)
s. amyloidosis
s. anemia (SA)
s. antibody deficiency
s. atelectasis
s. attack rate
s. buffer
s. carcinoma
s. coccidioidomycosis
s. coil
s. constriction
s. culture
s. degeneration
s. dextrocardia
s. disease
s. encephalitis
s. fixation
s. glaucoma
s. granule

s. hyperaldosteronism
s. hyperplasia
s. hypertrophic osteoarthropathy (SHO)
s. hypoadrenocorticism
s. hypogammaglobulinemia
s. immune response
s. immunodeficiency
s. infection
s. lysosome
s. methemoglobinemia
s. mucinosis
s. myeloid metaplasia
s. pulmonary hemosiderosis (SPH)
s. pyoderma
S. Reference Materials
s. refractory anemia
s. renal calculus
s. renal tubular acidosis
s. repair
s. sex character
s. structure
s. thrombus
s. trisomy
s. tuberculosis
s. union
second-order reaction
second-set
s.-s. graft rejection
s.-s. phenomenon
Secrétan syndrome
secretin
s. pancreozymin test
s. test
secretin-CCK stimulation test
secretion
cervical s.
s. rate (SR)
transport and s.
secretor
s. factor
s. gene
s. phenotype
s. trait
secretory
s. adenosis
s. carcinoma
s. component
s. cyst
s. granule
s. IgA
s. immunoglobulin
s. immunoglobulin A
s. otitis media (SOM)
s. stage
section
attached cranial s.
capture cross s.

cesarean s.
coronal s.
s. cutting
detached cranial s.
formalin-fixed tissue s.
s. freeze substitution technique
paraffin-embedded tissue s.
pituitary stalk s.
thin s.
sectioning
Albert-Linder bone s.
secular equilibrium
SED
spondyloepiphysial dysplasia
sedative
sediment
crystals in urine s.
stained urinary s. (SUS)
urinary s.
sedimentate
sedimentation
s. coefficient
s. equilibrium
erythrocyte s.
s. index
s. rate (SR)
s. technique
s. test
velocity-diffusion s.
s. velocity-diffusion
sedimentator
sedimented red cell (SRC)
sedimentometer
sedimentum
s. lateritium
sedoheptulose-7-phosphate
SEE
standard error of estimate
seeberi
Rhinosporidium s.
seg
segmented
segment
Okazaki s.
pairing s.
segmental glomerulonephritis
segmentation sphere
segmented (seg)
s. cell
s. granulocyte
s. hyalinizing vasculitis

s. leukocyte
s. neutrophil
segmenter
Segmentina
Segmentininae
segment long-spacing (collagen) (SLS)
segregation
segs
SeHCAT test
Seitelberger disease
Seitz filter
Selas filter
Seldinger technique
selectins
selection
s. against dominant mutations
s. against heterozygotes
s. against homozygotes
s. against recessive mutations
coefficient of s.
directional s.
natural s.
s. pressure
selective
s. medium
s. stain
selectivity ratio
selenite broth
selenite-cystine broth
selenium
s. assay
selenium-75
selenocyte
selenoid body
self-absorption
self-dose
self-infection
selfing
self-limited disease
Selivanoff
S. reagent
S. test
sella
empty s.
Selter disease
Selye syndrome
SEM
scanning electron microscope
semantics
semelincident
semen
s. analysis

S

NOTES

semen *(continued)*
    s. examination
    hyaluronidase unit for s. (HUS)
semenuria
semialdehyde
    glutamate s.
semiapochromatic objective
semicarbazide hydrochloride
semiconductor
    s. device
    extrinsic s.
    intrinsic s.
semidominance
semiinterquartile range
semilethal mutation
seminal
    s. fibrinolysin
    s. fluid
    s. vesical cyst
seminiferous
    s. epithelium
    s. tubule dysgenesis
seminoma
    spermacytic s.
seminomatous
seminuria
semipermeable membrane
semiquantitative
    s. analysis
    s. viral culture
semiquinone
Semisulcospina
Semliki Forest virus
Semple vaccine
Sendai virus
Senear-Usher
    S.-U. disease
    S.-U. syndrome
seneciosis
senile
    s. amyloidosis
    s. arteriosclerosis
    s. atrophy
    s. degeneration
    s. dwarfism
    s. ectasia
    s. elastosis
    s. fibroma
    s. hemangioma
    s. hip disease
    s. involution
    s. keratoderma
    s. keratoma
    s. keratosis
    s. melanoderma
    s. nephrosclerosis
    s. osteomalacia
    s. plaque

    s. sebaceous hyperplasia
    s. wart
senilis
    arcus s.
senior synonym
senna
sennoside
sense strand
sensitive
sensitivity
    acquired s.
    analytical s.
    antibiotic s.
    clinical s.
    contact s.
    culture and s. (C&S)
    diagnostic s.
    electrode s.
    idiosyncratic s.
    induced s.
    multiple chemical s.
    photoallergic s.
    phototoxic s.
    primaquine s.
    relative s.
    salt s.
sensitization
    active s.
    autoerythrocyte s.
    passive s.
    photodynamic s.
    s. response (SR)
sensitize
sensitized
    s. antigen
    s. cell
sensitizer
sensitizing
    s. dose
    s. injection
    s. substance
sensor
sentinel
    s. animal
    s. gland
    s. node
    s. pile
    s. tag
separating medium
separatory funnel
Sepsidae
sepsis, pl. **sepses**
    intestinal s.
    s. lenta
septa (*pl. of* septum)
septal
    s. defect (SD)

s. fibrosis of liver
s. fibrosis, liver
Septata
   S. intestinalis
septate mycelium
septemia
septic
   s. abortion
   s. disease
   s. embolus
   s. endocarditis
   s. fever
   s. infarct
   s. intoxication
   s. knee
   s. necrosis
   s. peritonitis
   s. phlebitis
   s. pneumonia
   s. shock
septicemia
   acute fulminating meningococcal s.
   anthrax s.
   cryptogenic s.
   puerperal s.
   typhoid s.
septicemic
   s. abscess
   s. plague
Septi-Chek culture system
septicopyemia
septicopyemic
septo-optic dysplasia
septum, pl. **septa**
   atrial s.
sequela, pl. **sequelae**
sequence
   insertion s.
   intervening s.
   s. ladder
   long terminal repeat s. (LTR)
   regulatory s.
   repeated DNA s.'s
   scanning s.
   termination s.
sequencer
   amino acid s.
sequential
   s. access
   s. analysis
   s. multichannel autoanalyzer (SMA)
sequester

sequestered antigen
sequestra (*pl. of* sequestrum)
sequestral
sequestration
   s. bronchopneumonia
   bronchopulmonary s.
   s. cyst
   s. dermoid
sequestrum, pl. **sequestra**
   primary s.
sequoiosis
sera (*pl. of* serum)
seralbumin
Sereny test
serial
   s. cardiac isoenzyme assay
   s. data transmission
   s. dilution
   s. operation
   s. passage
   s. thrombin time (STT)
sericata
   Phaenicia s.
Sericopelma
   S. communis
series, pl. **series**
   s. circuit
   erythrocytic s.
   gastrointestinal s. (GI series)
   granulocytic s.
   homologous s.
   lymphocytic s.
   monohistiocytic s.
   myeloid s.
   thrombocytic s.
serine
serocolitis
seroconversion
serocystic
serodiagnosis
   Leptospira s.
seroenteritis
seroepidemiology
serofast
serofibrinous
   s. effusion
   s. inflammation
   s. pericarditis
   s. pleurisy
serologic
   s. pipette
   s. test for syphilis (STS)

S

NOTES

serological
serologically
    s. defined (SD)
    s. defined antigen
serology
    AIDS s.
    Aspergillus s.
    bacterial s.
    Helicobacter pylori s.
    HIV I s.
    Lyme disease s.
    Mycoplasma s.
    pertussis s.
    s. test
seroma
seromucoid
    acid s.
    alpha-1 s.
α_1-seromucoid
seronegative
serophilic
seropositive
seropurulent
seropus
seroreversion
serosa
    polyemia s.
serosamucin
serosanguineous
    s. effusion
serositis
    multiple s.
serosity
serosynovial
serosynovitis
serotherapy
serothorax
serotonergic
serotonin
    s. assay
serotype
    heterologous s.
    homologous s.
serous
    s. acute inflammation
    s. acute synovitis
    s. atrophy
    s. cell
    s. cyst
    s. cystadenocarcinoma
    s. cystadenoma
    s. cystoma
    s. effusion
    s. fluid
    s. meningitis
    s. otitis media (SOM)
    s. pleurisy
serovaccination

serovar
serozyme
serpent
    s. infection
    s. worm
serpentine aneurysm
serpiginosum
    angioma s.
serpiginous
    s. keratitis
    s. ulcer
serpigo
serrate
Serratia
    S. indica
    S. kiliensis
    S. liquefaciens
    S. marcescens
    S. piscatorum
    S. plymuthica
    S. rubidaea
Serratieae
Sertoli
    S. cell
    S. cell tumor
Sertoli-cell-only syndrome
Sertoli-Leydig cell tumor
serum, pl. serums, sera (S)
    s. accelerator
    s. accelerator globulin
    s. accident
    s. agar
    aged s.
    s. agglutinin
    s. albumin (SA)
    s. alkaline phosphatase (SAP)
    s. alkaline phosphatase test
    s. amylase
    s. amylase test
    anallergenic s.
    anticholera s.
    anticomplementary s.
    antidiphtheric s.
    antiepithelial s.
    antihepatic s.
    antihuman lymphocyte s. (AHLS)
    antilymphocyte s. (ALS)
    antimacrophage s. (AMS)
    antimeningococcus s.
    anti-mouse lymphocyte s. (AMLS)
    antineutrophilic s. (ANS)
    antipertussis s.
    antiplague s.
    antiplatelet s.
    antipneumococcus s.
    antirabies s. (ARS)
    antireticular cytotoxic s. (ACS)
    antiscarlatinal s.

antistaphylococcus s.
antistreptococcus s.
antitetanic s. (ATS)
antithymocyte s. (ATS)
antitoxic s.
antivenomous s.
antiyphoid s.
s. bacterial test
s. bactericidal test
bacteriolytic s.
s. bilirubin (SB)
blood s.
s. broth
s. chemistry graft (SCG)
convalescent s.
Coombs s.
s. creatine kinase (SCK)
s. creatine phosphokinase (SCPK)
cytotrophic s.
s. defect (SD)
s. diagnosis
s. disease
dried human s.
endotheliolytic s.
s. enzyme
equine antihuman lymphoblast s.
  (EAHLS)
s. estriol
fetal bovine s. (FBS)
foreign s.
s. globulin (SG)
s. globulin test
s. glutamate oxaloacetate
  transaminase
s. glutamate pyruvate transaminase
s. glutamic-oxaloacetic transaminase
  (SGOT)
s. glutamic-pyruvic transaminase
  (SGPT)
guinea pig anti-insulin s. (GPAIS)
s. hepatitis (SH)
s. hepatitis virus
hereditary erythroblastic
  multinuclearity with a positive
  acidified s.
hereditary erythrocytic
  multinuclearity with positive
  acidified s. (HEMPAS)
heterologous s.
hog cholera s.
homologous s.
horse s. (HS)

human measles immune s.
human pertussis immune s.
human scarlet fever immune s.
s. hydroxybutyrate dehydrogenase
  (SHBD)
hyperimmune s.
immune s.
inactivated leukocytolytic s.
s. intoxication
s. iron (SI)
s. isocitric dehydrogenase (SICD)
liquid human s.
Löffler blood s.
measles convalescent s.
motile s.
muscle s.
s. nephritis
nephrotoxic s.
nonimmune s.
normal s.
normal blood s. (NBS)
normal horse s. (NHS)
normal human s. (NHS)
normal rabbit s. (NRS)
normal reference s. (NRS)
s. osmolality
pericardial s.
s. phosphatase
plague s.
polyvalent s.
pooled blood s.
s. precipitable iodine (SPI)
pregnant mare s. (PMS)
prophylactic s.
s. protein-bound iodine (SPBI)
s. protein electrophoresis (SPE)
s. protein electrophoresis test
s. prothrombin conversion
  accelerator (SPCA)
s. prothrombin conversion
  accelerator deficiency
s. prothrombin conversion
  accelerator factor
s. prothrombin time
rabbit antidog-thymus s. (RADTS)
rabbit antimouse-lymphocyte s.
rabbit antirat-lymphocyte s.
  (RARLS)
s. rash
s. reaction
salted s.
salvarsanized s.

NOTES

S

serum *(continued)*
    s. shock
    s. sickness
    specific s.
    streptococcus s.
    s. therapy
    s. thrombotic accelerator (STA)
    thyrotoxic s.
    s. urea nitrogen (SUN)
    s. uric acid (SUA)
    veronal-buffered saline:fetal
      bovine s. (VBS:FBS)
serumal
serum-fast
serum-neutralizing (SN)
serums (*pl. of* serum)
servomechanism
servomotor
seryl
sesame oil
sesquiterpene
sessile
    s. hydatid
    s. phagocyte
    s. polyp
set
    s. of idiotopes
    s. point
Setaria
setariasis
settled particulate
seven-segment display
severe (SV)
    s. combined immunodeficiency
    (SCID)
    s. combined immunodeficiency
    disease
    s. combined immunodeficient mice
severely subnormal (SSN)
Severinghaus electrode
Sever syndrome
Sevier-Munger stain
sex
    s. cell
    s. chromatin
    s. chromatin test (SCT)
    s. chromosome
    s. cords
    s. cord-stromal tumor
    s. determination
    s. differentiation
    s. factor
    heterogametic s.
    homogametic s.
    s. hormone (SH)
    s. pilus
sexalatus
    Physocephalus s.

sex-conditioned character
sexivalent
sex-limited character
sex-linked
    s.-l. character
    s.-l. gene
    s.-l. heredity
    s.-l. inheritance
sex-reversed mutation
sexually transmitted disease (STD)
sexual reproduction
Sézary
    S. cell
    S. erythroderma
    S. reticulosis
    S. syndrome
SF
    scarlet fever
Sf
    Svedberg flotation unit
SFP
    screen filtration pressure
SFT
    solitary fibrous tumor
S-G
    Sachs-Georgi
SG
    serum globulin
    skin graft
    specific gravity
SGAT
    salivary gland anlage tumor
signs (Sx)
SGOT
    serum glutamic-oxaloacetic transaminase
SGPT
    serum glutamic-pyruvic transaminase
SGV
    salivary gland virus
SH
    serum hepatitis
    sex hormone
    sinus histiocytosis
shadow
    s. cell
    s. corpuscle
    Gumprecht s.
    s. nucleus
    Ponfick s.
shadow-casting
Shaffer-Hartmann method
shaggy pericardium
shagreen
    s. patch
    s. skin
shake
    s. culture
    s. test

Shandon
>S. Candenza immunostainer
>S. cytospin chamber
>S. fixative

Sharpey
>perforating fibers of S.

Shaver disease

SHb
>sulfhemoglobin

SHBD
>serum hydroxybutyrate dehydrogenase

sheath
>giant cell tumor of tendon s. (GCTTS)

shedding
>virus s.

Sheehan syndrome

sheep
>s. blood agar
>s. cell agglutination test (SCAT)
>s. liver fluke
>s. red blood cell (SRBC)
>s. red cell (SRC)

sheep-pox
>s.-p. virus

sheet
>material safety data s. (MSDS)
>pleated s.

shell
>diffusion s.
>s. nail

Sherman-Bourquin unit of vitamin B$_2$

Sherman-Munsell unit

Sherman unit

Shichito disease

shield
>chloride s.
>gonadal s.
>s. to the left
>s. to the right
>syringe s.
>tabletop s.

shielding

shift
>antigenic s.
>bathochromic s.
>chemical s.
>chloride s.
>s. counter
>hyperchromic s.
>hypochromic s.
>hypsochromic s.

isohydric s.
>s. to the left
>regenerative blood s.
>s. register
>s. reticulocyte
>s. to the right
>Stokes s.

Shiga
>S. bacillus
>S. toxin

Shigella
>*S. alkalescens*
>*S. ambigua*
>*S. arabinotarda*
>*S. boydii*
>*S. ceylonensis*
>*S. dispar*
>*S. dysenteriae*
>*S. etousae*
>*S. flexneri*
>*S. madampensis*
>*S. newcastle*
>*S. paradysenteriae*
>*S. parashigae*
>*S. schmitzii*
>*S. shigae*
>*S. sonnei*
>*S. wakefield*

shigellosis

Shimadzu hemoglobin determination

shimamushi disease

shin
>saber s.

shingles

Shinowara-Jones-Reinhard (SJR)

ship fever

shipping
>s. fever
>s. fever virus

shirt-stud abscess

SHML
>sinus histiocytosis with massive lymphadenopathy

SHO
>secondary hypertrophic osteoarthropathy

shock
>anaphylactic s.
>anaphylactoid s.
>s. antigen
>s. artifact
>cardiogenic s.
>colloid s.

S

NOTES

shock *(continued)*
    endotoxic s.
    endotoxin s.
    faradic s.
    hemoclastic s.
    hemorrhagic s.
    histamine s.
    hypoglycemic s.
    hypovolemic s.
    insulin s.
    s. lung
    neurogenic s.
    osmotic s.
    peptone s.
    protein s.
    pseudoanaphylactic s.
    septic s.
    serum s.
    thyrotoxin s.
    toxic s.
    vasogenic s.
shocking dose
Shone anomaly
Shope
    S. fibroma
    S. fibroma virus
    S. papilloma
    S. papilloma virus
Shorr trichrome stain
short
    s. circuit
    s. incubation hepatitis
shortened
    s. bleeding time
    s. coagulation time
shortening
    abnormal s.
shotty breast
shower
    safety s.
shunt
    hexose monophosphate s. (HMPS)
    pentose s.
    portocaval s.
Shwachman-Diamond syndrome
Shwachman syndrome
Shwartzman reaction
Shy-Drager syndrome
SI
    International System of Units
    saturation index
    serum iron
    soluble insulin
    SI unit
SIADH
    syndrome of inappropriate antidiuretic
    hormone

    syndrome of inappropriate secretion of
    antidiuretic hormone
sialadenitis
sialadenoncus
sialadenosis
sialic acid
sialidase
    s. digestion
sialoblastoma
sialocele
sialolithiasis
sialometaplasia
    necrotizing s.
sialomucin
sialorrhea
Sialosyl-Tn antigen
Siamese twins
Sia test
sib
Sibine
Sibley-Lehninger (SL)
    S. unit
sibling species
sibship
Sicard syndrome
Sicariidae
sicca
    s. complex
    s. syndrome
siccant
siccative
siccolabile
siccostabile, siccostable
SICD
    serum isocitric dehydrogenase
sick building syndrome
sickle
    s. cell (SC)
    s. cell anemia
    s. cell crisis
    s. cell hemoglobin (Hb S)
    s. cell hemoglobin C disease
    s. cell hemoglobin D disease
    s. cell nephropathy
    s. cell test
    s. cell β-thalassemia
    s. cell thalassemia
    s. cell-thalassemia disease
    s. cell trait
sickled cell
Sickledex
    S. reagent
    S. test
sicklemia
Sicklequik test
sickling
    s. test

sickness
African horse s.
African sleeping s.
decompensation s.
decompression s.
green s.
Jamaican vomiting s.
radiation s.
serum s.
sleeping s.
side
s. effect
s. platelet aggregation test (SPAT)
side-chain theory
sideramine
sideroachrestic anemia
Siderobacter
sideroblast
sideroblastic anemia
Siderocapsa
Siderocapsaceae
siderochrome
Siderococcus
siderocyte
siderocyte stain
siderocytic granule
sideroderma
siderofibrosis
siderogenous
sideromycin
sideropenia
sideropenic
s. anemia
s. dysphagia
siderophage
siderophagocytosis
siderophil, siderophile
siderophilin
siderophilous
siderophore
siderosilicosis
siderosis
siderosome
siderotic
s. granule
s. nodule
SIDS
sudden infant death syndrome
sieve
molecular s.
sievert
Siggaard-Andersen alignment nomogram

sigma
s. bond
s. reaction (SR)
sigmavirus
sigmoiditis
sigmoidovesical fistula
sign
crescent s.
Cullen s.
dimple s.
groove s.
Higoumenakia s.
Mirchamp s.
Nikolsky s.
Romaña s.
scimitar s.
Vierra s.
vital s.'s (VS)
signal
analog s.
s. averaging
common mode s.
deflection s.
insufficient s. (IS)
s. level
s. node
signed
s. magnitude
s. rank test
signet
s. ring
s. ring adenocarcinoma
signet-ring
s.-r. cell
s.-r. cell carcinoma
significance
atypical squamous cells of
undetermined s. (ASCUS)
s. level
s. probability
test of s. (t)
significant
s. asymptomatic bacteriuria (SAB)
s. digits
not s. (NS)
not statistically s. (NSS)
statistically s. (SS)
SIL
squamous intraepithelial lesion
silanated slide
silane
silanization

NOTES

Silastic
silent
    s. mutation
    s. myocardial infarction
silhouette
    cardiac s.
silica
    s. gel
    s. granuloma
silicate
silicatosis
silicic acid
silicon
    s. dioxide
    s. granuloma
silicon-controlled
    s.-c. rectifier
    s.-c. switch
silicone
    s. implant
    s. lymphadenopathy
siliconoma
silicoproteinosis
silicosis
silver (Ag)
    s. cell
    s. impregnation
    s. nitrate
    s. nitrate stain
    s. nitroprusside test
    s. protein stain
    silver-ammoniacal s. (Ag-AS)
    S. syndrome
silver-ammoniacal
    silver-ammoniacal silver (Ag-AS)
    silver-ammoniacal silver stain
Silver-Russell
    S.-R. dwarfism
    S.-R. syndrome
silver/silver chloride electrode
Silverskiöld syndrome
Silvestrini-Corda syndrome
silvex
silylation
Simbu
    S. hepatitis
    S. virus
simian
    s. crease
    s. sarcoma virus (SSV)
    s. vacuolating virus No. 40
    s. virus (SV)
simicola
    Pneumonyssus s.
Simmonds disease
Simmons citrate agar
Simonea folliculorum
Simons disease

Simon septic factor
simple
    s. adenosis
    s. asphyxiant
    s. atrophy
    s. bone cyst
    s. fracture
    s. goiter
    s. hypertrophy
    s. lymphangiectasis
    s. microscope
    s. necrosis
    s. protein
    s. pulmonary eosinophilia
    s. random sample
    s. ulcer
    s. urethritis
simplex
    herpes s. (HS)
    toxoplasmosis, rubella,
      cytomegalovirus, and herpes s.
      (TORCH)
Sims-Huhner test
simulated
    s. hypertrophy
    S. Matrix Reference Materials
simulation
Simuliidae
Simulium
sin
sincalide
Sindbis
    S. fever
    S. virus
sinensis
    Clonorchis s.
sine wave
singer's node
single
    s. diffusion test
    s. (gel) diffusion precipitin test in
      one dimension
    s. (gel) diffusion precipitin test in
      two dimensions
    s. human leukocyte antigen
    s. immunodiffusion
    S. Use Diagnostic System (SUDS)
single-blind
single-phase
sinistrocardia
    isolated s.
sink
    heat s.
sinonasal undifferentiated carcinoma
    (SNUC)
sinuatum
    Entoloma s.
sinus, pl. sinus, sinuses

Aschoff-Rokitansky s.
dermal s.
s. histiocytosis (SH)
s. histiocytosis with massive
lymphadenopathy (SHML)
s. phlebitis
pilonidal s.
rhomboidal s.
Rokitansky-Aschoff s.
s. venosus remnant
sinusitis
sclerosing s.
sinusoid
sinusoidal
s. foam cell clusters
s. inflammation
Siphona irritans
Siphonaptera
Siphoviridae
Siphunculina
Sipple syndrome
sirenomelia
Sirius red
SIRS
soluble immune response suppressor
sister
s. chromatid
S. Joseph nodule
Sisyrosea
site
allosteric s.
antibody combining s.
antigen-binding s.
antigen combining s.
combining s.
immunologically privileged s.
implantation s.
privileged s.
receptor s.
in situ
carcinoma i. (CIS)
ductal carcinoma i. (DCIS)
endocrine ductal carcinoma i. (E-
DCIS)
endometrial carcinoma i. (ECIS)
isolated gland carcinoma i. (GCIS)
lobular i. (LIS)
lobular carcinoma i. (LCIS)
squamous cell carcinoma i.
surface carcinoma i. (SCIS)
tumor i. (TIS)
Siwe-Letterer disease

sixth venereal disease
size-exclusion chromatography
Sjögren
S. antibody
S. disease
S. syndrome
Sjögren-Larsson syndrome
SJR
Shinowara-Jones-Reinhard
SJR unit
skatole
skatoxyl
skein cell
skeinoid
s. fiber
skeletal muscle antibody
skeleton
s. hand
skeneitis, skenitis
Skevas-Zerfus disease
skew
skewed distribution
skewness
skin
alligator s.
s. biopsy
congenital localized absence of s.
(CLAS)
deciduous s.
s. dose
elastic s.
farmer's s.
fish s.
s. fungus culture
glabrous s.
s. graft (SG)
loose s.
s. mycobacteria culture
parchment s.
piebald s.
pig s.
porcupine s.
s. puncture
s. reaction
sailor's s.
shagreen s.
s. stone
s. tag
s. test dose (STD)
s. test unit (STU)
s. tumor
s. to tumor distance (STD)

NOTES

S

565

skin *(continued)*
    s. window test
    yellow s.
skinbound disease
Skinner classification
skin-puncture test
skin-reactive factor (SRF)
skin-sensitizing antibody (SSA)
skip
    s. areae
    s. lesion
skull
    cloverleaf s.
    maplike s.
    steeple s.
sky blue
SL
    Sibley-Lehninger
    streptolysin
    SL unit
sl
    slyke
SLA
    slide latex agglutination
slant culture
slaty anemia
SLE
    St. Louis encephalitis
    systemic lupus erythematosus
sleep
    NREM s.
sleeping sickness
SLEV
    St. Louis encephalitis virus
    St. Louis encephalitis virus serology
slide
    aminopropyltriethyloxysilane-coated
      glass s.
    s. latex agglutination (SLA)
    silanated s.
slide-wire potentiometer
sliding microtome
slit lamp
SLKC
    superior limbic keratoconjunctivitis
SLL
    small lymphocytic lymphoma
SLO
    streptolysin-O
slope culture
slot exhaust
slough
sloughing ulcer
slow
    s. fever
    s. neutron
    s. virus
    s. virus disease

"slow" hemoglobin
slow-moving protease (SMP)
slow-reacting
    s.-r. factor of anaphylaxis (SRF-A)
    s.-r. substance (SRS)
    s.-r. substance of anaphylaxis
      (SRS-A, SRSA)
SLR
    Streptococcus lactis R
SLS
    segment long-spacing (collagen)
Sluder syndrome
sludge
sludged blood
sluggish layer
slurry
Sly
    S. disease
    S. syndrome
slyke (sl)
SM
    streptomycin
    submucous
    suction method
SMA
    sequential multichannel autoanalyzer
    smooth-muscle actin
    SMA antibody
SMA-12 profile test
SMAC test
SMAF
    specific macrophage-arming factor
small
    s. calorie (c, cal)
    s. cell lung carcinoma (SCLC)
    s. cell sarcoma
    s. cell tumor
    s. cleaved cell
    s. intestine polyp
    s. intestine tumor
    s. lymphocytic lymphoma (SLL)
    s. non-cleaved cell (SNCC)
    s. nuclear ribonucleoproteins
      (SNRPs)
smallpox
    coherent s.
    confluent s.
    discrete s.
    fulminating s.
    hemorrhagic s.
    s. immunization
    inoculation s.
    malignant s.
    modified s.
    s. vaccine
    s. virus
    West Indian s.
Sm antigen

smart terminal
smear
>AFB s.
>air-dried s.
>alimentary tract s.
>s. background
>Bethesda Pap s.
>blood s.
>Breed s.
>bronchoscopic s.
>buccal s.
>buccal s. for sex chromatin evaluation
>buffy coat s.
>cervical s.
>colonic s.
>cul-de-sac s.
>cytologic s.
>cytospin slide centrifuge Gram-stained s.
>Diff-Quik s.
>duodenal s.
>ectocervical s.
>endocervical s.
>endometrial s.
>esophageal s.
>fast s.
>female genital tract cytologic s.
>FGT cytologic s.
>fungi s.
>gastric s.
>lateral vaginal wall s.
>*Legionella pneumophila* direct fA s.
>lower respiratory tract s.
>malaria s.
>nasal s.
>*Neisseria gonorrhoeae* s.
>oral s.
>pancervical s.
>Pap s.
>Papanicolaou s.
>peripheral blood s.
>s. preparation and staining for blood parasites
>sputum s.
>TB s.
>Tzanck s.
>urinary s.
>vaginal irrigation s. (VIS)
>VCE s.

smegma
>s. bacillus
>s. clitoridis
>s. embryonum
>s. preputii

smegmalith
***S*-methylmalonyl-CoA mutase**
Smith disease
Smith-Lemli-Opitz syndrome
Smith-Riley syndrome
Smith-Strang disease
smog
>photochemical s.

smoldering leukemia
SMON
>subacute myelo-optical neuropathy

smooth (S)
>s. bacterium
>s. colony
>s. leprosy
>s. muscle antibody

smoothing
smooth-muscle actin (SMA)
α-smooth-muscle actin
smooth-rough variation
SMP
>slow-moving protease

SMR
>somnolent metabolic rate
>standard mortality ratio

smudge cell
SMZL
>splenic marginal zone lymphoma

SN
>serum-neutralizing

snail
snakebite
snake venom (SV)
snap-frozen
SNB
>scalene node biopsy

SNCC
>small non-cleaved cell

Sneddon syndrome
Sneddon-Wilkinson disease
Snell law
Snook reticulum stain
SNOP
>Systematized Nomenclature of Pathology

snowshoe hare virus
SNRPs
>small nuclear ribonucleoproteins

NOTES

S

snub-nose dwarfism
SNUC
sinonasal undifferentiated carcinoma
Society
Musculoskeletal Tumor S. (MSTS)
sodium
s. bisulfite stain
s. cacodylate
s. chloride
s. chloride (6.5 %) broth
s. chloride (6.5 %) culture medium
s. chromate Cr 51
cloxacillin s.
colistimethate s.
dextrothyroxine s.
s. dodecyl sulfate
s. dodecyl sulfate-polyacrylamide
    gel electrophoresis (SDS-PAGE)
s. fluoroacetate
s. fluorosilicate
s. hexafluorosilicate
s. hydroxide stain
s. indigotin disulfonate
mercaptomerin s.
s. nitroprusside
oxacillin s.
plasma s. (P_{Na})
s. and potassium assays
rose bengal s.
sulfobromophathalein s.
s. test
s. thiosulfate stain
s. tungstoborate
tyropanoate s.
Yb-169 pentetate s.
soft
s. chancre
s. papilloma
s. sore
s. tissue calcification (STC)
s. tissue tumor
s. tubercle
s. ulcer
s. wart
software
SURGE s.
Sohval-Soffer syndrome
SOL, Sol
solution
space-occupying lesion
sol
metal s.
solid s.
solanine
solanocyte
Solanum
solar
s. elastosis

s. fever
s. keratosis
s. urticaria
soldier's patch
solenoid
Solenopotes capillatus
Solenopsis
solid
s. angle
s. carbon dioxide
s. carcinoma
s. edema
s. phase immunoassay
s. sol
s. state
s. teratoma
solidistic pathology
solid-phase radioimmunoassay
solitary
s. bone cyst
s. fibrous tumor (SFT)
s. osteocartilaginous exostosis
solubility
s. coefficient
s. product
s. test
solubilize
solubilizer
soluble (S)
s. antigen
s. immune response suppressor
    (SIRS)
s. insulin (SI)
s. interleukin-2 receptor
s. ribonucleic acid (SRNA)
s. specific substance
solute
total body s. (TBS)
solution (SOL, Sol)
ammoniacal silver s.'s
anticoagulant heparin s.
aqueous s.
azeotropic s.
Balamuth buffer s.
balanced salt s. (BSS)
Benedict s.
Bouin s.
buffered saline s. (BSS)
Burow s.
Cajal formol ammonium bromide s.
cleaning s.
Cytyc CytoLyt preservative s.
Cytyc Preservcyt preservative s.
Dakin s.
DAKO target retrieval s.
Delafield fixative s.
Diaphane s.
disclosing s.

Dragendorff s.
Earle s.
Fehling s.
Fonio s.
formaldehyde s.
formalin s.
formol ammonium bromide s.
Fowler s.
FU-48 Zenker fixative s.
Gallego differentiating s.
Gowers s.
Hartmann s.
Hayem s.
Hinfl s.
Histoclear slide processing s.
Hucker-Conn crystal violet s.
s. hybridization
hydrogen peroxide s.
ideal s.
isotonic sodium chloride s.
Karnovsky II s.
Krebs-Ringer s.
lactated Ringer s. (LRS)
Lange s.
Locke s.
Locke-Ringer s.
Lugol iodine s.
Lumi-Phos s.
mordant s.
nonideal s.
Orth s.
physiological saline s. (PSS)
physiologic saline s.
propidium iodide s.
pyridoxilated stroma-free
   hemoglobin s.
ribonuclease s.
Ringer s.
Ringer lactate s. (RLS)
Ruge s.
saline s.
saturated s. (SS)
Schallibaum s.
standard s.
TAC s.
Tellyesnicky fixative s.
test s. (TS)
Toison s.
volumetric s. (VS)
Weigert iodine s.
Zamboni s.
solvate

solvation
solve
solvent
   aprotic s.
   s. extraction
   protic s.
solvolysis
SOM
   secretory otitis media
   serous otitis media
somatic
   s. agglutinin
   s. antigen
   s. cell
   s. cell genetics
   s. chromosome
   s. death
   s. mutation
   s. mutation theory of cancer
   s. pairing
somatomammotropin
   chorionic s. (CS)
   human chorionic s. (hCS, hCSM)
   immunoradioassayable human
      chorionic s. (IRHCS)
somatomedins
somatosensory
somatostatinoma
somatostatin-producing small cell
somatostatin receptor
somatotroph adenoma
somatotropic
   s. hormone (STH)
somatotropin
somatotropin-releasing factor (SRF)
somnolent metabolic rate (SMR)
Somogyi
   S. effect
   S. method
   S. unit
sonicate
sonication
sonification
sonifier
sonify
Sonne-Duval bacillus
Sonne dysentery
soot wart
sooty capsule
sorbefacient
sorbent
sorbitol dehydrogenase

S

NOTES

sore
>canker s.
>cold s.
>fungating s.
>hard s.
>s. mouth
>oriental s.
>soft s.
>venereal s.

sorehead
soremouth
>s. virus

soremuzzle
Soret band
sorption
Sorsby syndrome
sorter
>fluorescence-activated cell s. (FACS)

SOS repair system
Sotos syndrome of cerebral gigantism
SOTT
>synthetic medium old tuberculin trichloroacetic acid (precipitated)

source
>flood s.
>s. language
>s. program
>s. statement

South
>S. African type porphyria
>S. American blastomycosis

Southern
>S. blot analysis
>S. blot technique
>S. blot test

soybean trypsin inhibitor (SBTI)
sp, pl. spp.
>species

space
>capsomer capsular s.
>s. charge
>intercristal s.
>intracristal s.
>intramembranous s.
>perinuclear s.
>Poiseuille s.

space-occupying lesion (SOL, Sol)
spacer
spade
>s. finger
>s. hand

SPAI
>steroid protein activity index

spallation product
Spanish influenza
SPARC-2
>Sun S.

sparganoma
sparganosis
Sparganum
>*S. proliferum*

sparganum
sparteine
spasm
>cadaveric s.
>epidemic transient diaphragmatic s.

spasmogen
spastic
>s. anemia
>s. colitis
>s. ileus

SPAT
>side platelet aggregation test

spatial isomerism
spatula
>Ayre s.
>Roux s.

SPBI
>serum protein-bound iodine

SPCA
>serum prothrombin conversion accelerator
>SPCA deficiency
>SPCA factor

SPE
>serum protein electrophoresis

Spearman rank correlation coefficient
special
>s. pathology
>s. reference method

specialist
specialized transduction
speciation
species (sp)
>sibling s.
>type s.

species-specific
>s.-s. antigen

specific
>s. absorptivity
>s. active immunity
>s. anergy
>s. antigen
>s. antiserum
>s. bactericide
>s. capsular substance
>s. coagulation factor deficiency
>s. disease
>s. dynamic action
>s. granule
>s. gravity (SG, sp gr)
>s. heat
>s. heat capacity
>s. hemolysin
>s. immune globulin (human)

s. ionization
s. macrophage-arming factor (SMAF)
s. opsonin
s. passive immunity
s. pathogen-free (SPF)
s. rate
s. reaction
s. rotation
s. serum
s. soluble polysaccharide
s. soluble substance (SSS)
s. soluble sugar
s. transduction

specificity
analytical s.
diagnostic s.
relative s.

specimen
bacteriologic s.
brush s.
clinical bacteriologic s.
cytologic s.
random urine s.
swab s.

spectinomycin
spectra (*pl. of* spectrum)
spectral
s. color
s. interference
s. overlap
s. resolution
s. response

spectrin
spectrofluorometer
spectrograph
mass s.

spectrometer
gamma s.
mass s.

γ-spectrometer
spectrometry
clinical s.
gamma s.
gas chromatography-mass s. (GC-MS)
isotope dilution-mass s.
mass s. (MS)

γ-spectrometry
spectrophotometer
AA s.
atomic absorption s.

spectrophotometric assay
spectrophotometry
atomic absorption s. (AAS)
flame emission s.
infrared s. (IRS)
ultraviolet/visible s.

spectroscope
direct vision s.

spectroscopy
clinical s.
emission s.
flame emission s. (FES)
infrared s.
nuclear magnetic resonance s.
Raman s.

spectrum, pl. **spectra, spectrums**
absorption s.
s. analyzer
antimicrobial s.
atomic s.
band s.
broad s.
clinical s.
continuous s.
emission s.
excitation s.
fiber s.
fluorescence s.
gamma-ray s.
line s.
toxin s.
wide s.

specular reflection
spelencephaly
Spelotrema
Spencer disease
Spen syndrome
sperm
s. crystal
muzzled s.
s. penetration assay

spermacytic seminoma
spermatic fistula
spermatid
spermatin
spermatocele
spermatocyst
spermatocyte
spermatogenesis

S

NOTES

spermatogenic
>   s. granuloma
>   s. maturation arrest

spermatogonium, pl. **spermatogonia**
spermatoid
spermatolysin
spermatolysis
spermatolytic
spermatoxin
spermatozoon, pl. **spermatozoa**
>   end piece of s.
>   middle piece of s.
>   neck of s.
>   outer dense fibers of s.
>   principal piece of s.

spermaturia
spermidine
spermin crystal
spermine
spermiogenesis
spermolith
spermolysis
spermotoxin
SPF
>   specific pathogen-free

sp gr
>   specific gravity

SPH
>   secondary pulmonary hemosiderosis

sphacelate
sphacelation
sphacelism
sphaceloderma
sphacelous
sphacelus
Sphaerophorus
>   *S. necrophorus*

sphenoiditis
spheno-occipital synchondrosis
sphenopetrosal synchondrosis
sphere
>   attraction s.
>   embryonic s.
>   Morgagni s.
>   prelytic s.
>   segmentation s.
>   vitelline s.

spherical polar coordinates
spherocyte
spherocytic
>   s. anemia
>   s. jaundice

spherocytosis
>   hereditary s. (HS)

spherophakia-brachymorphia syndrome
spheroplast
spherospermia
spherule

spherulin
sphincteral achalasia
sphincteritis
sphinganine
sphingenine
sphingolipidoses, sing. **sphingolipidosis**
sphingolipidosis
>   cerebral s.

sphingolipid storage disease
sphingolipodystrophy
sphingomyelin
>   s. lipidosis
>   s. phosphodiesterase

sphingomyelinase
sphingomyelinosis
sphingosine
SPI
>   serum precipitable iodine

spiculated
>   s. body

spicule
spider
>   s. angioma
>   arterial s.
>   black widow s.
>   brown recluse s.
>   s. cancer
>   s. cell
>   s. mole
>   s. nevus
>   s. pelvis
>   s. telangiectasia
>   vascular s.

spider-burst
spidery
Spiegler-Fendt
>   pseudolymphoma of S.-F.
>   S.-F. pseudolymphoma
>   S.-F. sarcoid

Spielmeyer acute swelling
Spielmeyer-Stock disease
Spielmeyer-Vogt disease
spike
spill
>   cellular s.
>   s. control
>   s. control kit
>   s. residue

spiloma
spilus
spina, pl. **spinae**
>   s. bifida
>   s. bifida aperta
>   s. bifida cystica
>   s. bifida manifesta
>   s. bifida occulta
>   s. ventosa

spinal
- s. cord concussion
- s. cord tumor
- s. embolism
- s. fluid
- s. fluid culture
- s. fluid leukocyte count

spindle
- achromatic s.
- s. attachment
- barbiturate s.
- bipolar s.
- s. cell
- s. cell carcinoma
- s. cell lipoma
- s. cell melanoma
- s. cell nevus
- s. cell sarcoma
- s. cell thymoma
- multipolar s.

spindling
spindly squamoid cell
spine
- cleft s.
- poker s.

spiniger
- *Heterodoxus* s.

spiracle
spiradenitis
spiradenoma
- eccrine s.

spiral
- Curschmann s.
- s. fracture
- Herxheimer s.
- s. hyphae
- s. wound (SW)

spiralis
- *Acuaria* s.

spiramycin
spirilla (*pl. of* spirillum)
Spirillaceae
spirillar dysentery
spirillosis
Spirillum
- *S. minor*
- *S. minus*

spirillum, pl. **spirilla**
- Obermeier s.

spirit lamp
Spirocerca lupi

Spirochaeta
- *S. daxensis*
- *S. eurystrepta*
- *S. marina*
- *S. plicatilis*
- *S. stenostrepta*

spirochetal
spirochete
- Becker stain for s.'s

spirochetemia
spirochetolysis
spirochetosis
spirogram
- forced expiratory s. (FES)

Spirolate broth
Spirometra
spironolactone test
Spirurata
Spirurida
Spiruridae
spiruroid
- s. larva migrans

Spiruroidea
Spitz nevus
SPL
- spontaneous lesion

splanchnic blood flow (SBF)
splanchnocystica
- dysencephalia s.

splanchnoptosia
splanchnoptosis
splanchnosclerosis
spleen
- accessory s.
- Banti s.
- diffuse waxy s.
- lardaceous s.
- sago s.
- sugar-coated s.
- waxy s.

splenauxe
Splendore-Hoeppli phenomenon
splenectopia
splenelcosis
splenemphraxis
splenic
- s. anemia
- s. anemia of infants
- s. hemangiosarcoma
- s. index
- s. leukemia

S

NOTES

splenic *(continued)*
    s. marginal zone lymphoma (SMZL)
    s. tumor
splenitis
    acute s.
splenocele
splenogonadal fusion
splenohepatomegalia
splenohepatomegaly
splenoma
splenomalacia
splenomedullary
splenomegalia
splenomegalic polycythemia
splenomegaly
    congestive s.
    Egyptian s.
    fibrocongestive s.
    hemolytic s.
splenomyelogenous
splenomyelomalacia
splenoncus
splenosis
splenotoxin
spliceosome
splicing
    gene s.
split
    s. gene
    s. pelvis
    s. renal function (SRF)
    s. renal function study (SRFS)
    s. renal function test
    s. tolerance
split-thickness skin graft (STSG)
splitting
    beam s.
split-virus vaccine
spodogenous
spodogram
spodography
spodophorous
Spondweni virus
spondylitis
    ankylosing s.
    rheumatoid ankylosing s.
    tuberculous s.
spondylocace
spondyloepiphysial, spondyloepiphyseal
    s. dysplasia (SED)
spondylolisthesis
spondylolisthetic
    s. pelvis
spondylolysis
spondylomalacia
spondylopathy
spondyloptosis

spondylopyosis
spondyloschisis
spondylosis
    cervical s.
    hyperostotic s.
    lumbar s.
spondylosyndesis
spongiform
    s. encephalopathy
    s. pustule of Kogoj
spongioblast
spongioblastoma
spongiocyte
spongioid
spongiosis
    status s.
spongiositis
spongy
    s. degeneration of infancy
    s. degenerative-type leukodystrophy
    s. nevus
spontaneous
    s. abortion
    s. agglutination
    s. amputation
    s. delivery (SD)
    s. generation
    s. lesion (SPL)
    s. mutation
    s. phagocytosis
    s. pneumothorax
sporadic
    s. diffuse goiter
    s. dysentery
    s. nodular goiter
sporadin
sporangia (*pl. of* sporangium)
sporangiophore
sporangiospore
sporangium, pl. sporangia
spore
    bacterial s.
    drumstick s.
    s. form
    fungal s.
    s. strip
sporicidal
sporicide
sporidium
sporoagglutination
sporoblast
sporocyst
Sporocystinea
sporodochium
sporogenesis
sporogenous
sporogeny
sporogony

sporont
sporophore
sporoplasm
sporotheca
Sporothrix
    S. schenckii
sporotrichosis
sporotrichosis serology
sporotrichositic chancre
Sporotrichum
    S. beurmanni
    S. gougerotii
    S. schenckii
Sporozoa
sporozoa (*pl. of* sporozoon)
sporozoan
Sporozoasida
Sporozoea
sporozoite
sporozooid
sporozoon, pl. **sporozoa**
sporular
sporulation
sporule
spot
    Bitot s.
    blood s.
    blue s.
    café au lait s.
    cherry red s.
    De Morgan s.
    electronic focal s.
    s. film
    Fordyce s.
    Koplik s.
    milk s.
    mongolian s.
    ruby s.
    Tardieu s.
    tendinous s.
    s. test
    s. test for infectious mononucleosis
    white s.
    yellow s. (YS)
spotted fever
spotty lobular necrosis
spp. (*pl. of* sp)
spray
    antistatic s.
Spray-Cyte slide fixative
spreading factor
spread plate

spring
    s. catarrhal conjunctivitis
    s. ophthalmia
sprinkler system
Sprinz-Nelson syndrome
sprue
    celiac s.
    nontropical s.
    tropical s. (TS)
spruelike syndrome
Spumavirinae
Spumavirus
spur
    s. cell
spuria
    placenta s.
spurious
    s. cast
    s. parasite
Spurway syndrome
sputum, pl. **sputa**
    s. aerogenosum
    s. cytology
    s. examination
    s. fungus culture
    globular s.
    green s.
    s. mycobacteria culture
    nummular s.
    prune-juice s.
    rusty s.
    s. smear
SQ
    subcutaneous
squalene
squama, pl. **squamae**
squamate
squamatization
squame
squamocolumnar junction
squamous
    s. cell
    s. cell carcinoma (SCC)
    s. cell carcinoma in situ
    s. cell index
    s. cell papilloma
    s. intraepithelial lesion (SIL)
    s. metaplasia
    s. metaplasia of amnion
    s. pearl
squamous cell index
square wave

NOTES

S

squarrose, squarrous
squill
>   red s.
SR
>   secretion rate
>   sedimentation rate
>   sensitization response
>   sigma reaction
>   systemic resistance
sr
>   steradian
SRBC
>   sheep red blood cell
SRC
>   sedimented red cell
>   sheep red cell
SRF
>   skin-reactive factor
>   somatotropin-releasing factor
>   split renal function
>   subretinal fluid
SRF-A
>   slow-reacting factor of anaphylaxis
SRFS
>   split renal function study
SRNA
>   soluble ribonucleic acid
SRS
>   slow-reacting substance
SRS-A
>   slow-reacting substance of anaphylaxis
SRSA
>   slow-reacting substance of anaphylaxis
S-R variation
SS
>   *Salmonella-Shigella*
>   saturated solution
>   statistically significant
>   subaortic stenosis
>   supersaturated
SSA
>   skin-sensitizing antibody
>   sulfosalicylic acid
SSD
>   sum of square deviations
SSKI
>   saturated solution of potassium iodide
SSN
>   severely subnormal
SSP
>   Sanarelli-Shwartzman phenomenon
SSPE
>   subacute sclerosing panencephalitis
SSS
>   scalded skin syndrome
>   specific soluble substance
SSV
>   simian sarcoma virus

ST
>   surface tension
STA
>   serum thrombotic accelerator
stab
>   stab culture
>   stab neutrophil
>   stab wound
stabilate
stabile
stability
stable
>   s. factor
>   s. factor deficiency
>   s. fly
stachybotryotoxicosis
stachyose
stack
Staclot Protein S test kit
stage
>   algid s.
>   Arneth s.
>   cold s.
>   defervescent s.
>   end s.
>   imperfect s.
>   incubative s.
>   s. of invasion
>   latent s.
>   menstrual s.
>   perfect s.
>   prodromal s.
>   proliferative s.
>   secretory s.
>   Tanner s.
>   tumor s.
staggered
staggers
staghorn calculus
staging
>   American Joint Committee on Cancer S. (AJCCS)
>   Butchart tumor s.
>   cancer s.
>   Clark malignant melanoma s.
>   Dukes s.
>   FAB tumor s.
>   FIGO classification of tumor s.
>   International Federation of Gynecology and Obstetrics classification of tumor s.
>   Jewett and Strong s.
>   malignant melanoma s.
>   TNM s.
>   tumor s.
stagnant
>   s. anoxia
>   s. hypoxia

Stagnicola
stagnora
stain

Abbott s. for spores
aceto-orcein s.
Achucárro s.
acid-fast s.
acid phosphatase s.
acid-Schiff s.
acridine orange s.
AE1 immunoperoxidase s.
AFB s.
Ag-AS s.
Albert s.
Alcian blue s.
alkaline phosphatase s.
Altmann anilin-acid fuchsin s.
3-amino-9-ethylcarbazole s.
ammonium silver carbonate s.
amyloid s.
antibody s.
antimony s.
argentaffin s.
arsenic s.
astrocyte s.
ATPase s.
auramine O fluorescent s.
auramine-rhodamine s.
azan s.
azure-eosin s.
B72.3 s.
bacterial s.
basic fuchsin-methylene blue s.
Bauer chromic acid leucofuchsin s.
Becker s. for spirochetes
Belke-Kleihauer s.
Bennhold Congo red s.
Ber-EP4 immunoperoxidase s.
Berg s.
Best carmine s.
Bethe s.
Betke s.
Bielschowsky s.
Biondi-Heidenhain s.
bipolar s.
Birch-Hirschfeld s.
Bodian copper-PROTARGOL s.
Borrel blue s.
Bowie s.
Brown-Brenn s.
Brown-Hopp tissue Gram s.
butyrate esterase s.

Cajal astrocyte s.
Cajal gold sublimate s.
calcofluor white s.
carbol-thionin s.
C-banding s.
CD79a s.
CEA immunoperoxidase s.
CEA-M s.
CEA-P s.
centromere banding s.
certified s.
chlorazol black E s.
chondroitin sulfate s.
ChrA immunoperoxidase s.
chromate s. for lead
chrome alum hematoxylin-
  phloxine s.
chymotrypsin s.
Ciaccio s.
colloidal iron s.
Congo red s.
contrast s.
cresyl blue brilliant s.
cresyl violet s.
Da Fano s.
Dane and Herman keratin s.
DAPI s.
Darrow red s.
Delafield hematoxylin s.
Del Rio Hortega s.
deoxyribonucleic acid s.
diaminobenzidine s.
diazo s. for argentaffin granules
Dieterle s.
differential s.
direct fluorescent antibody s.
DOPA s.
Dorner s.
double s.
D-PAS s.
DU-PAN-2 s.
Ehrlich acid hematoxylin s.
Ehrlich aniline crystal violet s.
Ehrlich triacid s.
Ehrlich triple s.
Einarson gallocyanin-chrome
  alum s.
elastica-van Gieson s.
elastic fiber s.
elastin s.
eosin s.
Eranko fluorescence s.

NOTES

stain *(continued)*
ethidium bromide s.
ferric ammonium sulfate s.
Feulgen s.
fibrin s.
Field rapid s.
Fink-Heimer s.
Fite s.
Fite-Faraco s.
Flemming triple s.
fluorescence plus Giemsa s.
fluorescent s.
Fontana-Masson silver s.
Fontana methenamine silver s.
Foot reticulin impregnation s.
Fouchet s.
Fraser-Lendrum s. for fibrin
Friedländer s. for capsules
fuchsin s.
fungal s.
Fungalase-F s.
G-banding s.
gentian orange s.
gentian violet s.
Giemsa chromosome banding s.
Gill #2 hematoxylin blue s.
Gimenez s.
Glenner-Lillie s. for pituitary
glycogen s.
glycolipid s.
glycoprotein s.
GMS s.
Golgi s.
Gomori aldehyde fuchsin s.
Gomori chrome alum hematoxylin-
phloxine s.
Gomori-Jones periodic acid-
methenamine-silver s.
Gomori methenamine-silver s.'s
(GMS)
Gomori nonspecific acid
phosphatase s.
Gomori nonspecific alkaline
phosphatase s.
Gomori one-step trichrome s.
Gomori silver impregnation s.
Gomori-Takamatsu s.
Goodpasture s.
Gordon and Sweet s.
Gram s.
Gram-Weigert s.
Gridley s. for fungi
Grimelius s.
Grocott-Gomori methenamine-
silver s.
Hale colloidal iron s.
Hansel s.
H&E s.

Heidenhain azan s.
Heidenhain iron hematoxylin s.
hematoxylin-eosin s.
hematoxylin-malachite green-basic
fuchsin s.
hematoxylin-phloxine B s.
hemosiderin s.
HHF-35 s.
Hirsch-Peiffer s.
Hiss s.
histochemical s.
Holmes s.
Hortega neuroglia s.
HRS4 MAb immunoperoxidase s.
Hucker-Conn s.
immunofluorescent s.
immunohistochemical s.
immunoperoxidase s.
India ink capsule s.
intravital s.
iodine s.
iron hematoxylin s.
Jenner s.
Jenner-Giemsa s.
Kasten fluorescent Feulgen s.
Kasten fluorescent PAS s.
Kenyon s.
keratin s.
Kinyoun carbol fuchsin s.
Kittrich s.
Kleihauer s.
Klinger-Ludwig acid-thionin s. for
sex chromatin
Klüver-Barrera Luxol fast blue s.
Kossa s.
Kronecker s.
LAP s.
Laquer s. for alcoholic hyalin
Lawless s.
lead hydroxide s.
Leishman s.
Lendrum inclusion body s.
Lendrum phloxine-tartrazine s.
Lepehne-Pickworth s.
leukocyte acid phosphatase s.
Leukostat s.
Leu-M1 immunoperoxidase s.
Levaditi s.
Levine alkaline Congo red s.
Lillie allochrome connective
tissue s.
Lillie azure-eosin s.
Lillie ferrous iron s.
Lillie sulfuric acid Nile blue s.
lipase 21 s.
lipase 105 s.
lipid s.
Lison-Dunn s.

Löffler caustic s.
Lugol s.
Luna-Ishak s.
Luxol fast blue s.
Macchiavello s.
MacNeal tetrachrome blood s.
malarial pigment s.
Maldonado-San Jose s.
Mallory s. for actinomyces
Mallory aniline blue s.
Mallory collagen s.
Mallory s. for hemofuchsin
Mallory iodine s.
Mallory phloxine s.
Mallory phosphotungstic acid
  hematoxylin s.
Mallory trichrome s.
Mallory triple s.
Mancini iodine s.
Mann methyl blue-eosin s.
Marchi s.
Masson argentaffin s.
Masson-Fontana ammoniacal
  silver s.
Masson trichrome s.
Maximow s. for bone marrow
Mayer acid alum hematoxylin s.
Mayer hemalum s.
Mayer mucicarmine s.
Mayer mucihematein s.
May-Grünwald s.
May-Grünwald-Giemsa s.
M-DES s.
meconium s.
Meissel s.
metachromatic s.
methenamine silver s.
methylene blue s.
methyl green-pyronin s.
Milligan trichrome s.
Movat pentachrome s.
Mowry colloidal iron s.
MSB trichrome s.
mucicarmine s.
mucopolysaccharide s.
multiple s.
Musto s.
MY-10 clone s.
myeloperoxidase s.
Nakanishi s.
naphthol-ASD chloroacetate
  esterase s.

Nauta s.
negative s.
Neisser s.
neutral s.
Nicolle s. for capsules
Nile blue fat s.
ninhydrin-Schiff s. for proteins
Nissl s.
nitroblue tetrazolium s.
Noble s.
Novelli s.
NSE s.
nuclear s.
nuclear fast red s.
oil red O s.
oligodendroglia s.
orcein s.
Orth s.
osmium tetroxide s.
oxalic acid s.
oxytalan fiber s.
Padykula-Herman s. for myosin
  ATPase
Paget-Eccleston s.
Palmgren silver impregnation s.
pancreatic islet s.
panoptic s.
Pap s.
Papanicolaou s.
PAPI s.
PAP immunoperoxidase s.
Pappenheim s.
paracarmine s.
Paragon blue s.
PAS s.
Perls Prussian blue s.
peroxidase s.
phloxine-tartrazine s.
phosphomolybdic acid s.
phosphotungstic acid s.
picric s.
picrocarmine s.
picro-Mallory trichrome s.
picronigrosin s.
plasma s., plasmic s.
plasmatic s.
plastic section s.
polychrome methylene blue s.
Pontamine sky blue s.
port-wine s.
positive s.
potassium metabisulfate s.

NOTES

579

stain *(continued)*
    potassium permanganate s.
    Protargol s.
    Prussian blue s.
    PTA s.
    PTAH s.
    Puchtler-Sweat s.
    Puchtler-Sweat s. for basement
        membranes
    Puchtler-Sweat s. for hemoglobin
        and hemosiderin
    pyrrol blue s.
    Q-banding s.
    quinacrine chromosome banding s.
    Rambourg chromic acid-
        phosphotungstic acid s.
    Rambourg periodic acid-chromic
        methenamine-silver s.
    Ranson pyridine silver s.
    R-banding s.
    reticulin s.
    reticulum s.
    rhodamine s.
    rhodanine s.
    Romanowsky blood s.
    Roux s.
    scarlet red s.
    Schaeffer-Fulton s.
    Schiff s.
    Schmorl ferric-ferricyanide
        reduction s.
    Schmorl picrothionin s.
    Schultz s.
    selective s.
    Sevier-Munger s.
    Shorr trichrome s.
    silver-ammoniacal silver s.
    silver nitrate s.
    silver protein s.
    Snook reticulum s.
    sodium bisulfite s.
    sodium hydroxide s.
    sodium thiosulfate s.
    Stirling modification of Gram s.
    Sudan black B fat s.
    supravital s.
    synaptophysin s.
    Taenzer s.
    Taenzer-Unna s.
    Takayama s.
    telomeric R-banding s.
    tetrachrome s.
    tetramethylbenzidine s.
    thiazine s.
    thioflavine T s.
    thionin s.
    Tilden s.
    Tizzoni s.

    T method s.
    Toison s.
    toluidine blue s.
    trichrome s.
    Truant auramine-rhodamine s.
    trypsin G-banding s.
    Turnbull blue s.
    Unna s.
    Unna-Pappenheim s.
    Unna-Taenzer s.
    uranyl acetate s.
    urate crystals s.
    van Ermengen s.
    van Gieson s.
    Verhoeff elastic tissue s.
    vimentin immunoperoxidase s.
    vital s.
    von Kossa s.
    Wachstein-Meissel s. for calcium-
        magnesium-ATPase
    Wade-Fite-Faraco s.
    Warthin-Starry silver s.
    Wayson s.
    Weigert s. for actinomyces
    Weigert s. for elastin
    Weigert s. for fibrin
    Weigert-Gram s.
    Weigert iron hematoxylin s.
    Weigert s. for myelin
    Weigert s. for neuroglia
    Weigert-Pal s.
    Weil myelin sheath s.
    Wilder s. for reticulum
    Williams s.
    Wright s.
    Ziehl s.
    Ziehl-Neelsen s.
stained urinary sediment (SUS)
Stainer
    CODE-ON Immunoslide S.
staining
    acid phosphatase s.
    alkaline phosphatase s.
    amyloid s.
    anti-GFAP s.
    astrocyte s.
    automated slide s.
    bacterial s.
    bipolar s.
    chondroitin sulfate s.
    deoxyribonucleic acid s.
    enterochromaffin s.
    fat s.
    fibrin s.
    fluorescent s.
    fungi s.
    glycogen s.
    glycolipid s.

glycoprotein s.
H and E s.
hematoxylin and eosin s.
hemosiderin s.
histologic s.
immunohistochemical s.
iodine s.
keratin s.
mast cell s.
mucopolysaccharide s.
oligodendroglia s.
phospholipid s.
progressive s.
regressive s.
reticulin s.
supravital s.
vital s.
stains-all
Stamey test
Stamnosoma
stand
    KINEX anatomic specimen s.
standard
s. acid reflux test (SART)
air quality s.
s. bicarbonate
certified s.
s. curve
s. deviation (SD)
s. electrode potential
s. enthalpy of formation
s. error (SE)
s. error of estimate (SEE)
s. free energy
s. hydrogen electrode
internal s.
s. morbidity ratio
s. mortality ratio (SMR)
Prader bead s.
primary s.
s. reduction potential
s. score
s. serologic test for syphilis
s. solution
s. state
s. temperature and pressure
s. temperature and pressure, dry (STPD)
s. test for syphilis (STS)
s. urea clearance
standardization
standardize

standardized
s. deviate
s. rate
standing plasma test
standstill
    cardiac s.
stannic
stannous
Stanton disease
staph
    staphylococcus
Staph-Ident test
Staph-Trac test
staphylococcal
s. clumping test (SCT)
s. enteritis
s. enterotoxin
s. pneumonia
s. scalded skin syndrome
staphylococcemia
staphylococci (*pl. of* staphylococcus)
staphylococcin
staphylococcolysin
staphylococcolysis
Staphylococcus
S. albus
S. aureus
S. aureus nasopharyngeal culture
S. aureus neutral proteinase
S. citreus
S. epidermidis
methicillin-resistant *S. aureus* (MRSA)
methicillin-resistant coagulase-negative *S.* (MRCNS)
methicillin-susceptible *S. aureus* (MSSA)
methicillin-susceptible coagulase-negative *S.* (MSCNS)
S. pyogenes aureus
S. saprophyticus
S. septicemia
staphylococcus, pl. **staphylococci (staph)**
s. antitoxin
s. vaccine
staphylohemia
staphylohemolysin
staphylokinase
staphylolysin
α-s.
alpha staphylolysin
β-s.

NOTES

S

staphylolysin *(continued)*
    beta staphylolysin
    δ s.
    delta staphylolysin
    ε s.
    epsilon staphylolysin
    γ s.
    gamma staphylolysin
staphyloma
staphylo-opsonic index
staphylotoxin
star
    venous s.
starch
    hydroxyethyl s.
    s. tolerance test
Stargardt disease
Starling law
start codon
starvation-induced protein breakdown
stasis, pl. stases
    bile s.
    s. cirrhosis
    s. dermatitis
    s. ulcer
Stasisia
stat
    s. test
state
    absorptive s.
    baseline steady s.
    carrier s.
    central excitatory s. (CES)
    central inhibitory s. (CIS)
    complement deficiency s.
    excited s.
    ground s.
    immunity deficiency s. (IDS)
    imperfect s.
    metastable s.
    oxidation s.
    perfect s.
    postabsorptive s.
    sample steady s.
    solid s.
    standard s.
    steady s.
    transition s.
statement
    assignment s.
    source s.
static
    s. gangrene
    s. storage allocation
statin
stationary phase
statistic
    Mann-Whitney rank sum s.

    test s.
    Wilcoxon signed rank s.
statistically significant (SS)
statistical symbol
statistics
status
    s. asthmaticus
    s. choreicus
    s. cribrosus
    s. criticus
    s. dysmyelinisatus
    s. dysraphicus
    s. epilepticus
    s. hemicranicus
    Karnofsky s.
    s. lacunaris
    s. lymphaticus
    s. marmoratus
    s. nervosus
    s. raptus
    s. spongiosis
    s. spongiosus
    s. thymicolymphaticus
    s. thymicus
Staub-Traugott effect
STC
    soft tissue calcification
STD
    sexually transmitted disease
    skin test dose
    skin to tumor distance
steady state
steady-state condition
steam-fitter's asthma
steapsin
stearate
stearic acid
stearin
steatitis
steatocystoma
    s. multiplex
steatohepatitis
steatolytic enzyme
steatomatosis
steatonecrosis
steatopyga, steatopygia
steatopygous
steatorrhea
steatosis
    s. cordis
    hepatic s.
steatozoon
Steele-Richardson-Olszewski syndrome
Steenbock unit
steeple skull
Stefan-Boltzmann law
stegnosis
Stegobium

Stegomyia
stegomyiae
>   *Myxococcidium s.*
Steinbrocker syndrome
Steiner syndrome
Steinert disease
Stein-Leventhal syndrome
Stelangium
Stellantchasmus
stellate
>   s. abscess
>   s. fracture
stem
>   s. cell
>   s. cell assay
>   s. cell leukemia
>   s. cell lymphoma
stemline
Stender dish
Stenoglossa
stenosal
stenosed
stenosis, pl. stenoses
>   aortic s. (AS)
>   buttonhole s.
>   calcific nodular aortic s.
>   congenital pyloric s.
>   coronary ostial s.
>   discrete subaortic s.
>   Dittrich s.
>   hypertrophic muscular subaortic s.
>   (HMSAS)
>   hypertrophic pyloric s. (HPS)
>   idiopathic hypertrophic subaortic s.
>   (IHSS)
>   infundibular s.
>   mitral s.
>   muscular subaortic s.
>   nodular calcific aortic s.
>   pulmonary s. (PS)
>   pulmonary artery s. (PAS)
>   pyloric s. (PS)
>   renal artery s. (RAS)
>   subaortic s. (SS)
>   subvalvar s.
>   supravalvar s.
>   supravalvular aortic s. (SAS,
>   SVAS)
>   tricuspid s.
>   valvular s.
stenothermal
stenotic

stenoxenous
step
>   s. function
>   rate-controlling s.
step-down transformer
Stephanofilaria stilesi
Stephanurus dentatus
step-up transformer
steradian (sr)
stercobilin
stercobilinogen
stercolith
stercoraceous ulcer
stercoral
>   s. abscess
>   s. appendicitis
>   s. fistula
>   s. ulcer
stercoroma
Sterculia
stereochemical isomerism
stereochemistry
stereocilia
stereognosis
stereoisomer
stereoisomerism
stereology
stereometer
stereometry
stereoscope
stereoscopic
>   s. microscope
>   s. radiography
stereospecific numbering
stereotactic brain biopsy
steric hindrance
sterigma, pl. sterigmata
sterile
>   s. abscess
>   s. cyst
sterility
>   s. culture
>   s. test broth
sterilization
>   discontinuous s.
>   fractional s.
>   intermittent s.
sterilize
sterilizer
>   gas s.
sternal
>   s. synchondrosis

NOTES

Sternberg disease
Sternberg-Reed cell
Sterneedle tuberculin test
sternocostal triangle
steroid
    anabolic s.
    s. fever
    s. hormone
    ketogenic s. (KGS)
    s. protein activity index (SPAI)
    s. saponin
steroid-binding
    s.-b. betaglobulin
steroid-21-hydroxylase
steroid-21-monooxygenase
steroidogenesis
steroid-receptor complex
sterol
    s. carrier protein
    s. glycoside
stetharteritis
stethomyitis
stethomyositis
Stevens-Johnson syndrome
Stewart-Morel syndrome
Stewart-Treves syndrome
STH
    somatotropic hormone
STI
    systolic time interval
stibine
stichochrome
    s. cell
Sticker disease
Stickler
    S. syndrome
sticky ends
Stieda disease
stigma, pl. **stigmas, stigmata**
    s. ventriculi
stilbene dye
stilbestrol
stilesi
    Stephanofilaria s.
still
    S. disease
    s. layer
stillbirth
    macerated s.
Still-Chauffard syndrome
Stilling syndrome
Stilling-Turk-Duane syndrome
stimulation
    paracrine s.
    repetitive s.
stimulator
    long-acting thyroid s. (LATS)
sting

stipple cell
stippled epiphysis
stippling
    basophilic s.
    Ziemann s.
Stirling modification of Gram stain
stitch abscess
STK
    streptokinase
St. Louis encephalitis (SLE)
    St. Louis encephalitis virus (SLEV)
    St. Louis encephalitis virus
      serology (SLEV)
STIPD
STM
    streptomycin
Stobo antigen
stochastic
stock
    s. culture
    s. strain
    s. vaccine
stoichiometry
stoke
Stokes
    S. law
    S. shift
Stokes-Adams (SA)
    S. disease
Stokvis-Talma syndrome
Stoll dilution egg count technique
stolon
stoma, pl. **stomata**
stomach
    bilocular s.
    drain-trap s.
    hourglass s.
    leather-bottle s.
    sclerotic s.
    trifid s.
    s. tumor
    wallet s.
    water-trap s.
stomal ulcer
stomata (*pl. of* stoma)
stomatitis, pl. **stomatitides**
    aphthous s.
    bovine papular s.
    gangrenous s.
    herpetic s.
    lead s.
    s. papulosa
    primary herpetic s.
    vesicular s.
    Vincent s.
stomatocyte
stomatocytosis
stomodeal

stomodeum
Stomoxys calcitrans
stone
    skin s.
    vein s.
stone-strippers' asthma
stool
    acholic s.
    s. fungus culture
    Gram stain of s.
    s. mycobacteria culture
    tarry s.
stopcock
stop codon
storage
    s. allocation
    s. capacity
    common s.
    compressed gas s.
    ether s.
    external s.
    internal s.
    s. limit
    s. location
    mass s.
    s. oscilloscope
    s. pool disease
    transport and s.
store
storiform
    s. neurofibroma
    s. pattern
Stormer viscosimeter
Stovall-Black method
STPD
    standard temperature and pressure, dry
    STPD conditions of gas
Strachan syndrome
straddling embolism
strain
    s. birefringence
    carrier s.
    cell s.
    HFR s.
    hypothetical mean s. (HMS)
    lysogenic s.
    pseudolysogenic s.
    recombinant s.
    reference s.
    stock s.
    type s.

strand
    complementary s.
    leading s.
    minus s.
    plus s.
    sense s.
    viral s.
strangulated hernia
strangulation
strap cell
Strassburg test
stratification
stratified
    s. random sample
    s. thrombus
Stratiomyidae
stratum malphigii
Stravigen immunohistochemical reagent
strawberry
    s. birthmark
    s. gallbladder
    s. gums
    s. mark
    s. nevus
strawberry-cream blood
stray light
streak
    s. culture
    s. gonad
    gonadal s.
    s. hyperostosis
    meningitic s.
    s. plate
streaming
    s. movement
street virus
Strengeria
strength
    dielectric s.
    ionic s.
    magnetic field s.
strep
    streptococcus
streptavidin-biotin-complex technique
streptavidin-biotin peroxidase method
strepticemia
Streptobacillus
    S. moniliformis
    S. pseudotuberculosis
streptocerciasis
Streptococcaceae

S

NOTES

streptococcal
   s. antigen test
   s. carditis
   s. cellulitis
   s. fibrinolysin
   s. pneumonia
   s. toxin immunization reaction
streptococcemia
Streptococcus
   S. agalactiae
   S. anaerobius
   S. anginosus-constellatus
   S. bovis
   S. cremoris
   S. durans
   S. equi
   S. equisimilis
   S. evolutus
   S. faecalis
   S. faecium
   group A *S.*
   group D *S.*
   group N *S.*
   S. hemolyticus
   S. intermedius
   S. lactis
   S. lactis R (SLR)
   S. liquefaciens
   S. M antigen
   S. MG
   S. MG-intermedius
   S. microaerophilic
   S. milleri
   S. mitis
   S. mutans
   S. pneumoniae
   S. pyogenes
   S. salivarius
   S. sanguis
   S. uberis
   S. viridans
   S. zooepidemicus
   S. zymogenes
streptococcus, pl. **streptococci (strep)**
   α s.
   alpha s.
   anaerobic s.
   anhemolytic s.
   Bargen s.
   beta s.
   beta hemolytic s.
   s. erythrogenic toxin
   Fehleisen s.
   γ s.
   gamma s.
   hemolytic s.
   β-hemolytic s. (BHS)
   s. MG

   microaerophilic s.
   nonhemolytic s.
   s. of Ostertag
   s. serum
   viridans s.
streptodornase (SD)
streptokinase (STK)
streptokinase-streptodornase
streptolysin (SL)
   s. O
   s. S
streptolysin-O (SLO)
Streptomyces
   S. madurae
   S. pelletieri
   S. somaliensis
Streptomycetaceae
streptomycin (SM, STM)
   s. unit
streptomycosis
streptosepticemia
Streptothrix
streptotrichosis
streptozyme
   s. test
stress
   s. protein
   s. reticulocyte
   s. ulcer
stria, pl. **striae**
   striae atrophicae
   striae cutis distensae
   striae gravidarum
   Wickham striae
striata
   area s.
striation
   basal s.
   tabby cat s.
   tigroid s.
striatonigral degeneration
stricture
   Hunner s.
   urethral s.
Strigeata
string
stringency
stringent response
strip
   reagent s.
   spore s.
stripped nucleus
stripping
   electrolytic s.
strobe light
strobila, pl. **strobilae**
strobilocercus

strobiloid
stroma, pl. stromata
    desmoplastic s.
    fibrocollagenous s.
    hyalinized s.
    mucinous s.
    Rollet s.
stromal
    s. endometriosis
    s. hyperplasia
    s. sarcoma
stromatin
stromatolysis
stromatosis
    endometrial s.
Strong bacillus
Strongylata
strongyle
Strongylidae
strongylina
    Ascarops s.
Strongyloidea
Strongyloides
    S. fulleborni
    S. stercoralis
strongyloidiasis
Strongyloididae
strongyloidosis
strongylosis
Strongylus
strontium
strontium-90
structural
    s. gene
    s. isomerism
    s. lesion
    s. protein
structure
    analogous s.
    s. collapse
    dipolar s.
    fine s.
    homologous s.
    list s.
    primary s.
    quaternary s.
    rudimentary s.
    secondary s.
    tertiary s.
    tuboreticular s.
struma, pl. strumae
    s. aberrata

s. colloides
Hashimoto s.
ligneous s.
s. lymphomatosa
s. maligna
s. medicamentosa
s. ovarii
Riedel s.
strumiform
strumipriva
    cachexia s.
strumitis
strumous
Strümpell disease
Strümpell-Leichtenstern disease
Strümpell-Lorrain disease
Strümpell-Marie disease
Strümpell-Westphal disease
struvite calculus
strychnine
    s. assay
Stryker-Halbeisen syndrome
STS
    serologic test for syphilis
    standard test for syphilis
STSG
    split-thickness skin graft
STT
    serial thrombin time
STU
    skin test unit
Stuart
    S. broth
    S. factor
Stuart-Power factor
Student-Newman-Keuls test
Student test
study
    case-control s.
    clinicopathologic s.
    cohort s.
    double-contrast s.
    dual-contrast s.
    erythrokinetic s.
    fat absorption s.
    ferrokinetics s.
    gene-arrangement s.
    haplotype association s.
    immunophenotypic s.
    prospective s.
    renal function s. (RFS)

NOTES

study *(continued)*
    retrospective s.
    split renal function s. (SRFS)
stump cancer
stunted
    s. embryo
    s. fetus
stupor
Sturge-Kalischer-Weber syndrome
Sturge syndrome
Sturge-Weber syndrome
STVA
    subtotal villose atrophy
stye
    meibomian s.
    zeisian s.
styloid
    s. process
styloiditis
stylosteophyte
Styloviridae
styptic
    chemical s.
    mechanical s.
    vascular s.
Stypven
    S. time
    S. time test
styrene
styrone
SUA
    serum uric acid
subacute
    s. abscess
    s. bacterial endocarditis (SBE)
    s. bronchopneumonia
    s. combined degeneration (SACD)
    s. combined degeneration (of spinal cord) (SCD)
    s. combined degeneration of the spinal cord
    s. combined sclerosis
    s. glomerulonephritis
    s. granulomatous thyroiditis
    s. hepatitis
    s. inclusion body encephalitis
    s. infective endocartitis
    s. inflammation
    s. meningitis
    s. myelomonocytic leukemia (MLS)
    s. myelo-optical neuropathy (SMON)
    s. necrotizing encephalopathy
    s. necrotizing myelitis
    s. nephritis
    s. sclerosing leukoencephalitis
    s. sclerosing panencephalitis (SSPE)
    s. spongiform encephalopathy

subadventitial fibrosis
subaortic stenosis (SS)
subarachnoid hemorrhage (SAH)
subareolar duct papillomatosis
subcellular
subclass
    immunoglobulin s.
subclassification
    Lukes-Butler histologic s.
subcorneal
    s. pustular dermatitis
    s. pustular dermatosis
subcortical arteriosclerotic encephalopathy
subcu, subcut, subq
    subcutaneous
subculture
subcutaneous (SC, SQ, subcu, subcut, subq)
    s. emphysema
    s. fat
    s. fat necrosis of newborn
    s. nodule
subdiaphragmatic abscess
subdural
    s. empyema
    s. hematoma
    s. hematorrhachis
    s. hygroma
subendocardial myocardial infarction
subependymal
    s. giant cell astrocytoma
    s. glioma
subependymoma
subepidermal
    s. abscess
    s. fibrosis
subepidermic bulla
suberosis
suberyl arginine
subfamily
subgenus
subgranular
subhepatic abscess
subicteric
subinfection
subinflammatory
subinvolution
subjective synonym
subkingdom
sublabial adhesion
subleukemia
subleukemic
    s. granulocytic leukemia
    s. lymphocytic leukemia
    s. monocytic leukemia
    s. myelosis
sublimation

sublingual cyst
subluxation
sublymphemia
submammary mastitis
submaxillary glycoprotein
submetacentric
submorphous
submucous (SM)
subnormal
 severely s. (SSN)
 s. temperature
suborder
subpapular
subperitoneal appendicitis
subphrenic abscess
subphylum
subplasmalemmal
 s. density
 s. microfilament
subpleural
subq (*var. of* subcu)
subretinal fluid (SRF)
subroutine
 recursive s.
subsclerotic
subscript
subscripted variable
subsinusoidal fibrosis
subspecies
substance
 alpha s.
 amount of s.
 antidiuretic s. (ADS)
 bacteriotropic s.
 beta s.
 blood group-specific s.'s A and B
 cement s.
 s. concentration
 controlled s.
 erythrocyte-sensitizing s. (ESS)
 exophthalmos-producing s. (EPS)
 fat-mobilizing s. (FMS)
 filar s.
 ground s.
 H s.
 hazardous s.
 hemolytic s.
 immunity s.
 methylene blue active s. (MBAS)
 pressor s.
 prostaglandin-like s. (PLS)
 rabbit aorta-contracting s.

 renal pressor s. (RPS)
 reticular s.
 sensitizing s.
 slow-reacting s. (SRS)
 soluble specific s.
 specific capsular s.
 specific soluble s. (SSS)
 threshold s.
 thromboplastic s.
 tumor polysaccharide s. (TPS)
 zymoplastic s.
α-substance
β-substance
substantia, pl. substantiae
 s. metachromaticogranularis
 s. nigra
 s. reticulofilamentosa
substernal goiter
substituent
substitute
 blood s.
 plasma s.
 Scott tap water s.
 volume s.
substitution
 s. product
 s. reaction
substrate
 defined s. (DS)
 s. level phosphorylation
 McGadey s.
subsynchronous
subtelocentric
subtotal villose atrophy (STVA)
subtribe
subungual
 s. abscess
 s. melanoma
subunit
 hCG-α s.
 hCG-β s.
 hCG-alpha s.
 hCG-beta s.
 s. vaccine
subvalvar stenosis
subvital mutation
succenturiata
 placenta s.
succinic acid
Succinivibrio
 S. dextrinosolvens
succinylcoenzyme A

S

NOTES

sucking louse
sucrase
sucrose
    s. hemolysis test
    s. intolerance
sucrose α-D-glucohydrolase
sucrosemia
sucrosuria
suction
    s. method (SM)
Suctoria
SUD
    sudden unexpected death
    sudden unexplained death
Sudan
    S. black B
    S. black B fat stain
    S. brown
    S. IV
    S. red III
    S. yellow
sudanophil
sudanophilia
sudanophilic
    s. leukodystrophy
sudanophobic
    s. zone
sudden
    s. cardiac death (SCD)
    s. coronary death (SCD)
    s. death syndrome (SDS)
    s. infant death syndrome (SIDS)
    s. unexpected death (SUD)
    s. unexpected, unexplained death
    (SUUD)
    s. unexplained death (SUD)
    s. unexplained infant death (SUID)
Sudeck
    S. atrophy
    S. disease
Sudeck-Leriche syndrome
sudor
    s. sanguineus
    s. urinosus
sudorikeratosis
sudoriparous abscess
SUDS
    Single Use Diagnostic System
sufficient
    s. condition
    not s. (NS)
    quantity not s. (QNS)
suffocation
suffocative goiter
suffusion
sugar
    s. acid
    blood s. (BS)

    s. broth
    fasting blood s. (FBS)
    invert s.
    postprandial blood s. (PPBS)
    reducing s.
    specific soluble s.
    s. tumor
sugar-coated spleen
sugar-icing liver
sugar water test screen
suggillation
    postmortem s.
suicide
    hot antigen s.
SUID
    sudden unexplained infant death
suid herpesvirus
sulfa
    s. drug
    s. film
sulfabenzamide
sulfacetamide
sulfadiazine
sulfaguanidine
sulfamerazine
sulfameter
sulfamethazine
sulfamethizole
sulfamethoxazole
sulfanilamide
sulfanilic acid
sulfapyridine
sulfatase
    iduronic s.
    phenol s.
    sulfatide s.
    L-sulfoiduronate s.
sulfate
    ammonium s.
    chondroitin s.
    colistin s.
    copper s.
    dermatan s.
    diethyl s.
    dimethyl s.
    heparan s.
    indoxyl s.
    keratan s.
    polymyxin B s.
    sodium dodecyl s.
sulfated acid mucopolysaccharide (SAM)
sulfatemia
sulfatiazole
sulfatidase
sulfatide
    cerebroside s.
    s. lipidosis
    s. sulfatase

sulfation
  s. factor
sulfhemoglobin (Hb S, SHb)
sulfhemoglobinemia
sulfhemoglobinuria
sulfhydryl group
sulfide
  dichlorodiethyl s.
sulfindigotic acid
sulfinic acid
sulfinpyrazone
sulfinyl
sulfisoxazole
sulfite
  s. oxidase
  s. oxidase deficiency
sulfmethemoglobin
sulfo
sulfobromophathalein sodium
S-sulfoglutathione
sulfolipid
sulfomucin
sulfonamide
  s. antagonist
  s. assay
sulfonate
  alkylbenzene s. (ABS)
  scarlet red s.
sulfonation
sulfone
sulfonic acid
sulfonmethane
sulfonyl
sulfonylurea assay
sulfoprotein
sulforhodamine B
sulfosalicylic
  s. acid (SSA)
  s. acid turbidity test
sulfoxide
  dimethyl s.
sulfur (S)
  s. bacterium
  s. dioxide
  s. dye
  s. granule
  s. trioxide
sulfuric acid
sulfurous acid
Sulkowitch
  S. reagent
  S. test

Sulzberger-Garbe syndrome
summer asthma
sum of square deviations (SSD)
SUN
  serum urea nitrogen
Sun SPARC-2
sup
  superficial
superacidity
superantigen
supercooled
superdistention
superdominance
superfemale
superficial (sup)
  s. burn
  s. implantation
  s. multicentric basal cell carcinoma
  s. spreading melanoma
  s. wound
superheated
superinduce
superinfection
superior
  s. limbic keratoconjunctivitis (SLKC)
  s. pulmonary sulcus tumor
  s. vena caval syndrome
  s. vena cava syndrome
Supermount slide fixative
supernatant
  postmitochondrial s. (PMS)
supernumerary
  s. kidney
  s. organ
superoxide
  s. assay
  s. dismutase
superparasite
superparasitism
superpigmentation
supersaturated (SS)
Superstitionia
supervoltage
supplemental inheritance
supplementary gene
supply
  power s.
support medium
suppressibility
suppression

S

NOTES

suppressor
    s. cell
    s. gene
    s. mutation
    soluble immune response s. (SIRS)
    s. T lymphocyte
    tRNA s.
suppressor-sensitive mutant
suppurant
suppurate
suppuration
suppurative
    s. acute appendicitis
    s. acute inflammation
    s. arthritis
    s. cerebritis
    s. cholangitis
    s. chronic inflammation
    s. chronic otitis media
    s. encephalitis
    s. granulomatous inflammation
    s. hepatitis
    s. keratitis
    s. mastitis
    s. necrosis
    s. nephritis
    s. pericarditis
    s. pleurisy
    s. pneumonia
    s. synovitis
suprapubic
    s. needle aspiration
    s. puncture
suprarenalis
    cachexia s.
suprasellar cyst
supravalvar stenosis
supravalvular aortic stenosis (SAS, SVAS)
supravergence (S)
supravital (SV)
    s. stain
    s. staining
suramin
surface
    s. carcinoma in situ (SCIS)
    s. tension (ST)
surface-active agent
surface-barrier detector
surface-oriented pinocytic activity
surfactant
    amniotic fluid pulmonary s.
    pulmonary s.
SURGE software
surgical
    s. defect
    s. emphysema

    s. pathology
    s. wound
surra
surveillance
    immune s.
    immunological s.
survey
    cross-sectional s.
    s. meter
    proficiency s.
    s. program
survival
    red blood cell s.
    s. time
SUS
    stained urinary sediment
susceptibility
    electric s.
    genetic s.
    magnetic s.
    s. testing
suspended particulate
suspension
sustentacular cell
Sutton
    S. disease
    S. nevus
    S. ulcer
suture granuloma
SUUD
    sudden unexpected, unexplained death
SV
    severe
    simian virus
    snake venom
    supravital
SV40
SV40-adenovirus hybrid
SVAS
    supravalvular aortic stenosis
Svedberg
    S. equation
    S. flotation unit (Sf)
    S. unit (S)
    S. unit of sedimentation coefficient (S)
SVR
    systemic vascular resistance
SW
    spiral wound
swab
    nasopharyngeal s.
    s. specimen
swamp
    s. fever
    s. fever virus
Swann antigen
swan-neck deformity

Sw^a antigen
swarm
swarming
sweat
    s. duct adenoma
    s. gland adenocarcinoma
    s. gland adenoma
    s. gland carcinoma
    s. gland tumor
    s. test
Swediaur disease
Sweet
    S. disease
    S. method
    S. syndrome
swelling
    albuminous s.
    brain s.
    Calabar s.
    cellular s.
    cloudy s.
    fugitive s.
    Neufeld capsular s.
    Spielmeyer acute s.
Swift disease
Swift-Feer disease
swimmer's itch
swimming
    s. pool conjunctivitis
    s. pool granuloma
swine
    s. encephalitis virus
    s. fever
    s. fever virus
    s. influenza
    s. influenza virus
    s. pest
    s. vesicular disease
swinepox
    s. virus
Swiss
    S. cheese endometrium
    S. cheese hyperplasia
    S. mouse leukemia virus
Swiss-type
    S.-t. agammaglobulinemia (SAG)
    S.-t. hypogammaglobulinemia
switch
    class s.
    double-pole double-throw s.
    double-pole single-throw s.
    silicon-controlled s.

Sx
    signs
    symptoms
syaloglycoprotein
sycoma
sycosis
Sydenham
    S. chorea
    S. disease
Sydney classification system
sylvatic plague
Sylvest disease
sym
    symptom
symbion
symbiont
symbiosis
symbiote
symbiotic
symbol
    hazard s.
    statistical s.
Symmers
    S. clay pipestem fibrosis
    S. disease
symmetric
    s. adenolipomatosis
    s. distribution
symmetrical gangrene
symmetry
    bilateral s.
    s. element
    s. group
    icosahedral s.
    s. operation
    s. plane
    radial s.
sympathetic
    s. chain
    s. imbalance
    s. ophthalmia
    s. ophthalmitis
sympathetoblastoma
sympathicectomy
sympathicoblastoma
sympathicogonioma
sympathiconeuritis
sympathicopathy
sympathicotonia
sympathicotripsy
sympathoblastoma
sympathogonioma

NOTES

sympathomimetic
sympexis
symphysis, gen. symphyses
symport
symptom (sym)
symptomatic
    s. fever
    s. myeloid metaplasia
    s. porphyria
    s. reaction
    s. ulcer
    s. varicocele
symptomatology
symptoms (Sx)
symtomatolytic
SYN
    synaptophysin
synapsis
synaptonemal complex
synaptophysin (SYN)
    s. stain
Syncephalastrum
syncephalus
synchondrosis
    spheno-occipital s.
    sphenopetrosal s.
    sternal s.
synchronism
    developmental s.
synchronized culture
synchronous
    s. counter
    s. data transmission
    s. neoplasm
syncyanin
syncytia (*pl. of* syncytium)
syncytial
    s. alteration
    s. endometritis
    s. trophoblast
syncytiotrophoblast
syncytiotrophoblastic cell
syncytium, pl. syncytia
syndactyly
syndesmitis
syndesmophyte
syndrome
    Aarskog s.
    Aarskog-Scott s.
    abdominal muscle deficiency s.
    Abercrombie s.
    Achard s.
    Achard-Thiers s.
    Achenbach s.
    acquired immunodeficiency s.
      (AIDS)
    acrofacial s.

acute respiratory distress s.
    (ARDS)
Adair-Dighton s.
addisonian s.
Adie s.
adrenal feminizing s.
adrenal gland virilizing s.
adrenogenital s. (AGS)
adult respiratory distress s. (ARDS)
Ahumada-Del Castillo s.
Aicardi s.
Albright s.
Albright-McCune-Sternberg s.
Aldrich s.
Alezzandrini s.
Allen-Masters s.
Alport s.
Alström s.
amenorrhea-galactorrhea s.
Amsterdam s.
Andersen s.
Angelucci s.
angio-osteohypertrophy s.
antibody deficiency s. (ADS)
antiphospholipid s.
Anton s.
aortic arch s. (AAS)
apallic s.
aplastic anemia s.
Argonz-Del Castillo s.
Arias s.
Arndt-Gottron s.
Arnold-Chiari s.
Arnold nerve reflex cough s.
arthritis-dermatitis s.
Ascher s.
Asherman s.
ataxia telangiectasia s.
autoerythrocyte sensitization s.
Avellis s.
Axenfeld s.
Ayerza s.
Baastrup s.
Babinski s.
Babinski-Fröhlich s.
Babinski-Nageotte s.
Babinski-Vaquez s.
bacterial overgrowth s.
Bäfverstedt s.
Balint s.
Baller-Gerold s.
Bamberger-Marie s.
Banti s.
Bardet-Biedl s.
bare lymphocyte s.
Barlow s.
Barré-Guillain s.
Barrett s.

Bart s.
Bartter s.
basal cell nevus s.
Bassen-Kornzweig s.
Bateman s.
Batten-Mayou s.
Bazex s.
Beau s.
Beckwith s.
Beckwith-Wiedemann s.
Behçet s.
Benedikt s.
Beradinelli s.
Bernard s.
Bernard-Horner s.
Bernard-Sergent s.
Bernard-Soulier s.
Bernhardt-Roth s.
Bernheim s.
Bertolotti s.
Besnier-Boeck-Schaumann s.
Bianchi s.
Biemond s.
bile salt deficiency s.
Björnstad s.
Blackfan-Diamond s.
Blatin s.
Bloch-Sulzberger s.
Bloom s.
blue diaper s.
Blum s.
body of Luys s.
Boerhaave s.
Bonnet-Dechaume-Blanc s.
Bonnevie-Ullrich s.
Bonnier s.
Böök s.
Börjeson s.
Börjeson-Forssman-Lehmann s.
Bouillaud s.
Bouveret s.
bowel bypass s.
Brachmann-de Lange s.
brain death s.
Brennemann s.
Briquet s.
Brissaud-Marie s.
Brissaud-Sicard s.
Bristowe s.
Brock s.
bronchiolitis obliterans s.
Brown-Séquard s.

Brugsch s.
Bruns s.
Brunsting s.
Buckley s.
Budd s.
Budd-Chiari s.
Bürger-Grütz s.
Burnett s.
Buschke-Ollendorf s.
Bywaters s.
Cacchi-Ricci s.
Caffey s.
Caffey-Silverman s.
Canada-Cronkhite s.
Capgras s.
Caplan s.
carcinoid s.
carotid sinus s.
Carpenter s.
Castleman s.
cat-cry s.
cat's-eye s.
Ceelen-Gellerstadt s.
cellular immunity deficiency s.
  (CIDS)
cerebellomedullary malformation s.
cerebrohepatorenal s.
cervical rib s.
Cestan s.
Cestan-Chenais s.
Cestan-Raymond s.
chancriform s.
Charcot s.
Charcot-Weiss-Barker s.
Charlin s.
Chauffard s.
Chauffard-Still s.
Chédiak-Higashi s. (CHS)
Chédiak-Steinbrinck-Higashi s.
Cheney s.
Chiari-Arnold s.
Chiari-Budd s.
Chiari-Frommel s. (CF)
Chiari II s.
Chilaiditi s.
CHILD s.
childhood hemolytic uremic s.
Chinese restaurant s. (CRS)
Chotzen s.
Christian s.
Christ-Siemens s.
Christ-Siemens-Touraine s.

NOTES

syndrome *(continued)*
    chromosomal breakage s.
    chromosomal malformation s.
    chronic brain s. (CBS)
    Churg-Strauss s.
    Citelli s.
    Clarke-Hadfield s.
    Claude s.
    Claude Bernard-Horner s.
    Clough-Richter s.
    Clouston s.
    Cockayne s.
    Coffin-Lowry s.
    Coffin-Siris s.
    Cogan s.
    cold agglutinin s.
    Collet s.
    Collet-Sicard s.
    combined immunodeficiency s.
    common variable
      immunodeficiency s.
    compartmental s.
    congenital rubella s.
    Conn s.
    Cornelia de Lange s.
    Costen s.
    Cotard s.
    Courvoisier-Terrier s.
    Crandall s.
    CREST s.
    Creutzfeldt-Jakob s.
    cri du chat s.
    Crigler-Najjar s.
    Cronkhite-Canada s.
    Crouzon s.
    Crow-Fukase s.
    CRST s.
    crush s.
    Cruveilhier-Baumgarten s.
    cryopathic hemolytic s.
    cryptophthalmus s.
    Curtis-Fitz-Hugh s.
    Curtius s.
    Cushing s.
    cutaneomucouveal s.
    Cyriax s.
    DaCosta s.
    Danbolt-Closs s.
    Dandy-Walker s.
    Danlos s.
    Debré-Semelaigne s.
    de Clerambault s.
    defibrination s.
    Degos s.
    Dejerine s.
    Dejerine-Klumpke s.
    Dejerine-Roussy s.
    Dejerine-Sottas s.

    de Lange s.
    Del Castillo s.
    dengue shock s.
    Dennie-Marfan s.
    De Sanctis-Cacchione s.
    De Toni-Fanconi s.
    Diamond-Blackfan s.
    DiGeorge s.
    Di Guglielmo s.
    Donohue s.
    Down s. (DS)
    Dresbach s.
    Dressler s.
    Duane s.
    Dubin-Johnson s.
    Dubin-Sprinz s.
    Dubreuil-Chambardel s.
    Duchenne s.
    Duchenne-Erb s.
    dumping s.
    Duplay s.
    Dupré s.
    Dyggve-Melchior-Clausen s.
    Dyke-Davidoff-Masson s.
    dysmyelopoietic s.
    dysplastic nevus s.
    dysuria-pyuria s.
    Eagle s.
    Eaton-Lambert s.
    ectopic ACTH s.
    Eddowes s.
    Edwards s.
    Edwards-Patau s.
    Ehlers-Danlos s. (EDS)
    Eisenlohr s.
    Eisenmenger s.
    Ekbom s.
    Ellis-van Creveld s.
    EMG s.
    empty sella s.
    endocrine polyglandular s.
    eosinophilia-myalgia s.
    Epstein s.
    Erb s.
    erythrodysesthesia s.
    Evans s.
    excited skin s.
    Faber s.
    Fallot s.
    Fanconi s.
    Fanconi-Zinsser s.
    Farber s.
    Farber-Uzman s.
    Felty s.
    fertile eunuch s.
    fetal alcohol s.
    fetal face s.
    fetal hydantoin s.

fetal trimethadione s.
Feuerstein-Mims s.
fibrinogen-fibrin conversion s.
Fiessinger-Leroy-Reiter s.
Figueira s.
first arch s.
Fisher s.
Fitz s.
Fitz-Hugh and Curtis s.
Fleischner s.
Flynn-Aird s.
focal dermal hypoplasia s.
Foix s.
folded-lung s.
Forbes-Albright s.
Forney s.
Foster Kennedy s.
Foville s.
fragile X s.
Fraley s.
Franceschetti s.
Franceschetti-Jadassohn s.
François s.
Fraser s.
Freeman-Sheldon s.
Frenkel anterior ocular traumatic s.
Frey s.
Friderichsen-Waterhouse s.
Friedmann vasomotor s.
Fröhlich s.
Froin s.
Frommel-Chiari s.
Fuchs s.
Furst-Ostrum s.
G s.
Gailliard s.
Gaisböck s.
Gamstorp s.
Ganser s.
Gardner s.
Gardner-Diamond s.
Gasser s.
gay lymph node s.
Gélineau s.
Gerhardt s.
Gerstmann s.
Gianotti-Crosti s.
Gilbert s.
Gilles de la Tourette s.
Glanzmann-Riniker s.
glomangiomatous osseous
  malformation s.

Goldberg-Maxwell s.
Goldenhar s.
Goldz-Gorlin s.
Goltz s.
Good s.
Goodpasture s.
Gopalan s.
Gorlin s.
Gorlin-Chaudhry-Moss s.
Gorlin-Goltz s.
Gorlin-Psaume s.
Gorman s.
Gougerot-Blum s.
Gougerot-Carteaud s.
Gowers s.
gracilis s.
Gradenigo s.
Graham Little s.
gray platelet s.
Gregg s.
Greig s.
Griscelli s.
Grönblad-Strandberg s.
Gruber s.
Gubler s.
Guillain-Barré s. (GB)
Gulf War s.
Gull-Sutton s.
Gunn s.
Haber s.
Hadfield-Clarke s.
Hakim s.
Hallermann-Streiff s.
Hallermann-Streiff-François s.
Hallervorden s.
Hallervorden-Spatz s.
Hallgren s.
Hallopeau-Siemens s.
Hamman s.
Hamman-Rich s.
hand-foot s.
Hanhart s.
Hanot-Chauffard s.
Hantavirus pulmonary s.
Harada s.
Hare s.
Harris s.
Hartnup s.
Hassin s.
Hayem-Widal s.
heart-hand s.
Heerfordt s.

S

NOTES

syndrome *(continued)*

Hegglin s.
Heidenhain s.
Helweg-Larssen s.
hemangioma-thrombocytopenia s.
hemolytic uremic s.
hemolytic-uremic s. (HUS)
Hench-Rosenberg s.
Henoch-Schonlein s.
Herlitz s.
Hermansky-Pudlak s.
herniated disk s. (HDS)
Herrmann s.
Hines-Bannick s.
Hirschowitz s.
Hoffmann-Werdnig s.
Holmes-Adie s.
Holt-Oram s.
Homén s.
Horner s.
Horton s.
Houssay s.
Hünermann s.
Hunt s.
Hunter s.
Hunter-Hurler s.
Hurler s. (HS)
Hutchinson-Gilford s.
Hutchison s.
hypereosinophilic s.
hyper-IgE s.
hyperimmunoglobulin E s.
hyperimmunoglobulin M s.
hyperviscosity s.
hypophysial s.
hypophysio-sphenoidal s.
idiopathic nephrotic s. (INS)
idiopathic respiratory distress s. (IRDS)
Imerslund-Grasbeck s.
immotile cilia s.
immunodeficiency s.
s. of inappropriate antidiuretic hormone (SIADH)
inappropriate antidiuretic hormone s. (IADHS)
s. of inappropriate secretion of antidiuretic hormone (SIADH)
Irvine s.
Ivemark s.
Jaccoud s.
Jackson s.
Jacod s.
Jadassohn-Lewandowski s.
Jahnke s.
Jeghers-Peutz s.
Jervell and Lange-Nielsen s.
Jeune s.

Job s.
Johnson-Dubin s.
Joseph s.
juvenile polyposis s.
Kallmann s.
Kandinskii-Clerambault s.
Kanner s.
Kartagener s.
Kasabach-Merritt s.
Kast s.
Kearns s.
Kennedy s.
Kiloh-Nevin s.
Kimmelstiel-Wilson s.
Kinsbourne s.
Klauder s.
Kleine-Levin s.
Klinefelter s. (KS)
Klippel-Feil s. (KFS)
Klippel-Trenaunay s.
Klippel-Trenaunay-Weber s.
Klumpke-Dejerine s.
Klüver-Bucy s.
Kniest s.
Kocher-Debré-Semelaigne s.
Koenig s.
Koerber-Salus-Elschnig s.
Korsakoff s.
Kostmann s.
Krabbe s.
Krause s.
Kunkel s.
Kuskokwim s.
Laband s.
Labbé neurocirculatory s.
Ladd s.
LAMB s.
Lambert-Eaton s.
Landry s.
Landry-Guillain-Barré s.
Larsen s.
Launois s.
Launois-Bensaude s.
Launois-Cléret s.
Laurence-Biedl s.
Laurence-Moon s.
Laurence-Moon-Bardet-Biedl s.
Laurence-Moon-Biedl s.
Lawford s.
Lawrence-Seip s.
lazy leukocyte s.
Lennox s.
Lenz s.
Leriche s.
Leri-Weill s.
Lermoyez s.
Lesch-Nyhan s.
Lévy-Roussy s.

Leyden-Möbius s.
Lhermitte-McAlpine s.
Libman-Sacks s.
Lichtheim s.
Li-Fraumeni cancer s.
Lightwood s.
Lignac s.
Lignac-Fanconi s.
linear sebaceous nevus s.
Lobstein s.
Löffler s.
Looser-Milkman s.
Lorain-Lévi s.
Louis-Bar s.
Lowe s.
Lowe-Terrey-MacLachlan s.
Lown-Ganong-Levine s.
Lucey-Driscoll s.
Lutembacher s.
Luys body s.
Lyell s.
lymphadenopathy s.
lymphoproliferative s.
MacKenzie s.
Macleod s.
Maffucci s.
malabsorption s.
male Turner s.
malformation s.
malignant carcinoid s.
Malin s.
Mallory-Weiss s.
mandibulofacial dysotosis s.
mandibulo-oculofacial s.
Marañón s.
Marchesani s.
Marchiafava-Micheli s.
Marcus Gunn s.
Marfan s.
Margolis s.
Marie s.
Marie-Bamberger s.
Marie-Robinson s.
Marinesco-Garland s.
Marinesco-Sjögren s.
Maroteaux-Lamy s.
Marshall s.
Martorell s.
Mauriac s.
Mayer Rokitansky-Küster s.
McCune-Albright s.
Meckel s.

Meckel-Gruber s.
megacystic s.
Meigs s.
Melchior s.
Melkersson s.
Melkersson-Rosenthal s.
Melnick-Needles s.
MEN s.
Ménétrier s.
Mengert shock s.
Ménière s.
Menkes s.
menopausal s.
metastatic carcinoid s.
methionine malabsorption s.
Meyenburg-Altherr-Uehlinger s.
Meyer-Betz s.
Meyer-Schwickerath and Weyers s.
Miescher s.
Mikulicz s.
milk alkali s.
Milkman s.
Millard-Gubler s.
minimal-change nephrotic s.
Minkowski-Chauffard s.
Minot-von Willebrand s.
Mirizzi s.
mixed cryoglobulin s.
Möbius s.
Monakow s.
Moore s.
Morel s.
Morgagni s.
Morgagni-Adams-Stokes s.
Morgagni-Stewart-Morel s.
Morquio s.
Morquio-Brailsford s.
Morquio-Ullrich s.
Morris s.
Morton s.
Morvan s.
Mosse s.
Mounier-Kuhn s.
Mucha-Habermann s.
Muckle-Wells s.
mucocutaneous lymph node s.
mucosal neuroma s.
Muir-Torre s.
multiple hamartoma s.
multiple lentigines s.
multiple mucosal neuroma s.
Münchausen s.

S

NOTES

syndrome *(continued)*
  Murchison-Sanderson s.
  myelodysplastic s.
  myeloproliferative s.'s
  myofascial s.
  Naegeli s.
  Naffziger s.
  nail-patella s.
  NAME s.
  Nelson s.
  nephritic s.
  nephrotic s. (NS)
  Netherton s.
  neurocutaneous phacomatosis s.
  neuroleptic malignant s.
  newborn respiratory s.
  Nezelof s.
  Noack s.
  Nonne-Milroy-Meige s.
  Noonan s.
  OAV s.
  ocular-mucous membrane s.
  oculobuccogenital s.
  oculocerebrorenal s.
  oculodentodigital s.
  oculovertebral s.
  ODD s.
  OFD s.
    orofaciodigital syndrome
  Ogilvie s.
  Omenn s.
  OMM s.
  Oppenheim s.
  organic brain s. (OBS)
  orofaciodigital s. (OFD syndrome)
  osteomyelofibrotic s.
  Ostrum-Furst s.
  otomandibular s.
  painful-bruising s.
  Pancoast s.
  papillary muscle s.
  Papillon-Léage and Psaume s.
  Papillon-Lefèvre s.
  paraneoplastic s.
  Parinaud oculoglandular s.
  parkinsonian s.
  parotitis s.
  Parry-Romberg s.
  Patau s.
  Paterson s.
  Paterson-Brown-Kelly s.
  Paterson-Kelly s.
  Pellizzi s.
  Pendred s.
  Pepper s.
  periodic s. (PS)
  Persian Gulf s.
  Peutz s.

  Peutz-Jeghers s.
  Pfaundler-Hurler s.
  Pfeiffer s.
  pharyngeal pouch s.
  Picchini s.
  Pick s.
  pickwickian s.
  PIE s.
  Pierre Robin s.
  Plummer-Vinson s.
  POEMS s.
  Poland s.
  Polhemus-Schafer-Ivemark s.
  polycystic ovary s.
  polysplenia s.
  postmenopausal s.
  postpump s. (PPS)
  postrubella s.
  Potter s.
  Prader-Willi s.
  premature senility s.
  primary fibromyalgia s.
  Profichet s.
  prune belly s.
  pseudothalidomide s.
  pseudo-Turner s.
  pterygium s.
  pulmonary dysmaturity s.
  Putnam-Dana s.
  radial aplasia-thrombocytopenia s.
  Raeder paratrigeminal s.
  Ramsay Hunt s.
  Raymond-Cestan s.
  Recklinghausen-Applebaum s.
  red cell fragmentation s.
  Refetoff s.
  Reichmann s.
  Reifenstein s.
  Reiter s.
  REM s.
  Rendu-Osler-Weber s.
  Renpenning s.
  respiratory distress s. (RDS)
  respiratory distress s. of the
   newborn
  Rett s.
  Reye s.
  Rh null s.
  Richards-Rundle s.
  Richter s.
  Rieger s.
  right ovarian vein s.
  Riley-Day s.
  Riley-Smith s.
  Roaf s.
  Roberts s.
  Robin s.
  Robinow s.

Roger s.
Rokitansky-Küster-Hauser s.
Romano-Ward s.
Romberg s.
Rosenbach s.
Rosenthal s.
Rosenthal-Kloepfer s.
Rosewater s.
Roth s.
Roth-Bernhardt s.
Rothmann-Makai s.
Rothmund s.
Rothmund-Thomson s.
Rotor s.
Rotter s.
Roussy-Dejerine s.
Roussy-Lévy s.
Rovsing s.
Rubinstein s.
Rubinstein-Taybi s.
Rud s.
rudimentary testis s.
Rundles-Falls s.
runting s.
Russell s.
Rust s.
Sabin-Feldman s.
Saethre-Chotzen s.
Sanchez Salorio s.
Sanfilippo s.
scalded skin s. (SSS)
scalenus anticus s.
Schafer s.
Schanz s.
Schaumann s.
Scheie s.
Schirmer s.
Schmid-Fraccaro s.
Schmidt s.
Schridde s.
Schroeder s.
Schüller s.
Schüller-Christian s.
Schultz s.
Schwartz s.
Sebright bantam s.
Seckel s.
Secrétan s.
Selye s.
Senear-Usher s.
Sertoli-cell-only s.
Sever s.

Sézary s.
Sheehan s.
Shwachman s.
Shwachman-Diamond s.
Shy-Drager s.
Sicard s.
sicca s.
sick building s.
Silver s.
Silver-Russell s.
Silverskiöld s.
Silvestrini-Corda s.
Sipple s.
Sjögren s.
Sjögren-Larsson s.
Sluder s.
Sly s.
Smith-Lemli-Opitz s.
Smith-Riley s.
Sneddon s.
Sohval-Soffer s.
Sorsby s.
Sotos s. of cerebral gigantism
Spen s.
spherophakia-brachymorphia s.
Sprinz-Nelson s.
spruelike s.
Spurway s.
staphylococcal scalded skin s.
Steele-Richardson-Olszewski s.
Steinbrocker s.
Steiner s.
Stein-Leventhal s.
Stevens-Johnson s.
Stewart Morel s.
Stewart-Treves s.
Stickler s.
Still-Chauffard s.
Stilling s.
Stilling-Turk-Duane s.
Stokvis-Talma s.
Strachan s.
Stryker-Halbeisen s.
Sturge s.
Sturge-Kalischer-Weber s.
Sturge-Weber s.
sudden death s. (SDS)
sudden infant death s. (SIDS)
Sudeck-Leriche s.
Sulzberger-Garbe s.
superior vena cava s.
superior vena caval s.

S

NOTES

syndrome *(continued)*

Sweet s.
Takayasu s.
Tapia s.
TAR s.
Taussig-Bing s.
Terry s.
testicular feminization s. (Tfm, TFS)
testicular regression s.
Thibierge-Weissenbach s.
third and fourth pharyngeal pouch s.
Thorn s.
thrombocytopenia-absent radius s.
thrombopathic s.
thrombotic thrombocytopenic purpura and hemolytic uremic s. (TTP-HUS)
Tietze s.
Timme s.
Tolosa-Hunt s.
TORCH s.
Tornwaldt s.
Torre s.
Torsten Sjögren s.
Touraine-Solente-Golé s.
toxic shock s.
Treacher Collins s.
triad s.
trichorhinophalangeal s.
trisomy 8 s.
trisomy 13 s.
trisomy 13-15 s.
trisomy 16-18 s.
trisomy 18 s.
trisomy 20 s.
trisomy 21 s.
trisomy 22 s.
trisomy C s.
trisomy D s.
trisomy E s.
Troisier s.
tropical splenomegaly s. (TSS)
Trousseau s.
tryptophan malabsorption s.
tumor lysis s.
Turcot s.
Turner s.
Uehlinger s.
Ullrich-Feichtiger s.
Ullrich-Turner s.
Ulysses s.
urogenital s.
Usher s.
uveo-encephalitic s.
van Buchem s.
van der Hoeve s.

Van der Woude s.
vasculocardiac s. of hyperserotonemia
Verner-Morrison s.
Vernet s.
vertebral basilar artery s.
vertebral crush-fracture s.
Villaret s.
Vinson s.
virilizing s.
virus-associated hemophagocytic s. (VAHS)
Vogt s.
Vogt-Koyanagi s.
Vohwinkel s.
Volkmann s.
von Willebrand s.
Waardenburg s.
Waldenström s.
Wallenberg s.
Ward-Romano s.
wasting s.
Waterhouse-Friderichsen s.
WDHA s.
Weber s.
Weber-Cockayne s.
Weber-Dubler s.
Wegener s.
Weil s.
Weill-Marchesani s.
Wells s.
Wermer s.
Werner s.
Wernicke s.
Wernicke-Korsakoff s.
West s.
Weyers oligodactyly s.
Weyers-Thier s.
whistling face s.
Widal s.
Wildervanck s.
Willebrand s.
Williams s.
Williams-Campbell s.
Wilson s.
Wilson-Mikity s.
Winter s.
Wiskott-Aldrich s.
Witkop-Von Sallmann s.
Wolff-Parkinson-White s.
Wolf-Hirschhorn s.
Wolfram s.
Wright s.
XO s.
XXY s.
XYZ s.
Young s.
Zellweger s.

Zieve s.
Zinsser-Cole-Engman s.
Zollinger-Ellison s.
synechia, pl. **synechiae**
s. pericardii
synencephalocele
syneresis
synergism
synergist
synergistic
synergy
Syngamidae
Syngamus
S. *laryngeus*
S. *trachea*
syngamy
syngeneic
s. graft
s. transplantation
syngenesioplastic transplantation
syngenesioplasty
syngenesiotransplantation
syngenic
syngraft
synkaryon
synonym
objective s.
senior s.
subjective s.
synophthalmia
synorchism
Synosternus
S. *pallidus*
synostosis
tribasilar s.
synotus
synovia
synovial
s. chondromatosis
s. cyst
s. fluid
s. fluid analysis
s. fluid examination
s. osteochondromatosis
s. sarcoma
synovioma
malignant s.
synovitis
acute serous s.
detritic s.
pigmented villonodular s. (PVNS)
proliferative s.

purulent s.
serous acute s.
suppurative s.
tendinous s.
vaginal s.
villonodular pigmented s.
syntax error
syntectic
syntenic
synteny
syntexis
synthase
glycogen (starch) s.
methionine s.
porphobilinogen s.
uroporphyrinogen I s.
synthesis
DNA s.
fatty acid s.
glycogen s.
protein s.
urea s.
synthetase
acetyl-CoA s.
acyl-CoA s.
alanyl RNA s.
argininosuccinate s.
glutathione s.
heme s. (HS)
methionyl-RNA s.
polydeoxyribonucleotide s.
tyrosyl-RNA s.
valyl-RNA s.
synthetic
s. dye
s. lethal
s. medium old tuberculin
trichloroacetic acid (precipitated)
(SOTT)
syntrophism
syntropic
Syphacia
S. *obvelata*
syphilemia
syphilid
gummatous s.
nodular s.
syphilimetry
syphilis
hemagglutination treponemal test
for s. (HATTS)
quaternary s.

NOTES

S

syphilis *(continued)*
    serologic test for s. (STS)
    standard test for s. (STS)
    Ternidens diminutus tertiary s.
    venereal disease-s. (VDS)
syphilitic
    s. abscess
    s. aneurysm
    s. aortitis
    s. fever
    s. meningitis
    s. meningoencephalitis
    s. nephritis
    s. osteochondritis
    s. periarteritis
    s. ulcer
syphiloma
    s. of Fournier
syphilomatous
syringadenoma
    papillary s.
syringe
    Roughton-Scholander s.
    s. shield
syringeal
syringitis
syringoadenoma
syringobulbia
syringocarcinoma
syringocele
syringocystadenoma
    s. papilliferum
syringocystoma
syringoencephalomyelia
syringoid
syringoma
    chondroid s.
syringomeningocele
syringomyelia
syringomyelocele
syringomyelus
syringopontia
syrinx
Syrphidae
Sysmex
    S. HS-330 robotic hematology
      system
    S. NE-8000 CBC analyzer
    S. R-1000 reticulocyte counter
system
    10-20 s.
    absolute s. of units
    AEC detection s.
    Ann Arbor staging s.
    API 20 Strep S.
    ASAP Biopsy S.
    avidin-biotin detection s.
    Bactalert s.

BACTEC blood culture s.
Bethesda S.
bicarbonate buffer s.
blood group s.'s
buffer s.
cell-free s.
centimeter-gram-second s.
CGS s.
Christopherson nuclear grading s.
complement s.
CRYO-VAC-A cryostat vacuum s.
Cyto-Rich cervical cytology
  monolayer s.
dichroic filter s.
Difco ESP testing s.
diffuse neuroendocrine s.
Duffy blood group s.
Edmondson tumor grading s.
Filtracheck-UTI disposable
  colormetric bacteriuria detection s.
Fuhrman s.
Halon s.
hematopoietic s.
Hybritech PSA determination s.
immune s.
indicator s.
Isolator blood culture s.
Jass staging s.
kallikrein s.
Kell blood group s.
Kidd blood group s.
kinin s.
Leitz image analysis s.
linnaean s. of nomenclature
Lutheran blood group s.
lymphoreticular s.
s. of macrophages
meter-kilogram-second s.
metric s.
microbiology identification s.'s
microsomal enzyme s.
MKS s.
mononuclear phagocyte s.
MSTS Staging S.
Munich tumor classification s.
Musculoskeletal Tumor Society
  Staging S.
myeloperoxidase s.
on-demand s.
operating s.
OptiMax immunostaining s.
portal s.
properdin s.
renin-angiotensin-aldosterone s.
reticuloendothelial s. (RES)
Roche Septi-Chek blood culture s.
Scarff-Bloom-Richardson tumor
  grading s.

Septi-Chek culture s.
Single Use Diagnostic S. (SUDS)
SOS repair s.
sprinkler s.
Sydney classification s.
Sysmex HS-330 robotic
  hematology s.
The Bethesda S. (TBS)
TNM cancer grading s.
turnkey s.
Uriscreen urine specimen bacteriuria
  detection s.
Vecta-Stain Elite ABC s.
Viratype In Situ S.
WAMPOLE ISOLATOR blood
  culture s.
Whitmore-Jewett tumor staging s.
systematic
  s. bacteriology
  s. error
systematized
  s. nevus
  S. Nomenclature of Pathology
    (SNOP)
systemic
  s. anaphylaxis

  s. arterial pressure (SAP)
  s. autoimmune disease
  s. calciphylaxis
  s. chondromalacia
  s. familial primary amyloidosis
  s. febrile disease
  s. histiocytosis
  s. hyalinosis
  s. lesion
  s. lupus erythematosus (SLE)
  s. myelitis
  s. poisoning
  s. resistance (SR)
  s. reticuloendotheliosis
  s. sclerosis
  s. vascular resistance (SVR)
systemoid
systolic
  s. hypertension
  s. time interval (STI)
Syva EMIT-II assay
syzygial
syzygium
syzygy
Szent-Györgyi reaction

S

NOTES

T
  temperature
  tesla
    T agglutination
    T agglutinogen
    T antigen
    T banding
    T and B lymphocyte subset assay
    T cell
    T cell antigen receptor
    T (cell) cytolytic (Tc)
    T (cell) cytotoxic (Tc)
    T cell-replacing factor (TRF)
    T cell-rich, B-cell lymphoma
      (TCRBCL)
    T cytotoxic cell
    T helper cell
    T lymphocyte
    T method stain
    T tubule
    T zone
T½, T 1/2, t½
  terminal half-life
T_3
  triiodothyronine
    reverse T_3
    T_3 uptake test
T_3 uptake
T_4 newborn screen
T_m
  maximal tubular excretory capacity of
    kidneys
T_{max}
  time of maximum concentration
T_{mg}
  maximal tubular reabsorption of glucose
t
  test of significance
    t test
t½ (*var. of* T½)
TA
  alkaline tuberculin
  therapeutic abortion
  titratable acid
  toxin-antitoxin
  tube agglutination
TA-4
  tumor-antigen 4
TAB
  typhoid, paratyphoid A and paratyphoid
    B
    TAB vaccine
tabanid
Tabanidae
Tabanus

tabby
  t. cat striation
tabes
  t. dorsalis
tabescence
tabescent
tabetic
tabetiform
tabic
tabid
table
  contingency t.
  decision t.
  Gaffky t.
  life t.
  truth t.
tablet
  graph t.
tabletop shield
TAC
  tetracaine, epinephrine, and cocaine
    TAC solution
Tac
  Tac antigen
Tacaribe
  T. complex of viruses
  T. virus
tache
  t. blanche
  t. laiteuse
tachetic
tachyphylaxis
tachyzoite
TAD
  thoracic asphyxiant dystrophy
tadpole cell
Taenia
    T. africana
    T. bremneri
    T. canina
    T. confusa
    T. diminuta
    T. echinococcus
    T. lata
    T. murina
    T. nana
    T. philippina
    T. saginata
    T. solium
    T. taeniaeformis
taenia
taeniaeformis
    Hydatigera t.
Taeniarhynchus
taeniasis

T

taeniid
Taeniidae
taenioid
Taeniorhynchus
Taenzer stain
Taenzer-Unna stain
TAF
  albumose-free tuberculin
  toxoid-antitoxin floccules
  trypsin-aldehyde-fuchsin
  tumor angiogenic factor
TAG
  tumor-associated glycoprotein
tag
    anal skin t.
    sentinel t.
    skin t.
TAG-72 antigen
T-agglutination
Tahyna virus
tail
    t. poikilocyte
    polyA t.
    polyadenylate t.
tailing
Takahara disease
Takata-Ara test
Takayama stain
Takayasu
    T. arteritis
    T. disease
    T. syndrome
TAL
  thymic alymphoplasia
talaje
    Alectorobius t.
talcosis
Talfan disease
tall-cell variant
Talma disease
TAM
  toxoid-antitoxin mixture
Tamm-Horsfall
    T.-H. mucoprotein
    T.-H. protein
tamponade
    cardiac t.
Tamulus
tan
tangent
Tangier disease
tanned
    t. red cell (TRC)
    t. red cell hemagglutination
      inhibition test
Tanner stage
tannic acid

TAO
  thromboangiitis obliterans
tape
    t. drive
    end of t.
    magnetic t.
    t. mark
    t. transport
tapeworm
    beef t.
    broad fish t.
    dwarf t.
    fish t.
    pork t.
    rat t.
Tapia syndrome
tapir mouth
TAR
    thrombocytopenia with absence of radius
      TAR syndrome
tar
    coal t.
    t. keratosis
TARA
    tumor-associated rejection antigen
tarantula
Tardieu
    T. ecchymoses
    T. petechiae
    T. spot
tare
target
    t. cell
    t. cell anemia
    t. lesion
    t. organ
Tarlov cyst
tarry
    t. cyst
    t. stool
tarsal cyst
tarsitis
tarsoepiphyseal aclasis
tarsomegaly
tarsophyma
tartaric acid
tart cell
tartrate
    t. resistant acid phosphatase
      (TRAcP)
    t. resistant leukocyte acid
      phosphatase
tartrate-inhibited acid phosphatase
tartrazine
Tarui disease
task
TAT
    tetanus antitoxin

thromboplastin activation test
total antitryptic activity
toxin-antitoxin
turn-around time

Tatlockia micdadei

tau

taurine

taurochenodeoxycholate

taurochenodeoxycholic acid

taurocholate

taurocholemia

taurocholic acid

taurodeoxycholic acid

taurolithocholic acid

Taussig-Bing
T.-B. disease
T.-B. syndrome

tautomer
keto-enol t.
proton t.
ring-chain t.
tautomerism
valence t.

taxa

taxis

taxon

taxonomic

taxonomy
numerical t.

Tay disease

Taylor disease

Tay-Sachs disease (TSD)

TB
toluidine blue
tracheobronchitis
tubercle bacillus
tuberculosis
TB smear

TBA
testosterone-binding affinity

TBC
tuberculosis

TBD
total body density

TBF
total body fat

TBG
thyroxine-binding globulin
TBG assay
TBG cap

TBGP
total blood granulocyte pool

TBH
total body hematocrit

TBI
thyroxine-binding index

TBII
TSH-binding inhibitory immunoglobulin

TBK
total body potassium

T/B lymphocyte assay

T and B lymphocyte subset assay

TBM
tuberculous meningitis

TBP
thyroxine-binding protein

TBPA
thyroxine-binding prealbumin

TB-RD
tuberculosis-respiratory disease

TBS
The Bethesda System
total body solute

TBT
tolbutamide test

TBV
total blood volume

TBW
total body water
total body weight

TC
to contain
temperature compensation
tetracycline
thermal conductivity
tissue culture
total cholesterol
TC detector
TC pipette

T$_4$(C)

Tc
T (cell) cytolytic
T (cell) cytotoxic
technetium
tetracycline
transcobalamin

^{99m}Tc, Tc-99m
technetium-99m
^{99m}Tc pentetic acid
^{99m}Tc red blood cell
^{99m}Tc serum albumin

TCA
trichloroacetic acid
TCA cycle

T

NOTES

TCBS
triosulfate-citrate-bile salts-sucrose
TCBS agar
TCD
tissue culture dose
TCD$_{50}$
median tissue culture dose
T-cell
T.-c. growth factor
T.-c. growth factor-1
T.-c. growth factor-2
T.-c. proliferation
T.-c. receptor (TCR)
TCH
total circulating hemoglobin
TCI
transient cerebral ischemia
TCID
tissue culture infective dose
TCID$_{50}$
median tissue culture infective dose
tissue culture infectious dose
TCIE
transient cerebral ischemic episode
TCM
tissue culture medium
Tc-99m (*var. of* ^{99m}Tc)
TCPI Rapid HIV test
TCR
T-cell receptor
TCRBCL
T cell-rich, B-cell lymphoma
tcRNA
translation control RNA
TCT
thrombin clotting time
thyrocalcitonin
TD
to deliver
tetanus-diphtheria
thymus-dependent
TD pipette
TDA
TSH-displacing antibody
T-dependent antigen
TDF
thoracic duct fistula
TDI
total-dose infusion
TDT
terminal deoxynucleotidyl transferase
TdT
terminal deoxynucleotidyl transferase
TdT immunostain
TDTH cell
TE
tissue-equivalent
total estrogen (excretion)

tear
Mallory-Weiss t.
teardrop cell
TeBG
testosterone-estradiol-binding globulin
Techmate 1000 immunostainer
technetium (Tc)
technetium-99m (^{99m}Tc, Tc-99m)
technical
technician
histologic t.
medical laboratory t.
technique
ABC t.
avidin-biotin immunoperoxidase t.
Brecher new methylene blue t.
Brown-Brenn t.
Carey Ranvier t.
Cattoretti t.
cellulose tape t.
Corbin t.
Dennis t.
DGGE t.
dilution-filtration t.
enzyme-assisted immunoassay t.
enzyme-multiplied immunoassay t.
(EMIT)
extracorporeal photophoresis t.
FA t.
Ficoll-Hypaque t.
flotation t.
fluorescent antibody t.
Highman Congo red t.
Hotchkiss-McManus PAS t.
immunofluorescence t.
immunohistochemical t.
immunoperoxidase t.
Jerne t.
Kato thick smear t.
Knott t.
Kohn one-step staining t.
Laurell t.
McMaster t.
membrane filter t.
Northern blot t.
Ouchterlony t.
PACONA t.
PAP t.
periodic acid-Schiff t.
peroxidase-antiperoxidase t.
plaque t.
pop-off t.
program evaluation and review t.
(PERT)
Rebuck skin window t.
Ritter-Oleson t.
roll-tube t.
saline t.

scintillation t.
sealed envelope t.
section freeze substitution t.
sedimentation t.
Seldinger t.
Southern blot t.
Stoll dilution egg count t.
streptavidin-biotin-complex t.
time diffusion t.
titration t.
Western blot t.
zinc sulfate centrifugal flotation t.

technologic life
technologist
medical t.
technology
Tectiviridae
TED
threshold erythema dose
thromboembolic disease
TEF
tracheoesophageal fistula
Teflon
teichoic
t. acid
t. acid antibody
Teladorsagia davtiani
telangiectasia
calcinosis cutis, Raynaud
phenomenon, sclerodactyly, and t.
(CRST)
calcinosis, Raynaud phenomenon,
esophageal motility disorders,
sclerodactyly, and t. (CREST)
cephalo-oculocutaneous t.
essential t.
hereditary hemorrhagic t. (HHT)
t. lymphatica
t. macularis eruptiva perstans
spider t.
t. verrucosa
telangiectasis, pl. **telangiectases**
telangiectatic
t. angioma
t. angiomatosis
t. cancer
t. fibroma
t. glioma
t. lipoma
t. osteogenic sarcoma
t. wart

telangiectodes
telangioma, pl. **teleangiomata**
telecytology
telencephalization
teleomorph
teleonomy
telepathology
tellurate
tellurite medium
tellurium assay
Tellyesnicky fixative solution
telocentric
telogen hair
telomere banding
telomeric R-banding stain
telopeptide
telophase
Telosporea
Telosporidia
TEM
transmission electron microscope
transmission electron microscopy
temperate
t. bacteriophage
t. phage
t. virus
temperature (T)
absolute t. (A)
ambient t.
body t.
t. coefficient (Q_{10})
t. compensation (TC)
critical t.
effective t. (ET)
eutectic t.
flash-point t.
ignition t.
maximal growth t.
maximum t.
melting t.
minimal growth t.
minimum t.
normal body t.
optimal growth t.
optimum t.
t. programming
room t.
subnormal t.
temperature-sensitive (t-s)
t.-s. mutant
t.-s. mutation
template

T

NOTES

temporal
- t. arteritis
- t. lobe epilepsy

temporary parasite

TEN
- toxic epidermal necrolysis

tendency
- central t.

tender line

tendinitis
- hypertrophic infiltrative t. (HIT)

tendinous
- t. spot
- t. synovitis

tendonitis

tendosynovitis

tendovaginitis
- radial styloid t.

Tenebrio

tenesmus

tenia

teniacide

teniafuge

tenial

teniasis

tenicide

teniform

tenifugal

tenifuge

tenioid

Teniposide

Tenney changes

tennis racket cell

tenonitis

tenontitis

tenontolemmitis

tenontothecitis

tenophyte

tenositis

tenostosis

tenosynovitis
- t. crepitans
- localized nodular t.
- pigmented villonodular t.
- villonodular pigmented t.
- villous t.

tenovaginitis

tension
- carbon dioxide t.
- t. cyst
- t. cyst of breast
- end-tidal CO_2 t.
- oxygen t.
- surface t. (ST)

tephromalacia

terahertz (THz)

teratoblastoma

teratocarcinoma

teratogen

teratogenesis

teratogenic

teratoid tumor

teratology

teratoma
- adult cystic t.
- benign t.
- cystic dermoid t.
- embryonal t.
- malignant t. (MT)
- malignant trophoblastic t. (MTT)
- monodermal t.
- solid t.
- triphyllomatous t.

teratomatous
- t. cyst

terminal
- t. addition enzyme
- amino t.
- t. banding
- t. bar
- carboxyl t.
- t. cisterna
- CRT t.
- t. deletion
- t. deoxynucleotidyl transferase (TDT, TdT)
- t. deoxyribonucleotidyl transferase
- t. endocarditis
- graphic t.
- t. half-life (T½, T 1/2, t½)
- t. hematuria
- t. ileitis
- t. latency
- t. leukocytosis
- smart t.
- t. web

terminalization

termination
- t. codon
- t. factor
- t. sequence

termini
- cohesive t.

termone

ternary acid

Ternidens
- *T. diminutus*
- *T. diminutus* tertiary syphilis

terpene

Terry syndrome

tertian
- t. fever
- t. malaria

tertiarism

tertiarismus

tertiary structure

Teschen
  T. disease
  T. virus
tesla (T)
test
  AAN t.
  abnormal glucose tolerance t.
    (AGTT)
  Abrams t.
  acetic acid and potassium
    ferrocyanide t.
  acetoacetic acid t.
  acetoin t.
  acetone t.
  acetowhite t.
  acid challenge t.
  acid clearance t. (ACT)
  acid elution t.
  acid hemolysin t.
  acidified serum t.
  acidity reduction t.
  acid-lability t.
  acidosis t.
  acid perfusion t.
  acid phosphatase t.
  acid phosphatase t. for semen
  acid reflux t.
  ACPA t.
  ACTH stimulation t.
  activated partial thromboplastin
    substitution t.
  active rosette t.
  Adamkiewicz t.
  Addis t.
  adhesion t.
  Adler t.
  adrenal ascorbic acid depletion t.
  adrenal function t.
  adrenalin t.
  adrenocortical inhibition t.
  adrenocorticotropic hormone
    stimulation t.
  adrenocorticotropic hormone
    suppression t.
  agglutination t.
  A/G ratio t.
  ALA t.
  AlaSTAT latex allergy t.
  albumin suspension t.
  aldolase t.
  aldosterone stimulation t.
  aldosterone suppression t.

  alizarin t.
  alkali denaturation t.
  alkaline phosphatase t.
  alkali tolerance t.
  alkaloid t.
  alkaptonuria t.
  Allen t.
  Allen-Doisy t.
  Almén t. for blood
  ΛL patch t.
  ALT t.
  Ames t.
  p-aminohippurate clearance t.
  α amino nitrogen t.
  aminopyrine breath t.
  ammoniacal silver nitrate t.
  ammonium chloride loading t.
  amylase t.
  Anderson-Collip t.
  Anderson and Goldberger t.
  androstenedione t.
  angiotensin I, II t.
  anion gap t.
  antibiotic sensitivity t.
  anti-*Chlamydia* antibody t.
  antichymotrypsin t.
  antideoxyribonuclease B titer t.
  antiglobulin t. (AGT)
  antihuman globulin t.
  anti-LA/SS-B t.
  anti-Ro/SS-A t.
  anti-Sm t.
  antistreptolysin-O t.
  antithrombin III t.
  antitoxoplasma antibody t.
  antitrypsin t.
  Anton t.
  Apt t.
  APTT t.
  arginine t.
  arginine insulin tolerance t. (AITT)
  Argo corn starch t.
  ART t.
  arylsulfatase t.
  Aschheim-Zondek t. (AZT)
  Ascoli t.
  ascorbate-cyanide t.
  ascorbic acid t.
  ASO t.
  Aspergillus antibody t.
  aspirin tolerance t.
  AST t.

NOTES

T

test *(continued)*
Astra profile t.
Astwood t.
atropine suppression t.
augmented histamine t. (AHT)
autohemolysis t.
Autolet blood glucose t.
automated reagin t. (ART)
Autopath QC t.
A-Z t.
Bachman t.
Bachman-Pettit t.
bacitracin disk t.
Baker acid hematein t.
Baker pyridine extraction t.
Barany caloric t.
barium t.
Barr body t.
basophil degranulation t.
Beard t.
BEI t.
Bence Jones protein t.
Benedict t.
Benedict t. for glucose
bentiromide t.
bentonite flocculation t. (BFT)
benzidine t.
Bernstein t.
Berson t.
Betke-Kleihauer t.
Bettendorff t.
Bial t.
bicarbonate titration t.
bile acid tolerance t.
bile esculin t.
bile esculin hydrolysis t.
bile pigment t.
bile salt breath t.
bile solubility t.
bilirubin tolerance t.
Binz t.
biuret t.
blind t.
blood urea nitrogen t.
Bloor t.
blot t.
Blount t.
Bloxam t.
Boas t.
Bonanno t.
borderline glucose tolerance t.
 (BGTT)
Bradshaw t.
breath analysis t.
bromocriptine suppression t.
bromphenol t.
bromsulphalein t.
brucella agglutination t.

BSFR t.
BSP excretion t.
buffy coat smear t.
butanol-extractable iodine t.
calcium oxalate t.
Calmette t.
CAMP t.
candida precipitin t.
capillary fragility t.
capon-comb-growth t.
carbohydrate fermentation t.
carbohydrate identification t.
carbohydrate utilization t.
carbon dioxide combining power t.
carbon 13-labeled ketoisocaproate
 breath t.
CA15-3 RIA t.
Carr-Price t.
Casoni intradermal t.
Castellani t.
catalase t.
catatorulin t.
catecholamine t.
cephalin-cholesterol flocculation t.
cephalin flocculation t.
cercarien-hullen-reaktion t.
ceruloplasmin t.
cervical mucus sperm penetration t.
cetylpyridium chloride t.
CF t.
CFF t.
C-glycoholic acid breath t.
Chagas disease serological t.
Chédiak t.
chemical inhibition isoamylase t.
chemiluminescence t.
Chemstrip BG t.
Chen t.
chenodeoxycholic acid t.
Chick-Martin t.
chi-squared t.
Chlamydiazyme t.
chlormerodrin accumulation t.
 (CAT)
cholecystokinin t.
cholesterol t.
cholesterol-lecithin flocculation t.
cholinesterase t.
chorionic gonadotropin t.
chromaffin reaction t.
chromogenic cephalosporin t.
chromogenic enzyme substrate t.
cis/trans t.
citrate t.
C lactose t.
Clark t.
Clauberg t.
Clinitest stool t.

clomiphene t.
clonidine suppression t.
CLOtest t.
coagulase t.
coagulation time t.
coccidioidin t.
cold agglutinin t.
cold hemolysin t.
colloidal gold t.
Coloscreen Self t.
comb-growth t.
combined pituitary function t.
compatibility t.
complement direct Coombs t.
complement-fixation t. (CFT)
complement lysis sensitivity t.
conglutinating complement
  absorption t. (CCAT)
Congo red t.
Coombs t. (CT)
copper-binding protein t.
copper reduction t.
coproporphyrin t.
Corner-Allen t.
cortisone-glucose tolerance t.
  (CGTT)
cortisone-primed oral glucose
  tolerance t. (COGTT)
C-peptide t.
C-reactive protein t.
creatine kinase t.
creatinine clearance t.
critical flicker fusion t.
C&S t.
CSF glutamine t.
cutaneous tuberculin t.
cutireaction t.
cyanide-ascorbate t.
cyanide-nitroprusside t.
cyclic AMP t.
cystic fibrosis t.
cystinuria t.
cytochrome oxidase t.
cytotropic antibody t.
DA pregnancy t.
Davidsohn differential absorption t.
Day t.
D-dimer t.
deferoxamine mesylate infusion t.
11-deoxycorticosterone t.
11-deoxycortisol t.
deoxyribonuclease t.

deoxyuridine suppression t.
dexamethasone suppression t. (DST)
dextrose t.
DFA-TP t.
  direct fluorescent antibody test -
  Treponema pallidum
DHEA t.
DHT t.
Diagnex Blue t.
diazepam breath t.
Dick t.
differential renal function t.
differential ureteral catheterization t.
dilution t.
dinitrophenylhydrazine t.
direct agglutination pregnancy t.
  (DAPT)
direct antiglobulin t. (DAGT)
direct bilirubin t.
direct Coombs t. (DCT)
direct fluorescent antibody t.
direct fluorescent antibody-
  Treponema pallidum t. (DFA-TP)
disaccharide tolerance t.
disk diffusion t.
dithionite t.
Dixon t.
DNase t.
Dold t.
Donath-Landsteiner t.
Donné t.
dot blot t.
double diffusion t.
double (gel) diffusion precipitin t.
  in one dimension
double (gel) diffusion precipitin t.
  in two dimensions
Dragendorff t.
Ducrey t.
Duke bleeding time t.
Dunnet multiple component t.
dye t. (DT)
dye exclusion t.
dye excretion t.
echinococcosis serological t.
edrophonium chloride t.
Ehrlich t.
electrophoresis t.
electrotransfer t.
Elek t.
Ellsworth-Howard t.
Emmens S/L t.

T

NOTES

test *(continued)*

enzyme-linked antibody t.
EP t.
E-rosette t.
erythrocyte adherence t.
erythrocyte fragility t.
erythropoietin t.
esculin hydrolysis t.
esophageal acid infusion t.
esterase t.
estradiol t.
ethanol gelation t.
euglobulin clot t. (ECT)
euglobulin lysis t.
ExacTech blood glucose meter t.
factor VIII-related antigen t.
FANA t.
Farber t.
Farr t.
fat absorption t.
febrile agglutination t.
fecal fat t.
fecal occult blood t.
Fehling t.
fermentation t.
fern t.
ferric chloride t.
ferric ferricyanide reduction t.
fetal hemoglobin t.
α-fetoprotein t.
Feulgen t.
Fevold t.
fibrinogen titer t.
fibrin-stabilizing factor t.
FIGLU excretion t.
filter paper microscopic t.
Filtracheck-UTI t.
Finn chamber patch t.
Fischer exact t.
Fishberg concentration t.
Fisher exact t.
Fleitmann t.
flocculation t.
fluorescent antibody t. (FAT)
fluorescent antinuclear antibody t.
fluorescent-treponemal antibody
  absorption t. (FTA-AB)
fluorescent treponemal antibody-
  absorption t.
foam stability t.
Folin t.
Folin-Looney t.
formiminoglutamic acid t. (FIGLU)
formol-gel t.
Foshay t.
Fouchet t.
fragility t.
Francis skin t.

Frei t.
Friedman t.
frog t.
fructose t.
FTA-ABS t.
Gaddum and Schild t.
galactose breath t.
galactose tolerance t.
gastric function t.
gastrin-calcium infusion
  stimulation t.
gastrin-protein stimulation t.
gastrin-secretin stimulation t.
Gastroccult t.
gastrointestinal blood loss t.
gastrointestinal protein loss t.
gel diffusion precipitin t.
gel diffusion precipitin t. in one
  dimension
gel diffusion precipitin t. in two
  dimensions
Geraghty t.
Gerhardt t. for acetoacetic acid
Gerhardt t. for urobilin in the
  urine
germ tube t.
Gibson-Cooke sweat t.
glucagon t.
glucose insulin tolerance t. (GITT)
glucose oxidase paper strip t.
glucose-6-phosphate
  dehydrogenase t.
glucose tolerance t. (GTT)
glutathione stability t.
glycogen storage t.
glycolic acid t.
glycosylated hemoglobin t.
glycyltryptophan t.
glyoxylic acid t.
Gmelin t.
Gofman t.
gold sol t.
gonadotropin t.
Gordon t.
Göthlin capillary fragility t.
G-6-PD t.
Graham-Cole t.
Gravindex pregnancy t.
guaiac t.
Gunning-Lieben t.
Günzberg t.
Guthrie t.
Gutzeit t.
Haagensen t.
Haenszel t.
Ham t.
Hamel t.
Hammarsten t.

hamster egg penetration t.
Hanger t.
haptoglobin t.
Harrison t.
Harris and Ray t.
heat coagulation t.
heat instability t.
heat precipitation t.
heavy-metal screening t.
Heinz body t.
Helisal rapid blood t.
hemadsorption virus t.
hemagglutination t.
hemagglutination-inhibition t. (HIT)
hematein t.
hemoccult t.
HemoQuant fecal blood t.
hemosiderinuria t.
Henry fructose t.
hepatic function t.
hepatitis B surface antigen t.
heterophil antibody t.
Hicks-Pitney thromboplastin
  generation t.
Hinton t.
hippuric acid excretion t.
Histalog t.
histamine flare t.
histoplasmin-latex t.
HIVAGEN t.
HIV-antibody t.
Hoffman t.
Hofmeister t.
Hogben t.
Hollander t.
homocystinuria t.
homogentisic acid t.
homovanillic acid t.
Hooker-Forbes t.
Hopkins-Cole t.
Hoppe-Seyler t.
Howard t.
Howell prothrombin t.
Huddleston agglutination t.
Huhner t.
human chorionic gonadotropin
  injection t.
human erythrocyte agglutination t.
  (HEAT)
HVA t.
hydroxybutyric t.
17-hydroxycorticosteroid t.

5-hydroxyindoleacetic t.
17-hydroxyprogesterone t.
ice water calorics t.
ICG excretion t.
icterus index t.
Ide t.
immune adhesion t.
immunoblot t.
immunofluorescence t.
immunoglobulin A, D, G, M t.
immunologic pregnancy t.
immunoperoxidase t.
implantation t. (IT)
IMViC t.'s
indican t.
indigo-carmine t.
indirect bilirubin t.
indirect Coombs t.
indirect fluorescent antibody t.
indirect hemagglutination t.
indole t.
indole, methyl red, Voges-
  Proskauer, and citrate t. (IMViC
  tests)
indophenol t.
inhibition t.
insulin clearance t.
insulin hypoglycemia t.
insulin sensitivity t. (IST)
insulin tolerance t. (ITT)
interference t.
intradermal t. (IT)
intraesophageal pH t.
intravenous glucose tolerance t.
  (IVGTT)
intravenous tolbutamide tolerance t.
  (IVTTT)
invasive activity t. (IAT)
iodine t.
iodine-azide t. (IAT)
iodine-131 uptake t.
iron-binding capacity t.
islet cell antibody screening t.
isocitrate dehydrogenase t.
isoiodeikon t.
isoniazid phenotype t.
isopropanol precipitation t.
Ito-Reenstierna t.
^{131}I uptake t.
^{131}I uptake t.
Ivy bleeding time t.
Jacquemin t.

T

NOTES

test *(continued)*
    Jaffe t.
    Jolles t.
    Jones-Cantarow t.
    Kahn t.
    Katayama t.
    ketogenic corticoids t.
    17-ketogenic steroid assay t.
    ketone body t.
    17-ketosteroid assay t.
    Kirby-Bauer t.
    Kleihauer acid elution t.
    Kleihauer-Betke t.
    Kober t.
    KOH t.
    Kolmer t.
    Kowarsky t.
    Krokiewicz t.
    Kruskal-Wallis t.
    Kunkel t.
    Kurzrok-Ratner t.
    Kveim t.
    Kveim-Stilzbach t. (KS)
    lactic dehydrogenase t.
    lactose tolerance t.
    Ladendorff t.
    Lancefield precipitation t.
    Landsteiner-Donath t.
    Lange colloidal gold t.
    LAP t.
    latex agglutination t.
    latex agglutination-inhibition t.
      (LAIT)
    latex fixation t.
    latex flocculation t. (LFT)
    latex slide agglutination t.
    LATS t.
      long-acting thyroid stimulating
        hormone test
    LE t.
    LE cell t.
    Lee-White clotting t.
    Legal t.
    leishmaniasis serological t.
    lepromin skin t.
    leucine aminopeptidase t.
    leukocyte adherence assay t.
    leukocyte bactericidal assay t.
    leukocyte esterase t. (LET)
    leukocyte histamine release t.
    Levinson t.
    levulose tolerance t.
    Liebermann-Burchard t.
    limulus lysate t.
    line t.
    lipase t.
    lipid t.
    lipoprotein electrophoresis t.

liver flocculation t.
liver function t. (LFT)
long-acting thyroid stimulating
    hormone t. (LATS test)
Lowenthal t.
Lücke t.
lupus band t.
lupus erythematosus cell t.
lymphocyte transfer t.
lymphocyte transformation t.
lysozyme t.
Machado-Guerreiro t.
macrophage migration inhibition t.
magnesium t.
malaria film t.
mallein t.
Malmejde t.
Mantoux skin t.
Master 2-step t.
mastic t.
maximal Histalog t.
Mazzotti t.
McNemar t.
McPhail t.
t. meal
Meinicke t.
melanin t.
melanogen t.
metabisulfite t.
metanephrine t.
methanol t.
methionine t.
3-methoxy-4-hydroxymandelic
    acid t.
methylene blue t.
methyl red t.
Metopirone t.
metrotrophic t.
metyrapone stimulation t.
MHA-TP t.
Microflow t.
microhemagglutination-*Treponema*
    pallidum t.
microimmunofluorescent t.
microprecipitation t.
microsomal thyroid antibody t.
Middlebrook-Dubos
    hemagglutination t.
migration inhibition t.
migration inhibitory factor t.
Millon-Nasse t.
mixed agglutination t.
mixed lymphocyte culture t.
MLC t.
mobilization t.
Molisch t.
Moloney t.
monocyte function t.

Mono-Diff t.
Monoscreen t.
Monospot t.
Monosticon Dri-Dot t.
Montenegro skin t.
Mörner t.
Mosenthal t.
motility t.
Motulsky dye reduction t.
mucin clot t.
mucopolysaccharide t.
mucoprotein t.
Mulder t.
multiple puncture tuberculin t.
mumps sensitivity t.
Murex *Candida albicans* CA50 t.
Murphy-Pattee t.
mutagenicity t.
MycoAKT latex bead
  agglutination t.
myoglobin t.
Napier formol-gel t.
NBT t.
neoprecipitin t. (NPT)
neutralization t. (NT)
niacin t.
Nickerson-Kveim t.
Nicklès t.
nitrate reduction t.
nitrate utilization t.
nitroblue tetrazolium t.
nitropropiol t.
nitroprusside t.
nitroso-indole-nitrate t.
nonprotein nitrogen t.
normal lymphocyte transfer t.
  (NLT)
Northern blot t.
Obermayer t.
Obermüller t.
occult blood t.
17-OH-corticoids t.
oleic acid uptake t.
one-tailed t.
ONPG t.
O&P t.
Optochin susceptibility t.
oral glucose tolerance t. (OGTT)
oral lactose tolerance t.
orcinol t.
osazone t.
osmotic fragility t.

Ouchterlony t.
ovarian ascorbic acid depletion t.
oxidase t.
oxidation-fermentation t.
oxytocin challenge t. (OCT)
Paget t.
pancreatic islet cell antibody t.
pancreozymin-secretin t.
Pandy t.
Pap t.
Papanicolaou smear t.
paper radioimmunosorbent t.
paracoagulation t.
parainfluenza antibody t.
partial thromboplastin time t.
PAS t.
passive cutaneous anaphylaxis t.
passive hemagglutination t.
patch t.
Paul t.
Paul-Bunnell t.
Paul-Bunnell-Barrett t.
pentagastrin t.
perchlorate discharge t.
periodic acid-Schiff t.
Perls t.
Petri t.
PharmChek seat patch drug
  detection t.
phenacetin breath t.
phenolphthalein t.
phenolsulfonphthalein t.
phentolamine t.
phenylketonuria t.
phenylpyruvic acid t.
phosphatase t.
phospholipid t.
phosphoric acid t.
photo-patch t.
phthalein t.
Piazza t.
picrate t.
Pirquet cutaneous tuberculin t.
pituitary function t.
P-K t.
PKU t.
placental and fetoplacental
  function t.'s
plant protease t. (PPT)
plasmacrit t.
plasma hemoglobin t.
platelet adhesiveness t.

T

NOTES

test *(continued)*
platelet aggregation t.
platelet retention t.
platelet survival t.
Porges-Meier t.
Porges-Salomon t.
porphyrin t.
Porter-Silber chromogens t.
Porteus maze t.
positive whiff t.
potassium hydroxide t.
P and P t.
PPD skin t.
Prausnitz-Küstner t.
precipitation t.
precipitin t.
Precision-G handheld blood
glucose t.
Precision QI-D handheld blood
glucose t.
predictive value of negative t.
predictive value of positive t.
pregnancy t.
presumptive heterophil t.
t. profile
prolactin t.
prostaglandin t.
protamine sulfate t.
protamine titration t.
protection t.
protein t.
protein-bound iodine t.
protein-bound iodine-131 t.
prothrombin consumption t.
prothrombin and proconvertin t.
prothrombin time t.
Protocult t.
protoporphyrin t.
provocative chelation t.
provocative Wassermann t.
pulmonary function t.
purine bodies t.
quantitation t.
Queckenstedt t.
quellung t.
Quick t.
QuickVue Chlamydia t.
quinine carbacrylic resin t.
Quinlan t.
rabbit t.
radioactive iodide uptake t.
radioactive iodine uptake t.
radioallergosorbent t. (RAST)
radioallergosorbent assay t. (RAST)
radioimmunosorbent t. (RIST)
radiosensitivity t. (RST)
RAI t.
RA latex fixation t.

random plasma glucose t.
rank sum t.
Rapid ANA II t.
rapid plasma reagin t.
RapiTex Hp t.
Rapoport t.
rat ovarian hyperemia t.
reactone red t.
red cell adherence t.
red cell survival t.
Reinsch t.
Reiter t.
Reiter protein complement-
fixation t. (RPCFT)
renal function t.
resorcinol t.
respiratory syncytial virus
antibody t.
respiratory syncytial virus
antigen t.
Reuss t.
Rh blocking t.
rheumatoid factor t.
riboflavin loading t.
rice-flour breath t.
Rimini t.
ring precipitin t.
Rinne t. (R)
RISA t.
Rocky Mountain spotted fever
antibody t.
Römer t.
Ropes t.
Rose t.
rose bengal radioactive (^{131}I) t.
Rosenbach t.
Rosenbach-Gmelin t.
rosette t.
Rose-Waaler t.
Ross-Jones t.
Rotazyme t.
Rothera nitroprusside t.
Rotter t.
Rous t.
Rowntree and Geraghty t.
RPR t.
rubella antibody t.
rubella HI t.
Rubin t.
Rubner t.
Rumpel-Leede t.
Sabin-Feldman dye t.
Sachs-Georgi t.
salicylic acid t.
saline agglutination t.
Sanford t.
Saundby t.
scarification t.

S-CCK-Pz t.
Schaffer t.
Schick t.
Schiller t.
Schilling t.
Schirmer t.
schistosomiasis serological t.
Schönbein t.
Schultz-Dale t.
Schumm t.
Schwarz t.
scratch t.
screening t.
secretin t.
secretin-CCK stimulation t.
secretin pancreozymin t.
sedimentation t.
SeHCAT t.
Selivanoff t.
Sereny t.
scrology t.
serum alkaline phosphatase t.
serum amylase t.
serum bacterial t.
serum bactericidal t.
serum globulin t.
serum protein electrophoresis t.
sex chromatin t. (SCT)
shake t.
sheep cell agglutination t. (SCAT)
Sia t.
sickle cell t.
Sickledex t.
Sicklequik t.
sickling t.
side platelet aggregation t. (SPAT)
signed rank t.
t. of significance (t)
silver nitroprusside t.
Sims-Huhner t.
single diffusion t.
single (gel) diffusion precipitin t.
  in one dimension
single (gel) diffusion precipitin t.
  in two dimensions
skin-puncture t.
skin window t.
SMAC t.
SMA-12 profile t.
sodium t.
solubility t.
t. solution (TS)

Southern blot t.
spironolactone t.
split renal function t.
spot t.
spot t. for infectious mononucleosis
Stamey t.
standard acid reflux t. (SART)
standard serologic t. for syphilis
standing plasma t.
Staph-Ident t.
Staph-Trac t.
staphylococcal clumping t. (SCT)
starch tolerance t.
stat t.
t. statistic
Sterneedle tuberculin t.
Strassburg t.
streptococcal antigen t.
streptozyme t.
Student t.
Student-Newman-Keuls t.
Stypven time t.
sucrose hemolysis t.
sulfosalicylic acid turbidity t.
Sulkowitch t.
sweat t.
t t.
Takata-Ara t.
tanned red cell hemagglutination
  inhibition t.
TCPI Rapid HIV t.
Tes-Tape urine glucose t.
tetrazolium t.
Thayer-Martin t.
thermostable opsonin t.
Thompson t.
Thormählen t.
Thorn t.
three-glass t.
thrombin time t.
thromboplastin activation t. (TAT)
thromboplastin generation t. (TGT)
thymol turbidity t.
thyroid function t. (TFT)
thyroid-stimulating hormone
  stimulation t.
thyroid suppression t.
thyroid uptake t.
thyrotropin-releasing hormone
  stimulation t.
thyroxine-binding index t.
TIBC t.

T

NOTES

test (continued)
  tine t.
  titratable acidity t.
  tolbutamide t. (TBT)
  tolbutamide tolerance t. (TTT)
  Töpfer t.
  total catecholamine t.
  TPH t.
  TPHA t.
  TPI t.
  transaminase t.
  transferrin t.
  treponemal immobilization t.
  Treponema pallidum
    hemagglutination t.
  Treponema pallidum
    immobilization t.
  TRH stimulation t.
  triiodothyronine resin uptake t.
  triiodothyronine suppression t.
  triple t.
  trypsin t.
  tryptophan load t.
  TSH stimulating t.
  TSH stimulation t.
  T_3U t.
  t. tube
  tube dilution t.
  tubeless gastric analysis t.
  tuberculin t.
  tuberculosis skin t.
  tumor skin t. (TST)
  T_3 uptake t.
  two-glass t.
  two-stage PT t.
  two-tail t.
  typhus antibody t.
  tyramine t.
  tyrosine t.
  Tzanck t.
  Uffelmann t.
  urea clearance t.
  urea nitrogen t.
  urease t.
  Uricult dipslide t.
  urinary concentration t.
  urine acetone t.
  Uriscreen t.
  urobilinogen t.
  uroporphyrin t.
  USR t.
  Valentine t.
  van Deen t.
  van den Bergh t.
  van der Velden t.
  vanillylmandelic acid t.
  Van Slyke t.
  varicella-zoster antibody t.

  VDRL t.
  ViraPap t.
  vitamin A clearance t.
  vitamin B_{12} absorption t.
  in vivo compatibility t.
  VMA t.
  Voges-Proskauer t.
  Volhard t.
  Vollmer t.
  VP t.
  Wagner t.
  Waldenström t.
  Wang t.
  Wassén t.
  Wassermann t.
  water-gurgle t.
  Watson-Schwartz t.
  Weber t.
  Webster t.
  Weil-Felix t.
  Welcozyme HIV 1&2 ELISA
    antibody t.
  Werner t.
  Westergren sedimentation rate t.
  Western blot t.
  Western immunoblot t.
  Wetzel t.
  wheal-and-erythema skin t.
  Wheeler-Johnson t.
  whiff t.
  Widal t.
  wire-loop t.
  Wormley t.
  Wurster t.
  xylose absorption t.
  D-xylose absorption t.
  xylose concentration t.
  D-xylose tolerance t.
  Yvon t.
  Zimmermann t.
  zinc flocculation t.
  zinc sulfate turbidity t.
  zinc turbidity t.
  Zollinger-Ellison t.
  zona-free hamster egg
    penetration t.
  Zsigmondy t.
testa
Testacealobosia
Tes-Tape urine glucose test
testcross
testes (*pl. of* testis)
testicular
  t. agenesis
  t. dysgenesis
  t. feminization
  t. feminization syndrome (Tfm,
    TFS)

t. hormone
t. regression syndrome
t. tubular adenoma
t. tumor

testing
 antibacterial agent susceptibility t.
 avidity t.
 bacterial susceptibility t.
 calcitonin t.
 Crithidia immunofluorescence t.
 histocompatibility t.
 hypothesis t.
 paternity t.
 point-of-care t.
 susceptibility t.

testis, pl. **testes**
 cryptorchid t.
 ectopic t.
 inverted t.
 movable t.
 obstructed t.
 t. redux
 retained t.
 rete t.
 retractile t.
 undescended t.

testitis
testoid hyperthecosis
testosterone
 free t.
 t. production rate (TPR)
testosterone-binding affinity (TBA)
testosterone-estradiol-binding globulin (TeBG)
TestPackChlamydia
Tet
 tetralogy of Fallot
tetanolysin
tetanospasmin
tetanotoxin
tetanus
 t. antibody
 t. antitoxin (TAT)
 t. antitoxin unit
 t. bacillus
 t. and gas gangrene antitoxins
 t. immune globulin
 t. immunoglobulin
 t. toxin
 t. toxin immunization reaction
 t. vaccine
tetanus-diphtheria (TD)

tetanus-perfringens antitoxin
Tete virus
tetracaine, epinephrine, and cocaine (TAC)
tetracarcinoma cell
tetrachlorethane poisoning
tetrachloride
 carbon t.
tetrachloroethylene
tetrachrome stain
tetracycline (TC, Tc)
 penicillin, streptomycin, and t. (PST)
tetrad
tetragonolobus
 peroxidase-conjugated lotus t.
tetrahedron chest
tetrahydrobiopterin
tetrahydrocannabinol
tetrahydrochloride
 3-3′-diaminobenzidine t.
tetrahydrocortisol
tetrahydrocortisone (THE)
tetrahydrodeoxycorticosterone (THDOC)
tetrahydro-11-deoxycortisol
tetrahydrofolate dehydrogenase
tetrahydrofolic acid
tetrahydrofuran
tetrahydropteroylglutamate methyltransferase
Tetrahymena pyriformis
tetralogy
 t. of Eisenmenger
 t. of Fallot (Tet, TF)
tetramastigote
tetramer
Tetrameres
tetramethyl acridine
tetramethylbenzidine
 t. chromogen
 t. stain
Tetramitidae
tetranitrate
 pentaerythritol t.
tetraplegia
tetraploid
tetraploidy
tetraptera
 Aspiculuris t.
tetrasomic
tetrasomy
tetrathionate enrichment broth

T

NOTES

Tetratrichomonas
    T. buccalis
    T. hominis
tetravalent
tetra-X chromosomal aberration
tetrazole
tetrazolium
    nitroblue t. (NBT)
    t. reduction (TR)
    t. reduction inhibition (TRI)
    t. test
tetrazonium salt
tetrodotoxin
tetrose
tetroxide
    dinitrogen t.
    osmium t.
tetter
    honeycomb t.
TF
    tetralogy of Fallot
    thymol flocculation
    tissue-damaging factor
    transfer factor
    tuberculin filtrate
    tubular fluid
TFA
    total fatty acids
Tfm
    testicular feminization syndrome
TFPI
    tissue factor pathway inhibitor
TFS
    testicular feminization syndrome
TFT
    thyroid function test
TG
    toxic goiter
TGA
    transposition of great arteries
TGAR
    total graft area rejected
Tg cell
TGE
    transmissible gastroenteritis
       TGE virus
TGFα
    transforming growth factor α
TGFβ
    transforming growth factor β
TGT
    thromboplastin generation test
    thromboplastin generation time
TGV
    thoracic gas volume
    transposition of great vessels
Th
    thorium

thalassanemia
thalassemia
    α-t.
    A_2 t.
    alpha t.
    alpha t. intermedia
    β-t.
    β-δ t.
    beta t.
    beta-delta t.
    F t.
    hemoglobin t.
    heterozygous t.
    homozygous t.
    t. intermedia
    α-t. intermedia
    Lepore t.
    t. major
    t. minor
    mixed t.
    sickle cell t.
    t. trait
thalassemia-sickle cell disease
thalidomide
thallic
thallitoxicosis
thallium
    t. assay
    t. poisoning
    t. sulfate
Thallophyta
thallophyte
thallospore
thallus
thanatophoric dwarfism
thanatopsy
thaumatropy
Thaumetopoea
Thaumetopoeidae
Thayer-Martin
    T.-M. agar
    T.-M. medium
    T.-M. test
Thaysen disease
THDOC
    tetrahydrodeoxycorticosterone
THE
    tetrahydrocortisone
thebaine
The Bethesda System (TBS)
theca
    t. cell
    t. cell-granuloma cell tumor
    t. cell tumor
    t. lutein tumor
thecal abscess
theca-lutein cyst
thecitis

thecoma
thecomatosis
Theiler
    T. disease
    T. mouse encephalomyelitis virus
    T. original virus
Theileria
theileriasis
Theileriidae
theileriosis
Thelazia
    T. callipaeda
thelaziasis
theliolymphocyte
thelium, pl. **thelia**
theloncus
Theobald Smith phenomenon
theophylline
    t. assay
theorem
    Bayes t.
    central limit t.
theoretical plate
theory
    Arrhenius-Madsen t.
    cellular immune t.
    clonal deletion t.
    clonal selection t.
    Cohnheim t.
    deletion t.
    Ehrlich side-chain t.
    emigration t.
    "fitter" cell t.
    Frerichs t.
    gametoid t.
    germ t.
    hematogenous t. of endometriosis
    information t.
    instructive t.
    lymphatic dissemination t. of
      endometriosis
    Metchnikoff t.
    monophyletic t.
    polyphyletic t.
    Ribbert t.
    side-chain t.
    somatic mutation t. of cancer
    Warburg t.
thèque
therapeutic
    t. abortion (TA)
    t. malaria

    t. phlebotomy
    t. pneumothorax
    t. ratio
therapia
    t. magna sterilisans
therapy
    alpha interferon t.
    anticoagulant t. (ACT)
    antimicrobial t.
    autoserum t.
    cancer management t.
    cytoreductive t.
    foreign protein t.
    glucocorticoid t.
    heterovaccine t.
    insulin coma t. (ICT)
    insulin shock t. (IST)
    α-interferon t.
    nonspecific t.
    plasma t.
    protein shock t.
    salvage t.
    serum t.
thermal
    t. conductivity (TC)
    t. conductivity detector
    t. death point
    t. death time
    t. equilibrium
    t. neutron
thermelometer
thermionic emission
thermistor
Thermoactinomyces
    T. candidus
    T. sacchari
    T. vulgaris
thermocouple thermometer
Thermocycler
thermodilution method
thermoduric
thermodynamic equilibrium
thermodynamics
thermogenic action
thermograph
thermolabile opsonin
Thermolospora viridis
thermoluminescence
thermoluminescent
    t. detector
    t. dosimeter
thermolysis

T

NOTES

thermometer
 air t.
 alcohol t.
 Beckmann t.
 bimetal t.
 Celsius t.
 centigrade t.
 differential t.
 Fahrenheit t.
 gas t.
 Kelvin t.
 liquid-in-glass t.
 maximum t.
 mercurial t.
 metallic t.
 metastatic t.
 minimum t.
 Rankine t.
 Réaumur t.
 recording t.
 resistance t.
 thermocouple t.
thermometry
thermophile
thermophilic
 t. actinomycete
 t. bacterium
thermophylic
thermoprecipitin reaction
thermoresistant
thermostabile
thermostable
 t. alkaline phosphatase
 t. body
 t. opsonin
 t. opsonin test
thermotaxis
thermotropism
thesaurismosis
thesaurocyte
theta
 t. antigen
 t. band
THF
 humoral thymic factor
thial
thiamin
 t. chloride unit
 t. hydrochloride unit
 phosphorylated t.
thiamine
 t. assay
 t. deficiency
thiamphenicol assay
Thiara
Thiaridae
thiazide diuretic

thiazin
 t. dye
thiazine stain
thiazole dye
Thibierge-Weissenbach syndrome
thickening
 hyaline t.
thick-layer autoradiography
thickness
 absorption-equivalent t. (AET)
 Breslow t.
 mean corpuscular t. (MCT)
Thiemann disease
thiemia
Thiersch canaliculi
thimerosal
thin-layer
 t.-l. chromatography (TLC)
 t.-l. electrophoresis (TLE)
 t.-l. immunoassay
thin-needle biopsy
ThinPrep
 T. cytologic preparation
 T. cytology
 T. slide process
thin section
thio acid
thioaldehyde
thiobarbiturate
thiocarbonyl group
thiochrome
thioctic acid
thiocyanate
 potassium t.
thioester
thioethanolamine
thioether
thioflavine
 t. S
 t. T
 t. T stain
thioglycolate
thioglycolic acid
thioglycollate
 t. broth
 t. medium
thioglycollate-135C broth
thioketone
thiol
thiolaminopropionic acid
thiolase
 acetoacetyl-CoA t.
thiolysis
thione
thionine
thionin stain
thioredoxin
thioridazine assay

thiosulfate
thiothixene
thiourea
thioxanthene tranquilizer
third
t. corpuscle
t. degree burn
t. degree frostbite
t. degree heart block
t. degree radiation injury
t. disease
t. and fourth pharyngeal pouch
syndrome
thixotropic
thixotropy
Thoma
T. counting chamber
T. fixative
Thompson test
Thomsen disease
Thoms method
Thomson disease
thoracic
t. aneurysm
t. asphyxiant dystrophy (TAD)
t. duct fistula (TDF)
t. fistula
t. gas volume (TGV)
t. goiter
t. index (TI)
thoracic-pelvic-phalangeal dystrophy
thorium (Th)
Thormählen test
thorn
t. apple crystal
T. syndrome
T. test
Thornwaldt (*var. of* Tornwaldt)
thorotrast
THPCOP
cyclophosphamide, THP-doxorubicin,
vincristine, prednisone
Thr
threonine
threads
mucous t.
threadworm
threatened abortion
three-day
t.-d. fever
t.-d. measles
three-glass test

three-part mitosis
three-phase current
three-point cross
threonin
threonine (Thr)
threonyl
threose
thresher's lung
threshold
t. body
t. dose
t. erythema dose (TED)
t. limit value (TLV)
mean cell t.
median detection t. (MDT)
renal t.
t. substance
throat
t. culture
putrid t.
thrombase
thrombasthenia
Glanzmann t.
Glanzmann-Naegeli t.
hereditary hemorrhagic t.
thrombi (*pl. of* thrombus)
thrombin
t. clotting time (TCT)
t. time (TT)
t. time test
thrombinogen
thrombinogenesis
thromboangiitis
t. obliterans (TAO)
thromboarteritis
t. purulenta
thromboasthenia
thromboblast
thromboclasis
thrombocyst
thrombocystis
thrombocytasthenia
thrombocyte
thrombocythemia
essential t.
hemorrhagic t.
primary t.
thrombocytic
t. leukemia
t. series
thrombocytin
thrombocytopathy

T

NOTES

thrombocytopenia
    autoimmune neonatal t.
    drug-induced t. (DIT)
    essential t.
    heparin-induced t. (HIT)
    immune t.
    isoimmune neonatal t.
    t. with absence of radius (TAR)
thrombocytopenia-absent radius syndrome
thrombocytopenic purpura (TP)
thrombocytopoiesis
thrombocytosis
thromboelastogram
thromboelastograph
thromboembolic disease (TED)
thromboembolism
    pulmonary t. (PTE)
thromboendarteritis
thromboendocarditis
thrombogen
thrombogene
thrombogenic
thromboglobulin
    beta t.
β-thromboglobulin
thromboid
thrombokatilysin
thrombokinase
thrombolic
thrombolus
thrombolymphangitis
thrombolysis
thrombolytic agent
thrombometer
thrombon
thrombonecrosis
    arteriolar t.
thrombopathic syndrome
thrombopathy
    constitutional t.
thrombopenia
thrombopenic anemia
thrombophilia
thrombophlebitis
    t. migrans
    migrating t.
    t. saltans
thromboplastic
    t. plasma component (TPC)
    t. substance
thromboplastid
thromboplastin
    t. activation test (TAT)
    t. antecedent deficiency
    automated activated partial t.
    t. generation test (TGT)
    t. generation time (TGT)

    RecombiPlasTin t.
    t. substitution test
    tissue t.
thromboplastinogen
thromboplastinogenase
thromboplastinogenemia
thrombopoiesis
thrombopoietin
thrombosed
    t. arteriosclerotic aneurysm
    t. hemorrhoid
thrombosin
thrombosis, pl. thromboses
    agonal t.
    atrophic t.
    cardiac t.
    cerebral t. (CT)
    coronary t. (CT)
    dilatation t.
    marantic t.
    marasmic t.
    mesenteric t.
    placental t.
    plate t.
    platelet t.
    portal vein t. (PVT)
    propagating t.
    puerperal t.
    renal vein t. (RVT)
    traumatic t.
    venous t.
thrombostasis
thrombosthenin
thrombotest
thrombotic
    t. gangrene
    t. infarct
    t. microangiopathy
    t. nonbacterial endocarditis
    t. occlusion
    t. phlegmasia
    t. thrombocytopenic purpura (TTP)
    t. thrombocytopenic purpura and hemolytic uremic syndrome (TTP-HUS)
thrombotonin
thromboxane
    t. A_2
    t. B_2
thrombozyme
thrombus, pl. thrombi
    agglutinative t.
    agonal t.
    antemortem t.
    ball t.
    ball-valve t.
    bile t.
    canalized t.

fibrin t.
globular t.
hyaline t.
infective t.
laminated t.
marantic t.
marasmic t.
mixed t.
mural t.
old t.
organized t.
pale t.
parietal t.
platelet t.
postmortem t.
recent t.
red t.
secondary t.
stratified t.
t. tumor
tumor t.
valvular t.
white t.
through-and-through myocardial infarction
thrush
t. fungus
thrust culture
thulium
thumb
hitchhiker t.
thumbprinting
Thy-1 antigen
Thygeson disease
thylacitis
thymic
t. abscess
t. agenesis
t. alymphoplasia (TAL)
t. carcinoma
t. dysplasia
t. humoral factor
t. hypoplasia
t. leukemia
t. lymphopoietic factor
t. replacing factor
t. reticulum cell
t. tumor
thymic-parathyroid aplasia
thymidine
t. diphosphate (dTDP)
t. monophosphate

t. triphosphate
tritiated t. (TTH)
thymidine-5'-phosphate
thymidylic acid
thymidylyl
thymin
thymine
t. dimer
t. ribonucleoside
t. ribonucleoside-5'-phosphate
thymine-2-deoxyriboside
thymitis
thymocyte
thymocytotoxic autoantibody
thymofibrolipoma
thymol
t. blue
t. flocculation (TF)
t. turbidity (TT)
t. turbidity test
thymolipoma
thymoliposarcoma
thymolphthalein
thymoma
epithelial t.
intrapulmonary spindle cell t.
lymphocytic t.
malignant t.
spindle cell t.
thymopathy
thymopoietin
thymosin
thymus-dependent (TD)
t.-d. antigen
thymus-independent antigen
thymus leukemia (TL)
thymus-leukemia antigen
thyristor
thyroadenitis
thyrocalcitonin (TCT)
thyrocardiac disease
thyrocele
thyrocolloid
thyroglobulin
thyroglossal
t. duct cyst
t. fistula
thyroid
t. antimicrosomal antibody
t. antithyroglobulin antibody
t. cachexia
t. crisis

NOTES

T

thyroid *(continued)*
 t. endocrine disorder
 t. follicle
 t. function test (TFT)
 medullary carcinoma of t.
 t. microsomal antibody
 t. stimulating hormone-releasing
  factor (TSH-RF)
 t. suppression test
 t. tumor
 t. uptake test
thyroidal clearance
thyroiditis
 acute t.
 autoimmune t.
 chronic t.
 chronic atrophic t.
 de Quervain t.
 focal lymphocytic t.
 giant cell t.
 granulomatous t.
 Hashimoto t.
 induced t.
 invasive fibrous t.
 ligneous t.
 parasitic t.
 Riedel t.
 subacute granulomatous t.
thyroid-stimulating
 t.-s. hormone (TSH)
 t.-s. hormone assay
 t.-s. hormone stimulation test
 t.-s. immunoglobulin (TSI)
thyroid-to-serum ratio (TSR)
thyrolingual cyst
thyrolytic
thyromegaly
thyroptosis
thyrosis
thyrotoxic
 t. complement-fixation factor
 t. encephalopathy
 t. heart disease
 t. myopathy
 t. serum
thyrotoxicosis
 t. factitia
thyrotoxin
 t. shock
thyrotrope
thyrotropic
 t. hormone (TTH)
thyrotropin
thyrotropin-producing adenoma
thyrotropin-receptor antibody
thyrotropin-releasing
 t.-r. factor (TRF)

 t.-r. hormone (TRH)
 t.-r. hormone stimulation test
thyroxine
 t. assay
 free (unbound) t. (FT_4)
 total t. (TT)
thyroxine-binding
 t.-b. albumin
 t.-b. globulin (TBG)
 t.-b. globulin assay
 t.-b. index (TBI)
 t.-b. index test
 t.-b. prealbumin (TBPA)
 t.-b. protein (TBP)
thyroxine-specific activity (T_4SA)
thyrse
 en t.
Thysanosoma actinoides
THz
 terahertz
TI
 thoracic index
 time interval
 tricuspid incompetence
 tricuspid insufficiency
TIA
 transient ischemic attack
TIBC
 total iron-binding capacity
  TIBC test
tibia, pl. tibiae
 saber t.
tibial tuberosity
TIC
 trypsin-inhibitory capacity
ticarcillin
tick
 t. fever
 t. paralysis
tick-borne
 t.-b. encephalitis (Central European
  subtype)
 t.-b. encephalitis (Eastern subtype)
 t.-b. encephalitis virus
 t.-b. virus
TID
 titrated initial dose
tide
 acid t.
 alkaline t.
 fat t.
TIE
 transient ischemic episode
Tierfellnaevus
tiering
 parakeratotic t.
Tietze syndrome
Tietz-Fiereck method

tiger heart
tigroid striation
TIL
    tumor-infiltrating lymphocyte
Tilden stain
Tillaux disease
tilorone
TILS
    tumor-infiltrating lymphocyte
time
    absolute retention t. (ART)
    access t.
    activated coagulation t. (ACT)
    activated partial thromboplastin t.
      (APTT, aPTT)
    bleeding t. (BT)
    blood-clot lysis t. (BLT)
    calcium t.
    cell cycle t.
    circulation t. (CT)
    clot lysis t. (CLT)
    clot retraction t.
    clotting t. (CT)
    coagulation t. (CT)
    compile t.
    corrected retention t.
    dead t.
    decimal reduction t.
    t. diffusion technique
    doubling t.
    Duke method of bleeding t.
    electrode response t.
    euglobulin clot lysis t. (ECLT)
    euglobulin lysis t. (ELT)
    execution t.
    t. of flight
    gastric emptying t. (GET)
    generation t.
    grain count halving t.
    helium equilibration t. (HET)
    t. interval (TI)
    Ivy method of bleeding t.
    Kaolin-clotting t.
    kaolin partial thromboplastin t.
      (KPTT)
    lag t.
    t. of maximum concentration (T_{max})
    mean circulation t. (MCT)
    mean generation t.
    occlusion t. (OT)
    operating t.
    partial thromboplastin t. (PTT)

    particle transport t. (PTT)
    plasma clotting t.
    plasma-iron disappearance t. (PIDT)
    prolonged bleeding t.
    prolonged coagulation t.
    prothrombin t. (PT)
    prothrombin consumption t. (PCT)
    reaction t. (RT)
    recalcification t.
    recovery t.
    relative retention t.
    resolving t.
    retention t.
    Russell viper venom clotting t.
    RV t.
    serial thrombin t. (STT)
    serum prothrombin t.
    shortened bleeding t.
    shortened coagulation t.
    Stypven t.
    survival t.
    thermal death t.
    thrombin t. (TT)
    thrombin clotting t. (TCT)
    thromboplastin generation t. (TGT)
    tissue thromboplastin inhibition t.
    turn-around t. (TAT)
    wash t.
    wheal reaction t. (QRZ)
    whole-blood clotting t.
timer
time-sharing
time-tension index (TTI)
Timme syndrome
timothy bacillus
TIN
    tubulointerstitial nephropathy
Tinca
tinctable
tinction
tinctorial
tincture of iodine
tinea
    t. amiantacea
    t. barbae
    t. capitis
    t. ciliorum
    t. circinata
    t. corporis
    t. cruris
    t. favosa
    t. glabrosa

T

NOTES

tinea *(continued)*
t. imbricata
t. inguinalis
t. kerion
t. manus
t. manuum
t. nigra
t. pedis
t. sycosis
t. tonsurans
t. tropicalis
t. unguium
t. versicolor
tine test
tingibility
tingible
tingible-body macrophage
tint
TIS
tumor in situ
tissue
aberrant t.
adipose t.
areolar connective t.
bile pigment demonstration in t.
bilirubin demonstration in t.'s
brown adipose t.
"bursa-equivalent" t.
cancellous t.
connective t.
t. culture (TC)
t. culture dose (TCD)
t. culture infectious dose ($TCID_{50}$)
t. culture infective dose (TCID)
t. culture medium (TCM)
diffuse lymphatic t.
t. factor
t. factor pathway inhibitor (TFPI)
t. glycogen
granulation t.
gut-associated lymphoid t. (GALT)
hard t.
hematopoietic t.
hemoglobin demonstration in t.
hormone demonstration in t.
inflammation of connective t. (ICT)
lead demonstration in t.
t. lymph
mucosa-associated lymphoid t. (MALT)
myeloid t.
paraffin-embedded t. (PET)
t. processing
t. thromboplastin
t. thromboplastin inhibition time
t. tolerance dose (TTD)

tuberculosis granulation t.
t. typing
tissue-coding factor (TSF)
tissue-damaging factor (TF)
tissue-equivalent (TE)
tissue-specific antigen
titan yellow
titer
agglutination t.
AH t.
antibody t.
antideoxyribonuclease B t.
antihyaluronidase t. (AHT)
anti-Rh t.
antistreptolysin-O t.
ASO t.
California encephalitis virus t.
CF antibody t.
Chlamydia group t.
cold agglutinin t.
Coxsackievirus A, B virus t. (C virus)
cryptococcal antigen t.
Cryptococcus antibody t.
cysticercosis t.
differential agglutination t. (DAT)
eastern equine encephalitis virus t.
fibrin t.
hemagglutination t. (HT)
influenza A and B t.
lymphogranuloma venereum t.
mumps antibody t.
poliomyelitis I, II, III t.
psittacosis t.
Q fever t.
Salmonella t.
titrant
titratable
t. acid (TA)
t. acidity test
titrated initial dose (TID)
titration
coulometric t.
potentiometric t.
t. technique
titrator
Cotlove t.
titrimetric
Tityus serrulatus
Tizzoni stain
Tj antigen
TKD
tokodynamometer
TKG
tokodynagraph
TL
thymus leukemia
TL antigen

TLC
    thin-layer chromatography
    total L-chain concentration
TLD
    tumor lethal dose
T/LD$_{100}$
    minimum dose causing death or
      malformation of 100% of fetuses
TLE
    thin-layer electrophoresis
TLV
    threshold limit value
Tm cell
TMV
    tobacco mosaic virus
T/natural killer cell lymphoma
TNF
    tumor necrosis factor
TNM
    (primary) tumor, (regional lymph) nodes,
      (remote) metastases
      TNM cancer grading system
      TNM staging
T-nodule
TNTC
    too numerous to count
TO
    no evidence of primary tumor
    original tuberculin
      TO virus
to
    t. contain (TC)
    t. deliver (TD)
TOA
    tubo-ovarian abscess
toad toxin
tobacco mosaic virus (TMV)
Tobie, von Brand, and Mehlman
    diphasic medium
tobramycin
tocainide
Todd
    T. body
    T. unit (TU)
Todd-Hewitt broth
toe
    clubbed t.
    Hong Kong t.
    webbed t.
Togaviridae
togavirus
toggle

Toison
    T. solution
    T. stain
Tokelau ringworm
tokodynagraph (TKG)
tokodynamometer (TKD)
tolbutamide
    t. test (TBT)
    t. tolerance test (TTT)
tolerance
    drug t.
    glucose t. (GT)
    high dose t.
    immunological t.
    immunologic high dose t.
    t. interval
    nonresponder t.
    split t.
tolerogen
tolerogenic
tolnaftate
Tolosa-Hunt syndrome
toluene 2,4-diisocyanate
toluic acid
toluidine
    alkaline t. blue O
    t. blue (TB)
    t. blue O
    t. blue stain
toluol
toluylene red
tome
Tommaselli disease
tone
toner
tongue
    bifid t.
    black hairy t.
    cleft t.
    t. worm
tonicity
toning
    gold t.
tonofibril
tonofilament
tonometer
tonsillaris
    cynanche t.
tonsillitis
too numerous to count (TNTC)
Tooth disease
Töpfer test

T

NOTES

tophaceous
    t. gout
tophus, pl. **tophi**
    gouty t.
topical calciphylaxis
topoisomerase II enzyme
topopathogenesis
TOPV
    trivalent oral poliovirus vaccine
TORCH
    toxoplasmosis, rubella, cytomegalovirus,
      and herpes simplex
    TORCH syndrome
Tornwaldt, Thornwaldt
    T. abscess
    T. disease
    T. syndrome
torocyte
torose, torous
torque
torr
Torre syndrome
torsion
    t. injury
    t. of testis
Torsten Sjögren syndrome
torticollis
    congenital t.
Torula
    T. capsulatus
    T. histolytica
torular meningitis
toruloidea
    Hendersonula t.
toruloma
Torulopsis
    T. glabrata
torulopsosis
torulosis
tosylate
total
    t. acidity (A, a)
    t. antitryptic activity (TAT)
    t. blood granulocyte pool (TBGP)
    t. blood volume (TBV)
    t. body clearance (Q_B)
    t. body density (TBD)
    t. body fat (TBF)
    t. body hematocrit (TBH)
    t. body potassium (TBK)
    t. body solute (TBS)
    t. body water (TBW)
    t. body weight (TBW)
    t. calcium assay
    t. catecholamine test
    t. cell count
    t. cholesterol (TC)
    t. circulating hemoglobin (TCH)

    t. estriol
    t. estrogen (excretion) (TE)
    t. exchangeable potassium
      measurement
    t. fatty acids (TFA)
    t. graft area rejected (TGAR)
    t. hematuria
    t. internal reflection
    t. iron-binding capacity (TIBC)
    t. L-chain concentration (TLC)
    t. necrosis
    t. oxidant
    t. peripheral resistance (TPR)
    t. protein (TP)
    t. pulmonary resistance
    t. pulmonary vascular resistance
      (TPVR)
    t. resistance (TR)
    t. response (TR)
    t. ridge count (TRC)
    t. serum prostatic acid phosphatase
      (TSPAP)
    t. serum protein (TSP)
    t. thyroxine (TT)
    t. urinary gonadotropin (TUG)
total-dose infusion (TDI)
totipotency
totipotent
totipotential cell
Touraine-Solente-Golé syndrome
Tourette disease
Touton
    T. giant cell
toxalbumin
toxanemia
toxaphene
Toxascaris leonina
toxemia
    preeclamptic t. (PET)
    t. of pregnancy
toxemic
    t. jaundice
toxic
    t. adenoma
    t. anemia
    t. chemical handling
    t. cirrhosis
    t. cyanosis
    t. dermatitis
    t. epidermal necrolysis (TEN)
    t. equivalent
    t. erythema
    t. glycosuria
    t. goiter (TG)
    t. granulation
    t. granule
    t. hemoglobinuria
    t. idiopathy

t. megacolon
t. methemoglobinemia
t. nephrosis
t. shock
t. shock syndrome
t. unit (TU)
t. waste
toxicant
toxicemia
toxicity
acetaminophen hepatic t.
aspirin t.
EP t.
toxicogenic conjunctivitis
toxicologic
toxicologist
toxicology
analytical t.
clinical t.
environmental t.
forensic t.
industrial t.
toxicopathic
toxicosis
toxigenic
t. bacterium
toxigenicity
toxin
animal t.
anthrax t.
Bacillus anthracis t.
bacterial t.
bee venom t.
botulinum t.
botulinus t., botulismotoxin
cholera t.
Clostridium difficile t.
Coley t.
diagnostic diphtheria t.
Dick test t.
dinoflagellate t.
diphtheria t.
erythrogenic t.
extracellular t.
intracellular t.
normal t.
plant t.
scarlet fever erythrogenic t.
Schick test t.
Shiga t.
t. spectrum

streptococcus erythrogenic t.
tetanus t.
toad t.
t. unit (TU)
toxin-antitoxin (TA, TAT)
toxinic
toxinogenic
toxinogenicity
toxinology
toxinosis
toxipathic
toxipathy
Toxocara
T. canis
T. cati
T. mystax
toxocariasis
toxoid
alum-precipitated t. (APT)
toxoid-antitoxin
t.-a. floccules (TAF)
t.-a. mixture (TAM)
toxoid-antitoxoid
toxon
toxoneme
toxonosis
toxophil
toxophore
toxophorous
Toxoplasma
T. gondii
T. pyrogenes
Toxoplasmatidae
Toxoplasmea
toxoplasmin
toxoplasmosis
acquired t. in adults
congenital t.
t., rubella, cytomegalovirus, and herpes simplex (TORCH)
t. serology
TP
thrombocytopenic purpura
total protein
tryptophan
tube precipitin
tuberculin precipitation
TPA
Treponema pallidum agglutination
TPC
thromboplastic plasma component

T

NOTES

TPCF
>*Treponema pallidum* complement-
>   fixation

TPH
>transplacental hemorrhage
>*Treponema pallidum* hemagglutination
>   TPH test

TPHA test

TPI
>*Treponema pallidum* immobilization
>   TPI assay
>   TPI test

TPIA
>*Treponema pallidum* immobilization
>   (immune) adherence

TPR
>testosterone production rate
>total peripheral resistance

TPS
>tumor polysaccharide substance

TPT
>typhoid-paratyphoid (vaccine)

TPVR
>total pulmonary vascular resistance

TR
>tetrazolium reduction
>total resistance
>total response
>tuberculin R (new tuberculin)

Tr
>trace

tra
>transfer
>   t. operon

trabecula, pl. trabeculae
>trabeculae of bone
>trabeculae carneae

trabecular
>t. adenocarcinoma
>t. adenoma
>t. carcinoma
>t. pattern

trabeculation

trace (Tr)
>t. alternant
>t. element
>t. routine

tracé discontinu

tracer

tracheal aspiration

tracheitis

trachelematoma

trachelocystitis

trachelomyitis

trachelopanus

trachelophyma

tracheoaerocele

tracheobiliary fistula

tracheobronchial dyskinesia

tracheobronchitis (TB)

tracheobronchomegaly

tracheoesophageal fistula (TEF)

tracheomalacia

tracheomegaly

tracheopathia
>t. osteoplastica

tracheopathy

trachitis

trachoma
>t. body
>t. virus

trachoma-inclusion conjunctivitis (TRIC)

Trachybdella bistriata

trachychromatic

tracing

TRAcP
>tartrate resistant acid phosphatase

tract
>female genital t. (FGT)

tractellum

traction
>t. aneurysm
>t. atrophy
>t. diverticulum

trait
>secretor t.
>sickle cell t.
>thalassemia t.

trance
>death t.

tranquilizer
>major t.
>minor t.
>phenothiazine t.
>thioxanthene t.

trans **activation**

transaldolase

transaminase
>aspartate t.
>erythrocyte glutamic oxaloacetic t.
>   (EGOT)
>glutamate-pyruvate t.
>glutamic-oxaloacetic t.
>hepatic t.
>serum glutamate oxaloacetate t.
>serum glutamate pyruvate t.
>serum glutamic-oxaloacetic t.
>   (SGOT)
>serum glutamic-pyruvic t. (SGPT)
>t. test
>valine t.

transamination

transcapsidation

transcarbamoylase
>ornithine t.

transcobalamin (Tc)

transconfiguration
transcortin
transcript
    primary t.
transcriptase
    reverse t.
transcription
    inhibitors of t.
    reverse t.
    t. unit
transcriptional promoter
transduce
transducer
transductant
transduction
    abortive t.
    complete t.
    general t.
    generalized t.
    high frequency t.
    low frequency t.
    specialized t.
    specific t.
transepidermal water loss (TWL)
transfection
transfer (tra)
    t. factor (TF)
    t. function
    t. gene
    group t.
    t. host
    t. operon
    passive t.
    t. pipette
    replication and t. (RTF)
    t. RNA (tRNA)
transferase
    deoxynucleotidyl t.
    hypoxanthine guanine
      phosphoribosyl t. (HGPRT)
    terminal deoxynucleotidyl t. (TDT,
      TdT)
    terminal deoxyribonucleotidyl t.
    UDP-glucuronyl t.
transference
    passive t.
transferred
    t. antigen-cell-bound antibody
      reaction
    t. antigen-transferred antibody
      reaction

transferrin
    t. assay
    t. saturation
    t. test
transformant
transformation
    asbestos t.
    bacterial t.
    cell t.
    globular-fibrous t.
    human lymphocyte t. (hLT)
    logit t.
    lymphocyte t.
    lymphocytic t.
    malignant t.
    nodular t. of the liver
    probit t.
    pseudoxanthomatous t.
transformed lymphocyte
transformer
    high-voltage t.
    step-down t.
    step-up t.
    voltage-regulating t.
transforming
    t. agent
    t. gene
    t. growth factor
    t. growth factor α (TGFα)
    t. growth factor β (TGFβ)
    t. growth factor alpha
    t. growth factor beta
transfusion
    autologous t.
    coagulation factor t.
    exchange t.
    t. hepatitis
    intrauterine t.
    leukocyte t.
    massive t.
    t. nephritis
    platelet t.
    predeposit autologous t.
    t. reaction
    reciprocal t.
transfusion-associated graft-vs-host
  disease
transgenic mice
transglutaminase
transient
    t. agammaglobulinemia
    t. albuminuria

NOTES

transient *(continued)*
    t. cerebral ischemia (TCI)
    t. cerebral ischemic episode (TCIE)
    t. derepression
    t. equilibrium
    t. hypogammaglobulinemia
    t. hypogammaglobulinemia of infancy
    t. ischemic attack (TIA)
    t. ischemic episode (TIE)
transistor
    field effect t.
    insulated gate field effect t.
    junction field effect t.
    metal oxide semiconductor field effect t.
    unijunction t.
transistor-transistor logic
transition
    isomeric t. (IT)
    t. mutation
    t. state
    t. zone
transitional
    t. cell carcinoma
    t. cell papilloma
    t. cell tumor
    t. leukocyte
transketolase assay
translation
    t. control RNA (tcRNA)
    formula t. (FORTRAN)
translator
translocation
    autosome t.
    balance t.
    chromosome t.
    t. factor
    insertional t.
    reciprocal t.
    robertsonian t.
    t. trisomy
translucent
transmandibular projection
transmethylase
transmethylation
transmissible
    t. dementia
    t. enteritis
    t. gastroenteritis (TGE)
    t. gastroenteritis of swine
    t. gastroenteritis virus of swine
    t. mink encephalopathy
    t. plasmid
    t. turkey enteritis virus
transmission
    asynchronous data t.
    t. electron microscope (TEM)

    t. electron microscopy (TEM)
    horizontal t.
    serial data t.
    synchronous data t.
    vertical t.
transmittance
    peak t.
transmogrification
    placental t.
transmogrify
transmural myocardial infarction
transmutation
transparent
transpeptidase
    glutamyl t.
transphosphorylase
transplacental hemorrhage (TPH)
transplant
transplantation
    allogenic t.
    t. antigen
    autologous t.
    bone marrow t. (BMT)
    heterotopic t.
    homotopic t.
    orthoptic t.
    syngeneic t.
    syngenesioplastic t.
transport
    active t.
    carrier-mediated t.
    direct t.
    t. disease
    effective oxygen t. (EOT)
    indirect t.
    lipid t.
    t. medium
    membrane t.
    passive t.
    primary active t.
    secondary active t.
    t. and secretion
    t. and storage
    tape t.
transposable element
transpose
transposition
    corrected t. (CT)
    t. of great arteries (TGA)
    t. of great vessels (TGV)
transposon
transsynaptic
    t. chromatolysis
    t. degeneration
transubstantiation
transudate
    acute inflammatory t.
transudation

transudative inflammation
transurethral
- t. prostatectomy (TURP)
- t. resection (TUR)

transvector
transverse
- t. fracture
- t. myelitis
- t. myelopathy

transversion mutation
Tr^a antigen
Trapp formula
Trapp-Häser formula
Traube
- T. corpuscle
- T. plug

trauma, pl. traumata
traumatic
- t. abnormality
- t. anemia
- t. aneurysm
- t. atrophy
- t. bone cyst
- t. fever
- t. hemolysis
- t. herpes
- t. neuroma
- t. progressive encephalopathy
- t. thrombosis

trazodone
TRC
- tanned red cell
- total ridge count

Treacher Collins syndrome
treatment
- isoserum t.
- preventive t.
- prophylactic t.

trefoil peptide
trehala
trehalose
Trematoda
trematode
- prosostomate t.

tremelloid
tremellose
tremens
- delirium t. (DT)

tremor
- epidemic t.

trench
- t. fever

- t. foot
- t. mouth

Treponema
- _T. buccale_
- _T. calligyrum_
- _T. carateum_
- direct fluorescent antibody test - _T. pallidum_ (DFA-TP test)
- _T. genitalis_
- _T. macrodentium_
- _T. microdentium_
- _T. mucosum_
- _T. orale_
- _T. pallidum_
- _T. pallidum_ agglutination (TPA)
- _T. pallidum_ complement-fixation (TPCF)
- _T. pallidum_ hemagglutination (TPH)
- _T. pallidum_ hemagglutination test
- _T. pallidum_ immobilization (TPI)
- _T. pallidum_ immobilization assay
- _T. pallidum_ immobilization (immune) adherence (TPIA)
- _T. pallidum_ immobilization reaction
- _T. pallidum_ immobilization test
- _T. pertenue_
- _T. pintae_
- _T. refringens_
- _T. scoliodontum_
- _T. vincentii_

treponema-immobilizing antibody
treponemal
- t. antibody
- t. immobilization test

treponematosis
tresis
Trevor disease
TRF
- T cell-replacing factor
- thyrotropin-releasing factor

TRH
- thyrotropin-releasing hormone
  - TRH stimulation test

TRI
- tetrazolium reduction inhibition

triac
triacetin
triacetylglycerol
triacetyloleandomycin
triacylglycerol lipase
triad
- acute compression t.

T

NOTES

triad *(continued)*
    adrenomedullary t.
    Andersen t.
    Beck t.
    Hutchinson t.
    portal t.
    t. syndrome
trials
    clinical t.
triamcinolone
triangle
    sternocostal t.
triangular wave
triarylmethane dye
Triatoma
triatomic
triatomid
Triatominae
triatriatum
    cor t.
tribasic
    t. acid
    t. potassium phosphate
tribasilar synostosis
tribe
TRIC
    trachoma-inclusion conjunctivitis
tricarboxylic
    t. acid
    t. acid cycle
Tricercomonas
trichatrophia
trichilemmal cyst
trichilemmoma
Trichina
trichina
Trichinella
    T. spiralis
trichinelliasis
Trichinellicae
Trichinelloidea
trichinellosis
trichiniasis
trichiniferous
trichinization
trichinoscope
trichinosis
    t. serology
trichinous
    t. embolism
trichite
trichitis
trichlorfon
trichloride
    acetylene t.
    vinyl t.
trichloroacetic acid (TCA)
1,1,1-trichloroethane

1,1,2-trichloroethane
trichloroethylene
(2,4,5-trichlorophenoxy)acetic acid
Trichobilharzia
trichoblastoma
    desmoplastic t.
trichocephaliasis
Trichocephalus
    T. trichiura
trichochrome
trichocyst
Trichodectes
trichodectis
    Cryptocystis t.
Trichoderma
trichoepithelioma
    desmoplastic t.
    hereditary multiple t.
    t. papillosum multiplex
trichofolliculoma
trichoid
tricholemmoma
Tricholoma
    T. pardinum
Tricholomapardinum
trichomonacide
trichomonad
Trichomonadidae
Trichomonas
    T. buccalis
    T. hominis
    T. intestinalis
    T. preparation
    T. pulmonalis
    T. tenax
    T. vaginalis
trichomoniasis
    t. vaginitis
trichomycosis
    t. axillaris
    t. chromatica
    t. favosa
    t. rubra
trichonodosis
trichophytic
trichophytid
trichophytin
Trichophyton
    T. concentricum
    T. crateriforme
    T. epilans
    T. equinum
    T. ferrugineum
    T. gallinae
    T. glabrum
    T. gourvilii
    T. gypseum
    T. megninii

T. mentagrophytes
T. purpureum
T. rosaceum
T. rubrum
T. sabouraudi
T. schoenleinii
T. simii
T. sulfureum
T. tonsurans
T. verrucosum
T. violaceum
trichophytosis
t. barbae
t. capitis
t. corporis
t. cruris
t. unguium
Trichopleuris
Trichoprosopon
Trichoptera
trichorhinophalangeal syndrome
trichorrhexis nodosa
trichosomatous
Trichosporon
T. beigelii
T. cutaneum
T. giganteum
T. pedrosianum
trichosporosis
trichostrongyle
trichostrongyliasis
Trichostrongylidae
Trichostrongyloidea
trichostrongylosis
Trichostrongylus
T. axei
T. brevis
T. colubriformis
T. instabilis
T. orientalis
T. probolurus
T. vitrinus
Trichothecium
T. roseum
trichotoxin
trichrome stain
trichuriasis
Trichuris
T. trichiura
Trichuroidea
tricresol
tricresyl phosphate

Tricula
tricuspid
t. atresia
t. incompetence (TI)
t. insufficiency (TI)
t. stenosis
tricyclic antidepressant
trident hand
tridermoma
triene
triethanolamine
trifid stomach
trifluoride-methanol
boron t.
triglyceride
t. assay
long-chain t. (LCT)
medium-chain t.
plasma t.
trigonitis
trigonum, pl. trigona
t. sternocostale
trihexosidase
ceramide t.
triiodothyronine (T₃)
t. assay
free T₃
t. resin uptake (T₃RU)
t. resin uptake test
reverse t. (rT₃)
t. by RIA
t. suppression test
triketohydrindene reaction
triloba
placenta t.
trilobate placenta
trilocular heart
trimastigote
trimer
trimethoprim
trimethoxyamphetamine
trimethylamine
trimethylaminuria
trimming resistor
trimorphic
trimorphism
trimorphous
2,4,6-trinitrotoluene
trinocular microscope
tri-o-cresyl phosphate
Triodontophorus
T. diminutus

NOTES

triol
trioleandomycin
triolein I 131
triose
triosephosphate
    t. dehydrogenase
    t. isomerase
    t. isomerase assay
    t. isomerase deficiency
triosulfate-citrate-bile salts-sucrose
   (TCBS)
2,6,8-trioxypurine
tripartita
    placenta t.
triphasic wave
triphenylmethane
    t. dye
Triphleps insidiosus
triphosphatase
    adenosine t. (ATPase)
triphosphate
    adenosine t. (ATP)
    cytidine t. (CTP)
    cytosine t. (CTP)
    deoxythymidine t. (dTTP)
    guanosine t. (GTP)
    inosine t.
    thymidine t.
    uridine t. (UTP)
triphyllomatous teratoma
triple
    t. bond
    t. phosphate
    t. point
    t. sugar iron (TSI)
    t. sugar iron agar
    t. symptom complex
    t. test
triple-blind
triplet
    t. code
    coding t.
    nonsense t.
triple-X chromosomal aberration
triploid
triploidy
tris(hydroxymethyl) aminomethane
trisomic cell
trisomy
    chromosome t.
    t. C syndrome
    double t.
    t. D syndrome
    t. E syndrome
    partial t.
    primary t.
    secondary t.
    t. 8 syndrome

    t. 13 syndrome
    t. 13-15 syndrome
    t. 16-18 syndrome
    t. 18 syndrome
    t. 20 syndrome
    t. 21 syndrome
    t. 22 syndrome
    translocation t.
tristate logic
tristearin
trisymptome
trit
    triturate
triterpene
triterpenoid saponin
tritiated
    t. thymidine (TTH)
tritici
    Pyemotes t.
tritium
triton tumor
Triton-X 100
Tritrichomonas
triturate (trit)
trivalent oral poliovirus vaccine (TOPV)
tRNA
    transfer RNA
    tRNA suppressor
Troglotrema salmincola
Troglotrematidae
Troisier
    T. ganglion
    T. node
    T. syndrome
Trojan Horse inhibitor
Trombicula
    T. akamushi
    T. alfreddugèsi
    T. autumnalis
    T. deliensis
    T. irritans
    T. pallida
    T. scutellaris
    T. tsalsahuatl
    T. vandersandi
trombiculiasis
trombiculid
    t. mite
Trombiculidae
Trombidiidae
Trombidoidea
tromethamine
tropeolins
trophedema
trophic
    t. gangrene
    t. lesion

t. nucleus
t. ulcer
trophoblast
syncytial t.
trophoblastic
t. disease
t. neoplasia
trophoblastoma
trophochromatin
trophochromidia
trophodermatoneurosis
trophoneurosis
facial t.
Romberg t.
trophoneurotic
t. leprosy
trophonucleus
trophoplasm
trophoplast
trophotaxis
trophozoite
trophy
tropical
t. abscess
t. anemia
t. bubo
t. diarrhea
t. disease
t. mask
t. measles
t. splenomegaly syndrome (TSS)
t. sprue (TS)
t. typhus
tropicalis
adenitis t.
Tropicorbis
tropism
viral t.
tropocollagen
tropoelastin
tropomyosin
troponin
Trousseau-Lallemand body
Trousseau syndrome
TRU
turbidity-reducing unit
T₃RU
triiodothyronine resin uptake
Truant auramine-rhodamine stain
true
t. aneurysm

t. diverticulum
t. hypertrophy
truncate
truncation
trunk duplication
truth table
Try
trypan
t. blue
t. red
trypanicidal
trypanicide
trypanid
trypanocidal
trypanocide
Trypanoplasma
Trypanosoma
T. ariarii
T. brucei
T. castellani
T. cruzi
T. gambiense
T. hominis
T. nigeriense
T. rangeli
T. rhodesiense
T. triatomae
T. ugandense
trypanosomatid
Trypanosomatidae
trypanosome
trypanosomiasis
African t.
American t.
Brazilian t.
Gambian t.
Rhodesian t.
trypanosomic
trypanosomicidal
trypanosomicide
trypanosomid
tryparsamide
Trypetidae
trypomastigote
trypsin
t. assay
t. G-banding stain
t. inhibitor
t. test
trypsin-aldehyde-fuchsin (TAF)
α₁-trypsin inhibitor
trypsin-inhibitory capacity (TIC)

NOTES

643

trypsinization
trypsinogen
tryptamine
tryptic
    t. activity
    t. soy agar
trypticase
    t. soy agar (TSA)
    t. soy broth (TSB)
    t. soy with agar broth
    t. soy yeast (TSY)
tryptone
tryptonemia
tryptophan (TP)
    t. load test
    t. malabsorption syndrome
tryptophanemia
tryptophanuria
tryptophyl
TS
    test solution
    tropical sprue
t-s
    temperature-sensitive
        t-s mutation
TSA
    trypticase soy agar
T$_4$SA
    thyroxine-specific activity
TSB
    trypticase soy broth
TSD
    Tay-Sachs disease
tsetse
    t. fly
TSF
    tissue-coding factor
TSH
    thyroid-stimulating hormone
        TSH stimulating test
        TSH stimulation test
TSH-binding inhibitory immunoglobulin (TBII)
TSH-displacing antibody (TDA)
TSH-releasing hormone
TSH-RF
    thyroid stimulating hormone-releasing factor
TSI
    thyroid-stimulating immunoglobulin
    triple sugar iron
        TSI agar
TSP
    total serum protein
TSPAP
    total serum prostatic acid phosphatase
TSR
    thyroid-to-serum ratio

TSS
    tropical splenomegaly syndrome
TST
    tumor skin test
TSTA
    tumor-specific transplantation antigen
T-strain mycoplasma
T-suppressor cell
tsutsugamushi
    t. disease
    t. fever
TSY
    trypticase soy yeast
TT
    thrombin time
    thymol turbidity
    total thyroxine
T$_4$:TBG Ratio
TTD
    tissue tolerance dose
TTH
    thyrotropic hormone
    tritiated thymidine
TTI
    time-tension index
TTP
    thrombotic thrombocytopenic purpura
TTP-HUS
    thrombotic thrombocytopenic purpura and hemolytic uremic syndrome
TTT
    tolbutamide tolerance test
TU
    Todd unit
    toxic unit
    toxin unit
    tuberculin unit
tubal
    t. abortion
    t. infantilism
    t. pregnancy
tube
    t. agglutination (TA)
    Babcock t.
    t. cast
    cathode ray t. (CRT)
    t. culture
    t. dilution test
    Eppendorf t.
    germ t.
    glow modulator t.
    indicator t.
    Isolator lysis-centrifugation t.
    NIXIE t.
    photomultiplier t.
    t. precipitin (TP)
    roll t.
    test t.

vacuum t.
voltage-regulator t.
Wintrobe hematocrit t.
tubeless gastric analysis test
tuberc
    tuberculosis
tubercle
    anatomical t.
    t. bacillus (TB)
    caseous t.
    dissection t.
    fibrous t.
    Ghon t.
    hard t.
    hyaline t.
    postmortem t.
    prosector's t.
    sebaceous t.
    soft t.
tubercula (*pl. of* tuberculum)
tubercular
tuberculate
tuberculated
tuberculation
tuberculid
    nodular t.
    papular t.
    papulonecrotic t.
    rosacea-like t.
tuberculin
    albumose-free t. (TAF)
    alkaline t. (TA)
    t. filtrate (TF)
    Koch old t.
    old t. (OT)
    original t. (TO)
    t. precipitation (TP)
    purified protein derivative of t.
    t. reaction
    t. R (new tuberculin) (TR)
    t. test
    t. unit (TU)
    vacuum t. (VT)
    t. zymoplastiche (TZ)
tuberculin-type
    t.-t. hypersensitivity
    t.-t. reaction
tuberculitis
tuberculization
tuberculochemotherapeutic
tuberculocidal
tuberculoderma

tuberculofibroid
tuberculoid
    t. granuloma
    t. leprosy
tuberculoma
tuberculo-opsonic index
tuberculoprotein
tuberculosis (TB, TBC, tuberc)
    acute miliary t.
    adult t.
    anthracotic t.
    arrested t.
    attenuated t.
    basal t.
    central nervous system t.
    cerebral t.
    childhood type t.
    cutaneous t.
    t. cutis
    t. cutis luposa
    t. cutis orificialis
    t. cutis verrucosa
    dermal t.
    disseminated t.
    endobronchial t.
    extrapulmonary t.
    gastrointestinal t.
    general t.
    t. granulation tissue
    healed t.
    inactive t.
    laryngeal t.
    t. lymphadenitis
    miliary t.
    open t.
    pericardial t.
    pleural t.
    postprimary t.
    primary t.
    pulmonary t.
    reinfection t.
    secondary t.
    t. skin test
    t. ulcerosa
    t. vaccine
tuberculosis-respiratory disease (TB-RD)
tuberculostat
tuberculostatic
tuberculostearic acid
tuberculous
    t. abscess
    t. bronchopneumonia

NOTES

tuberculous *(continued)*
    t. infiltration
    t. lymphadenitis
    t. meningitis (TBM)
    t. nephritis
    t. osteomyelitis
    t. pericarditis
    t. peritonitis
    t. rheumatism
    t. scrofuloderma
    t. spondylitis
    t. wart
tuberculum, pl. **tubercula**
    t. arthriticum
    tubercula dolorosa
    t. sebaceum
    t. syphiliticum
tuberiferous
tuberose
tuberosity
    ischial t.
    pubic t.
    tibial t.
tuberous
    t. sclerosis
Tubifera
tubocurarine
tuboendometrioid metaplasia
tubo-ovarian
    t.-o. abscess (TOA)
    t.-o. varicocele
tubo-ovaritis
tuboreticular structure
tubovillous adenoma
tubular
    t. adenoma
    t. aneurysm
    t. carcinoma
    t. cyst
    t. fluid (TF)
    t. interstitial nephritis
    t. nephrosis
    t. pit
tubule
    T t.
tubulin
    beta t.
β-tubulin
    neuron-associated class III β-t.
tubulocyst
tubulodermoid
tubulointerstitial
    t. nephritis
    t. nephropathy (TIN)
tubulonecrosis
tubuloneogenesis
tubulopapillary carcinoma
tubulorrhexis

tuffstone body
tufted phalanx
tuftsin
    t. deficiency
TUG
    total urinary gonadotropin
tularemia
    t. agglutinins
    enteric tularemia
    oculoglandular t.
    pneumonia t.
    typhoidal t.
    ulceroglandular t.
tularemic
    t. chancre
    t. conjunctivitis
tumefacient
tumefaction
tumefy
tumentia
tumescence
tumescent
tumeur d'emblée
tumid
tumor
    acinar cell t.
    acinic cell t.
    acute splenic t.
    adenoid t.
    adenomatoid odontogenic t.
    adipose t.
    adrenal t.
    adrenocortical rest t.
    adult granulosa cell t. (AGCT)
    ameloblastic adenomatoid t.
    amyloid t.
    t. aneuploidy
    t. angiogenesis
    t. angiogenic factor (TAF)
    angiomatoid t.
    t. antigen (T antigen)
    aortic body t.
    Askin t.
    astrocytic t.
    Bednar t.
    benign epithelial breast t.
    bladder t. (BT)
    blood t.
    bone t.
    borderline t.
    brain t. (BT)
    breast t.
    Brenner t.
    Brooke t.
    brown t.
    t. burden
    Burkitt t.
    Buschke-Löwenstein t.

calcifying epithelial odontogenic t. (CEOT)
t. of Capella
carcinoid t.
carotid body t.
t. cell
t. cell kinetics
cellular t.
central nervous system t.
cerebellopontine angle t.
chemoreceptor t.
chondromatous giant cell t.
chromaffin t.
clear cell "sugar" t.
Codman t.
collision t.
colon t.
composite t.
compound t.
connective t.
Dabska t.
dendritic cell t.
dermal duct t.
dermoid t.
desmoid t.
desmoplastic small round-cell t. (DSRCT)
ductus deferens t.
dysembryoplastic neuroepithelial t.
eccrine t.
ectomesenchymal chondromyxoid t. (ECT)
eighth nerve t.
t. embolism
t. embolus
embryonal t.
embryonic t.
endobronchial t.
endodermal sinus t.
endometrioid t.
Erdheim t.
esophageal t.
Ewing t.
extragonadal germ cell t.
extrarenal rhabdoid t. (ERRT)
eye t.
fallopian tube t.
fecal t.
Fechner t.
feminizing t.
fibroid t.
gastrointestinal autonomic nerve t.

gastrointestinal stromal t. (GIST)
gemistocytic t.
germ cell t. (GCT)
giant cell t.
giant cell t. of bone
giant cell t. of lung
giant cell t. of tendon sheath (GCTTS)
glomus jugulare t.
Godwin t.
gonadal stromal t.
t. grading
granular cell t.
granulosa cell t. (GCT)
granulosa-theca cell t.
Grawitz t.
Gubler t.
heart t.
heterologous t.
hilar cell t. of ovary
histoid t.
homologous t.
Hürthle cell t.
hylic t.
inflammatory myofibroblastic t. (IMT)
innocent t.
interdigitating dendritic cell t.
interstitial cell t. of testis
islet cell t.
juvenile granulosa cell t. (JGCT)
juxtaglomerular cell t. (JCT)
Koenen t.
Krukenberg t.
Landschutz t.
t. lethal dose (TLD)
Leydig cell t.
Leydig-Sertoli cell t.
Lindau t.
lipophyllodes t.
low malignant potential t.
lung t.
t. lysis syndrome
malignant breast t.
malignant mixed mesodermal t. (MMMT)
malignant mixed müllerian t.
t. marker
mast cell t.
melanotic neuroectodermal t.
melanotic neuroectodermal t. of infancy

T

NOTES

tumor *(continued)*
Merkel cell t.
mesonephroid t.
metastatic t.
mixed epithelial-mesenchymal t.
mixed mesodermal t.
mixed t. of salivary gland
mixed t. of skin
monoclonal t.
mucoepidermoid t.
müllerian t.
myofibroblastic mammary stromal t.
t. necrosis
necrosis t.
t. necrosis factor (TNF)
t. necrosis factor-beta
Nelson t.
neuroectodermal t.
no evidence of primary t. (TO)
oil t.
oncocytic hepatocellular t.
organoid t.
ovarian granulosa cell t.
ovarian serous borderline t.
  (OSBT)
Pancoast t.
pancreatic t.
papillary t.
paraffin t.
parathyroid t.
pearl t.
peripheral neuroectodermal t.
  (PNET)
phantom t.
phyllodes t.
pilar t. of scalp
Pindborg t.
pituitary t.
placental site trophoblastic t.
polyclonal t.
t. polysaccharide substance (TPS)
pontine angle t.
potato t. of neck
(primary) t., (regional lymph)
  nodes, (remote) metastases (TNM)
primitive neuroectodermal t.
  (PNET)
t. promoter
prostatic t.
pseudosarcomatous
  myofibroblastic t. (PMT)
ranine t.
Rathke pouch t.
Recklinghausen t.
t. registry
renal t.
rete cell t.
retinal anlage t.

Rous t.
salivary gland t.
salivary gland anlage t. (SGAT)
sand t.
Sertoli cell t.
Sertoli-Leydig cell t.
sex cord-stromal t.
t. in situ (TIS)
skin t.
t. skin test (TST)
small cell t.
small intestine t.
soft tissue t.
solitary fibrous t. (SFT)
spinal cord t.
splenic t.
t. stage
t. staging
stomach t.
sugar t.
superior pulmonary sulcus t.
t. suppressor gene
sweat gland t.
teratoid t.
testicular t.
theca cell t.
theca cell-granuloma cell t.
theca lutein t.
thrombus t.
t. thrombus
thymic t.
thyroid t.
transitional cell t.
triton t.
turban t.
ulcerogenic t.
urethral t.
uterine t.
vaginal t.
villous t.
t. virus
vulvar t.
Warthin t.
WHO histologic classification of
  ovarian t.'s
Wilms t.
Yaba t.
yolk sac t.
Zollinger-Ellison t.
tumoraffin
tumoral calcinosis
tumor-antigen 4 (TA-4)
tumor-associated
  t.-a. antigen
  t.-a. glycoprotein (TAG)
  t.-a. rejection antigen (TARA)
tumor-associated rejection antigen
  (TARA)

tumorigenesis
    foreign body t.
tumorigenic
tumor-infiltrating lymphocyte (TIL, TILS)
tumorlet
tumorous
tumor-specific
    t.-s. antigen
    t.-s. transplantation antigen (TSTA)
TUNEL
    in situ DNA nick end labeling
Tunga penetrans
tungiasis
Tungidae
tungsten
    t. arc lamp
    t. halogen lamp
tungstic acid
tunica albuginea
TUR
    transurethral resection
turban tumor
Turbatrix
    T. aceti
turbid
turbidimeter
turbidimetric
    t. immunoassay
turbidimetry
turbidity
    thymol t. (TT)
turbidity-reducing unit (TRU)
turbinal varix
Türck degeneration
Turcot syndrome
turgescence
turgescent
turgid
Türk
    T. cell
    T. irritation leukocyte
turkey
    t. meningoencephalitis virus
    t. red
Turlock virus
turn-around time (TAT)
Turnbull
    T. blue
    T. blue stain
Turner syndrome
turnkey system

turnover
    t. number
    plasma iron t. (PIT)
TURP
    transurethral prostatectomy
turpentine oil
turricephaly
T$_3$U test
TWAR-stain
twin
    conjoined t.'s
    corporea lutea t.
    t. crystal
    dichorionic placenta t.'s
    dizygotic t.'s
    fraternal t.'s
    heterokaryotic t.'s
    identical t.'s
    incomplete conjoined t.'s
    monoamniotic placenta t.'s
    monochorionic diamniotic
        placenta t.
    monozygotic t.'s
    parasitic t.
    placenta t.
    t. placenta
    Siamese t.'s
TWL
    transepidermal water loss
two-dimensional
    t.-d. chromatography
    t.-d. immunoelectrophoresis
two-emulsion autoradiography
two-glass test
Twort-d'Herelle phenomenon
Twort phenomenon
two's complement
two-sided alternative
two-slide method
two-stage PT test
two-tail test
Ty
    typhoid
tylosis, pl. tyloses
    t. palmaris et plantaris
tympanic cell
tympanosclerosis
Tymphonotonus
tyndallization
type
    blood t.
    t. culture

T

NOTES

type *(continued)*
    t. 1, 2, 3, 4 dextrocardia
    hypertyrosinemia, Oregon t.
    t. I, II cells
    t. I, II error
    t. III hypersensitivity reaction
    intratubular germ cell neoplasia of
      the unclassified t. (IGGNU)
    t. IS mucopolysaccharidosis
    t. IVA, B mucopolysaccharidosis
    t. I–VIII mucopolysaccharidosis
    t. species
    t. strain
    wild t.
typhinia
typhlectasis
typhlenteritis
typhlitis
typhloenteritis
typhlomegaly
typhoid (Ty)
    typhoid bacillus
    typhoid bacteriophage
    typhoid cholera
    typhoid fever
    typhoid immunization reaction
    typhoid, paratyphoid A and
      paratyphoid B (TAB)
    provocation typhoid
    typhoid septicemia
typhoidal tularemia
typhoid-paratyphoid A and B vaccine
typhoid-paratyphoid (vaccine) (TPT)
typholysin
typhosepsis
typhous
typhus
    amarillic t.
    t. antibody test
    endemic murine t.
    t. epidemic
    epidemic louse-borne t.
    louse-borne t.
    mite t.
    murine t.
    recrudescent t.

    scrub t.
    tropical t.
    t. vaccine
typing
    ABO t.
    ABO-Rh t.
    bacteriophage t.
    blood t.
    HLA t.
    primed lymphocyte t.
    Rh t.
    $Rh_o(D)$ t.
    tissue t.
tyramine test
Tyroglyphidae
Tyroglyphus
    T. longior
    T. siro
tyroid
tyroketonuria
tyroma
tyropanoate sodium
Tyrophagus putrescentiae
tyrosine
    t. assay
    t. crystal
    t. phosphorylation
    t. test
tyrosinemia
tyrosinosis
tyrosinuria
tyrosis
tyrosyl
tyrosyl-RNA synthetase
tyrosyluria
tyrothricin
Tyzzer disease
Tyzzeria
TZ
    tuberculin zymoplastiche
Tzanck
    T. cell
    T. smear
    T. test
T-zone dysplasia

U
    unit
        U fibers
U6 riboprobe
UA
    unaggregated
    urinalysis
    uterine aspiration
UBBC
    unsaturated vitamin B_{12}-binding capacity
UBF
    uterine blood flow
UBG
    urobilinogen
UBI
    ultraviolet blood irradiation
ubiquinol
ubiquinone
ubisemiquinone
UC
    ulcerative colitis
    ultracentrifugal
    urea clearance
U-cell lymphoma
UCG
    urinary chorionic gonadotropin
UCHL1 antibody
UCHL1ᵃ antibody
UCL3D3 antibody
UCP
    urinary coproporphyrin
UD
    urethral discharge
UDP
    uridine diphosphate
N-acetyl->UDP-*N*-acetyl-D-galactosamine
N-acetyl->UDP-*N*-acetyl-D-glucosamine
UDP-bilirubin glucuronosyltransferase
UDP-galactose
UDP-glucose
UDP-glucose-hexose-1-phosphate
        UDP-g.-h.-p. uridylyltransferase
        UDP-g.-h.-p. uridylyl-transferase
        assay
UDP-glucuronate
UDP-glucuronate:bilirubin-
    glucuronosyltransferase
UDP-glucuronic acid
UDP-glucuronyl transferase
UDP-L-iduronate
UDP-iduronic acid
UDP-xylose
UEA-1
    Ulex europaeus agglutinin I
Uehlinger syndrome

UFA
    unesterified fatty acid
Uffelmann test
Uganda S virus
Uhl anomaly
UIBC
    unsaturated iron-binding capacity
UIF
    undegraded insulin factor
UIP
    usual interstitial pneumonitis
UL
    undifferentiated lymphoma
ulcer
        acute hemorrhagic u.
        amebic u.
        amputating u.
        aphthous u.
        Barrett u.
        Buruli u.
        chancroidal u.
        chronic u.
        cockscomb u.
        cold u.
        constitutional u.
        corneal u.
        creeping u.
        Curling u.
        Cushing u.
        decubitus u.
        diabetic u.
        diphtheritic u.
        distention u.
        duodenal u.
        elusive u.
        Fenwick-Hunner u.
        focal u.
        gastric u. (GU)
        groin u.
        gummatous u.
        hard u.
        healed u.
        hemorrhagic u.
        herpetic u.
        Hunner u.
        indolent u.
        inflamed u.
        Lipschütz u.
        lupoid u.
        marginal u.
        Marjolin u.
        Meleney u.
        penetrating u.
        peptic u. (PU)
        perambulating u.

U

ulcer *(continued)*
 perforated gastric u.
 perforating u.
 phagedenic u.
 phlegmonous u.
 rodent u.
 serpiginous u.
 simple u.
 sloughing u.
 soft u.
 stasis u.
 stercoraceous u.
 stercoral u.
 stomal u.
 stress u.
 Sutton u.
 symptomatic u.
 syphilitic u.
 trophic u.
 varicose u.
 venereal u.
 warty u.
 Zambesi u.
ulcera (*pl. of* ulcus)
ulcerate
ulcerated
ulceration
 aphthous u.
ulcerative
 u. colitis (UC)
 u. cystitis
 u. dermatosis
 u. inflammation
 u. scrofuloderma
ulcerogenic
 u. tumor
ulceroglandular
 u. tularemia
ulceromembranous
ulcerosa
 blepharitis u.
ulcerous
ULCL4D12 antibody
ulcus, pl. **ulcera**
 u. ambulans
 u. terebrans
 u. venereum
 u. vulvae acutum
ulegyria
ulerythema
 u. ophryogenes
Ulex
 U. europaeus
 U. europaeus agglutinin I (UEA-1)
Ullmann line
Ullrich-Feichtiger syndrome
Ullrich-Turner syndrome

ULN
 upper limits of normal
ulodermatitis
uloid
ultimate principle
ultimobranchial body
ultimum moriens
ultracentrifugal (UC)
ultracentrifugation
ultracentrifuge
 analytic u.
ultracytostome
ultrafilter
ultrafiltrate
ultrafiltration hemodialyzer
ultrahigh vacuum
ultramicroanalysis
ultramicrotome
ultrasonication
ultrasonic nebulizer (USN)
ultrastructure
ultrathin section
ultraviolet
 u. blood irradiation (UBI)
 u. burn
 u. fluorescent dosimeter
 u. light
 u. light-induced mutation
 u. microscope
 u. radiation
ultraviolet/visible spectrophotometry
ultravirus
ultropaque method
Ulysses syndrome
umbilical
 u. cyst
 u. fistula
 u. hernia
 u. polyp
umbrella cell
Umbre virus
UN
 urea nitrogen
unaggregated (UA)
unattended laboratory operation
unbiased estimate
unbound thyroxine-binding globulin (UTBG)
uncertainty principle
Uncinaria
 U. americana
 U. duodenalis
uncinariasis
uncinate epilepsy
unclassified
 arbovirus group u.

uncompensated
    u. acidosis
    u. alkalosis
uncomplemented
unconditional jump
unconjugated
    u. bilirubin
    u. estriol
uncouplers
    oxidative phosphorylation u.
undecaprenol
    u. phosphate
undegraded insulin factor (UIF)
underflow
understain
Underwood disease
undescended testis
undetermined nitrogen
undifferentiated
    u. adenocarcinoma
    u. cell adenoma
    u. epidermoid carcinoma
    u. lymphoma (UL)
    u. sarcoma
    u. squamous cell carcinoma
    u. type fever
undifferentiation
Undritz anomaly
undulant fever
undulating membrane
undulipodium
unesterified fatty acid (UFA)
unguium
    achromia u.
unheated serum reagin (USR)
Uniblue A
unicameral bone cyst
unicellular
    u. sclerosis
unicentral
unicentric blastoma
unidirectional
uniflagellate
unifocal eosinophilic granuloma
unijunction transistor
unilocular
    u. echinococcosis
    u. hydatid
    u. hydatid cyst
unimodal
union
    faulty u.

    primary u.
    secondary u.
    vicious u.
un-ionized hemoglobin (HHb)
uniovular
unipolar
uniport
unit (U)
    α u.
    absolute u.
    alexin u.
    Allen-Doisy u.
    alpha u.'s
    amboceptor u.
    androgen u.
    Ångstrom u. (A)
    antigen u.
    antitoxin u. (AU)
    antivenene u.
    atomic mass u. (amu)
    atomic weight u. (awu)
    base u.'s
    Behnken u. (R)
    Bessey-Lowry u. (BLU)
    Bethesda u.
    biological standard u.
    bird u.
    BLB u.
    Bodansky u. (BU)
    Bowers-McComb u.
    British thermal u. (BTU)
    cat u.
    u. cell
    centimeter-gram-second u.
    central processing u.
    CGS u.
    chlorophyll u.
    chorionic gonadotropin u.
    Clauberg u.
    colony-forming u.
    complement u.
    Corner-Allen u.
    corpus luteum hormone u.
    Dam u.
    dial u.
    digitalis u.
    diphtheria antitoxin u.
    dog u.
    Ehrlich u. (EU)
    electromagnetic u. (emu)
    electrostatic u. (ESU)
    enzyme u. (EU)

U

NOTES

unit (*continued*)
    equine gonadotropin u.
    estradiol benzoate u.
    estrone u.
    Fishman-Lerner u.
    Florey u.
    G u. of streptomycin
    Gutman u.
    heat u. (HU)
    hemagglutinating u. (HU)
    hemolysin u.
    hemolytic u.
    heparin u.
    Holzknecht u. (H)
    Hounsfield u. (H)
    Howell u.
    immunizing u. (IU)
    u. inheritance
    insulin u.
    u. of intermedin
    international u. (IU)
    international benzoate u. (IBU)
    International System of u.'s (SI)
    Jenner-Kay u.
    kallikrein-inhibiting u. (KIU)
    Karmen u. (KU)
    King u.
    King-Armstrong u. (KAU)
    L u. of streptomycin
    u. of luteinizing activity
    Mache u. (MU)
    map u.
    u. of mass
    u. membrane
    meter-kilogram-second u.
    MKS u.
    Montevideo u. (MU)
    mouse u. (m.u., mu, μ)
    mouse uterine u. (MUU)
    Oxford u.
    u. of oxytocin
    pantothenic acid u.
    u. of penicillin
    peripheral resistance u. (PRU)
    phosphatase u.
    physiologic u.
    plaque-forming u. (PFU)
    u. of progestational activity
    progesterone u.
    prolactin u.
    protein nitrogen u. (PNU)
    radiation measuring u.
    rat u. (RU)
    resistance u. (RU)
    riboflavin u.
    Russell u.
    Sherman u.
    Sherman-Bourquin u. of vitamin B$_2$

    Sherman-Munsell u.
    SI u.
    Sibley-Lehninger u.
    SJR u.
    skin test u. (STU)
    SL u.
    Somogyi u.
    S u. of streptomycin
    Steenbock u.
    streptomycin u.
    Svedberg u. (S)
    Svedberg flotation u. (Sf)
    tetanus antitoxin u.
    thiamin chloride u.
    thiamin hydrochloride u.
    u. of thyrotrophic activity
    Todd u. (TU)
    toxic u. (TU)
    toxin u. (TU)
    transcription u.
    tuberculin u. (TU)
    turbidity-reducing u. (TRU)
    u. of vasopressin
    vitamin A u.
    vitamin B$_1$ hydrochloride u.
    vitamin B$_2$ u.
    vitamin B$_6$ u.
    vitamin C u.
    vitamin D u.
    vitamin E u.
    vitamin K u.
    u. of wavelength
    u. of weight
    Wohlgemuth u.
unitarian hypothesis
unit-erythroid
    colony-forming u. (CFU-E)
unit membrane
    asymmetric u. m.
univalent antibody
univariate analysis
universal donor
universalis
    alopecia u.
univitelline
unknown etiology
Unna
    U. disease
    U. mark
    U. stain
Unna-Pappenheim stain
Unna-Taenzer stain
unorganized virus
unpack
unresolved
    u. hepatitis
    u. lobar pneumonia

unresponsiveness
    immunologic u.
unsaturated
    u. hydrocarbon
    u. iron-binding capacity (UIBC)
    u. vitamin B_{12}-binding capacity
    (UBBC)
unstable
    u. hemoglobin
    u. hemoglobin disease
    u. hemoglobin hemolytic anemia
ununited fracture
unusual isolates/fastidious organisms
Unverricht disease
unwinding protein
UP
    uroporphyrin
U/P
    urine-plasma ratio
update
UPG
    uroporphyrinogen
UPI
    uteroplacental insufficiency
upper
    u. limits of normal (ULN)
    u. respiratory disease (URD)
    u. respiratory infection (URI)
    u. respiratory tract infection
    (URTI)
up-regulation
upsilon, Ψ
upstream
uptake
    absolute iodine u. (AIU)
    oxygen u.
    radioactive iodine u. (RAIU, RIU)
    triiodothyronine resin u. (T_3RU)
uptime
urachal
    u. cyst
    u. fistula
uracil
uracrasia
uranin
uranium nephritis
uranyl acetate stain
uraroma
urarthritis
urate
    u. calculus
    u. crystal

    u. crystals stain
    De Galantha method for u.'s
    monosodium u. (MSU)
uratemia
uratohistechia
uratoma
uratosis
uraturia
Urbach-Oppenheim disease
Urbach-Wiethe disease
urban plague
URD
    upper respiratory disease
urea
    u. agar
    u. clearance (C/u/, UC)
    u. clearance test
    u. cycle
    u. nitrogen (UN)
    u. nitrogen assay
    u. nitrogen or plasma
    u. nitrogen test
    u. synthesis
Ureaplasma
    U. urealyticum
    U. urealyticum genital culture
ureapoiesis
urease
    Helicobacter pylori u.
    u. test
    u. test broth
urecchysis
uredema
urelcosis
uremia
    hypercalcemic u.
uremic
    u. cachexia
    u. colitis
    u. coma
    u. eclampsia
    u. encephalopathy
    u. inflammation
    u. lung
    u. pericarditis
    u. pneumonia
    u. pneumonitis
uremigenic
ureotelic
ureter
    bifid u.

U

NOTES

ureteral
    u. hyperperistalsis
    u. ileus
    u. peristalsis disorder
ureterectasia
ureteritis
    u. cystica
    u. glandularis
ureterocele
ureterocutaneous fistula
ureterohydronephrosis
ureterolith
ureterolithiasis
ureterolysis
ureteropelvic obstruction
ureteropyelitis
ureteropyelonephritis
ureteropyosis
ureterostenosis
ureterostoma
ureterovaginal fistula
ureterovesical obstruction
urethan
urethral
    u. caruncle
    u. discharge (UD)
    u. diverticulum
    u. hematuria
    u. obstruction
    u. stricture
    u. tumor
urethratresia
urethrism
urethritis
    follicular u.
    granular u.
    nongonococcal u. (NGU)
    nonspecific u. (NSU)
    u. petrificans
    posterior u.
    simple u.
urethrocele
urethrocystitis
urethrophyma
urethrostenosis
urethrovaginal fistula
URF
    uterine relaxing factor
urhidrosis
URI
    upper respiratory infection
uric .
    u. acid
    u. acid assay
    u. acid calculus
    u. acid crystal
    u. acid infarct
uricacidemia

uricemia
uricolytic index
uricosuria
uricosuric
Uricult dipslide test
uridine
    u. diphosphate (UDP)
    u. monophosphate
    u. triphosphate (UTP)
uridine-5′-phosphate
uridrosis
uridylic acid
uridyltransferase
    hexose-1-phosphate u.
uridylyl
uridylyltransferase
    UDP-glucose-hexose-1-phosphate u.
urinal
urinalysis (UA)
urinary
    u. amylase
    u. calculus
    u. cast
    u. chorionic gonadotropin (UCG)
    u. concentration test
    u. coproporphyrin (UCP)
    u. cyst
    u. estriol
    u. fistula
    u. free cortisol
    u. nitrogen
    u. obstruction
    u. sand
    u. sediment
    u. smear
    u. tract disease
    u. tract infection (UTI)
urine
    u. acetone test
    ammoniacal u.
    black u.
    chylous u.
    cloudy u.
    crude u.
    u. cytology
    diabetic u.
    febrile u.
    feverish u.
    u. fungus culture
    gouty u.
    honey u.
    maple syrup u.
    milky u.
    u. mycobacteria culture
    nebulous u.
    u. osmolality
    pregnancy u. (PU)
    reducing substances in u.

residual u.
u. sediment crystal
u. specimen collection
u. urea nitrogen (UUN)
u. urobilinogen (UU)
urinemia
urine-plasma ratio (U/P)
urinoma
urinometer
urinometry
urinophilous
urinoscopy
urinous
Uriscreen
U. test
U. urine specimen bacteriuria
detection system
uroammoniac
urobenzoic acid
urobilin assay
urobilinemia
urobilinogen (UBG)
u. assay
fecal u. (FU)
u. test
urine u. (UU)
urobilinogenuria
urobilinuria
urocanic acid
urocele
urocheras
urochrome
urocortisol
urocrisia
urocyanin
urocyanogen
urocyanosis
urocystitis
uroedema
uroerythrin
urofuscohematin
urogenital
u. disorder
u. fistula
u. syndrome
uroglaucin
urogram
excretory u. (XU)
urogravimeter
urohemolytic coefficient
urokinase
urolith

urolithiasis
urolithic
urometer
uromucoid assay
uroncus
Uronema caudatum
uronephrosis
uronic acid
uronophile
uronoscopy
uropepsin
uropepsinogen assay
urophanic
urophein
uroporphyria
uroporphyrin (UP)
u. assay
u. test
uroporphyrinogen (UPG)
u. decarboxylase
u. III cosynthase
u. 1 synthase
uroporphyrinogen-I-synthase
uroporphyrinuria
uropsammus
uroreaction
urorosein
urorubin
urorubrohematin
uroschesis
uroscopic
uroscopy
urosemiology
urosepsin
uroseptic
urothelium
urotoxic coefficient
uroureter
uroxanthin
ursodeoxycholic acid
URTI
upper respiratory tract infection
urticaria
aquagenic u.
cholinergic u.
cold u.
congelation u.
factitious u.
giant u.
u. gigans
u. gigantea
u. perstans

U

NOTES

urticaria *(continued)*
>   u. pigmentosa
>   pressure u.
>   solar u.
>   u. tuberosa

urticate

urticating caterpillar

Uruma virus

useful life

Usher syndrome

USN
>   ultrasonic nebulizer

USR
>   unheated serum reagin
>   USR test

ustilaginism

Ustilago
>   *U. maydis*
>   *U. zeae*

usual interstitial pneumonitis (UIP)

uta

UTBG
>   unbound thyroxine-binding globulin

uterine
>   u. aspiration (UA)
>   u. blood flow (UBF)
>   u. calculus
>   u. colic
>   u. leiomyoma
>   u. relaxing factor (URF)
>   u. tumor

uteritis

in utero

utero
>   dead fetus in u. (DFU)

uterolith

utero-ovarian varicocele

uteroperitoneal fistula

uteroplacental insufficiency (UPI)

uterus
>   bifid u.
>   male rudimentary u.

UTI
>   urinary tract infection

utilization
>   ketone body u.
>   net protein u. (NPU)

UTP
>   uridine triphosphate

utricular cyst

utriculitis

utrophin marker

UU
>   urine urobilinogen

UUN
>   urine urea nitrogen

uveitis
>   lens-induced u.
>   phacoanaphylactic u.

uveo-encephalitic syndrome

uveomeningitis

uveoparotid fever

uviofast

uvioresistant

uviosensitive

uvulitis

V
>V antigen
>factor V
>V factor

V$_{CO_2}$
>carbon dioxide output

V-2 carcinoma

VA
>vacuum aspiration
>volt-ampere

vaccenic acid

vaccina

vaccinal

vaccinate

vaccination
>roseola v.

vaccinator

vaccine
>adjuvant v.
>aqueous v.
>attenuated v.
>autogenous v.
>Bacillus Calmette-Guérin v.
>BCG v.
>brucella strain 19 v.
>Calmette-Guérin v.
>cholera v.
>Cox v.
>crystal violet v.
>diphtheria toxoid, tetanus toxoid, and pertussis v.
>duck embryo v. (DEV)
>duck embryo origin v.
>Flury strain v.
>foot-and-mouth disease virus v.
>*Haemophilus pertussis* v. (HPV)
>Haffkine v.
>hepatitis B v.
>heterogenous v.
>high-egg-passage v.
>hog cholera v.
>human diploid cell rabies v. (HDCV)
>inactivated poliovirus v.
>influenza virus v.
>killed v. (KV)
>killed measles virus v. (KMV)
>live oral poliovirus v.
>low-egg-passage v.
>v. lymph
>measles, mumps, and rubella v. (MMR)
>measles virus v.
>multivalent v.
>mumps virus v.
>oil v.
>oral poliovirus v. (OPV)
>Pasteur v.
>pertussis v.
>plague v.
>pneumococcal v.
>poliomyelitis v.
>poliovirus v.
>polyvalent v.
>rabies v.
>rabies v., Flury strain egg-passage
>RhoGAM v.
>rickettsia v., attenuated
>Rocky Mountain spotted fever v.
>rubella virus v., live
>Sabin v.
>Salk v.
>Semple v.
>smallpox v.
>split-virus v.
>staphylococcus v.
>stock v.
>subunit v.
>TAB v.
>tetanus v.
>trivalent oral poliovirus v. (TOPV)
>tuberculosis v.
>typhoid-paratyphoid A and B v.
>typhus v.
>v. virus
>whooping cough v.
>yellow fever v.

vaccinia
>v. gangrenosa
>generalized v.
>progressive v.
>v. vaccinia
>v. virus

vaccinia-immune globulin (VIG)

vaccinial

vacciniform

vaccinist

vaccinization

vaccinogen

vaccinogenous

vaccinoid
>v. reaction

vaccinostyle

vaccinum

vacuo
>in v.

vacuolar
>v. degeneration
>v. nephrosis

vacuolated

vacuolating
    v. agent
    v. virus
vacuolation
vacuole
    v. alteration phagocytosis
    autophagic v.
    condensing v.
    contractile v.
    cytoplasmic v.
    digestion v.
    heterophagic v.
    plasmocrine v.
    rhagiocrine v.
vacuolization
    cytoplasmic v.
    nuclear v.
vacuome
vacuum
    v. aspiration (VA)
    v. breaker
    v. distillation
    v. flask
    v. gauge
    high v.
    permeability of v.
    permittivity of v.
    v. tube
    v. tuberculin (VT)
    v. tube voltmeter (VTVM)
    ultrahigh v.
vagabond
    v. disease
    v. melanosis
vagina
    congenital absence of v. (CAV)
    v., ectocervix, and endocervix
      (VCE)
vaginal
    v. adenosine
    v. adenosis
    v. atresia
    v. irrigation smear (VIS)
    v. pool
    v. synovitis
    v. tumor
vaginalitis
vaginismus
vaginitis, pl. **vaginitides**
    v. adhesiva
    adhesive v.
    v. cystica
    desquamative inflammatory v.
    v. emphysematosa
    emphysematous v.
    granular v.
    v. senilis
vaginomycosis

Vaginulus plebeius
Vagitest
Vahlkampfia
VAHS
    virus-associated hemophagocytic
      syndrome
Val
    valine
valence
    v. electron
    v. tautomer
Valentine test
valeric acid
valgus deformity
valine (Val)
    v. aminotransferase
    v. transaminase
valinemia
valinuria
valley fever
valproic acid
Valsalva maneuver
value
    absolute v.
    acetyl v.
    acid v.
    buffer v.
    buffer v. of the blood
    cot v.
    crot v.
    D v.
    GC v.
    globular v.
    iodine v.
    normal v.
    P v.
    predictive v.
    reference v.
    rot v.
    threshold limit v. (TLV)
valve
    cleft leaflet, mitral v.
    cleft leaflet, tricuspid v.
    congenital v.
    mitral v.
valvular
    v. atresia
    v. disease of heart (VDH)
    v. endocarditis
    v. incompetence
    v. stenosis
    v. thrombus
    v. tissue embolus
valvulitis
    rheumatic v.
valvulotomy
valyl
valyl-RNA synthetase

van
- v. Bogaert disease
- v. Buchem syndrome
- v. Buren disease
- v. Deen test
- v. den Bergh test
- v. der Hoeve syndrome
- v. der Velden test
- v. der Waals equation
- v. der Waals forces
- V. der Woude syndrome
- v. Diest criteria
- v. Ermengen stain
- v. Gieson stain
- V. Slyke apparatus
- V. Slyke and Cullen method
- V. Slyke formula
- V. Slyke test

vanadium
vancomycin
vanillic acid
vanillism
vanillylmandelic
- v. acid (VMA)
- v. acid test

vapor
- combustible v.
- v. pressure
- v. pressure depression osmometer

vaporization
vaporize
vapor-phase chromatography (VPC)
Vaquez disease
Vaquez-Osler disease
var
- variant

variable
- v. autotransformer
- v. capacitor
- dependent v.
- dichotomous v.
- double-precision v.
- dummy v.
- endogenous v.
- exogenous v.
- fixed-point v.
- floating-point v.
- independent v.
- label v.
- v. number tandem repeats (VNTRs)
- ordinal v.
- pointer v.

- random v.
- v. region
- v. resistor
- subscripted v.

variance
- analysis of v. (ANOVA)
- multivariate analysis of v. (MANOVA)
- phenotypic v.

variant (var)
- floral v.
- v. hemoglobin
- inherited albumin v.
- L-phase v.
- tall-cell v.

variate
- binary v.

variation
- coefficient of v. (CV)
- contingent negative v.
- meristic v.
- microbial v.
- negative v. (NV)
- rough-smooth v.
- R-S v.
- smooth-rough v.
- S-R v.

varication
variceal
varicella
- v. encephalitis
- v. virus

varicellation
varicella-zoster (VZ)
- v. antibody test
- v. virus (VSV, VZV)
- v. virus culture
- v. virus serology

varicelliform
- v. eruption

varicelloid
varices (*pl. of* varix)
variciform
varicocele
- ovarian v.
- symptomatic v.
- tubo-ovarian v.
- utero-ovarian v.

varicoid
varicole
varicophlebitis

V

NOTES

varicose
- v. aneurysm
- v. ulcer
- v. vein

varicosis, pl. varicoses
varicosity
varicule
variegate porphyria
variety
variola
- v. benigna
- v. hemorrhagica
- v. major
- v. maligna
- v. miliaris
- v. minor
- v. pemphigosa
- v. sine eruptione
- v. vaccine
- v. vera
- v. verrucosa
- v. virus

variolar
variolate
variolation
variolic
varioliform
variolization
varioloid
variolous
variolovaccine
varix, pl. varices
- v. anastomoticus
- aneurysmal v.
- cirsoid v.
- esophageal varices
- lymph v.
- turbinal v.

varus deformity
vascular
- v. anomaly
- v. birthmark
- v. hemophilia
- v. keratitis
- v. leiomyoma
- v. myxoma
- v. nevus
- v. polyp
- v. resistance (VR)
- v. ring
- v. sclerosis
- v. spider
- v. styptic

vasculare
- poikiloderma atrophicans v.

vascularization
- corneal v.

vascularized

vasculature
vasculitis
- cutaneous v.
- hypersensitivity v.
- leukocytoclastic v.
- livedo v.
- necrotizing v.
- nodular v.
- segmented hyalinizing v.

vasculocardiac syndrome of hyperserotonemia
vasculomyelinopathy
vasculotoxic
vasitis
- v. nodosa

vasoactive
- v. intestinal peptide (VIP)
- v. intestinal polypeptide (VIP)

vasoconstriction
vasodepressor material (VDM)
vasodilatation
vasoexcitor material (VEM)
vasoformative
vasogenic shock
vasomotor
- v. hypotonia
- v. paralysis
- v. rhinitis (VMR)

vasoparalysis
vasoparesis
vasopressin (VP)
- arginine v. (AVP)

vasorum
- *Haemostrongylus* v.

vasospasm
vasospastic
VATER
- vertebral defects, anal atresia, tracheoesophageal fistula with esophageal atresia, and radial and renal anomalies
- VATER complex

VBS:FBS
- veronal-buffered saline:fetal bovine serum

VCA
- viral capsid antigen

VCE
- vagina, ectocervix, and endocervix
- VCE smear

VD
- venereal disease

VDBR
- volume of distribution of bilirubin

VDEL
- Venereal Disease Experimental Laboratory

VDG
venereal disease-gonorrhea
VDH
valvular disease of heart
VDM
vasodepressor material
VDRL
Venereal Disease Research Laboratory
VDRL test
VDS
venereal disease-syphilis
Vectabond reagent
Vecta-Stain
V.-S. Elite ABC system
V.-S. immunohistochemical reagent
V.-S. Universal Elite ABC kit
V.-S. Universal Quick kit
vection
vector
biological v.
cloning v.
electric field v.
expression v.
mechanical v.
v. product
recombinant v.
vectorial
VEE
Venezuelan equine encephalomyelitis
V. virus
vegetans
pyoderma v.
vegetation
bacterial v.
verrucous v.
vegetative
v. bacteriophage
v. endocarditis
v. multiplication
vehicle
veil
aqueduct v.
veiled cell
Veillonaceae
Veillonella
V. *alcalescens*
V. *discoides*
V. *orbiculus*
V. *parvula*
V. *reniformis*
V. *vulvovaginitidis*

vein
key v.
v. stone
varicose v.
veined
Vejovis
velamen, pl. **velamina**
v. vulvae
velamentous
Vel antigen
vellicate
vellication
velocity
v. coefficient
wave v.
velocity-diffusion
sedimentation v.
v. sedimentation
velogenic
velopharyngeal insufficiency
VEM
vasoexcitor material
Vena
Ven antigen
veneniferous
venenous
venereal
v. disease (VD)
V. Disease Experimental Laboratory (VDEL)
v. disease-gonorrhea (VDG)
V. Disease Research Laboratory (VDRL)
v. disease-syphilis (VDS)
v. lymphogranuloma
v. sore
v. ulcer
v. wart
venereology
venereum
lymphogranuloma v. (LGV)
lymphopathia v.
Venezuelan
V. equine A encephalomyelitis virus
V. equine encephalitis
V. equine encephalomyelitis (VEE)
V. equine encephalomyelitis virus (VEE virus)
venin
Venn diagram
venofibrosis

V

NOTES

venom
    antisnake v. (ASV)
    cobra v.
    kokoi v.
    Malayan pit viper v.
    Protac v.
    Russell viper v.
    snake v. (SV)
    viper v. (VV)
veno-occlusive disease of the liver
venosclerosis
venostasis
    visual evoked potential
venous
    v. blood
    v. claudication
    v. congestion
    v. embolism
    v. gangrene
    v. hematocrit (VH)
    v. insufficiency
    mixed v. (MV)
    v. pressure
    v. star
    v. thrombosis
ventilation
    local exhaust v.
ventricle
ventricose
ventricosus
    Haemodipsus v.
    Pediculoides v.
ventricular
    v. aneurysm
    v. bigeminy
    v. diverticulum
    v. hypertrophy
    v. septal defect (VSD)
ventriculoradial dysplasia
ventriculus
ventroptosia
ventroptosis
VEPA
    vincristine, cyclophosphamide,
      prednisone, doxorubicin (Adriamycin)
      VEPA and bleomycin (VEPA-B)
VEPA-B
    VEPA and bleomycin
vera
    myeloid metaplasia with
      polycythemia v. (PCV-M)
verapamil
verbascose
verdoglobin
verdohemochrome
verdohemoglobin
verdoperoxidase

vergeture
Verhoeff elastic tissue stain
Vermes
vermicidal
vermicide
vermicular
vermicule
vermiculose
vermiculus
vermiform
vermifugal
vermifuge
vermilion
vermin
verminal
vermination
verminous
    v. abscess
    v. colic
vermis
vernal
    v. conjunctivitis
    v. encephalitis
Verner-Morrison syndrome
Vernet syndrome
Verneuil
    V. disease
    V. neuroma
vernier dial
Verocay body
veronal buffer
**veronal-buffered saline:fetal bovine
    serum (VBS:FBS)**
verruca, pl. **verrucae**
    v. acuminata
    v. digitata
    v. filiformis
    v. glabra
    v. mollusciformis
    v. necrogenica
    v. peruana
    v. plana
    v. plana juvenilis
    v. plana senilis
    v. plantaris
    seborrheic v.
    v. seborrheica
    v. senilis
    v. simplex
    v. virus
    v. vulgaris
verrucal
    v. atypical endocarditis
    v. nonbacterial endocarditis
verruciform
verruciformis
    acrokeratosis v.

verrucopapillary
  v. alteration
  v. external genital lesion
verrucose
verrucosis
  lymphostatic v.
verrucous
  v. carcinoma
  v. carditis
  v. endocarditis
  v. hyperplasia
  v. nevus
  v. papilloma
  v. scrofuloderma
  v. vegetation
  v. xanthoma
verruga
Verse disease
versicolor
vertebral
  v. arthritis
  v. basilar artery syndrome
  v. crush-fracture syndrome
  v. polyarthritis
  v. defects, anal atresia,
    tracheoesophageal fistula with
    esophageal atresia, and radial and
    renal anomalies (VATER)
vertical
  v. growth phase
  v. transmission
Verticillium
  V. graphii
verumontanitis
very
  v. high density lipoprotein (VHDL)
  v. high frequency
  v. large scale integration (VLSI)
  v. late activation (VLA)
  v. low density lipoprotein (VLDL,
    VLDLP)
vesica, pl. **vesicae**
  malacoplakia vesicae
vesical
  v. blood fluke
  v. calculus
  v. diverticulum
  v. dysplasia
  v. fistula
  v. hematuria
vesicle
  acrosomal v.

  germinal v.
  micropinocytotic v.
  phospholipid v.
  pinocytotic v.
vesicobullous
vesicocolic fistula
vesicocutaneous fistula
vesicointestinal fistula
vesicolithiasis
vesicopustular
vesicopustule
vesicoureteral reflux
vesicouterine fistula
vesicovaginal fistula
vesicovaginorectal fistula
vesicular
  v. acute inflammation
  v. chromatin pattern
  v. emphysema
  v. exanthema
  v. exanthema of swine virus
  v. granulomatous inflammation
  v. keratitis
  v. mole
  v. nucleus
  v. stomatitis
  v. stomatitis virus (VSV)
vesiculate
vesiculated
vesiculation
vesiculiform
vesiculin
vesiculitis
vesiculocavernous
vesiculopapular
vesiculoprostatitis
vesiculopustular
vesiculose
vesiculous
Vesiculovirus
vessel
  aberrant renal v.
  blood v.
  pinocytotic v.
  transposition of great v.'s (TGV)
vestibular anus
vestigial
vesuvin
VH
  venous hematocrit
  viral hepatitis

NOTES

VHD
viral hematodepressive disease
VHDL
very high density lipoprotein
Vi
Vi agglutination
Vi antibody
Vi antigen
VIA
virus-inactivating agent
viability
viable cell count
vibration second (v.s.)
Vibrio
V. alginolyticus
V. bubulus
V. cholerae
V. cholerae-asiaticae
V. coli
V. comma
V. danubicus
V. eltor
V. fecalis
V. fetus
V. finkleri
V. ghinda
V. group F (EF-6)
V. jejuni
V. massauah
V. metschnikovii
V. niger
V. parahaemolyticus
V. phosphorescens
V. proteus
V. septicus
V. sputorum
V. tyrogenus
V. vulnificus
vibrio
Celebes v.
cholera v.
El Tor v.
Nasik v.
nonagglutinating v.
paracholera v.
vibrion
Vibrionaceae
vibriosis
vicarious
v. hemoptysis
v. hypertrophy
Vicia
V. graminea
vicinal
vicine
vicious union

victoria
v. blue
v. orange
Vidal disease
vidarabine
videocamera
Ikegami v.
Vierra sign
view
radius of v.
VIG
vaccinia-immune globulin
Villaret syndrome
villi (*pl. of* villus)
villiform configuration
villoglandular
villoma
villonodular
v. pigmented synovitis
v. pigmented tenosynovitis
villositis
villous
v. adenoma
v. atrophy
v. carcinoma
v. papilloma
v. polyp
v. tenosynovitis
v. tumor
villus, pl. villi
abnormal chorionic villi
chorionic villi
mature abnormal chorionic villi
vimentin
v. antibody
v. immunoperoxidase stain
VIN
vulvar intraepithelial neoplasia
Vincent
V. angina
V. disease
V. organism
V. stomatitis
V. white mycetoma
vincristine
v., cyclophosphamide, prednisone, doxorubicin (Adriamycin) (VEPA)
v. neuropathy
vindesine, etoposide, procarbazine, prednisone, bleomycin (FEPP-B)
vinegar acid
Vinson syndrome
vinyl
v. chloride
v. chloride disease
v. polymers
v. trichloride
violaceous

violet
>   amethyst v.
>   aniline gentian v. (AGV)
>   Bensley safranin acid v.
>   Bernthsen methylene v.
>   chrome v.
>   cresyl v. (CV)
>   crystal v.
>   gentian v. (GV)
>   hexamethyl v.
>   Hoffman v.
>   Lauth v.
>   methyl v.
>   methylene v.
>   pentamethyl v.

viomycin
viosterol
VIP
>   vasoactive intestinal peptide
>   vasoactive intestinal polypeptide
>   voluntary interruption of pregnancy

viper
>   Russell v.
>   v. venom (VV)

vipoma
viral
>   v. capsid antigen (VCA)
>   v. culture
>   v. dysentery
>   v. encephalomyelitis
>   v. envelope
>   v. gastroenteritis
>   v. hemagglutination
>   v. hematodepressive disease (VHD)
>   v. hemorrhagic fever
>   v. hemorrhagic fever virus
>   v. hepatitis (VH)
>   v. hepatitis type A, B, C, D, E
>   v. inclusion
>   v. meningitis
>   v. neutralization
>   v. pericarditis
>   v. pneumonia
>   v. probe
>   v. respiratory infection (VRI)
>   v. strand
>   v. tropism
>   v. wart

ViraPap test
Viratype In Situ System
Virchow
>   V. crystal

>   V. disease
>   V. hydatid
>   V. law
>   V. node
>   V. psammoma

viremia
virgin
virginal
virginity
viricidal
viricide
viridans streptococcus
virilism
>   adrenal v.
>   congenital adrenal v. (CAV)

virilization
>   adrenal v.

virilizing syndrome
virion
virogene
viroid
virologist
virology
viropexis
virucidal
virucide
virucopria
virulence
virulent
>   v. bacteriophage

viruliferous
viruria
virus
>   2060 v.
>   Abelson murine leukemia v.
>   v. A, B hepatitis
>   adeno-associated v. (AAV)
>   adenosatellite v.
>   African horse sickness v.
>   African swine fever v.
>   AIDS-related v. (ARV)
>   Akabane v.
>   AKT1 v.
>   Aleutian mink disease v.
>   amphotropic v.
>   animal v.
>   v. animatum
>   APC v.
>   apeu v.
>   Argentine hemorrhagic fever v.
>   attenuated v.
>   Aujeszky disease v.

V

NOTES

virus *(continued)*
    Australian X disease v.
    Australian X encephalitis v.
    avian encephalomyelitis v.
    avian erythroblastosis v.
    avian infectious laryngotracheitis v.
    avian influenza v.
    avian leukosis-sarcoma v.
    avian lymphomatosis v.
    avian myeloblastosis v.
    avian myelocytomatosis v. (AMV2)
    avian neurolymphomatosis v.
    avian pneumoencephalitis v.
    avian sarcoma v.
    avian viral arthritis v.
    B v.
    B19 v.
    bacterial v.
    Bittner v.
    biundulant milk fever v.
    BK v.
    v. blockade
    bluecomb v.
    bluetongue v.
    Borna disease v.
    Bornholm disease v.
    bovine leukemia v. (BLV)
    bovine leukosis v.
    bovine papular stomatitis v.
    bovine virus diarrhea v.
    v. bronchopneumonia
    Brunhilde v.
    Bunyamwera v.
    Bwamba fever v.
    C v.
        Coxsackievirus A, B virus titer
    CA v.
    Cache Valley v.
    California v.
    California encephalitis v.
    canarypox v.
    canine distemper v.
    Capim v.
    Caraparu v.
    cat distemper v.
    cattle plague v.
    Catu v.
    CELO v.
    Central European encephalitis v. (CEEV)
    Central European tick-borne encephalitis v.
    C group v.
    Chagres v.
    chicken embryo lethal orphan v.
    chickenpox v.
    chikungunya fever v.
    Coe v.

cold v.
Colorado tick fever v.
Columbia S. K. v.
common cold v.
contagious ecthyma (pustular dermatitis) v. of sheep
contagious pustular stomatitis v.
cowpox v.
Crimean-Congo hemorrhagic fever v.
Crimean hemorrhagic fever v.
croup-associated v.
cytomegalic inclusion disease v.
cytopathogenic v.
δ v.
defective v.
dengue v.
diphasic meningoencephalitis v.
diphasic milk fever v.
distemper v.
DNA v.
dog distemper v.
duck hepatitis v.
duck influenza v.
duck plague v.
eastern equine encephalomyelitis v.
EB v.
Ebola v.
EBV v.
ECBO v.
ECDO v.
ECHO v.
ECMO v.
ecotropic v.
ECSO v.
ecthyma infectiosum v.
ectromelia v.
EEE v.
EMC v.
emerging v.
encephalitis v.
encephalomyocarditis v.
enteric cytopathogenic bovine orphan v. (ECBO virus)
enteric cytopathogenic human orphan v. (ECHO virus)
enteric cytopathogenic monkey orphan v. (ECMO virus)
enteric cytopathogenic swine orphan v. (ECSO virus)
enteric orphan v.
entomopox v.
enzootic encephalomyelitis v.
ephemeral fever v.
epidemic gastroenteritis v.
epidemic keratoconjunctivitis v.
epidemic myalgia v.
epidemic parotitis v.

epidemic pleurodynia v.
Epstein-Barr v. (EBV)
equine abortion v.
equine arteritis v.
equine coital exanthema v.
equine encephalomyelitis v.
equine infectious anemia v.
equine influenza v.
equine rhinopneumonitis v.
exanthem subitum v.
FA v.
feline ataxia v. (FAV)
feline leukemia v. (FeLV)
feline panleukopenia v.
feline rhinotracheitis v.
fibromatosis v. of rabbits
fibrous bacterial v.
fifth disease v.
filamentous bacterial v.
filterable v.
filtrable v.
fixed v.
Flury strain rabies v.
FMD v.
foamy v.
foot-and-mouth disease v.
fowl erythroblastosis v.
fowl lymphomatosis v.
fowl myeloblastosis v.
fowl neurolymphomatosis v.
fowl plague v.
fowlpox v.
fox encephalitis v.
Friend leukemia v.
GAL v.
gallus adeno-like v.
gastroenteritis v. type A
gastroenteritis v. type B
German measles v.
Germiston v.
goatpox v.
Graffi v.
green monkey v.
Gross leukemia v.
Guama v.
Guaroa v.
HA1 v.
HA2 v.
hand-foot-and-mouth disease v.
Hantaan v.
hard pad v.
helper v.

hemadsorption v., type 1, 2
hepatitis v.
hepatitis A v. (HAV)
hepatitis B v. (HBV)
hepatitis C v. (HCV)
hepatitis D v.
hepatitis delta v. (HDV)
v. hepatitis of ducks
hepatitis E v. (HEV)
herpangina v.
herpes v.
herpes-like v. (HLV)
herpes simplex v. (HSV)
herpes-type v. (HTV)
herpes zoster v.
hog cholera v.
horsepox v.
human immunodeficiency v. (HIV)
human papilloma v.
human T cell leukemia-
  lymphoma v. (HTLV)
human T-cell
  lymphoma/leukemia v.
human T-cell lymphotropic v.
human T-cell lymphotropic v. type
  I (HTLV-I)
human T-cell lymphotropic v. type
  II (HTLV-II)
human T-cell lymphotropic v. type
  III (HTLV-III)
human T lymphotrophic v.
Ibaraki v.
IBR v.
v. III of rabbits
Ilhéus v.
inclusion conjunctivitis v.
infantile gastroenteritis v.
infectious arteritis v. of horses
infectious bovine rhinotracheitis v.
infectious bronchitis v. (IBV)
infectious ectromelia v.
infectious hepatitis v.
infectious papilloma v.
infectious porcine
  encephalomyelitis v.
influenza v.
insect v.
iridescent v.
Itaqui v.
Jamestown Canyon v.
Japanese B encephalitis v.
JC v.

V

NOTES

669

virus *(continued)*
 JH v.
 Junin v.
 K v.
 Kelev strain rabies v.
 v. keratoconjunctivitis
 Kilham rat v.
 Kisenyi sheep disease v.
 Koongol v.'s
 Korean hemorrhagic fever v.
 Kumba v.
 Kyasanur Forest disease v.
 La Crosse v.
 lactate dehydrogenase v.
 lactic dehydrogenase v. (LDV)
 Lansing v.
 Lassa v.
 latent rat v.
 LCM v.
 Leon v.
 lepori pox v.
 louping-ill v.
 Lucké v.
 Lunyo v.
 lymphadenopathy-associated v. (LAV)
 lymphocytic choriomeningitis v.
 lymphogranuloma venereum v.
 Machupo v.
 maedi v.
 malignant catarrhal fever v.
 Maloney leukemia v.
 mammary cancer v. of mice
 mammary tumor v. (MTV)
 mammary tumor v. of mice
 Marburg v.
 Marek disease v.
 Marituba v.
 marmoset v.
 masked v.
 Mason-Pfizer v.
 Mayaro v.
 measles v.
 medi v.
 Mengo v.
 milker's nodule v.
 mink enteritis v.
 MM v.
 Mokola v.
 molluscum contagiosum v.
 molluscum sebaceum v.
 Moloney v.
 Moloney leukemogenic v. (MLV)
 Moloney sarcoma v. (MSV)
 monkey B v.
 monkeypox v.
 mouse encephalomyelitis v.
 mouse hepatitis v.

 mouse leukemia v. (MLV)
 mouse mammary tumor v. (MMTV)
 mouse parotid tumor v.
 mouse poliomyelitis v.
 mousepox v.
 mouse thymic v.
 mucosal disease v.
 mumps v.
 murine sarcoma v. (MSV)
 Murray Valley encephalitis v.
 Murutucu v.
 MVE v.
 myxomatosis v.
 Nairobi sheep disease v.
 naked v.
 ND v.
 Nebraska calf scours v.
 Neethling v.
 negative strand v.
 Negishi v.
 neonatal calf diarrhea v.
 neurotropic v.
 Newcastle disease v. (NDV)
 non-A, non-B hepatitis v.
 nonbacterial gastroenteritis v.
 nonoccluded v.
 Norwalk v.
 Ntaya v.
 occluded v.
 Omsk hemorrhagic fever v.
 oncogenic v.
 o'nyong-nyong fever v.
 orf v.
 Oriboca v.
 ornithosis v.
 Oropouche v.
 orphan v.
 Pacheco parrot disease v.
 panleukopenia v. (PLV)
 panleukopenia v. of cats
 pantropic v.
 papilloma v.
 pappataci fever v.
 papular stomatitis v. of cattle
 parainfluenza v.
 parapox v.
 paravaccinia v.
 parrot v.
 Patois v.
 pharyngoconjunctival fever v.
 phlebotomus fever v.
 plant v.
 pneumonia v. of mice (PVM)
 v. pneumonia of pigs
 pneumonitis v.
 v. poliomyelitis
 poliomyelitis v.

polyoma v.
porcine hemagglutinating
  encephalomyelitis v.
Powassan v.
pox v.
progressive pneumonia v.
pseudocowpox v.
pseudolymphocytic
  choriomeningitis v.
pseudorabies v.
psittacosis v.
PVM v.
quail bronchitis v.
Quaranfil v.
rabbit fibroma v.
rabbit myxoma v.
rabbitpox v.
rabies v.
rabies v., Flury strain
rabies v., Kelev strain
rat v. (RV)
Rauscher leukemia v.
REO v.
reservoir of v.
respiratory enteric orphan v.
respiratory exanthematous v.
respiratory infection v.
respiratory syncytial v. (RSV)
Rida v.
Rift Valley fever v.
rinderpest v.
RNA tumor v.
roseola infantum v.
Ross River v.
Rous-associated v. (RAV)
Rous sarcoma v. (RSV)
Rs v.
Rubarth disease v.
rubella v. (RV)
rubeola v.
Russian autumn encephalitis v.
Russian spring-summer
  encephalitis v.
Salisbury common cold v.
salivary v.
salivary gland v. (SGV)
sandfly fever v.
San Miguel sea lion v.
Semliki Forest v.
Sendai v.
serum hepatitis v.
v. shedding

sheep-pox v.
shipping fever v.
Shope fibroma v.
Shope papilloma v.
Simbu v.
simian v. (SV)
simian sarcoma v. (SSV)
simian vacuolating v. No. 40
Sindbis v.
slow v.
smallpox v.
snowshoe hare v.
soremouth v.
Spondweni v.
St. Louis encephalitis v. (SLEV)
strect v.
swamp fever v.
swine encephalitis v.
swine fever v.
swine influenza v.
swinepox v.
Swiss mouse leukcmia v.
Tacaribe v.
Tahyna v.
temperate v.
Teschen v.
Tete v.
TGE v.
Theiler mouse encephalomyelitis v.
Theiler original v.
tick-borne v.
tick-borne encephalitis v.
TO v.
tobacco mosaic v. (TMV)
trachoma v.
transmissible gastrocntcritis v. of
  swinc
transmissible turkey enteritis v.
tumor v.
turkey meningoencephalitis v.
Turlock v.
Uganda S v.
Umbre v.
unorganized v.
Uruma v.
vaccine v.
vaccinia v.
vacuolating v.
varicella v.
varicella-zoster v. (VSV, VZV)
variola v.
VEE v.

NOTES

virus *(continued)*
    Venezuelan equine
      encephalomyelitis virus
  Venezuelan equine A
  encephalomyelitis v.
  Venezuelan equine
  encephalomyelitis v. (VEE virus)
  verruca v.
  vesicular exanthema of swine v.
  vesicular stomatitis v. (VSV)
  viral hemorrhagic fever v.
  visceral disease v.
  visna v.
  VS v.
  WEE v.
    western equine encephalomyelitis
    virus
  Wesselsbron v.
  Wesselsbron disease v.
  western equine encephalomyelitis v.
  (WEE virus)
  West Nile encephalitis v.
  v. X disease
  xenotropic v.
  Yaba monkey v.
  yellow fever v.
  Zika v.
virus-associated hemophagocytic
  syndrome (VAHS)
virus-inactivating agent (VIA)
virus-neutralizing (VN)
virusoid
virus-transformed cell
VIS
  vaginal irrigation smear
visceral
  v. disease virus
  v. inversion
  v. larva migrans
  v. leishmaniasis
  v. lymphomatosis
  v. pleurisy
visceromegaly
visceroptosia
visceroptosis
viscerotomy
viscerotrophic reflex
viscid
viscidosis
viscometer
viscosimeter
  Ostwald v.
  Stormer v.
viscosimetry
viscosity
  absolute v.
  dynamic v.
  kinematic v.

viscous
visible light
Visiprep Solid-Phase Extraction Vacuum
  Manifold
visna
  v. virus
visual evoked potential (venostasis)
vital
  v. dye
  v. red
  v. signs (VS)
  v. stain
  v. staining
vitamin
  v. A
  v. A and carotene assays
  v. A clearance test
  v. A unit
  v. A_1
  v. A_1aldehyde
  v. A_2
  v. B complex
  v. B_c
  v. B_x
  v. B_1
  v. B_1 hydrochloride unit
  v. B_2
  v. B_2 unit
  v. B_3
  v. B_6
  v. B_6 assay
  v. B_6 unit
  v. B_7
  v. B_{12}
  v. B_{12} unsaturated binding capacity
  v. B_{12} absorption test
  v. B_{12} assay
  v. C unit
  v. D assay
  v. D intoxication
  v. D unit
  v. D_3
  v. deficiency
  v. deficiency anemia
  v. E assay
  v. E unit
  v. K assay
  v. K unit
  v. K_1
  v. K_1 oxide
  v. K_2
  v. K_3
  microbial v.
vitaminoid action
Vitek GPI
vitellarium
vitellin
vitelline sphere

vitellointestinal cyst
vitiation
vitiligines
vitiliginous
vitiligo, pl. vitiligines
    circumnevic v.
vitiligoidea
vitreous humor
in vitro
vitulorum
    Neoascaris v.
vivax
    v. fever
    v. malaria
vivipara
    Probstymayria v.
Viviparidae
Viviparus
in vivo
vivum
    contagium v.
VLA
    very late activation
    VLA antigen
VLDL, VLDLP
    very low density lipoprotein
VLSI
    very large scale integration
VM
    voltmeter
VMA
    vanillylmandelic acid
    VMA test
VMR
    vasomotor rhinitis
VN
    virus-neutralizing
VNTRs
    variable number tandem repeats
Voges-Proskauer (VP)
    V.-P. broth
    V.-P. reaction
    V.-P. test
Vogt-Koyanagi syndrome
Vogt-Spielmeyer disease
Vogt syndrome
Vohwinkel syndrome
vol
volatile
    v. oil
    v. organic substances assay
    v. screen

volatility
volatilization
vole bacillus
Volhard test
Volkmann
    V. contracture
    V. disease
    V. syndrome
Vollmer test
volt
    electron v. (ev)
    giga electron v.
    kilo electron v. (kev)
    megaelectron v. (MeV)
    million electron v.'s (mev)
voltage
    anode v.
    v. divider
    v. drop
    high v.
    v. regulator
    ripple v.
voltage-regulating transformer
voltage-regulator tube
voltage-to-frequency converter
voltammetry
volt-ampere (VA)
voltmeter (VM)
    digital v.
    vacuum tube v. (VTVM)
volt-ohm-milliammeter
volt-ohm-millimeter (VOM)
Voltolini disease
volume
    blood v.
    cell v. (CV)
    central blood v. (CBV)
    circulating blood v. (CBV)
    v. coefficient
    v. conduction
    conductivity cell v. (CCV)
    corrected blood v. (CBV)
    v. of distribution of bilirubin
    (VDBR)
    effective circulating blood v.
    (ECBV)
    extracellular v. (ECV)
    extracellular fluid v. (ECFV, EFV)
    fluid v. (FV)
    v. index
    intracellular fluid v. (IFV)
    intrathoracic gas v. (IGV)

V

NOTES

volume *(continued)*
    mean cell v. (MCV)
    mean corpuscular v. (MCV)
    minute v. (MV)
    packed cell v. (PCV)
    v. of packed red cells (VPRC)
    placental residual blood v. (PRBV)
    plasma v. (PV)
    pulmonary capillary blood v.
    red blood cell v. (RBCV, VRBC)
    red cell v. (RCV)
    regional cerebral blood v. (RCBV)
    retention v.
    reticulocyte mean corpuscular v.
     (MCVr)
    v. substitute
    thoracic gas v. (TGV)
    total blood v. (TBV)
    weight per v. (w/v)
volumetric
    v. flask
    v. pipette
    v. solution (VS)
voluntary interruption of pregnancy
    (VIP)
Volutella
    V. cinerescens
volutin
Volvox
volvulosis
volvulus
    gastric v.
VOM
    volt-ohm-millimeter
vomica
vomicose
vomit
vomiting
    epidemic v.
vomitus
    colonic v.
von
    v. Bechterew disease
    v. Clauss method
    v. Economo disease
    v. Gierke disease
    v. Hippel disease
    v. Hippel-Lindau disease
    v. Jaksch disease
    v. Kossa calcium assay
    v. Kossa method
    v. Kossa stain
    v. Meyenburg complex
    v. Meyenburg disease
    v. Recklinghausen disease
    v. Willebrand antigen
    v. Willebrand disease (VW)
    v. Willebrand factor

    v. Willebrand factor antigen
    v. Willebrand factor assay
    v. Willebrand factor multimer
     assay
    v. Willebrand syndrome
Voorhoeve disease
Vorticella
VP
    vasopressin
    Voges-Proskauer
    VP reaction
    VP test
VP16
VPC
    vapor-phase chromatography
VPRC
    volume of packed red cells
VR
    vascular resistance
VRBC
    red blood cell volume
VRI
    viral respiratory infection
Vrolik disease
VS
    vital signs
    volumetric solution
    VS virus
v.s.
    vibration second
VSD
    ventricular septal defect
VSV
    varicella-zoster virus
    vesicular stomatitis virus
VT
    vacuum tuberculin
VTVM
    vacuum tube voltmeter
vulgaris
    acne v.
    psoriasis v.
vulpis
    Crenosoma v.
vulva, pl. **vulvae**
    kraurosis vulvae
    multinucleated atypia of the v.
     (MAV)
vulvar
    v. dystrophy
    v. intraepithelial neoplasia (VIN)
    v. tumor
vulvitis
    chronic atrophic v.
    chronic hypertrophic v.
    leukoplakic v.
vulvovaginal anus
vulvovaginitis

VV
    viper venom
VW
    von Willebrand disease
Vw antigen

VZ
    varicella-zoster
VZV
    varicella-zoster virus
    VZV culture

NOTES

V

W
    watt
    Weber
w
    watt
Waardenburg syndrome
Wachstein-Meissel stain for calcium-magnesium-ATPase
Wade-Fite-Faraco stain
Wagner
    W. disease
    W. test
Wako NEFA test kit
Waldenström
    W. disease
    W. macroglobulinemia
    W. purpura
    W. syndrome
    W. test
Waldeyer
    W. ring
    W. ring lymphoma
Walker
    W. carcinoma
    W. carcinosarcoma
wall
    anterior w. (AW)
    cell w.
    cross w.
Wallenberg syndrome
wallerian degeneration (WD)
wallet stomach
Walsh average
Walthard
    W. cell rest
WAMPOLE ISOLATOR blood culture system
wandering
    w. abscess
    w. cell
    w. goiter
    w. liver
    w. organ
    w. pacemaker
    w. pneumonia
Wangiella
Wang test
warble
    w. fly
Warburg theory
Ward-Romano syndrome
Wardrop disease
warfarin
    w. assay

warm
    w. agglutinin
    w. antibody
    w. autoantibody
    w. hemagglutinin
warm-cold hemolysin
wart
    anatomical w.
    anogenital w.
    cattle w.
    common w.
    digitate w.
    fig w.
    filiform w.
    flat w.
    genital w.
    infectious w.
    moist w.
    mosaic w.
    necrogenic w.
    pitch w.
    plane w.
    plantar w.
    pointed w.
    postmortem w.
    prosector's w.
    seborrheic w.
    senile w.
    soft w.
    soot w.
    telangiectatic w.
    tuberculous w.
    venereal w.
    viral w.
Wartenberg disease
Warthin-Finkeldey
    W.-F. type polykaryocyte
Warthin-Finkeldey-type giant cell
Warthin-Starry
    W.-S. method
    W.-S. silver stain
Warthin tumor
wartpox
warty
    w. dyskeratoma
    w. horn
    w. ulcer
wash
    Gravlee jet w.
    w. time
washed
    w. red blood cells
    w. red cells (WRC)

W

washing
    bronchial w.
    w. cytology
washout pipette
WASP
  World Association of Societies of
  Pathology
Wassén test
wasserhelle
    w. cell
    w. hyperplasia
Wassermann
    W. antibody
    W. antigen
    W. reaction (WR, Wr)
    W. test
Wassermann-fast
Wassilieff disease
waste
    chemical w.
    infectious w.
    w. product
    radioactive w.
    toxic w.
wasting
    w. disease
    w. syndrome
water
    w. aspirator
    w. bacterium
    w. bath
    w. conductivity
    extracellular w. (ECW)
    w. gas
    gentian aniline w.
    w. immersion
    interstitial w. (ISW)
    w. intoxication
    intracellular w. (ICW)
    w. in oil (W/O)
    oil in w. (O/W)
    total body w. (TBW)
water-clear cell
water-clear-cell hyperplasia
water-gurgle test
Waterhouse-Friderichsen syndrome
watering-can
    w.-c. perineum
    w.-c. scrotum
waterpox
water-soluble scarlet
water-trap stomach
watery diarrhea, hypokalemia,
  achlorhydria (WDHA)
watsoni
    Cladorchis w.
    Watsonius w.
Watsonius watsoni

Watson-Schwartz test
watt (W, w)
watt-second (ws)
wave
    acid w.
    alkaline w.
    w. amplitude
    w. analyzer
    diphasic w.
    monophasic w.
    w. number
    periodic w.
    polyphasic w.
    sawtooth w.
    sine w.
    square w.
    triangular w.
    triphasic w.
    w. velocity
waveform
waveguide
wavelength
    w. accuracy
    w. repeatability
wax
    grave w.
waxy
    w. cast
    w. degeneration
    w. finger
    w. kidney
    w. liver
    w. spleen
    w. urinary cast
Wayson stain
WB
    whole blood
    Willowbrook (virus)
Wb
    weber
WBC
    white blood cell
WBC/hpf
    white blood cells per high power field
WBF
    whole-blood folate
WBH
    whole-blood hematocrit
WC
    white cell
    white (cell) cast
WC′
    whole complement
WCC
    white cell count
WD
    wallerian degeneration

WDCA
  well-differentiated carcinoma
WDHA
  watery diarrhea, hypokalemia,
    achlorhydria
    WDHA syndrome
WDLL
  well-differentiated lymphocytic
    lymphoma
WE
  western encephalitis
  western encephalomyelitis
weakly
  w. positive (WP)
  w. reactive (WR, Wr)
wear-and-tear
  w.-a.-t. pigment
  w.-a.-t. pigmentation
web
  cell w.
  esophageal w.
  laryngeal w.
  terminal w.
Webb antigen
webbed
  w. finger
  w. neck
  w. toe
webbing
Weber (W)
  W. syndrome
  W. test
weber (Wb)
Weber-Christian disease
Weber-Cockayne syndrome
Weber-Dubler syndrome
Weber-Rendu-Osler disease
Webster test
weddellite calculus
WEE
  western equine encephalomyelitis
  WEE virus
Wegener
  W. granulomatosis
  W. syndrome
Wegner
  W. disease
  W. line
Weibel-Palade body
Weichselbaum diplococcus
Weidel reaction

Weigert
  W. iodine solution
  W. iron hematoxylin
  W. iron hematoxylin stain
  W. stain for actinomyces
  W. stain for elastin
  W. stain for fibrin
  W. stain for myelin
  W. stain for neuroglia
Weigert-Gram stain
Weigert-Pal stain
weighing
weight (wt)
  atomic w.
  fat-free dry w. (FFDW)
  fat-free wet w. (FFWW)
  gram-molecular w. (GMW)
  high birth w. (HBW)
  high molecular w. (HMW)
  ideal body w. (IBW)
  low birth w. (LBW)
  low molecular w. (LMW)
  molar w.
  molecular w. (MW)
  w. per volume (w/v)
  total body w. (TBW)
weighted average
Weil
  W. disease
  W. myelin sheath stain
  W. syndrome
Weil-Felix (WF)
  W.-F. reaction (WFR)
  W.-F. test
Weil-Felix agglutinins
Weill-Marchesani syndrome
Weinberg reaction
Weinman medium
Weir Mitchell disease
Welch bacillus
**Welcozyme HIV 1&2 ELISA antibody
  test**
welder's
  w. conjunctivitis
  w. lung
Welker method
well-differentiated
  w.-d. carcinoma (WDCA)
  w.-d. lymphocytic lymphoma
    (WDLL)
Wells syndrome
welt

W

NOTES

wen
Wenckebach disease
Werdnig-Hoffmann disease
Werlhof disease
Wermer syndrome
Werner
    W. syndrome
    W. test
Werner-His disease
Werner-Schultz disease
Wernicke
    W. encephalopathy
    W. syndrome
Wernicke-Korsakoff (WK)
    W. encephalopathy
    W. syndrome
Wesenberg-Hamazaki body
Wesselsbron
    W. disease
    W. disease virus
    W. fever
    W. virus
West
    W. African fever
    W. Indian smallpox
    W. Nile encephalitis virus
    W. Nile fever
    W. syndrome
Westergren
    W. sedimentation rate
    W. sedimentation rate method
    W. sedimentation rate test
western
    W. blot
    W. blot analysis
    W. blot technique
    W. blot test
    w. encephalitis (WE)
    w. encephalomyelitis (WE)
    w. equine ·encephalitis
    w. equine encephalitis virus
      serology
    w. equine encephalomyelitis (WEE)
    w. equine encephalomyelitis virus
      (WEE virus)
    w. immunoblot test
Westphal disease
Westphal-Strümpell
    W.-S. disease
    W.-S. pseudosclerosis
wet
    w. gangrene
    w. mount
    w. pleurisy
wetting agent
Wetzel test
Weyers oligodactyly syndrome
Weyers-Thier syndrome

WF
    Weil-Felix
WFR
    Weil-Felix reaction
WGA
    wheat germ agglutinin
whartonitis
wheal
    w. reaction time (QRZ)
wheal-and-erythema
    w.-a.-e. reaction
    w.-a.-e. skin test
wheal-and-flare reaction
wheat
    w. broth
    w. germ agglutinin (WGA)
Wheatstone bridge
Wheeler-Johnson test
whetstone crystal
whewellite calculus
whey
    litmus w.
whiff test
Whipple
    W. disease
    W. method
whipworm
    w. infection
whistling face syndrome
white
    w. bile
    w. blood cell (WBC)
    w. blood cell cast
    w. blood cell count
    w. blood cells per high power
      field (WBC/hpf)
    w. blood cell urinary cast
    w. cell (WC)
    w. (cell) cast (WC)
    w. cell count (WCC)
    w. corpuscle
    W. disease
    w. gangrene
    w. graft
    w. infarct
    w. leg
    methylene w.
    w. muscle disease
    w. patch
    w. piedra
    w. spot
    w. spot disease
    w. thrombus
whitehead
whitepox
whitlow
    herpetic w.
    melanotic w.

Whitmore
- W. bacillus
- W. disease

Whitmore-Jewett tumor staging system
Whitten effect
WHO histologic classification of ovarian tumors
whole
- w. blood (B, WB)
- w. complement (WC')
- w. ragweed extract (WRE)

whole-arm fusion
whole-blood
- w.-b. clotting time
- w.-b. folate (WBF)
- w.-b. hematocrit (WBH)

whole blood (B, WB)
whole-body titration curve
whooping cough
- w. c. vaccine

Whytt disease
Wickham striae
Widal
- W. reaction
- W. syndrome
- W. test

wide
- w. field eyepiece
- w. spectrum

width
- red cell diameter w. (RDW)
- red cell distribution w.
- reticulocyte distribution w. (RDW)
- reticulocyte hemoglobin distribution w. (HDW)

Wilcoxon signed rank statistic
wild
- w. type
- w. yeast

Wilder stain for reticulum
Wildervanck syndrome
wild-type gene
Wilkie disease
Wilkins-Chilgren agar
Willebrand syndrome
Williams
- W. factor
- W. stain
- W. syndrome

Williams-Campbell syndrome
Willis disease
Willowbrook (virus) (WB)

Wilms tumor
Wilson
- W. disease
- W. method
- W. syndrome

Wilson-Mikity syndrome
Winckel disease
windage
wind contusion
window
Windscheid disease
Winiwarter-Buerger disease
Winkler disease
winter
- w. dysentery of cattle
- w. itch
- W. syndrome

Winton disease
Wintrobe
- W. hematocrit tube
- W. and Landsberg method
- macromethod of W.
- W. sedimentation rate
- W. sedimentation rate method

wire-loop
- w.-l. lesion
- w.-l. test

wire-wound resistor
wiry
Wiskott-Aldrich syndrome
Wistar rat
withering crypt appearance
within normal limits (WNL)
Witkop disease
Witkop-Von Sallmann syndrome
WK
- Wernicke-Korsakoff

WMR
- work metabolic rate

WNL
- within normal limits

W/O
- water in oil

wobble hypothesis
Wohlfahrtia
- *W. magnifica*
- *W. opaca*
- *W. vigil*

wohlfahrtiosis
Wohlfart-Kugelberg-Welander disease
Wohlgemuth unit
Wolfe breast carcinoma

W

NOTES

Wolff-Chaikoff effect
wolffian
    w. cyst
    w. duct carcinoma
    w. rest
Wolff-Parkinson-White syndrome
Wolff-Parkinson-White (syndrome) (WPW)
Wolf-Hirschhorn syndrome
Wolf-Orton body
Wolfram syndrome
Wolman disease
Wood
    W. glass
    W. lamp
    W. light
woodcutter's encephalitis
woolsorter's disease
Woringer-Kolopp disease
working distance
work metabolic rate (WMR)
workup
World Association of Societies of Pathology (WASP)
worm
    w. abscess
    Bancroft filarial w.
    dragon w.
    serpent w.
    tongue w.
Wormley test
wort broth
wound
    abraded w.
    avulsed w.
    w. botulism
    contused w.
    w. culture
    w. fever
    gunshot w.
    incised w.
    lacerated w.

    missile w.
    mutilating w.
    penetrating w.
    perforating w.
    spiral w. (SW)
    stab w.
    superficial w.
    surgical w.
woven bone
WP
    weakly positive
WPW
    Wolff-Parkinson-White (syndrome)
WR, Wr
    Wassermann reaction
    weakly reactive
Wr^a
    Wright antigen
    Wr^a antigen
Wratten filter
WRC
    washed red cells
WRE
    whole ragweed extract
Wright
    W. antigen (Wr^a)
    W. stain
    W. syndrome
wrinkled nucleus
ws
    watt-second
wt
    weight
Wuchereria
    W. bancrofti
    W. malayi
    W. pacifica
wuchereriasis
Wurster test
w/v
    weight per volume
Wyeomyia

X
homeopathic symbol for decimal scale of potencies
magnification
X chromatin
X chromatin body
X chromosome
X factor
X karyotype

Xa
antifactor Xa
xanchromatic
xanthelasma
generalized x.
x. palpebrarum
xanthelasmoidea
xanthematin
xanthemia
xanthene dye
xanthine
xanthinuria
xanthiuria
xanthoastrocytoma
pleomorphic x. (PXA)
xanthochromatic
xanthochromia
xanthochromic
xanthocyte
xanthoderma
xanthoerythrodermia perstans
xanthogranuloma
adult-type x. (AXG)
juvenile x. (JXG)
necrobiotic x.
xanthogranulomatous
x. bursitis
x. cholecystitis
x. pyelonephritis
xanthoma
x. cell
x. disseminatum (XD)
fibrous x.
normolipemic x. planum
x. palpebrarum
x. planum
x. tuberosum
x. tuberosum simplex
verrucous x.
xanthomatosis
biliary x.
cerebrotendinous x.
normal cholesteremic x.
xanthomatous
x. deposition
Xanthomonas

xanthopsia
xanthopsydracia
xanthopterin
xanthosine monophosphate
xanthosine-5'-phosphate
xanthosis
xanthous
xanthurenic
x. acid
x. aciduria
xanthurenic acid
xanthuria
xanthylic acid
x-axis
XD
xanthoma disseminatum
XDP
xeroderma pigmentosum
xenobiotic
xenodiagnosis
xenogeneic
x. graft
xenogenetic
xenogenic
xenogenous
xenograft
xenology
xenon
xenon-127
xenon-133
xenoparasite
Xenopsylla
X. astia
X. brasiliensis
X. cheopis
Xenopus
X. laevis
xenotropic virus
xeransis
xerantic
xerocytosis
xeroderma
x. pigmentosum (XDP, XP)
xeronosus
xerophthalmia
xerosis
xerostomia
xerotic
Xg antigen
X-inactivation
xiphoiditis
XLD
xylose-lysine-deoxycholate
XLD agar

X

X-linked
- X.-l. agammaglobulinemia
- X.-l. character
- X.-l. dominant inheritance
- X.-l. familial hypophosphatemia
- X.-l. gene
- X.-l. heredity
- X.-l. human androgen receptor (HUMARA)
- X.-l. hypogammaglobulinemia
- X.-l. ichthyosis
- X.-l. infantile hypogammaglobulinemia
- X.-l. lymphoproliferative disease
- X.-l. recessive inheritance

XM
- crossmatch

XO
- XO gonadal dysgenesis
- XO karyotype
- XO syndrome

XP
- xeroderma pigmentosum

x-ray
- x-r. crystallography
- x-r. microscope

XS
- excess

XT
- exotropia

XU
- excretory urogram

Xu
- x-unit

x-unit (Xu)

XX
- XX gonadal dysgenesis
- XX karyotype

XXX karyotype
XX/XY sex chromosome pattern
XXY
- XXY karyotype
- XXY syndrome

XY
- XY gonadal dysgenesis
- XY karyotype

xylene
- x. cyanol FF

xylidine
- ponceau D x.

xylitol dehydrogenase
xyloketose
xylol
xylose
- x. absorption test
- x. concentration test

D-xylose
- D-x. absorption test
- D-x. tolerance test

xylose-lysine-deoxycholate (XLD)
- x.-l.-d. agar

xylosuria
xylulose
L-xylulose
- L-x. dehydrogenase
- L-x. reductase

xylulosuria
L-xylulosuria
xysma
XYY karyotype
X-Y-Z beam scanning method coordinate
XYZ syndrome

Y

Y body
Y chromatin
Y chromosome
fragment Y

Yaba

Y. monkey virus
Y. tumor

yaws

crab y.
forest y.

y-axis

Yb

ytterbium

Yb-169 pentetate sodium

yeast

bakers' y.
dried y.
y. extract agar
y. fungus
imperfect y.
perfect y.
trypticase soy y. (TSY)
wild y.

yellow

acridine y.
alizarin y.
y. atrophy of liver
y. body
brilliant y.
butter y.
chrome y.
y. corallin
corralin y.
fast y.
y. fat
y. fever (YF)
y. fever vaccine
y. fever virus
y. hepatization

hydrazine y.
Leipzig y.
lemon y.
martius y.
metanil y.
metaniline y.
methyl y.
y. nail
Paris y.
y. skin
y. spot (YS)
Sudan y.
titan y.

yellowish

light green SF y.

Yersinia

Y. *enterocolitica*
Y. *enterocolitica* antibody
Y. *pestis*
Y. *pestis* antibody
Y. *pseudotuberculosis*

Yersinieae

YF

yellow fever

yield

quantum y.

Y-linked character

Yokogawa fluke

yolk

y. sac carcinoma
y. sac tumor

Yorke autolytic reaction

Young syndrome

YS

yellow spot

YSI 2300 STAT glucose and lactate analyzer

Yt^a antigen

ytterbium (Yb)

Yvon test

ζ (*var. of* zeta)
    ζ sedimentation rate (ZSR)
    ζ sedimentation ratio (ZSR)

Z
    Z line
    Z score

Zahn
    Z. infarct
    line of Z.
    Z. line
    striae of Z.

Zahorsky disease
Zambesi ulcer
Zamboni
    Z. fluid
    Z. solution

Zappert counting chamber
z-axis
Z/D
    zero defects

ZE
    Zollinger-Ellison

zebra body
Zebrina
zeisian stye
Zeiss
    Z. Axiophot fluorescent microscope
    Z. Axioplan microscope
    Z. LSM-10 laser microscope
    Z. transmission electron microscope

zellballen pattern
Zellen
    helle Z.

Zellweger syndrome
Zenker
    Z. degeneration
    Z. diverticulum
    Z. dysplasia
    Z. fixative
    Z. fluid
    Z. necrosis

zeolite
zero
    absolute z.
    z. defects (Z/D)

zero-order reaction
zeta, ζ
    z. potential
    z. sedimentation ratio method

zetacrit
zidovudine
Ziehen-Oppenheim disease
Ziehl-Neelsen
    Z.-N. method
    Z.-N. stain

Ziehl stain
Ziemann
    Z. dots
    Z. stippling

Zieve syndrome
ZIG
    zoster immune globulin

Zika
    Z. fever
    Z. virus

Zimmermann
    Z. corpuscle
    Z. elementary particle
    Z. granule
    pericyte of Z.
    Z. reaction
    Z. test

zinc
    z. assay
    z. flocculation test
    z. formalin
    z. phosphide
    z. sulfate centrifugal flotation technique
    z. sulfate flotation method
    z. sulfate turbidity test
    z. turbidity test

zincalism
Zinsser-Brill disease
Zinsser-Cole-Engman syndrome
ziram
zirconium (Zr)
    z. granuloma

zoite
Zollinger-Ellison (ZE)
    Z.-E. syndrome
    Z.-E. test
    Z.-E. tumor

zona
    z. dermatica
    z. epithelioserosa
    z. facialis
    z. ignea
    z. medullovasculosa
    z. ophthalmica
    z. serpiginosa

zona-free hamster egg penetration test
zonal necrosis
zonate
zone
    antibody excess z.
    epileptogenic z.
    equivalence z.
    flame intensity z.
    focal z.

Z

zone *(continued)*
    Golgi z.
    hemorrhoidal z.
    hyperesthetic z.
    mantle z.
    sudanophobic z.
    T z.
    transition z.
zoning
zonula
    z. adherens
    z. occludens
zonular keratitis
zooanthroponoses
zooanthroponosis
zoofulvin
Zoogloea
zoograft
zooid
Zoomastigina
Zoomastigophorasida
Zoomastigophorea
zoomylus
zoonosis
    enteric helminthic z.
zoonotic
    z. infection
    z. potential
zooparasite
zoophilic
zoophyte
zooprophylaxis
zoospermia

zootoxin
zoster
    z. encephalomyelitis
    z. immune globulin (ZIG)
Zr
    zirconium
Zsigmondy test
ZSR
    ζ sedimentation rate
    ζ sedimentation ratio
    ZSR method
Zuberella
zuckergussleber
Zygomycetes
zygomycosis
zygonema
zygosperm
zygospore
zygote
zygotene
zygotoblast
zygotomere
Zymobacterium
zymodeme
zymogen
    z. granule
zymogenic cell
zymogram
Zymomonas
zymoplastiche
    tuberculin z. (TZ)
zymoplastic substance
zymosan

Appendix 1
Culture Media

agar cutter
agar diffusion method
agar plate count
Apathy gum syrup medium
ascitic agar
Bactalert FAN culture medium
bacterial agar method
Balamuth culture medium
bile salt agar
bile-esculin agar
birdseed agar
bismuth-sulfite agar
blood agar
blood agar plate
Boeck-Drbohlav-Locke egg-serum
    medium
Bordet-Gengou potato blood agar
boric acid broth
brain-heart infusion agar
brain-heart infusion broth medium
brilliant green bile salt agar
carbohydrate broth
casein agar
Casman broth
CB agar
chocolate blood agar
chopped meat broth
chopped meat medium
Christensen urea agar
citrate agar
citrate agar gel electrophoresis
clearing medium
Columbia blood agar
Columbia medium
contrast medium
cornmeal agar
Cryo-Gel embedding medium
culture medium
cystine trypticase agar
Czapek solution agar
Czapek-Dox agar
Czapek-Dox medium
decarboxylase broth
deep agar
deoxycholate-citrate agar
deoxyribonuclease agar
dermatophyte test medium

dispersive medium
DNase agar
Eagle basal medium
Eagle minimum essential medium
egg-yolk agar
Eijkman lactose broth
EMB agar
Emmon modification of Sabouraud dex-
    trose agar
enrichment medium
eosin-methylene blue agar
ethyl violet azide broth
Farrant medium
French proof agar
glucose-format broth
glycerin broth
glycerin-potato broth
glycerol gelatin medium
GN broth
Gram-negative broth
haricot broth
Hektoen enteric agar
hippurate broth
indole-nitrate broth
inhibitory mold agar
inosite-free broth
iron broth
Kitasato broth
Kliger iron agar
Koser citrate broth
lactose-litmus broth
laked blood agar
Lash casein hydrolysate-serum medium
lauryl sulfate broth
lead broth
Loeffler blood culture medium
Loeffler coagulated serum medium
Löwenstein-Jensen medium
lysine-iron agar
MacConkey agar
MacConkey broth
malachite green broth
malt agar
malt extract broth
Martin broth
Martin-Lester agar
Middlebrook agar

Middlebrook broth
minimum essential medium
mounting medium
MR-VP broth
Mueller-Hinton agar
Mueller-Hinton broth
mycobiotic agar
nitrate agar
nitrate broth
Novy, MacNeal, and Nicolle medium
nutrient agar
nutrient broth
nutrient medium
oatmeal-tomato paste agar
OF medium
oxidation-fermentation medium
Parietti broth
passive medium
Petragnani medium
Pfeiffer blood agar
phenylalanine agar
phenylethyl alcohol blood agar
Pike streptococcal broth
potato dextrose agar
PVA lacto-phenol medium
rabbit blood agar
radiopaque medium
Rees culture medium
refracting medium
rice-Tween agar
Rosenow veal-brain broth
Sabhi agar
Sabouraud dextrose and brain heart in-
    fusion agar
Salmonella-Shigella agar
Schaedler blood agar
selective medium
selenite broth
selenite-cystine broth
separating medium
serum agar

serum broth
sheep blood agar
Simmons citrate agar
sodium chloride (6.5 %) broth
sodium chloride (6.5 %) culture
    medium
Spirolate broth
sterility test broth
Stuart broth
sugar broth
support medium
synthetic medium old tuberculin
    trichloroacetic acid (precipitated)
TCBS agar
tellurite medium
tetrathionate enrichment broth
Thayer-Martin agar
Thayer-Martin medium
thioglycollate broth
thioglycollate medium
thioglycollate-135C broth
tissue culture medium
Tobie, von Brand, and Mehlman dipha-
    sic medium
Todd-Hewitt broth
transport medium
triple sugar iron agar
tryptic soy agar
trypticase soy agar
trypticase soy broth
trypticase soy with agar broth
TSI agar
urea agar
urease test broth
Voges-Proskauer broth
Weinman medium
wheat broth
Wilkins-Chilgren agar
wort broth
XLD agar
xylose-lysine-deoxycholate agar

Appendix 2
Laboratory Tests

yeast extract agar
1,25-dihydroxycholecalciferol assay
11-deoxycorticosterone test
11-deoxycortisol test
^{131}I (radioactive iodine) uptake test
17-hydroxycorticosteroid test
17-hydroxyprogesterone test
17-ketogenic steroid assay test
17-ketosteroid assay test
17-OH-corticoid test
25-hydroxyvitamin D assay
3-amino-9-ethylcarbazole stain
3-methoxy-4-hydroxymandelic acid test
5-hydroxyindoleacetic acid assay
5-hydroxyindolcacetic test
A-Z test (Aschheim-Zondek test)
AAN test (amino acid nitrogen test)
Abbé test plate
Abbott stain for spores
ABO typing
ABO-Rh typing
Abrams test
abscess aerobic culture
absolute eosinophil count
absolute retention time
absorbency index
access time
acetaminophen assay
acetic acid and potassium ferrocyanide
    test
aceto-orcein stain
acetoacetic acid test
acetoin test
acetone test
acetowhite test
acetylcholinesterase assay
Achucárro stain
acid challenge test
ACT (acid clearance test)
acid clearance test
acid elution test
acid hemolysin test
acid perfusion test
acid phosphatase assay
acid phosphatase stain
acid phosphatase test
acid phosphatase test for semen

acid reflux test
acid stain
acid-base diagram
acid-base nomogram
acid-fast stain
acid-lability test
acid-Schiff stain
acidified serum test
acidity reduction test
acidophilic index
acidosis test
ACPA test (anticytoplasmic antibody
    test)
Acridine orange stain
ACTH stimulation test (adrenocorti-
    cotropic hormone stimulation test)
Actinomyces culture
ACT (activated coagulation time)
activated partial thromboplastin substi-
    tution test
activated partial thromboplastin time
activation analysis
active rosette test
Adamkiewicz test
Addis count
Addis test
adenovirus culture
ADH assay (antidiuretic hormone as-
    say)
adhesion test
Adler test
adrenal antibody
adrenal ascorbic acid depletion test
adrenal function test
adrenalin test
adrenocortical inhibition test
adrenocorticotropic hormone stimula-
    tion test
adrenocorticotropic hormone suppres-
    sion test
AE1 immunoperoxidase stain
AEC detection system
aerobic and anaerobic blood culture
AFB smear
AFB stain
A/G test
albumin-globulin test

Ag-AS stain
agar plate count
agglutination test
agglutination titer
AH assay
AH titer
AIDS serology
air-dried smear
AL patch test
ALA test
AlaSTAT latex allergy test
Albert stain
albumin suspension test
albumin test
albumin-globulin ratio test
Alcian blue stain
alcohol assay
aldolase assay
aldolase test
aldosterone assay
aldosterone stimulation test
aldosterone suppression test
alimentary tract smear
alizarin test
alkali denaturation test
alkali tolerance test
alkaline phosphatase assay
alkaline phosphatase stain
alkaline phosphatase test
alkaloid test
alkaptonuria test
Allen test
Allen-Doisy test
alloantigen-D antibody
Almén test for blood
alpha amino nitrogen test
AFP test
ALT test
Altmann aniline-acid fuchsin stain
American Type Culture Collection
Ames assay
Ames test
amino acid screen
amino acid nitrogen test
aminopyrine breath test
ammoniacal silver nitrate test
ammonium chloride loading test
ammonium silver carbonate stain
amniotic fluid analysis
amylase test
amylase-creatinine clearance
amyloid stain
anaerobic bacteria culture

analysis of variance
analytic cytology
Anderson and Goldberger test
Anderson-Collip test
androstenedione test
angiotensin I, II test
animal cell culture
anion gap test
anti-*Chlamydia* antibody test
anti-deoxyribonuclease B titer test
anti-DNA antibody assays
anti-DNase B assay
anti-LA/SS-B test
anti-Rh titer
anti-Ro/SS-A test
anti-sialosyl-Tn antigen
anti-Sm test
anti-smooth muscle antibody assay
antibiotic sensitivity test
antibody detection
antibody identification
antibody stain
antibody titer
antichymotrypsin test
anticytoplasmic antibody test
antideoxyribonuclease-B titer
antigen-binding region
antigenic assay
AGT (antiglobulin test)
antiglobulin test
antihuman globulin test
antihyaluronidase titer
antimitochondrial antibody assays
antinuclear antibody assay
antiparietal cell antibody assays
antistreptolysin-O test
antistreptolysin-O titer
antithrombin III test
antithrombin test
antitoxoplasma antibody test
antitrypsin test
antitryptic index
Anton test
APTT test
argentaffin stain
AITT test
arginine test
Argo corn starch test
Arneth count
Arneth index
arsenic stain
ART (automated reagin test)
automated reagin test

arterial line culture
arylsulfatase test
ASAP Biopsy System
ascariasis serological test
Aschheim-Zondek test
Ascoli test
ascorbate-cyanide test
ascorbic acid test
ASO test
ASO titer
Aspergillus antibody test
Aspergillus serology
aspirin tolerance test
AST test
ASTRA profile test
astrocyte stain
Astwood test
ATPase stain
atropine suppression test
attenuated culture
AHT (augmented histamin test)
augmented histamine test
auramine O fluorescent stain
auramine-rhodamine stain
autohemolysis test
Autolet blood glucose test
automated cell image analysis
automated multiphasic screening
automated reagin test
Autopath QC test
avidin-biotin detection system
azan stain
AZT (Ascheim-Zondek test)
azure-eosin stain
B72.3 stain
babesiosis serological test
Bachman-Pettit test
bacitracin disk test
background count
Bactalert FAN culture medium
BACTEC blood culture system
bacterial antigen detection method
bacterial culture
bacterial killing assay
bacterial serology
bacterial stain
bacteriological index
bacteriophage typing
Baker acid hematein test
Baker pyridine extraction test
Balamuth culture medium
Barany caloric test
barium test

Barr body test
basic fuchsin-methylene blue stain
basophil degranulation test
Bauer chromic acid leucofuchsin stain
Beard test
Beaver direct smear method
Becker antigen
Becker stain for spirochetes
Beckman assay
BEI test
Belke-Kleihauer stain
Bence Jones protein test
Benedict test
Benedict test for glucose
Bennhold Congo red stain
bentiromide test
BFT (bentonite flocculation test)
bentonite flocculation test
benzidine test
Ber-EP4 immunoperoxidase stain
Berg stain
Bernstein test
Berson test
Best carmine stain
Bethe stain
Bethesda Pap smear
Betke stain
Betke-Kleihauer test
Bettendorff test
Beutler test
Bial test
bicarbonate titration test
bicolor guaiac test
Bielschowsky stain
bile acid tolerance test
bile esculin test
bile fluid examination
bile pigment test
bile salt breath test
bile solubility test
bile-esculin hydrolysis test
bilirubin tolerance test
Binz test
biochemical profile
biologic assay
biological assay
Biondi-Heidenhain stain
biotin streptavidin detection method
bipolar stain
Birch-Hirschfeld stain
biuret test
blastogenesis assay
blastomycosis serology

bleeding time
blind test
block diagram
blood cell count
blood count
blood culture
blood gas analysis
blood smear
blood typing
blood urea nitrogen test
blood volume nomogram
blood-clot lysis time
Bloor test
blot test
Blount test
Bloxam test
Boas test
Bodian copper-PROTARGOL stain
body fluid analysis
Bonanno test
bone marrow aspiration and biopsy
bone marrow biopsy
bone marrow differential count
BGTT (borderline glucose tolerance test)
borderline glucose tolerance test
Borrel blue stain
Bouin fluid
Bowie stain
Bowie stain
Boyden chamber assay device
Bradshaw test
breakpoint analysis
breast biopsy
breath analysis test
Breed smear
Breslow malignant melanoma assay
Broders tumor index
bromocriptine suppression test
bromphenol test
bromsulphalein test
bronchial aspirate anaerobic culture
bronchial washings cytology
bronchoscopic smear
Brown-Brenn stain
Brown-Hopp tissue Gram stain
brucella agglutination test
brushings cytology
BSFR test
BSP excretion test
buccal smear
buccal smear for sex chromatin evaluation

buffy coat smear study
buffy coat smear test
burn culture
burn index
butanol extractable iodine assay
butanol-extractable iodine test
butyrate esterase stain
C lactose test
C-banding stain
C-F test
C-glycoholic acid breath test
C-peptide test
C-reactive protein assays
C-reactive protein test
C_1q immune Complex detection
CA 19–9 assay
CA125 assay
CA15-3 RIA test
Cache Valley virus
Cajal astrocyte stain
Cajal gold sublimate stain
calcitonin assay
calcium ionized assay
calcium oxalate test
calcium time
calcofluor white stain
California encephalitis virus titer
Callison fluid
Calmette test
CAMP test
Candida precipitin test
candidiasis serologic test
capillary fragility test
capon-comb-growth test
carbamazepine assay
carbohydrate antigen
carbohydrate fermentation test
carbohydrate identification test
carbohydrate metabolism index
carbohydrate utilization test
carbol fuchsin stain
carbol-thionin stain
carbon 13-labeled ketoisocaproate breath test
carbon dioxide combining power test
carboxyhemoglobin assay
cardiac index
Cardiac T Rapid assay
Carr-Price test
cartesian nomogram
Casoni intradermal test
Castellani test
catalase test

catatorulin test
catecholamine test
CD4/CD8 count
CEA assay
CEA immunoperoxidase stain
CEA-M stain
CEA-P stain
cell block preparation
cell count
cell culture
cell cycle time
cell volume profile
cell wall defective bacteria culture
cell-mediated lympholysis assay
centigram
centimeter-gram-second system
centromere banding stain
cephalic index
cephalin flocculation test
cephalin-cholesterol flocculation test
cerebrospinal fluid analysis
cerebrospinal fluid assays
cerebrospinal fluid culture
cerebrospinal fluid cytology
ceruloplasmin test
cervical culture
cervical mucus sperm penetration test
    (Penetrak)
cervical smear
cervical/vaginal cytology
cetylpyridium chloride test
CF antibody titer
CF test
CFF test
Chagas disease serological test
Chédiak test
chemical inhibition isoamylase test
chemiluminescence test
chemistry profile
chemotherapeutic index
Chemstrip bG test
Chen test
chenodeoxycholic acid test
chi-squared test
Chick-Martin test
Chlamydia culture
Chlamydia group titer
Chlamydia trachomatis direct FA test
Chlamydiazyme EIA assay
Chlamydiazyme test
chlorazol black E stain
CAT (chlormerodrin accumulation test)
chlormerodrin accumulation test

cholecystokinin test
cholesterol test
cholesterol-lecithin flocculation test
cholinesterase test
chondroitin sulfate stain
chorioallantoic culture
chorionic gonadotropin test
ChrA immunoperoxidase stain
chromaffin reaction test
chromate stain for lead
chromatogram
chrome alum hematoxylin-phloxine
    stain
chromogenic cephalosporin test
chromogenic enzyme substrate test
chromosome analysis
chymotrypsin stain
Ciaccio fluid
Ciaccio stain
circulation time
cis/trans test
citrate test
Clark test
Clarke fluid
Clauberg test
clean-catch urine culture
clinicopathologic analysis
Clinitest stool test
clomiphene test
clonidine suppression test
cloning inhibitory factor
clonogenic assay
Clostridium difficile toxin assay
clot retraction time
clot-lysis time
CLOtest test
clotting time
CMV culture
coagulase test
coagulation factor
coagulation factor assay
coagulation time test
coagulogram
Coblentz test method
cocaine metabolite assay
coccidioidin test
cold agglutinin screen
cold agglutinin test
cold agglutinin titer
cold hemolysin test
colloidal gold test
colloidal iron stain
colonic smear

colony-forming unit-culture
color index
Color Index
Coloscreen Self test
Colour Index
comb-growth test
combined pituitary function test
compartmental analysis
compatibility test
competitive protein-binding assay
compile time
complement binding assay
complement chemotactic factor
complement direct Coombs test
Coombs test
CT (Coombs test)
CFT (complement-fixation test)
complement-fixation test
complement lysis sensitivity test
complete blood count
compressed spectral assay
concentration test
cone biopsy
CCAT (conglutinating complement absorption test)
conglutinating complement absorption test
Congo red stain
Congo red test
conjunctival culture
conjunctival fungus culture
continuous flow culture
contrast stain
Coombs test
copper reduction test
copper-binding protein test
coproporphyrin assay
coproporphyrin test
cord blood screen
Corner-Allen test
coronary prognostic index
corrected retention time
corrected reticulocyte count
cortisol assay
CGTT (cortisone-glucose tolerance test)
cortisone-glucose tolerance test
COGTT (cortisone-primed oral glucose tolerance test)
cortisone-primed oral glucose tolerance test
Corynebacterium diphtheriae throat culture
cosyntropin test

Covalink MicroElisa culture plate
Coxsackie A virus titer
Coxsackie B virus titer
creatine kinase test
creatinine clearance test
cresyl blue brilliant stain
cresyl violet stain
critical flicker fusion test
critical path analysis
crowded cell index
cryocrit
cryptococcal antigen titer
Cryptococcus antibody titer
crystal-induced chemotactic factor
C&S test
CSF glutamine test
CT-guided stereotactic biopsy
cul-de-sac smear
Cult-Dip Plus bacteriologic culture
culture and sensitivity test
culture media
cutaneous tuberculin test
cutireaction test
cyanide-ascorbate test
cyanide-nitroprusside test
cyclic AMP test
cyst fluid cytology
cystic fibrosis test
cysticercosis titer
cystinuria test
Cyto-Rich cervical cytology monolayer system
cytochrome oxidase test
cytologic screening
cytologic smear
cytology
cytomegalic inclusion disease cytology
cytomegalovirus culture
cytometric image analysis
cytospin analysis
cytospin slide centrifuge Gram-stained smear
cytotropic antibody test
D-dimer assay
D-dimer test
D-PAS stain
D-xylose absorption test
D-xylose tolerance test
Da Fano stain
DA pregnancy test
Dale-Laidlaw clotting time method
Dane and Herman keratin stain
DAPI stain

Darrow red stain
Davidsohn differential absorption test
Day test
De Castro fluid
dead time
DeBakey aortic assay
decimal reduction time
deferoxamine mesylate infusion test
degenerative index
Del Rio Hortega stain
Delafield hematoxylin stain
deoxyribonuclease test
deoxyribonucleic acid stain
deoxyuridine suppression test
depramine assay
dermatophyte test medium
DST (dexamethasone suppression test)
dexamethasone suppression test
dextrose test
DFA-TP test
ECT (euglobulin clot test)
FAT (fluorescent antibody test)
DAPT (direct agglutination pregnanct test)
DAGT (direct antiglobulin test)
DHEA test
DHT test
Diagnex Blue test
diaminobenzidine stain
diazepam breath test
diazo stain for argentaffin granules
Dick test
Dieterle stain
Diff-Quik smear
differential agglutination titer
differential count
differential leukocyte count
differential renal function test
differential stain
differential ureteral
catheterization test
differential white blood count
dilution test
dinitrophenylhydrazine test
direct agglutination pregnancy test
direct agglutination test
direct antiglobulin test
direct bilirubin test
DCT (direct Coombs test)
direct Coombs test
direct culture
direct fluorescent antibody stain
direct fluorescent antibody test

direct fluorescent antibody test—*Treponema pallidum*
direct fluorescent antibody—*Treponema pallidum* test
direct fluorescent assay
disaccharide tolerance test
discriminant analysis
disk diffusion test
displacement analysis
dithionite test
Dixon test
DNase test
Dold test
Donath-Landsteiner test
Donné test
DOPA stain
Dorner stain
dot blot test
double antibody immunoassay
double antibody method
double antibody precipitation
double antibody sandwich assay
double diffusion test
double (gel) diffusion precipitin test in one dimension
double (gel) diffusion precipitin test in two dimensions
double stain
doubling time
doxepin hydrochloride assay
Dragendorff test
drug abuse screen
drug screening assay
DT (dye test)
Du-pan2 stain
Ducrey test
Ducry intradermal test
Duffy antibodies, Fy^a, Fy^b
Duffy antigen
Duffy blood group system
Duke bleeding time
Duke bleeding time test
Duke method of bleeding time
Dunnet multiple component test
duodenal smear
dye exclusion test
dye excretion test
dye test
E erythrocyte rosette assay
E-rosette test
EAC rosette assay
ear culture
eastern equine encephalitis virus titer

EBV culture
echinococcosis serological test
ectocervical smear
edrophonium chloride test
edrophonium test
effusion cytology
Ehrlich acid hematoxylin stain
Ehrlich aniline crystal violet stain
Ehrlich test
Ehrlich triacid stain
Ehrlich triple stain
Einarson gallocyanin-chrome alum
  stain
elastica-van Gieson stain
elastin stain
elective culture
electroblot analysis
electropherogram
electrophoresis test
electrophoretogram
electrotransfer test
Elek test
ELISA titer assay
Ellsworth-Howard test
Emmens S/L test
endemic index
endocervical smear
endometrial cytology
endometrial smear
endometrium anaerobic culture
enrichment culture
Entamoeba histolytica serological test
enterovirus culture
enzyme-linked antibody test
enzyme-linked immunosorbent assay
eosin stain
eosinophil count
eosinophil smear
eosinophilic index
EP test
Epics Profile flow cytometer
Epstein-Barr virus antibody assay
Epstein-Barr virus culture
Epstein-Barr virus serology
Eranko fluorescence stain
Erlanger and Gasser peripheral nerve
  assay
erythrocyte adherence test
erythrocyte fragility test
erythrocyte, antibody, and complement
  rosette assay
erythrocytic series
erythropoietin test

esculin hydrolysis test
esophageal acid infusion test
esophageal smear
ESR assay
esterase test
estradiol test
estrogen receptor assay
ethanol gelation test
ethidium bromide stain
euglobulin clot lysis time
euglobulin clot test
euglobulin lysis test
euglobulin lysis time
ExacTech blood glucose meter test
excisional biopsy
execution time
exfoliative cytology
extracellular fluid volume
factor assay
factor VIII-related antigen test
FANA test
Farber test
Farr test
Farrant mounting fluid
fast smear
fat absorption test
fat, fecal test
fatty acid profile
febrile agglutination test
fecal leukocyte count
fecal occult blood test
Fehling test
female genital tract cytologic smear
fermentation test
fern test
ferric ammonium sulfate stain
ferric chloride test
ferric ferricyanide reduction test
ferritin assay
fetal hemoglobin test
Feulgen stain
Feulgen test
Fevold test
FGT cytologic smear
fibrin degradation products method
fibrin stain
fibrin titer
fibrin-split product
fibrin-stabilizing factor test
fibrinogen method
fibrinogen titer test
Field rapid stain
FIGLU excretion test

filament-nonfilament count
filariasis peripheral blood preparation
filariasis serological test
filter paper microscopic test
Filtracheck-UTI disposable colormetric bacteriuria detection system
fine needle aspiration biopsy
Fink-Heimer stain
Finn chamber patch test
Fischer exact test
Fishberg concentration test
Fisher exact test
Fite-Faraco stain
flask culture
Flaujeac factor
flecainide
Fleitmann test
Flemming triple stain
flocculation test
flow cytometric reticulocyte analysis
fluorescence plus Giemsa stain
fluorescent antibody darkfield
fluorescent antibody technique
fluorescent antibody test
fluorescent antinuclear antibody test
fluorescent cytoprint assay
fluorescent gonorrhea test cytologic smear
fluorescent stain
fluorescent treponemal antibody-absorption test
fluorescent-treponemal antibody absorption test
foam stability test
folded-cell index
Folin-Looney test
Fontana methenamine silver stain
Fontana-Masson silver stain
Foot reticulin impregnation stain
forced expiratory spirogram
formiminoglutamic acid test
formol-gel test
Forssman antigen-antibody reaction
Foshay test
Fouchet stain
Fouchet test
Fourier analysis
fragility test
Francis skin test
Fraser-Lendrum stain for fibrin
free thyroxine index
free triiodothyronine index
Frei test

Friedländer stain for capsules
Friedman test
frog test
fructose assay
fructose test
FSH assay
FSH-RH assay
FTA-ABS test
fuchsin stain
fungal antibody screen
fungal stain
Fungalase-F stain
fungi smear
fungus culture
G-6-PD test
G-banding stain
Gaddum and Schild test
galactose assay
galactose breath test
galactose tolerance test
gastric analysis
gastric aspirate cell count
gastric emptying time
gastric function test
gastric smear
gastrin assay
gastrin-calcium infusion stimulation test
gastrin-protein stimulation test
gastrin-secretin stimulation test
Gastroccult test
gastrointestinal blood loss test
gastrointestinal protein loss test
gastrointestinal series
gel diffusion precipitin test
gel diffusion precipitin tests in one dimension
gel diffusion precipitin tests in two dimensions
Gendre fluid
gene frequency
gene mapping
gene-arrangement study
generation time
genetic abnormality analysis
genetic linkage analysis
genetic mapping
genetic marker
genetic screening
genetic susceptibility
genital culture
gentian orange stain
gentian violet stain
Geraghty test

Gerhardt test for acetoacetic acid
Gerhardt test for urobilin in the urine
germ tube test
GGT assay
Gibson-Cooke sweat test
Giemsa chromosome banding stain
Gill hematoxylin stain
Gill #2 hematoxylin blue stain
Gimenez stain
GITT (glucose insulin tolerance test)
Glenner-Lillie stain for pituitary
glial fibrillary acidic protein
glucagon test
glucose insulin tolerance test
glucose oxidase paper strip test
glucose tolerance test
glucose-6-phosphate dehydrogenase
 screen
glucose-6-phosphate dehydrogenase test
glutathione stability test
glycine assay
glycogen stain
glycogen storage test
glycolic acid test
glycolipid stain
glycoprotein stain
glycosylated hemoglobin test
glycyltryptophan test
glyoxylic acid test
Gmelin test
GMS stain
Gofman test
gold sol test
Golgi stain
Gomori aldehyde fuchsin stain
Gomori chrome alum hematoxylin-
 phloxine stain
Gomori methenamine-silver stain
Gomori nonspecific acid phosphatase
 stain
Gomori nonspecific alkaline phosphatase stain
Gomori one-step trichrome stain
Gomori silver impregnation stain
Gomori trichrome stain
Gomori-Jones periodic
 acid-methenamine-silver stain
Gomori-Takamatsu stain
gonadotropin test
gonorrhea culture
Goodpasture stain
Gordon and Sweet stain
Gordon test

Göthlin capillary fragility test
Graham-Cole test
grain count halving time
Gram iodine
gram ion
Gram method
Gram stain
Gram stain of stool
Gram-negative broth
Gram-positive identification
Gram-Sure reagent
Gram-Weigert stain
granulocytic series
graphic analysis
Gravindex pregnancy test
gravity-settling culture
grid index
grid ratio
Gridley stain for fungi
Grimelius argyrophil stain method
Grimelius stain
Grocott-Gomori methenamine-silver
 stain
group A Beta-hemolytic streptococci
 throat culture
GSC (gravity settling culture)
GTT (glucose tolerance test)
guaiac test
guinea pig kidney absorption test
Gunning-Lieben test
Günzberg test
Guthrie bacterial inhibition assay
Guthrie test
Gutzeit test
Haagensen test
Haenszel test
hair analysis
Hale colloidal iron stain
halothane assay
Ham test
Hamel test
Hammarsten test
hamster egg penetration assay
hamster egg penetration test
Hanger test
hanging-block culture
hanging-drop culture
Hansel stain
haptoglobin test
Harris and Ray test
Harris test
Harrison test
HATTS test

HDL cholesterol assay
HDRA (histoculture drug response assay)
H&E stain
head space analysis
HEAT (human erythrocyte agglutination test)
heat coagulation test
heat instability test
heat labile test
heat precipitation test
heavy metal screen
heavy metal screening test
Heidenhain azan stain
Heidenhain iron hematoxylin stain
Heinz body stain
Heinz body test
Helicobacter pylori serology
Helicobacter pylori urease test and culture
Helisal rapid blood test
helium equilibration time
Helly fluid
hemadsorption virus test
hemagglutination assay
hemagglutination inhibition assay
hemagglutination test
hemagglutination titer
hemagglutination treponemal test for syphilis (HATTS)
hemagglutination-inhibition test
hematein test
hematopenic index
hematoxylin and eosin stain
hematoxylin-eosin stain
hematoxylin-malachite green-basic fuchsin stain
hematoxylin-phloxine B stain
hemoccult test
hemoglobin F assay
hemoglobin H assay
hemogram
hemolytic index
hemolytic plaque assay
HemoQuant fecal blood test
hemosiderin stain
hemosiderinuria test
Henry fructose test
hepatic function test
hepatitis B surface antigen test
hepatitis C serology
hepatitis D serology
herpes cytology

herpes simplex virus culture
herpes simplex virus isolation
heterophil antibody test
heterophil antigen reaction
hexachlorophene assay
HHF-35 stain
Hicks-Pitney thromboplastin generation test
Hinton test
hippuric acid excretion test
Hirsch-Peiffer stain
Hiss stain
Histalog test
histamine flare test
histamine test
histochemical stain
histoculture drug response assay (HDRA)
Histoplasma antibody assay
histoplasmin-latex test
histoplasmosis serology
HIT (hemagglutination-inhibition test)
HIV culture
HIV I serology
HIV-antibody test
HIVAGEN test
HLA typing
Hoffman test
Hofmeister test
Hogben test
Hollander test
Holmes stain
homocystinuria test
homogentisic acid test
homologous series
homovanillic acid test
Hooker-Forbes test
Hopkins-Cole test
Hoppe-Seyler test
hormonal evaluation
Hortega neuroglia stain
Howard test
Howell prothrombin test
HRS4 MAb immunoperoxidase stain
HSV simplex culture
Hucker-Conn stain
Huddleston agglutination test
Huhner test
human chorionic gonadotropin injection test
human erythrocyte agglutination test
human immunodeficiency virus culture
human papillomavirus DNA probe test

HVA test
hydroxybutyric test
hydroxyproline index
hypercoagulable state coagulation
    screen
hypersensitivity pneumonitis serology
IAT (invasive activity test, iodine-azide
    test)
ice water calorics test
ICG excretion test
icteric index
icterus index test
Ide test
idiogram
IgG index
image analysis
image cytology
image display and analysis
immune adherence hemagglutination
    assay
immune adhesion test
immune assay
immune complex assay
immunoblot test
immunochemical assay
immunoconcentration assay
immunoenzymometric assay
immunofluorescence assay
immunofluorescence test
immunofluorescent assay
immunofluorescent stain
immunoglobulin A, D, G, M test
immunohistochemical stain
immunologic pregnancy test
immunoperoxidase stain
immunoperoxidase test
immunoradiometric assay
implantation test
impression preparation
IMViC test (indole, methyl red, Voges-
    Proskauer, and citrate tests)
in vivo compatibility test
index case
index of refraction
index register
India ink capsule stain
India ink preparation
India ink stain
indican test
indigo-carmine test
indirect assay
indirect bilirubin test
indirect Coombs test

indirect fluorescent antibody test
indirect fluorescent rabies antibody test
indirect hemagglutination test
indole test
indole, methyl red, Voges-Proskauer,
    and citrate tests
indophenol test
infectious mononucleosis screening test
infertility screen
influenza A and B titer
influenza virus culture
inhibition test
inhibitor assay
insulin clearance test
insulin hypoglycemia test
insulin sensitivity test
insulin tolerance test
inter-α-globulin
interference test
International Normalized Ratio
International Sensitivity Index
intracellular fluid volume
intradermal test
intraesophageal pH test
intravascular coagulation screen
intravenous glucose tolerance test
intravenous tolbutamide tolerance test
intravital stain
invasive activity test
iodine stain
iodine test
iodine-131 uptake test
iodine-azide test
ionogram
ionopherogram
iron hematoxylin stain
iron index
iron stain
iron-binding capacity test
islet cell antibody screening test
isocitrate dehydrogenase test
isoiodeikon test
Isolator blood culture system
isoniazid phenotype test
isopropanol precipitation test
IST (insulin sensitivity test)
IT (implantation test, intradermal test)
ITT (insulin tolerance test)
Ito-Reenstierna test
IVGTT (intravenous glucose tolerance
    test)
IVTTT (intravenous tolbutamide toler-
    ance test)

Ivy bleeding time test
Ivy method of bleeding time
Ivy template bleeding time
Jacquemin test
Jaffe assay
Jaffe test
Jansky human blood group classification
Jenner stain
Jenner-Giemsa stain
Jerne plaque assay
Jolles test
Jones-Cantarow test
juxtaglomerular granulation index
Kahn test
kaolin partial thromboplastin time
kaolin clotting time
karyopyknotic index
Kasten fluorescent Feulgen stain
Kasten fluorescent PAS stain
Katayama test
Kato thick smear technique
Kell blood group system
Kenyon stain
keratin stain
ketogenic corticoids test
ketone bodies tests
Kidd blood group system
kidney profile
kidney stone analysis
KINEX anatomic specimen stand
Kinyoun carbol fuchsin stain
Kirby-Bauer test
Kittrich stain
Kleihauer acid elution test
Kleihauer stain
Kleihauer-Betke test
Klinger-Ludwig acid-thionin stain for sex chromatin
Klüver-Barrera Luxol fast blue stain
Knodell histological activity index
Kober test
Kobert test
KOH preparation
KOH test
Kolmer test
Kolmer test with Reiter protein
Kossa stain
Kovats index
Kowarsky test
Krebs leukocyte index
Krokiewicz test
Kronecker stain

Kruskal-Wallis test
KS test (Kveim-Stilzbach test)
Kunkel test
Kurzrok-Ratner test
Kveim test
Kveim-Stilzbach test
labeling index
lactic dehydrogenase test
Lactobacillus bulgaricus factor
lactose tolerance test
Ladendorff test
lag time
LAIT (latex agglutination-inhibition test)
Laki-Lorand factor
Lancefield precipitation test
Landsteiner-Donath test
Lange colloidal gold test
LAP stain
LAP test
Laquer stain for alcoholic hyalin
large vessel hematocrit
lateral vaginal wall smear
latex agglutination test
latex agglutination-inhibition test
latex fixation test
latex flocculation test
latex screen
latex slide agglutination test
LATS test
Lawless stain
LDL cholesterol assay
LE cell test
lead hydroxide stain
lecithin-sphingomyelin ratio determination
Lee-White clotting test
Lee-White clotting time
Lee-White clotting time method
left-to-right ratio
Legal test
Legionella pneumophila culture
Legionella pneumophila direct FA smear
Leishman stain
leishmaniasis serological test
Leitz image analysis system
Lendrum inclusion body stain
Lendrum phloxine-tartrazine stain
Lepehne-Pickworth stain
lepromin skin test
Leptospira culture
Leptospira serodiagnosis

LET (leukocyte esterase test)
Leu-M1 immunoperoxidase stain
leucine aminopeptidase test
leukocyte acid phosphatase stain
leukocyte adherence assay test
leukocyte bactericidal assay test
leukocyte differential count
leukocyte esterase test
leukocyte histamine release test
leukogram
leukopenic index
Leukostat stain
leukotactic assay
Levaditi stain
Levine alkaline Congo red stain
Levinson test
levulose tolerance test
LFT (liver function test, latex flocculation test)
Liebermann-Burchard test
Lillie allochrome connective tissue stain
Lillie azure-eosin stain
Lillie ferrous iron stain
Lillie sulfuric acid Nile blue stain
Limulus amebocyte lysate assay
limulus lysate test
Limulus test
line test
lipase 105 stain
lipase 21 stain
lipase test
lipid profile
lipid test
lipoprotein electrophoresis test
Lison-Dunn stain
liver flocculation test
liver function test
liver profile
Loeffler blood culture medium
Loeffler caustic stain
long-acting thyroid stimulating hormone test
long-acting thyroid-stimulator hormone assay
Löwenthal test
lower respiratory tract smear
Lücke test
Lugol stain
Luna-Ishak stain
lupus band test
lupus erythematosus cell test
Lutheran blood group system
Luxol fast blue stain

Lyme disease serology
lymph node biopsy
lymphocyte microcytotoxicity assay
lymphocyte transfer test
lymphocyte transformation test
lymphocytic series
lymphogranuloma venereum titer
lymphoid series
lysozyme test
M-DES stain
Macchiavello stain
Machado-Guerreiro test
MacNeal tetrachrome blood stain
macrophage migration inhibition test
magnesium test
malaria film test
malaria smear
malarial pigment stain
Maldonado-San Jose stain
malignant catarrhal fever virus
mallein test
Mallory aniline blue stain
Mallory collagen stain
Mallory iodine stain
Mallory phloxine stain
Mallory phosphotungstic acid hematoxylin stain
Mallory stain for actinomyces
Mallory stain for hemofuchsin
Mallory trichrome stain
Mallory triple stain
Malmejde test
Mancini iodine stain
Mann methyl blue-eosin stain
Mantoux skin test
Marchi stain
Masson argentaffin stain
Masson trichrome stain
Masson-Fontana ammoniacal silver stain
Master 2-step test
maturation index
maximal Histalog test
Maximow stain for bone marrow
May-Grünwald-Giemsa stain
Mayer acid alum hematoxylin stain
Mayer hemalum stain
Mayer mucicarmine stain
Mayer mucihematein stain
Mazzotti test
McNemar test
McPhail test
mean circulation time

mean circulatory hematocrit
mean generation time
median detection threshold
Meinicke test
Meissel stain
melanin test
melanogen test
metabisulfite test
metacarpal index
metachromatic stain
metanephrine test
methanol test
methenamine silver stain
methionine test
methyl green-pyronin stain
methyl red test
methylene blue stain
methylene blue test
Metopirone test
metrotrophic test
metyrapone stimulation test
metyrapone test
MHA-TP test
microbiological assay
microdiffusion analysis
Microflow test
microhemagglutination assay
microhemagglutination-*Treponema pallidum* test
microimmunofluorescent test
microlymphocytotoxicity assay
microprecipitation test
microsomal thyroid antibody test
microtoxicity assay
Middlebrook-Dubos hemagglutination test
Mielke bleeding time
migration inhibition test
migration inhibitory factor test
Milligan trichrome stain
Millon-Nasse test
mitosis-karyorrhexis index
mitotic index
mixed agglutination test
mixed culture
mixed leukocyte culture
mixed lymphocyte culture reaction
mixed lymphocyte culture test
MLC test
mobilization test
Molisch test
Moloney test
Mono-Diff test

monocyte function test
monohistiocytic series
Monoscreen test
Monospot test
Monosticon Dri-Dot test
Montenegro skin test
Mörner test
Mosenthal test
motility test
Motulsky dye reduction test
Movat pentachrome stain
Mowry colloidal iron stain
MSB trichrome stain
mucicarmine stain
mucin clot test
mucopolysaccharide stain
mucopolysaccharide test
mucoprotein test
Mulder test
multiphasic screening
multiple-puncture tuberculin test
multiple stain
multivariate analysis of variance
mumps antibody titer
mumps sensitivity test
mumps serology
mumps skin test antigen
mumps virus culture
Murex *Candida albicans* CA50 test
Murphy-Pattee test
muscle biopsy
Musto stain
mutagenicity test
MY-10 clone stain
MycoAKT latex bead agglutination test
mycobacteria culture
Mycoplasma serology
myeloid series
myeloperoxidase stain
myoglobin test
Nakanishi stain
naphthol-ASD chloroacetate esterase stain
Napier formol-gel test
nasal smear
nasopharyngeal culture
Nauta stain
NBT test
needle aspiration cytology
needle culture
Neisser stain
Neisseria gonorrhoeae culture
Neisseria gonorrhoeae smear

neonatal screening
neoprecipitin test
nephelometric inhibition assay
net protein utilization
neutral stain
neutralization test
newborn screen
niacin test
Nickerson-Kveim test
Nickerson-Kveim test reaction
Nicklès test
Nicolle stain for capsules
Nile blue fat stain
ninhydrin-Schiff stain for proteins
nipple discharge cytology
Nissl stain
nitrate reduction test
nitrate utilization test
nitroblue tetrazolium stain
nitroblue tetrazolium test
nitropropiol test
nitroprusside test
nitroso-indole-nitrate test
NLT (normal lymphocyte transfer test)
Noble stain
Nocardia culture
nomogram
nonpermissive culture media
nonprotein nitrogen test
normal lymphocyte transfer test
Northern blot analysis
Northern blot test
Novelli stain
NPT (neoprecipitin test)
NSE stain
NT (neutralization test)
nuclear fast red stain
nuclear stain
nucleoplasmic index
Obermayer test
Obermüller test
occlusion time
occult blood test
OCT (oxytocin challenge test)
ocular cytology
oil red O stain
oleic acid uptake test
oligodendroglia stain
one-tailed test
ONPG test
O&P test
opsonic index
Optochin susceptibility test

oral cavity cytology
oral glucose tolerance test
oral lactose tolerance test
oral smear
OraSure HIV-1 Oral Specimen Collection Device
orcein stain
orcinol test
organ culture
Orth fluid
osazone test
osmium tetroxide stain
osmotic fragility test
Ouchterlony test
ovarian ascorbic acid depletion test
oxalic acid stain
oxidase test
oxidation-fermentation test
oxyhemogram
oxytalan fiber stain
oxytocin challenge test
P and P test (prothrombin and proconvertin test)
P blood group
p-aminohippurate clearance test
P-K test (Prausnitz-Küstner test)
Padykula-Herman stain for myosin ATPase
Paget test
Paget-Eccleston stain
Palmgren silver impregnation stain
pancervical smear
pancreatic islet cell antibody test
pancreatic islet stain
pancreozymin-secretin test
Pandy test
panoptic stain
PAP immunoperoxidase stain
Pap smear
Pap stain
Pap test
Papanicolaou smear
Papanicolaou smear test
Papanicolaou stain
paper radioimmunosorbent test
PAPI stain
Pappenheim stain
paracarmine stain
paracoagulation test
Paragon blue stain
parainfluenza antibody test
parainfluenza viral serology
parainfluenza virus culture

parasite screen
partial thromboplastin time test
particle transport time
PAS stain
PAS test
passive cutaneous anaphylaxis test
passive hemagglutination test
patch test
Paul test
Paul-Bunnell test
penicillinase test
pentagastrin test
perchlorate discharge test
pericardial fluid examination
periodic acid-Schiff (method, reaction, stain, technique, test)
peripheral blood preparation
peripheral blood smear
peritoneal fluid examination
Perls Prussian blue stain
Perls test
permissive culture media
peroxidase stain
pertussis serology
Petri test
phagocytic cell immunocompetence profile
phagocytic index
PharmChek seat patch drug detection test
phenacetin breath test
phenobarbital assay
phenolphthalein test
phenolsulfonphthalein test
phentolamine test
phenylalanine test
phenylalanine tolerance index
phenylketonuria test
phenylpyruvic acid test
phloxine-tartrazine stain
phosphatase test
phosphate excretion index
phospholipid test
phosphomolybdic acid stain
phosphoric acid test
phosphotungstic acid stain
photo-patch test
photopeak detection efficiency
phthalein test
phytohemagglutinin assay
Piazza test
picrate test
picric stain

picro-Mallory trichrome stain
picrocarmine stain
picronigrosin stain
pinworm preparation
Pirquet cutaneous tuberculin test
pituitary function test
PKU test
placental and fetoplacental function tests
plant protease test
plaque-forming cell assay
plasma clotting time
plasma hemoglobin test
plasma protein fraction
plasma stain
plasma-iron disappearance time
plasmacrit test
plasmatic stain
plasmic stain
plasminogen activator inhibitor assay
plastic section stain
plate culture
platelet adhesion test
platelet adhesiveness test
platelet aggregation test
platelet count
platelet retention test
pleural fluid examination
polarogram
polychrome methylene blue stain
polyethylene glycol precipitation assay
Pontamine sky blue stain
Porges-Meier test
Porges-Salomon test
porphyrin test
Porter-Silber chromogens test
Porteus maze test
positive stain
positive whiff test
potassium hydroxide test
potassium metabisulfate stain
potassium permanganate stain
PPD skin test
PPT (plant protease test)
Prausnitz-Kustner test
precipitation test
precipitin test
Precision QI-D handheld blood glucose test
Precision-G handheld blood glucose test
predictive value of negative test
predictive value of positive test
pregnancy test

prenatal screening
presumptive heterophil test
primary culture
primed lymphocyte typing
progesterone receptor assay
program evaluation and review technique
prolactin test
proliferative index
prolonged bleeding time
prolonged coagulation time
proportional count
prostaglandin test
protamine sulfate test
protamine titration test
Protargol stain
protection test
protein assay
protein bound iodine assay
protein separation method
protein synthesis
protein test
protein-bound iodine test
protein-bound iodine-131 test
prothrombin and proconvertin test
prothrombin consumption test
prothrombin consumption time
prothrombin time
prothrombin time test
prothrombokinase factor
Protocult test
protoporphyrin test
provocative chelation test
provocative Wassermann test
Prower-Stuart factor
Prussian blue stain
PSFR assay
psittacosis titer
PTA stain
PTAH stain
PTH assay
Puchtler-Sweat stain
Puchtler-Sweat stain for basement
    membranes
Puchtler-Sweat stain for hemoglobin
    and hemosiderin
pulmonary function test
punch biopsy
pure culture
purified protein derivative
purified protein derivative of tuberculin
purified protein derivative-standard
purine bodies test

pyknotic index
pyrrol blue stain
Q fever titer
Q-banding stain
qualitative analysis
quantitation test
quantitative analysis
Queckenstedt test
quellung test
Quick test
QuickVue Chlamydia test
quinacrine chromosome banding stain
quinine carbacrylic resin test
Quinlan test
R-banding stain
RA latex fixation test
rabbit test
Radford nomogram
radioactive iodide uptake test
radioactive iodine uptake test
radioallergosorbent assay test
RAST (radioallergosorbent test)
radiochromatogram
radioenzymatic assay
radioimmunoprecipitation assay
radioimmunosorbent test
radioisotopic culture
radioligand assay
radioreceptor assay
radiosensitivity test
RAI test (radioactive iodine)
Raji cell radioimmune assay
Rambourg chromic acid-phospho-
    tungstic acid stain
Rambourg periodic acid-chromic
    methenamine-silver stain
random plasma glucose test
random urine specimen
rank sum test
Ranson pyridine silver stain
Rapid ANA II test
rapid plasma reagin test
RapiTex Hp test
Rapoport test
radioallergosorbent assay test
radioallergosorbent test
rat ovarian hyperemia test
ratio scale
reaction time
reactone red test
recalcification time
red blood cell count
red cell adherence test

red cell count
red cell survival test
red test
Rees culture medium
Rees-Ecker fluid
refractive index
Reid index
Reinsch test
Reiter protein complement-fixation test
relative retention time
relative value index
renal function test
renal venous renin assay
renin assay
reptilase-R time
resolving time
resorcinol test
respiratory syncytial virus antibody test
respiratory syncytial virus antigen test
respiratory syncytial virus culture
respiratory syncytial virus serology
Response GM granulocyte count
retention index
retention time
reticulin stain
reticulocyte count
reticulocytic production index
reticulum stain
Reuss test
Rh blocking test
Rh typing
rheumatoid factor reaction
rheumatoid factor test
$Rh_o(D)$ typing
rhodanine stain
riboflavin loading test
rice-flour breath test
Rimini test
ring precipitin test
Rinne test
Rio-rad protein assay
RISA test
RIST (radioimmunosorbent test)
Roche Septi-Chek blood culture system
Rocky Mountain spotted fever antibody
   test
Rocky Mountain spotted fever serology
Romanowsky blood stain
Römer test
Ropes test
rose bengal radioactive (^{131}I) test
Rose-Waaler test
Rosenbach-Gmelin test

rosette test
Ross-Jones test
rotavirus serology
Rotazyme test
Rothera nitroprusside test
Rotter test
Rous test
routine test dilution
Roux stain
Rowntree and Geraghty test
RPCFT (Reiter protein complementa-
   tion-fixation test)
RPR test
RST (radiosensitivity test)
RSV culture
rubella antibody test
rubella HI test
rubella serology
rubella virus culture
rubeola serology
Rubner test
Rumpel-Leede test
Russell viper venom clotting time
Russell viper venom time
RV time
S-CCK-Pz test
Sabin-Feldman dye test
Sachs-Georgi test
salicylic acid test
saline agglutination test
Salmonella titer
Sanford test
SART test
saturation analysis
saturation index
Saundby test
scalene node biopsy
scarification test
scarlet red stain
SCAT (sheep cell agglutination test)
scatter diagram
scattergram
Schaeffer-Fulton stain
Schaffer test
Schick test
Schick test toxin
Schiff stain
Schiller test
Schilling blood count
Schilling index
Schilling test
Schirmer test
schistosomiasis serological test

Schmorl ferric-ferricyanide reduction
   stain
Schmorl picrothionin stain
Schönbein test
Schultz stain
Schultz-Dale test
Schumm test
Schwarz test
scintillation count
scratch test
screening test
SCT (sex chromatin test, staphylococcal
   clumping test)
secondary culture
secretin pancreozymin test
secretin-CCK stimulation test
sedimentation index
sedimentation test
SeHCAT test
selective stain
Selivanoff test
semen analysis
semiquantitative analysis
semiquantitative viral culture
Septi-Chek culture system
sequential analysis
Sereny test
serial cardiac isoenzyme assay
serial thrombin time
serodiagnosis
serologic test for syphilis
serology test
serum alkaline phosphatase test
serum amylase test
serum bacterial test
serum bactericidal test
serum globulin test
serum protein electrophoresis test
serum prothrombin time
Sevier-Munger stain
sex chromatin test
shake culture
shake test
sheep cell agglutination test
Shorr trichrome stain
shortened bleeding time
shortened coagulation time
Sia test
sickle cell test
Sickledex test
Sicklequik test
sickling test
side platelet aggregation test

siderocyte stain
Siggaard-Andersen alignment nomogram
signed rank test
silver-ammoniacal silver stain
silver nitrate stain
silver nitroprusside test
silver protein stain
silver-ammoniacal silver stain
Sims-Huhner test
single diffusion test
single (gel) diffusion precipitin test in
   one dimension
single (gel) diffusion precipitin test in
   two dimensions
single human leukocyte antigen
skin fungus culture
skin mycobacteria culture
skin test
skin test unit
skin window test
skin-puncture test
skin-reactive factor
slant culture
slope culture
SMA-12 profile test
SMAC test
smear background
smear preparation and staining for
   blood parasites
Snook reticulum stain
sodium bisulfite stain
sodium chloride (6.5 %) culture
   medium
sodium hydroxide stain
sodium test
sodium thiosulfate stain
solubility test
Southern blot analysis
Southern blot test
SPAT (side platelet aggregation test)
SPCA factor
sperm penetration assay
spinal fluid culture
spinal fluid leukocyte count
spirogram
spironolactone test
splenic index
split renal function test
spodogram
sporotrichosis serology
spot test
spot test for infectious mononucleosis

sputum culture
sputum cytology
sputum fungus culture
sputum mycobacteria culture
sputum smear
squamous cell index
St. Louis encephalitis virus serology
stab culture
Staclot Protein S test kit
Stamey test
standard serologic tests for syphilis
standard test for syphilis
standing plasma test
Staph-Ident test
Staph-Trac test
staphyloopsonic index
staphylococcal clumping test
Staphylococcus aureus nasopharyngeal culture
starch tolerance test
stem cell assay
stereotactic brain biopsy
sterility culture
sterility test broth
Sterneedle tuberculin test
steroid protein activity index
Stirling modification of Gram stain
stock culture
Stoll dilution egg count technique
stool culture
stool fungus culture
stool mycobacteria culture
Strassburg test
streak culture
streptococcal antigen test
streptozyme test
Student-Newman-Keuls test
Stypven time
Stypven time test
sucrose hemolysis test
Sudan black B fat stain
Sudan black stain
sugar water test screen
Sulkowitch test
superoxide assay
supravital stain
swab specimen
sweat test
synaptophysin stain
synchronized culture
synovial fluid analysis
synovial fluid examination

systolic time interval
Syva EMIT-II assay
T and B lymphocyte subset assay
TAT (thromboplastin activation test)
T method stain
t test
T_3 uptake test
T_3U test
T_4 newborn screen
Taenzer-Unna stain
Takata-Ara test
Takayama stain
tanned red cell hemagglutination inhibition test
T/B lymphocyte assay
TB smear
TBT (tolbutamide test)
TCPI Rapid HIV test
telomeric R-banding stain
Tes-Tape urine glucose test
test of significance
test profile
test solution
test statistic
tetrachrome stain
tetramethylbenzidine stain
tetrazolium test
TFT (thyroid function test)
TGT (thromboplastin generation test)
Thayer-Martin test
thermal death time
thermostable opsonin test
thiazine stain
thin-needle biopsy
ThinPrep cytologic preparation
ThinPrep cytology
thioflavine T stain
thionin stain
Thompson test
Thormählen test
Thorn test
three-glass test
throat culture
thrombin clotting time
thrombin time
thrombin time test
thrombocytic series
thromboelastogram
thromboplastin activation test
thromboplastin generation test
thromboplastin generation time
thromboplastin substitution test
thrust culture

thymol turbidity test
thyroid function test
thyroid suppression test
thyroid uptake test
thyroid-stimulating hormone assay
thyroid-stimulating hormone stimulation test
thyrotropin-releasing hormone stimulation test
thyroxine assay
thyroxine-binding globulin assay
thyroxine-binding index
thyroxine-binding index test
TIBC test
Tilden stain
time diffusion technique
time of maximum concentration
time-tension index
tine test
tissue culture
tissue culture medium
tissue thromboplastin inhibition time
tissue typing
titratable acidity test
Tizzoni stain
Toison stain
tolbutamide tolerance test
toluidine blue stain
Töpfer test
total body hematocrit
total catecholamine test
total cell count
total protein
total ridge count
total serum protein
total thyroxine
toxoplasmosis serology
TPH test
TPHA test
TPI assay
TPI test
transaminase test
transferred antigen-cell-bound antibody reaction
transferred antigen-transferred antibody reaction
transferrin test
Treponema pallidum hemagglutination test
Treponema pallidum immobilization assay
Treponema pallidum immobilization test

treponemal immobilization test
TRH stimulation test
trichinosis serology
Trichomonas preparation
trichrome stain
triiodothyronine resin uptake test
triiodothyronine suppression test
triple test
Truant auramine-rhodamine stain
trypsin G-banding stain
trypsin test
tryptophan load test
TSH stimulating test
TSH stimulation test
TST (tumor skin tumor)
TTT (tolbutamide tolerance test)
tube culture
tube dilution test
tubeless gastric analysis test
tuberculin test
tuberculoopsonic index
tuberculosis skin test
tumor skin test
Turnbull blue stain
TWAR-stain
two-glass test
two-stage PT test
two-tailed test
type culture
typhus antibody test
typing
tyramine test
tyrosine test
Tzanck smear
Tzanck test
Uffelmann test
unheated serum reagin test
univariate analysis
Unna-Pappenheim stain
Unna-Taenzer stain
uranyl acetate stain
urate crystals stain
urea clearance test
urea nitrogen test
ureaplasma urealyticum genital culture
urease test
urease test broth
uricolytic index
Uricult dipslide test
urinary concentration test
urinary smear
urine acetone test
urine culture

urine cytology
urine fungus culture
urine mycobacteria culture
urine specimen collection
Uriscreen test
urobilinogen test
uroporphyrin test
Uriscreen urine specimen bacteriuria
   detection system
vaginal irrigation smear
Valentine test
van Deen test
van den Bergh test
van der Velden test
van Ermengen stain
van Gieson stain
Van Slyke test
vanillylmandelic acid test
varicella-zoster antibody test
varicella-zoster virus culture
varicella-zoster virus serology
VCE smear
VDRL test
Vecta-Stain Elite ABC system
Vecta-Stain Universal Elite ABC kit
Vecta-Stain Universal Quick kit
Venn diagram
venous hematocrit
Verhoeff elastic tissue stain
viable cell count
vimentin immunoperoxidase stain
viral culture
ViraPap test
vital stain
vitamin A clearance test
vitamin B_{12} absorption test
vitamin B_6 assay
VMA test
Voges-Proskauer test
volatile organic substances assay
volatile screen
Volhard test
Vollmer test
volume index
von Kossa calcium assay
von Kossa stain
von Willebrand factor multimer assay
VP test
VZV culture
Wachstein-Meissel stain for
   calcium-magnesium-ATPase
Wade-Fite-Faraco stain
Wagner test

Wako NEFA test kit
Waldenström test
WAMPOLE ISOLATOR blood culture
   system
Wang test
Warthin-Starry silver stain
wash time
washing cytology
Wasséen test
Wassermann test
water-gurgle test
Watson-Schwartz test
Wayson stain
Weber test
Webster test
Weigert iron hematoxylin stain
Weigert stain for actinomyces
Weigert stain for elastin
Weigert stain for fibrin
Weigert stain for myelin
Weigert stain for neuroglia
Weigert-Gram stain
Weigert-Pal stain
Weil myelin sheath stain
Weil-Felix test
Welcozyme HIV 1&2 ELISA antibody
   test
Werner test
Westergren sedimentation rate test
Western blot analysis
Western blot test
western equine encephalitis virus serol-
   ogy
Western immunoblot test
Wetzel test
wheal reaction time
wheal-and-erythema skin tests
Wheeler-Johnson test
whiff test
white blood cell count
white cell count
whole-blood clotting time
whole-blood hematocrit
Widal test
Wilder stain for reticulum
Williams stain
wire loop test
Wormley test
wound culture
Wright stain
Wurster test
xylose absorption test
xylose concentration test

xylose test
Yvon test
Zamboni fluid
Zenker fluid
zeta sedimentation ratio method
zetacrit
Ziehl stain
Zimmermann test

zinc flocculation test
zinc turbidity test
zinc-sulfate turbidity test
Zollinger-Ellison test
zona-free hamster egg penetration
  test
Zsigmondy test
zymogram

Show-Hong Duh, Ph.D., D.A.B.C.C. / Gladys Alonsozana, M.D.

Reference range values are for apparently healthy individuals and often overlap significantly with values for persons who are sick. Actual values may vary significantly due to differences in assay methodologies and standardization. Institutions may also set up their own reference ranges based on the particular populations that they serve; thus there can be regional differences. Consequently, values reported by individual laboratories may differ from those listed in this appendix.

All values are given in conventional and SI units. However, where the SI units have not been widely accepted, conventional units are used. In case of the heterogenous nature of the materials measured or uncertainty of the exact molecular weight of the compounds, the SI system cannot be followed, and mass per volume is used as the unit of concentration.

ABBREVIATIONS

ACD, acid-citrate-dextrose; **CHF**, congestive heart failure; **Cit**, citrate; **CNS**, central nervous system; **CSF**, cerebrospinal fluid; **cyclic AMP**, adenosine 3': 5'- cyclic phosphate; **EDTA**, ethylenediaminetetraacetic acid; **HDL**, high-density lipoprotein; **Hep**, heparin; **LDL-C**, low-density lipoprotein-cholesterol; **Ox**, oxalate; **RBC**, red blood cell(s); **RIA**, radioimmunoassay; **SD**, standard deviation

REFERENCES

Reference Intervals. In: Tietz Textbook of Clinical Chemistry. 2nd ed. Burtis CA, Ashwood ER, eds. Philadelphia: WB Saunders, 1994.

Hematologic Values. In: Clinical Hematology and Fundamentals of Hemostasis. 2nd ed. Harmening DM, ed. Philadelphia: FA Davis, 1992.

National Cholesterol Education Program. Report of the expert panel on detection, evaluation, and treatment of high blood cholesterol in adults. Arch Intern Med 1988;148:36-69.

Department of Pathology. Clinical Chemistry Laboratory: 'Reference Range Values in Clinical Chemistry. Professional services manual. Baltimore: University of Maryland Medical System, 1993.

Triglyceride, High Density Lipoprotein, and Coronary Heart Disease. National Institutes of Health Consensus Statement, NIH Consensus Development Conference, 1992;10 (2).

Tests	Conventional Units	SI Units
Acetaminophen, serum or plasma (Hep or EDTA)		
Therapeutic	10–30 μg/mL 66–199 μmol/L	
Toxic	>200 μg/mL	>1324 μmol/L
Acetone		
Serum		
Qualitative	Negative	Negative
Quantitative	0.3–2.0 mg/dL	3–20 mg/L
Urine		
Qualitative	Negative	Negative
N-Acetylprocainamide, serum or plasma (Hep or EDTA); trough		
Therapeutic	5–30 μg/mL	18–108 μmol/L
Toxic	>40 μg/mL	>144 μmol/L
Acid hemolysis test (Ham)	No hemolysis	No hemolysis
Adrenocorticotropin (ACTH), plasma		
6 AM	10–80 pg/mL	10–80 ng/L
6 PM	<50 pg/mL	<50 ng/L
Alanine aminotransferase (see Transaminase)		
Albumin		
Serum		
Adult	3.5–5.0 g/dL	35–50 g/L
>60 y	3.4–4.8 g/dL	34–48 g/L
	Avg. of 0.3 g/dL higher in upright individuals	Avg. of 3 g/L higher in upright individuals
Urine		
Qualitative	Negative	Negative
Quantitative	10–100 mg/24 h	10–100 mg/24 h
CSF	10–30 mg/dL	100–300 mg/L
*Aldolase, serum	0–11 U/L (30°C)	Same
Aldosterone		
Serum		
Supine	3–10 ng/dL	0.08–0.3 nmol/L
Standing		
Male	6–22 ng/dL	0.17–0.61 nmol/L
Female	5–30 ng/dL	0.14–0.8 nmol/L
Urine	3–20 μg/24 h	8.3–55 nmol/24 h
Alpha amino nitrogen		
Serum	3.0–5.5 mg/dL	2.1–3.9 mmol/L
Urine	50–200 mg/24 h	3.6–14.3 nmol/24 h
Amikacin, serum or plasma (EDTA)		
Therapeutic		
Peak	25–35 μg/mL	43–60 μmol/L
Trough		
Less severe infection	1–4 μg/mL	1.7–6.8 μmol/L
Life-threatening infection	4–8 μg/mL	6.8–13.7 μmol/L
Toxic		
Peak	>35–40 μg/mL	>60–68 μmol/L
Trough	>10–15 μg/mL	>17–26 μmol/L
δ-Aminolevulinic acid, urine	1.3–7.0 mg/24 h	10–53 μmol/24 h
Amitriptyline, serum or plasma (Hep or EDTA); trough (≥12 h after dose)		

*Test values are method dependent.

Tests	Conventional Units	SI Units
Therapeutic	120–250 ng/mL	433–903 nmol/L
Toxic	>500 ng/mL	>1805 nmol/L
Ammonia nitrogen		
Plasma	15–45 µg/dL	11–32 µmol/L
Urine	140–1500 mg/d	10–107 mmol/d
Amylase		
Serum	25–125 mIU/mL	25–125 U/L
Urine	1–17 U/h	Same
Amylase/creatinine clearance ratio	1–4%	0.01–0.04
Anion gap	8–16 mEq/L	8–16 mmol/L
Arsenic		
Whole blood (Hep)	0.2–6.2 µg/dL	0.03–0.83 µmol/L
Chronic poisoning	10–50 µg/dL	1.33–6.65 µmol/L
Acute poisoning	60–930 µg/dL	7.98–124 µmol/L
Urine, 24 h	5–50 µg/d	0.07–0.67 µmol/d
Ascorbic acid, blood	0.4–1.5 mg/dL	23–85 µmol/L
Aspartate aminotransferase (see Transaminase)		
Base excess, blood	0 ± 2 mEq/L	0 ± 2 mmol/L
Bicarbonate, serum	23–29 mEq/L	23–29 mmol/L
Bile acids, serum	0.3–3.0 mg/dL	3.0–30.0 mg/L
Bilirubin		
Serum		
Adults		
Conjugated	0.0–0.3 mg/dL	0–5 µmol/L
Unconjugated	0.01–1.1mg/dL	0–19 µmol/L
Delta	0–0.2 mg/dL	0–3 µmol/L
Total	0.2–1.3 mg/L	3–22 µmol/L
Neonates		
Conjugated	0–0.6 mg/dL	0–10 µmol/L
Unconjugated	0.6–10.5 mg/dL	10–180 µmol/L
Total	1.0–10.5 mg/dL	1.7–180 µmol/L
Urine, qualitative	Negative	Negative

Bone marrow, differential cell count	Range (%)	Average (%)	Range	Average
Myeloblasts	0.3–5.0	2.0	0.003–0.05	0.02
Promyelocytes	1.0–8.0	5.0	0.01–0.08	0.05
Myelocytes				
Neutrophilic	5.0–19.0	12.0	0.05–0.19	0.12
Eosinophilic	0.5–3.0	1.5	0.005–0.03	0.015
Basophilic	0.0–0.5	0.3	0.00–0.005	0.003
Metamyelocytes	13.0–32.0	22.0	0.13–0.32	0.22
Polymorphonuclear neutrophils	7.0–30.0	20.0	0.07–0.30	0.20
Polymorphonuclear eosinophils	Range (%) 0.5–4.0	Average (%) 2.0	Range 0.005–0.04	Average 0.02
Polymorphonuclear basophils	0.0–0.7	0.2	0.00–0.007	0.002
Lymphocytes	3.0–17.0	10.0	0.03–0.17	0.10
Plasma cells	0.0–2.0	0.4	0.00–0.02	0.004
Monocytes	0.5–5.0	2.0	0.005–0.05	0.02
Reticulum cells	0.1–2.0	0.2	0.001–0.02	0.002
Megakaryocytes	0.3–3.0	0.4	0.003–0.03	0.004
Pronormoblasts	1.0–8.0	4.0	0.01–0.08	0.04
Normoblasts	7.0–32.0	18.0	0.07–0.32	0.18

*Test values are method dependent.

Tests	Conventional Units		SI Units
Cadmium, whole blood (Hep)	0.1–0.5 µg/dL		0.89–4.45 nmol/L
Toxic	10–300 µg/dL		0.89–26.70 µmol/L
Cadmium, urine, 24 h	<15 µg/d		<0.13 µmol/d
Calcium, serum	8.4–10.2 mg/dL		2.1–2.6 mmol/L
	(Slightly higher in children)		(Slightly higher in children)
Calcium, ionized, serum	4.65–5.28 mg/dL		1.16–1.32 mmol/L
Calcium, urine			
Low-calcium diet	<150 mg/24 h		<3.8 nmol/24 h
Usual diet; trough	<250 mg/24 h		<6.3 nmol/24 h
Carbamazepine, serum or plasma (Hep or EDTA)			
Therapeutic	8–12 µg/mL		34–51 µmol/L
Toxic	>15 µg/mL		>63 µmol/L
Carbon dioxide, total, serum/ plasma (Hep)	22–29 mmol/L (lower in children)		Same
Carbon dioxide tension (Pco_2), blood	35–45mm Hg		35–45 mm Hg
Carbon monoxide as carboxyhemoglobin (HbCO), whole blood (EDTA)			
Nonsmokers	0.5–1.5% total Hb		0.005–0.015 HbCO fraction
Smokers			
1–2 packs/d	4–5% total Hb		0.04–0.05 HbCO fraction
>2 packs/d	8–9% total Hb		0.08–0.09 HbCO fraction
Toxic	>20% total Hb		>0.20 HbCO fraction
Lethal	>50% total Hb		>0.5 HbCO fraction
Carotene, serum	40–200 µg/dL		0.74–3.72 µmol/L
*Catecholamines, urine			
Epinephrine	<10 µg/24 h		<55 nmol/24 h
Norepinephrine	<100 µg/24 h		<590 nmol/24 h
Total free catecholamines	4–126 µg/24 h		24–745 nmol/24 h (as norepinephrine)
Total metanephrines	0.1–1.6 mg/24 h		0.5–8.1 µmol/24 h (as metanephrine)
Cell counts (Coulter)			
Erythrocytes			
Males	$4.7–6.1 \times 10^6$/µL		$4.7–6.1 \times 10^{12}$/L
Females	$4.2–5.4 \times 10^6$/µL		$4.2–5.4 \times 10^{12}$/L
Children (varies with age)	$3.8–5.5 \times 10^6$/µL		$3.8–5.5 \times 10^{12}$/L
Leukocytes			
Total	$4.8–10.8 \times 10^3$/µL		$4.8–10.8 \times 10^9$/L
Differential	*Percentage*	*Absolute*	
Myelocytes	0	0/µL	0/L
Band neutrophils	3–5	150–400/µL	$150–400 \times 10^6$/L
Segmented neutrophils	54–62	3000–5800/µL	$3000–5800 \times 10^6$/L
Lymphocytes	25–33	1500–3000/µL	$1500–3000 \times 10^6$/L
Monocytes	3-7	300–500/µL	$300–500 \times 10^6$/L
Eosinophils	1–3	50–250/µL	$50–250 \times 10^6$/L
Basophils	0-0.75	15–50/µL	$15–50 \times 10^6$/L
Platelets	$150–450 \times 10^3$/µL	$150–450 \times 10^9$/L	
Reticulocytes	25,000–75,000/µL	$25–75 \times 10^9$/L	
	0.5–1.5% of erythrocytes		
Cells, CSF	<5/µL (all mononucleocytes)		Same

*Test values are method dependent.

Tests	Conventional Units	SI Units
*Ceruloplasmin, serum	23–44 mg/dL	230–440 mg/L
Chloramphenicol, serum or plasma (Hep or EDTA); trough		
Therapeutic	10–25 μg/mL	31–77 μmol/L
Toxic	>25 μg/mL	>77 μmol/L
Chloride		
Serum	96–106 mmol/L	Same
Sweat		
Normal	0–30 mmol/L	Same
Cystic fibrosis	60–200 mmol/L	Same
Urine, 24 h (vary greatly with Cl intake)		
Infant	2–10 mmol/d	Same
Child	14–50 mmol/d	Same
Adults	110–250 mmol/d	Same
CSF	120–130 mmol/L (20 mmol/L higher than serum)	Same
Cholesterol, serum	Recommended desirable range: <200 mg/dL	Recommended desirable range: <5.2 mmol/L
	Borderline range: 200–239 mg/dL	Borderline range: 5.2–6.2 mmol/L
Cholinesterase		
Serum	0.5–1.3 pH units	0.5–1.3 pH units
Erythrocytes	0.5–1.0 pH unit	0.5–1.0 pH unit
*Chorionic gonadotropin, β-subunit (β-hCG)		
Serum or plasma (EDTA)		
Male and nonpregnant female	<3.0 IU/L	Same
Female, postconception		
7-10 d	>3.0 IU/L	Same
30 d	100–5000 IU/L	Same
40 d	>2000 IU/L	Same
10 wk	50,000–140,000 IU/L	Same
14 wk	10,000–50,000 IU/L	Same
Trophoblastic disease	>100,000 IU/L	Same
Urine, 24 h		
Male and nonpregnant female	0 IU/d	Same
Pregnancy (wk)		
6th	13,000 U/d (mean)	Same
8th	30,000 U/d (mean)	Same
12–14th	105,000 U/d (mean)	Same
16th	46,000 U/d (mean)	Same
Thereafter	5,000–20,000 U/d (mean)	Same
Clonazepam, serum or plasma (Hep or EDTA); trough		
Therapeutic	15–60 ng/mL	48–190 nmol/L
Toxic	>80 ng/mL	>254 nmol/L
Coagulation tests		
Antithrombin III (synthetic substrate)	80–120% of normal	0.8–1.2 of normal
Bleeding time (Duke)	0–6 min	0–6 min
Bleeding time (Ivy)	1–6 min	1–6 min
Bleeding time (template)	2.3–9.5 min	2.3–9.5 min
Clot retraction, qualitative	Begins in 30–60 min Complete in 24 h	Begins in 30–60 min Complete in 24 h

*Test values are method dependent.

Tests	Conventional Units	SI Units
Coagulation time (Lee-White)	5–15 min (glass tubes) 19–60 min (siliconized tubes)	5–15 min (glass tubes) 19–60 min (siliconized tubes)
Cold hemolysin test (Donath-Landsteiner)	No hemolysis	No hemolysis
Complement components		
Total hemolytic complement activity, plasma (EDTA)	75–160 U/mL or >33% of plasma CH50	75–160 kU/L Fraction of CH50 : >0.33
Total complement decay rate (functional), plasma (EDTA)	10–20% Deficiency: >50%	Fraction decay rate: 0.10–0.20 >0.50
$C1_q$, serum	5.1–7.9 mg/dL	51–79 mg/L
$C1_r$, serum	2.2–4.6 mg/dL	22–46 mg/L
$C1_s$(C1 esterase), serum	2.1–4.1 mg/dL	21–41 mg/L
C2, serum	1.9–2.5 mg/dL	19–25 mg/L
C3, serum	83–177 mg/dL	830–1770 mg/L
C4, serum	12–36 mg/dL	120–360 mg/L
C5, serum	3.8–9.0 mg/dL	38–90 mg/L
C6, serum	4.0–7.2 mg/dL	40–72 mg/L
C7, serum	4.9–7.0 mg/dL	49–70 mg/L
C8, serum	4.3–6.3 mg/dL	43–63 mg/L
C9, serum	4.7–6.9 mg/dL	47–69 mg/L
Coombs' test		
Direct	Negative	Negative
Indirect	Negative	Negative
Copper		
Serum		
Males	70–140 µg/dL	11–22 µmol/L
Females	85–155 µg/dL	13–24 µmol/L
Urine	0–50 µg/24 h	0–0.80 µmol/24 h
Corpuscular values of erythrocytes (values are for adults; in children, values vary with age)		
Mean corpuscular hemoglobin (MCH)	27–31 pg	0.42–0.48 fmol
Mean corpuscular hemoglobin concentration (MCHC)	33–37 g/dL	330–370 g/L
Mean corpuscular volume (MCV)	80-96 µ³ 80-96 fL	
Cortisol		
Plasma		
8 AM	5–23 µg/dL	138–635 nmol/L
4 PM	3–16 µg/dL	82–441 nmol/L
10 PM	<50% of 8 AM value	<0.5 of 8 AM value
Free, urine	10–100 µg/24 h	27.6–276 mmol/24 h
Creatine		
Serum	0.2–0.8 mg/dL	15–61 µmol/L
Urine		
Males	0–40 mg/24 h	0–0.30 mmol/24 h
Females	0–100 mg/24 h (Higher in children and pregnant women)	0–0.76 mmol/24 h (Higher in children and pregnant women)
*†Creatine kinase, serum (CK, CPK)		
White		
Male	60–320 U/L (37°C)	Same

*Test values are method dependent.

†Test values are race dependent.

Tests	Conventional Units	SI Units
Female	50–200 U/L (37°C)	Same
Black		
Male	130–450 U/L (37°C)	Same
Female	60–270 U/L (37°C)	Same
*Creatine kinase MB isoenzyme, serum	0–5 ng/mL	Same
*Creatinine enzymatic		
Serum or plasma, adult		
Male	0.7–1.3 mg/dL	62–115 µmol/L
Female	0.6–1.1 mg/dL	53–97 µmol/L
Urine		
Male	14–26 mg/kg body weight/24 h	0.12–0.23 mmol/kg body weight/24h
Female	11–20 mg/kg body weight/24 h	0.10–0.18 mmol/kg body weight/24 h
*Creatinine clearance, enzymatic		
Males	90–139 mL/min/1.73 m²	0.87–1.34 mL/s/m²
Females	80–125 mL/min/1.73 m²	0.77–1.2 mL/s/m²
Cryoglobulins, serum	0	0
Cyanide		
Serum		
Nonsmokers	0.004 mg/L	0.15 µmol/L
Smokers	0.006 mg/L	0.23 µmol/L
Nitroprusside therapy	0.01–0.06 mg/L	0.38–2.30 µmol/L
Toxic	>0.1 mg/L	>3.84 µmol/L
Whole blood (Ox)		
Nonsmokers	0.016 mg/L	0.61 µmol/L
Smokers	0.041 mg/L	1.57 µmol/L
Nitroprusside therapy	0.05–0.5 mg/L	1.92–19.20 µmol/L
Toxic	>1 mg/L	>38.40 µmol/L
Cyclic AMP		
Plasma (EDTA)		
Males	4.6–8.6 ng/mL	14–26 nmol/L
Females	4.3–7.6 ng/mL	13–23 nmol/L
Urine, 24 h	0.3–3.6 mg/d or 0.29–2.1 mg/g creatinine	1.0–10.9 µmol/d or 100–723 µmol/mol creatinine
Cystine or cysteine, urine, qualitative	Negative	Negative
*C-Peptide, serum	0.78–1.89 ng/mL	0.26–0.62 nmol/L
*C-Reactive protein, serum		
Cord blood	1–35 µg/dL 10–350 µg/L	
Adult	6.8–820 µg/dL	68–8200 µg/L
*≠Cyclosporine, whole blood		
Therapeutic, trough	100–200 ng/mL	83–166 nmol/L
Dehydroepiandrosterone, urine	<15% of total 17–ketosteroids	<15% of total 17–ketosteroids
Males	0.2–2.0 mg/24 h	0.7–6.9 µmol/24 h
Females	0.2–1.8 mg/24 h	0.7–6.2 µmol/24 h
Desipramine, serum or plasma (Hep or EDTA); trough (12 h after dose)		
Therapeutic	75–300 ng/mL	281–1125 nmol/L
Toxic	>400 ng/mL	>1500 nmol/L
Diazepam, serum or plasma (Hep or EDTA); trough		
Therapeutic	100–1000 ng/mL	0.35–3.51 µmol/L

*Test values are method dependent.
≠Actual therapeutic range should be adjusted for individual patient.

Tests	Conventional Units	SI Units
Toxic	>5000 ng/mL	>17.55 µmol/L
Digitoxin, serum or plasma (Hep or EDTA); 6 h after dose		
Therapeutic	20–35 ng/mL	26–46 nmol/L
Toxic	>45 ng/mL	>59 nmol/L
Digoxin, serum or plasma (Hep or EDTA); 12 h after dose		
Therapeutic		
CHF	0.8–1.5 ng/mL	1.0–1.9 nmol/L
Arrhythmias	1.5–2.0 ng/mL	1.9–2.6 nmol/L
Toxic		
Adult	>2.5 ng/mL	>3.2 nmol/L
Child	>3.0 ng/mL	>3.8 nmol/L
Disopyramide, serum or plasma (Hep or EDTA); trough		
Therapeutic arrhythmias		
Atrial	2.8–3.2 µg/mL	8.3–9.4 µmol/L
Ventricular	3.3–7.5 µg/mL	9.7–22 µmol/L
Toxic	>7 µg/mL >20.7 µmol/L	
Doxepin, serum or plasma (Hep or EDTA); trough (≥ 12 h after dose)		
Therapeutic	30–150 ng/mL	107–537 nmol/L
Toxic	>500 ng/mL	>1790 nmol/L
Electrophoresis, CSF	Predominantly albumin	Predominantly albumin
Estrogens, urine		
Males		
Estrone	3–8 µg/24 h	11–30 nmol/24 h
Estradiol	0–6 µg/24 h	0–22 nmol/24 h
Estriol	1–11 µg/24 h	3–38 nmol/24 h
‡Total	4–25 µg/24 h	14–90 nmol/24 h
Females		
Estrone	4–31 µg/24 h	15–115 nmol/24 h
Estradiol	0–14 µg/24 h	0–51 nmol/24 h
Estriol	0–72 µg/24 h	0–250 nmol/24 h
‡Total	5–100 µg/24 h (Markedly increased during pregnancy)	18–360 nmol/24 h (Markedly increased during pregnancy)
Ethanol, whole blood (Ox) or serum		
Depression of CNS	>100 mg/dL	>21.7 mmol/L
Fatalities reported	>400 mg/dL	>86.8 mmol/L
Ethosuximide, serum or plasma (Hep or EDTA); trough		
Therapeutic	40–100 µg/mL	283–708 µmol/L
Toxic	>150 µg/mL	>1062 µmol/L
Euglobulin lysis time	2–6 h at 37°C	2–6 h at 37°C
Factor VIII and other coagulation factors	70–150% of normal	0.70–1.5 of normal
Fibrin split products (Thrombo–Wellco test)	<10 µg/mL	<10mg/L
Fibrinogen	200–400 mg/dL	5.9–11.7 µmol/L

‡Assuming a mixture of estrone, estradioles, and estriol in a molecular proportion of 2:1:2.

Tests	Conventional Units	SI Units
Fibrinolysins	0	Same
Partial thromboplastin time, activated (APTT)	20–35 sec	Same
Prothrombin consumption	Over 80% consumed in 1 h	Over 0.80 consumed in 1 h
Prothrombin content	100% (calculated from prothrombin time)	1.0 (calculated from prothrombin time)
Prothrombin time (one stage)	12.0–14.0 sec	Same
Tourniquet test	Ten or fewer petechiae in a 2.5 cm circle after 5 min	Same
Fat, fecal, F, 72 h		
Infant, breast–fed	<1 g/d	Same
0–6 y	<2 g/d	Same
Adult	<7 g/d	Same
Adult (fat–free diet)	<4 g/d	Same
§Fatty acids, total, serum	190–420 mg/dL	7–15 mmol/L
Nonesterified, serum	8–25 mg/dL	0.30–0.90 mmol/L
Ferritin, serum		
Males	20–250 ng/mL	20–250 µg/L
Females	10–120 ng/mL (higher if postmenopausal)	10–120 µg/L (higher if postmenopausal)
Ferritin values of <20 ng/mL (20 µg/L) have been reported to be generally associated with depleted iron stores		
Fibrinogen, plasma	200–400 mg/dL	5.9–11.7 µmol/L
Fluoride		
Plasma (Hep)	0.01–0.2 µg/mL	0.5–10.5 µmol/L
Urine	0.2–1.1 µg/mL	10.5–57.9 µmol/L
Urine, occupational exposure	<8 µg/mL	<421 µmol/L
Folate, serum	2.2–17.3 ng/mL	5.0–39.2 nmol/L
Erythrocytes	169–707 ng/mL	451–1602 nmol/L
*Follicle-stimulating hormone (FSH), serum		
Males	2.0–17.7 mIU/mL	2.0–17.7 IU/L
Females		
Follicular phase	3.6–16.0 mIU/mL	Same
Midcycle peak	8.1–28.9 mIU/mL	Same
Luteal phase	1.8–11.7 mIU/mL	Same
Postmenopause	22.9–167 mIU/mL	Same
Gastrin, serum		
Males	<100 pg/mL	<100 ng/L
Females	<75 pg/mL	<75 ng/L
Gentamicin, serum or plasma (EDTA)		
Therapeutic		
Peak		
Less severe infection	5–8 µg/mL	10.4–16.7 µmol/L
Severe infection	8–10 µg/mL	16.7–20.9 µmol/L
Trough		
Less severe infection	<1 µg/mL	<2.1 µmol/L
Moderate infection	<2 µg/mL	<4.2 µmol/L
Severe infection	<2–4 µg/mL	<4.2–8.4 µmol/L
Toxic		
Peak	>10–12 µg/mL	>21–25 µmol/L
Trough	>2–4 µg/ml	>4.2–8.4 µmol/L

*Test values are method dependent.
§"Fatty acids" include a mixture of different aliphatic acids of varying molecular weight; a mean molecular weight of 284 daltons has been assumed.

Tests	Conventional Units	SI Units
Glucose (fasting)		
Blood	60–100 mg/dL	3.33–5.55 mmol/L
Plasma or serum	70–115 mg/dL	3.89–6.38 mmol/L
Glucose, 2 h postprandial, serum	<120 mg/dL	<6.7 mmol/L
Glucose, urine		
Quantitative	<500 mg/24 h	<2.8 mmol/24 h
Qualitative	Negative	Negative
Glucose, CSF	50–75 mg/dL (20 mg/dL less than serum)	2.8–4.2 mmol/L (1.1 mmol/L less than serum)
*Glucose-6-phosphate dehydrogenase (G-6-PD) in erythrocytes, whole blood (ACD, EDTA, or Hep)	12.1 ± 2.1 U/g Hb (SD) 351 ± 60.6 U/10^{12} RBC	0.78 ± 0.13 mU/mol Hb 0.35 ± 0.06 nU/RBC
	4.11 ± 0.71 U/mL RBC	4.11 ± 0.71 kU/L RBC
*γ-Glutamyltransferase		
Males	≤50 U/L (37°C)	Same
Females	≤30 U/L (37°C)	Same
Glutethimide, serum		
Therapeutic	2–6 µg/mL	9–28 µmol/L
Toxic	>5 µg/mL	>23 µmol/L
Growth hormone, serum	0–10 ng/mL	0–10 µg/L
Haptoglobin, serum	26–185 mg/dL	260–1850 mg/L
Haptoglobin (as hemoglobin binding capacity)	40–336 mg/dL	0.4–36 g/L
HDL-cholesterol (HDL-C), serum or plasma (EDTA)	Recommended desirable range: >40 mg/dL	Recommended desirable range: >1.04 mmol/L
Borderline: 35–40 mg/dL		
Hematocrit		
Males	42–52%	0.42–0.52
Females	37–47%	0.37–0.47
Newborns	53–65%	0.53–0.65
Children (varies with age)	30–43%	0.30–0.43
Hemoglobin (Hb)		
Males	14.0–18.0 g/dL	2.17–2.79 mmol/L
Females	12.0–16.0 g/dL	1.86–2.48 mmol/L
Newborns	17.0–23.0 g/dL	2.64–3.57 mmol/L
Children (varies with age)	11.2–16.5 g/dL	1.74–2.56 mmol/L
Hemoglobin, fetal	≥1 y old: <2% of total Hb	≥1 y old: <2% of total Hb
Hemoglobin, plasma	0–5.0 mg/dL	0–0.8 µmol/L
Hemoglobin and myoglobin, urine, qualitative	Negative	Negative
Hemoglobin electrophoresis, whole blood (EDTA, Cit or Hep)		
HbA	96–98.6%	0.96–0.986 Hb fraction
HbA$_{1c}$	5.3–7.5%	0.053–0.075 Hb fraction
HbA$_2$	1.5–3.5%	0.015–0.035 Hb fraction
HbF	<2%	<0.02 Hb fraction
Homogentisic acid, urine, qualitative	Negative	Negative
*Hydroxybutyric dehydrogenase serum (HBD)	0–180 mU/mL (30°C)	0–180 U/L (30°C)
17-Hydroxycorticosteroids		
Plasma	8–18 µg/dL	0.22–0.50 µmol/L

*Test values are method dependent.

Tests	Conventional Units	SI Units
Urine		
Males	3–9 mg/24 h	8.3–25 µmol/24 h (as cortisol)
Females	2–8 mg/24 h	5.5–22 µmol/24 h (as cortisol)
5-Hydroxyindoleacetic acid, urine		
Qualitative	Negative	Negative
Quantitative	2–6 mg/24 h	10.4–31.2 µmol/24 h
Imipramine, serum or plasma (Hep or EDTA); trough (≥12 h after dose)		
Therapeutic	125–250 ng/mL	446–893 nmol/L
Toxic	>500 ng/mL	>1785 nmol/L
*Immunoglobulins, serum		
IgG	723–1685 mg/dL	7.2–16.9 g/L
IgA	69–382 mg/dL	0.69–3.8 g/L
IgM	63–277 mg/dL	0.63–2.8 g/L
IgD	0–8 mg/dL	0–80 mg/L
IgE	0–380 IU/mL 0–380 kIU/L	
Immunoglobulin G (IgG), CSF	0.5–6.1 mg/dL	0.5–6.1 g/L
Insulin, plasma (fasting)	5–25 µU/mL 36–179 pmol/L	
*Iron, serum		
Males	65–170 µg/dL	11.6–30.4 µmol/L
Females	50–170 µg/dL	9.0–30.4 µmol/L
Iron binding capacity, serum		
Total 250–450 mg/24 h	45–81 µmol/L43–73	43–73
Saturation	20–55%	0.20–0.55
*Isoenzymes, serum by agarose gel electrophoresis		
Fraction 1	14–26% of total	0.14–0.26 fraction of total
Fraction 2	29–39% of total	0.29–0.39 fraction of total
Fraction 3	20–26% of total	0.20–0.26 fraction of total
Ketosteroids, urine		
Males	8–20 mg/24 h	28–70 µmol/24 h
Females	6–15 mg/24 h (decrease with age)	21–52 µmol/24 h (decrease with age)
L-Lactate		
Plasma (NaF)		
Venous	4.5–19.8 mg/dL	0.5–2.2 mmol/L
Arterial	4.5–14.4 mg/dL	0.5–1.6 mmol/L
Whole blood (Hep), at bed rest		
Venous	8.1–15.3 mg/dL	0.9–1.7 mmol/L
Arterial	3–7 mg/dL	0.36–0.75 mmol/L
Urine, 24 h	496–1982 mg/d	5.5–22 mmol/d
CSF	<25.5 mg/dL <2.8 mmol/L	
*Lactate dehydrogenase (LDH)		
Total (L→P), 37°C, serum		
Newborn	290–775 U/L Same	
Neonate	545–2000 U/L	Same
Infant	180–430 U/L Same	
Child	110–295 U/L Same	
Adult	100–190 U/L Same	
>60 y	110–210 U/L Same	

*Test values are method dependent.

Tests	Conventional Units	SI Units
Fraction 4	8–16% of total	0.08–0.16 fraction of total
Fraction 5	6–16% of total	0.06–0.16 fraction of total
*Lactate dehydrogenase, CSF	10% of serum value	0.10 fraction of serum value
LDL-cholesterol (LDL–C), calculated, serum or plasma (EDTA)	Recommended desirable range for adults: <130 mg/dL	<3.37 mmol/L
Lead,		
Whole blood (Hep)	<10 µg/dL	<0.48 µmol/L
Urine, 24 h	<80 µg/d	<0.39 µmol/d
Lecithin–sphingomyelin (L/S) ratio, amniotic fluid	2.0–5.0 indicates probable fetal lung maturity; > 3.5 in diabetics	Same
*Leucine aminopeptidase, serum	14–40 mU/mL (30°C)	14–40 U/L (30°C)
Lidocaine, serum or plasma (Hep or EDTA); 45 min after bolus dose		
Therapeutic	1.5–6.0 µg/mL	6.4–26 µmol/L
Toxic		
CNS, cardiovascular depression	6–8 µg/mL	26–34.2 µmol/L
Seizures, obtundation, decreased cardiac output	>8 µg/mL	>34.2 µmol/L
*Lipase, serum	23–208 U/L (37°C)	23–208 U/L (37°C)
Lithium, serum or plasma (Hep or EDTA); 12 h after last dose		
Therapeutic	0.6–1.2 mEq/L	0.6–1.2 mmol/L
Toxic	>2 mEq/L	>2 mmol/L
Lorazepam, serum or plasma (Hep or EDTA), therapeutic	50–240 ng/mL	156–746 nmol/L
*Luteinizing hormone (LH), serum		
Males	0.9–10.6 mIU/mL	0.9–10.6 IU/L
Females		
Follicular phase	1.1–11.1 mIU/mL	1.1–11.1 IU/L
Midcycle peak	17.5–72.9 mIU/mL	17.5–72.9 IU/L
Luteal phase	0.4–15.1 mIU/mL	0.4–15.1 IU/L
Postmenopausal	6.8–46.6 mIU/mL	6.8–46.6 IU/L
Magnesium		
Serum	1.3–2.1 mEq/L	0.65–1.05 mmol/L
	1.6–2.5 mg/dL	16–25 mg/L
Urine	6.0–10.0 mEq/24 h	3.0–5.0 mmol/24 h
Mercury		
Whole blood (EDTA)	0.6–59 µg/L	<0.29 µmol/L
Urine, 24 h	<20 µg/d	<0.1 µmol/d
Toxic	>150 µg/d	>0.75 µmol/d
Metanephrines (see Catecholamines)		
Methemoglobin (MetHb, hemoglobin), whole blood (EDTA, Hep or ACD)	0.06–0.24 g/dL or 0.78 ± 0.37% of total Hb (SD)	9.3–37.2 µmol/L or Mass fraction of total Hb: 0.008 ± 0.0037 (SD)
Methotrexate, serum or plasma (Hep or EDTA)		
Therapeutic	Variable	Variable

*Test values are method dependent.

Tests	Conventional Units	SI Units
Toxic		
post IV infusion	24 h <5 µmol/L	Same
48 h	<0.5 µmol/L	Same
72 h	<0.05 µmol/L	Same
Myelin basic protein, CSF	<2.5 mg/mL	<2.5 µg/L
Nortriptyline, serum or plasma		
(Hep or EDTA);		
trough (≥12 h after dose)		
Therapeutic	50–150 ng/mL	190–570 nmol/L
Toxic	>500 ng/mL	>1900 nmol/L
*5′-Nucleotidase, serum	2–17 U/L	Same
Occult blood, feces, random	Negative (<2 mL blood/ 150 g stool/d)	Negative (<13.3 mL blood/ kg stool/d)
Qualitative, urine, random	Negative	Negative
Osmolality		
Serum	275–295 mOsm/kg serum water	285–295 mmol/kg serum water
Urine	50–1200 mOsm/kg water	38–1400 mmol/kg water
Ratio, urine/serum	1.0–3.0, 3.0–4.7 after 12 h fluid restriction	Same
Osmotic fragility of erythrocytes	Begins in 0.45–0.39% NaCl	Begins in 77–67 mmol/L NaCl
	Complete in 0.33– 0.30% NaCl	Complete in 56–51 mmol/L NaCl
Oxazepam, serum or plasma		
(Hep or EDTA),		
therapeutic	0.2–1.4 µg/mL	0.70–4.9 µmol/L
Oxygen, blood		
Capacity	16–24 vol% (varies with hemoglobin)	7.14–10.7 mmol/L (varies with hemoglobin)
Content		
Arterial	15–23 vol%	6.69–10.3 mmol/L
Venous	10–16 vol%	4.46–7.14 mmol/L
Saturation		
Arterial and capillary	95–98% of capacity	0.95–0.98 of capacity
Venous	60–85% of capacity	0.60–0.85 of capacity
Tension		
pO_2 arterial and capillary	83–108 mm Hg	Same
Venous	35–45 mm Hg	Same
P50, blood	25–29 mm Hg (adjusted to pH 7.4)	3.33–3.86 kPa
Pentobarbital, serum or plasma		
(Hep or EDTA);		
trough		
Therapeutic		
Hypnotic	1–5 µg/mL	4–22 µmol/L
Therapeutic coma	20–50 µg/mL	88–221 µmol/L
Toxic	>10 µg/mL	>44 µmol/L
pH		
Blood, arterial	7.35–7.45	Same
Urine	4.6–8.0 (depends on diet)	Same
Phenacetin, plasma (EDTA)		
Therapeutic	1–30 µg/mL	6–167 µmol/L
Toxic	50–250 µg/mL	279–1395 µmol/L

*Test values are method dependent.

Tests	Conventional Units	SI Units
Phenobarbital, serum or plasma (Hep or EDTA); trough		
Therapeutic	15–40 µg/mL	65–170 µmol/L
Toxic		
Slowness, ataxia, nystagmus	35–80 µg/mL	151–345 µmol/L
Coma with reflexes	65–117 µg/mL	280–504 µmol/L
Coma without reflexes	>100 µg/mL	>430 µmol/L
Phenolsulfonphthalein excretion (PSP), urine	28–51% in 15 min	0.28–0.51 in 15 min
	13–24% in 30 min	0.13–0.24 in 30 min
	9–17% in 60 min	0.09–0.17 in 60 min
	3–10% in 2 h	0.03–0.10 in 2 hr
	(After injection of 1 mL PSP intravenously)	(After injection of 1 mL PSP intravenously)
Phenylalanine, serum	0.8–1.8 mg/dL	48–109 µmol/L
Phenylpyruvic acid, urine, qualitative	Negative	Negative
Phenytoin, serum or plasma (Hep or EDTA); trough		
Therapeutic	10–20 µg/mL	40–79 µmol/L
Toxic	>20 µg/mL	>79 µmol/L
*Phosphatase, acid, prostatic, serum		
RIA	<3.0 ng/mL	<3.0 µg/L
*Phosphatase, alkaline		
Leukocyte	Total score: 14–100	Total score: 14–100
Serum (ALP)	20–90 mU/mL (30°C)	20–90 U/L (30°C)
	(Values are higher in children)	(Values are higher in children)
Phosphate, inorganic, serum		
Adults	2.7–4.5 mg/dL	0.87–1.45 mmol/L
Children	4.5–5.5 mg/dL	1.45–1.78 mmol/L
Phosphatidylglycerol (PG), amniotic fluid		
Fetal lung immaturity	Absent	Same
Fetal lung maturity	Present	Same
Phospholipids, serum	125–275 mg/dL	1.25–2.75 g/L
Phosphorus, urine	0.4–1.3 g/24 h	12.9–42 mmol/24 h
Porphobilinogen, urine		
Qualitative	Negative	Negative
Quantitative	<2.0 mg/24 h	<9 µmol/24 h
Porphyrins, urine		
Coproporphyrin	34–230 µg/24 h	52–351 nmol/24 h
Uroporphyrin	<50 µg/24 h	<60 nmol/24 h
Potassium, plasma (Hep)		
Males	3.5–4.5 mEq/L	3.5–4.5 mmol/L
Females	3.4–4.4 mEq/L	3.4–4.4 mmol/L
Potassium		
Serum		
Premature		
Cord	5.0–10.2 mEq/L	5.0–10.2 mmol/L
48 h	3.0–6.0 mEq/L	3.0–6.0 mmol/L
Newborn, cord	5.6–12.0 mEq/L	5.6–12.0 mmol/L
Newborn	3.7–5.9 mEq/L	3.7–5.9 mmol/L
Infant	4.1–5.3 mEq/L	4.1–5.3 mmol/L
Child	3.4–4.7 mEq/L	3.4–4.7 mmol/L

*Test values are method dependent.

Tests	Conventional Units	SI Units
Adult	3.5–5.1 mEq/L	3.5–5.1 mmol/L
Urine, 24 h	25–125 mEq/d, varies with diet	25–125 mmol/d; varies with diet
CSF	70% of plasma level or 2.5–3.2 mEq/L; rises with plasma hyperosmolality	0.70 of plasma level or 2.5–3.2 mmol/L; rises with plasma hyperosmolality
Pregnanediol, urine		
Males	0–1.9 mg/24 h	0–5.9 µmol/24 h
Females		
Follicular phase	<2.6 mg/24 h	<8 µmol/24 h
Luteal phase	2.6–10.6 mg/24 h	8–33 µmol/24 h
Postmenopausal phase	0.2–1.0 mg/24 h	6.2–3.1 µmol/24 h
Pregnanetriol, urine	0.4–2.5 mg/24 h in adults	1.2–7.5 µmol/24 h in adults
Pressure, CSF	70–180 mm H_2O	Same
Primidone, serum or plasma (Hep or EDTA); trough		
Therapeutic	5–12 µg/mL	23–55 µmol/L
Toxic	>15 µg/mL	>69 µmol/L
Procainamide, serum or plasma (Hep or EDTA); trough		
Therapeutic	4–10 µg/mL	17–42 µmol/L
Toxic (also consider effect of metabolite (NAPA)	>10–12 µg/mL	>42–51 µmol/L
*Prolactin, serum		
Males	1.58–23.12 ng/mL	1.58–23.12 µg/L
Females	<0.6–27.33 ng/mL	<0.6–27.33 µg/L
Propoxyphene, plasma (EDTA)		
Therapeutic	0.1–0.4 µg/mL	0.3–1.2 µmol/L
Toxic	>0.5 µg/mL	>1.5 µmol/L
Propranolol, serum or plasma (Hep or EDTA); trough		
Therapeutic	50–100 ng/mL	193–386 nmol/L
*Protein, serum		
Total	6.4–8.3 g/dL	64–83 g/L
Albumin	3.9–5.1 g/dL	39–51 g/L
Globulin		
α_1	0.2–0.4 g/dL	2–4 g/L
α_2	0.5–0.9 g/dL	5–9 g/L
β	0.6–1.1 g/dL	6–11 g/L
γ	0.7–1.7 g/dL	7–17 g/L
Protein		
Urine		
Qualitative	Negative	Negative
Quantitative	50–80 mg/24 h (at rest)	Same
CSF, total	15–40 mg/dL	150–400 mg/dL
Protoporphyrin, free, erythrocyte	17–77 µg/dL packed RBC	0.3–1.37 µmol/L packed RBC
Pyruvate, blood	0.3–0.9 mg/dL	34–103 µmol/L
Quinidine, serum or plasma (Hep or EDTA); trough		
Therapeutic	2–5 µg/mL	6–15 µmol/L
Toxic	>6 µg/mL	>18 µmol/L

*Test values are method dependent.

Tests	Conventional Units	SI Units
Salicylates, serum or plasma (Hep or EDTA); trough		
Therapeutic	150–300 µg/mL	1.09–2.17 mmol/L
Toxic	>500 µg/mL	>3.62 mmol/L
Sedimentation rate		
Wintrobe		
Males	0–10 mm in 1 h	0–5 mm/h
Females	0–20 mm in 1 h	0–15 mm/H
Westergren		
Males	0–15 mm in 1 h	0–15 mm/h
Females	0–20 mm in 1 h	0–20 mm/h
Sodium		
Serum or plasma (Hep)		
Premature		
Cord	116–140 mEq/L	116–140 mmol/L
48 h	128–148 mEq/L	128–148 mmol/L
Newborn, cord	126–166 mEq/L	126–166 mmol/L
Newborn	134–144 mEq/L	134–144 mmol/L
Infant	139–146 mEq/L	139–146 mmol/L
Child	138–145 mEq/L	138–145 mmol/L
Adult	136–146 mEq/L	136–146 mmol/L
Urine, 24 h	40–220 mEq/d (diet dependent)	40–220 mmol/d (diet dependent)
Sweat		
Normal	10–40 mEq/L	10–40 mmol/L
Cystic fibrosis	70–190 mEq/L	70–190 mmol/L
Specific gravity	1.002–1.030	Same
Sulfates, inorganic, serum	0.8–1.2 mg/dL	83–125 µmol/L
*Testosterone, plasma		
Males	300–1000 ng/dL	10.4–34.7 nmol/L
Females	20–75 ng/dL	0.69–2.6 nmol/L
Pregnant females	3–4 times the adult level	Same
Theophylline, serum or plasma (Hep or EDTA)		
Therapeutic		
Bronchodilator	8–20 µg/mL	44–111 µmol/L
Prem. apnea	6–13 µg/mL	33–72 µmol/L
Toxic	>20 µg/mL	>110 µmol/L
Thiocyanate		
Serum or plasma (EDTA)		
Nonsmoker	1–4 µg/mL	17–69 µmol/L
Smoker	3–12 µg/mL	52–206 µmol/L
Therapeutic after nitroprusside infusion	6–29 µg/mL	103–499 µmol/L
Urine		
Nonsmoker	1–4 mg/d	17–69 µmol/d
Smoker	7–17 mg/d	120–292 µmol/d
Thiopental, serum or plasma (Hep or EDTA); trough		
Hypnotic	1.0–5.0 µg/mL	4.1–20.7 µmol/L
Coma	30–100 µg/mL	124–413 µmol/L
Anesthesia	7–130 µg/mL	29–536 µmol/L
Toxic concentration	>10 µg/mL	>41 µmol/L
*Thyroid-stimulating hormone (TSH), serum	0.32–5 µIU/L	0.32–5 mIU/L

*Test values are method dependent.

Tests	Conventional Units	SI Units
Thyroxine (T_4) serum	5–12 µg/dL (varies with age, higher in children and pregnant women)	65–155 nmol/L (varies with age, higher in children and pregnant women)
Thyroxine, free, serum	0.8–2.3 ng/dL	10.3–31 pmol/L
Thyroxine binding globulin (TBG), serum (as thyroxine)	1.5–3.4 mg/dL	15–34 mg/L
Tobramycin, serum or plasma (Hep or EDTA)		
Therapeutic		
Peak		
Less severe infection	5–8 µg/mL	11–17 µmol/L
Severe infection	8–10 µg/mL	17–21 µmol/L
Trough		
Less severe infection	<1 µg/mL	<2 µmol/L
Moderate infection	<2 µg/mL	<4 µmol/L
Severe infection	<2–4 µg/mL	<4–9 µmol/L
Toxic		
Peak	>10–12 µg/mL	>21–26 µmol/L
Trough	>2–4 µg/mL	>4–9 µmol/L
*Transaminase, serum		
AST (asparate aminotransferase, SGOT)	5–40 U/L (37°C)	Same
ALT (alanine aminotransferase, SGPT)	7–56 U/L (37°C)	Same
Transferrin, serum		
Newborn	130–275 mg/dL	1.30–2.75 g/L
Adult	220–400 mg/dL	2.20–4.00 g/L
>60 y	180–380 mg/dL	1.80–3.80 g/L
Triglycerides, serum, fasting		
Males	40–160 mg/dL	0.45–1.81 mmol/L
Females	35–135 mg/dL	0.4–1.53 mmol/L
Triiodothyronine, total (T_3) serum	150–250 ng/dL	1.54–3.08 nmol/L
*Triiodothyronine (T_3) uptake, resin (T_3RU)	24–34% uptake	0.24–0.34 uptake
Urea nitrogen, serum	7–18 mg/dL	2.5–6.4 mmol Urea/L
Urea nitrogen/creatinine ratio, serum	12:1 to 20:1	48–80 urea/creatinine mole ratio
Uric acid		
Serum, enzymatic		
Male	4.5–8.0 mg/dL	0.27–0.47 mmol/L
Female	2.5–6.2 mg/dL	0.15–0.37 mmol/L
Child	2.0–5.5 mg/dL	0.12–0.32 mmol/L
*Urine	250–750 mg/24 h (with normal diet)	1.48–4.43 mmol/24 h (with normal diet)
Urobilinogen, urine	0.1–0.8 Ehrlich unit/2 h	Same
	0.5–4.0 mg/24 h	Same
Valproic acid, serum or plasma (Hep or EDTA); trough		
Therapeutic	50–100 µg/mL	347–693 µmol/L
Toxic	>100 µg/mL	>693 µmol/L

*Test values are method dependent.

Tests	Conventional Units	SI Units
Vancomycin, serum or plasma (Hep or EDTA)		
Therapeutic		
Peak	20–40 µg/mL	14–28 µmol/L
Trough	5–10 µg/mL	3–7 µmol/L
Toxic	>80–100 µg/mL	>55–69 µmol/L
Vanillylmandelic acid (VMA), urine (4-hydroxy-3-methoxymandelic acid)	1.4–6.5 mg/24 h	7–33 µmol/d
Viscosity, serum	1.4–1.8 times water	Same
Vitamin A, serum	30–80 µg/dL	1.05–2.8 µmol/L
Vitamin B$_{12}$, serum	100–700 pg/mL	74–516 pmol/L
Vitamin E, serum		
Normal	5–18 µg/mL	11.6–46.4 µmol/L
Therapeutic	30–50 µg/mL	69.6–116 µmol/L
Zinc, serum	70–150 µg/mL	10.7–22.9 µmol/L

Tests	Conventional Units	SI Units
Vancomycin, serum or plasma (Hep or EDTA)		
Therapeutic		
Peak	20–40 µg/mL	14–28 µmol/L
Trough	5–10 µg/mL	3–7 µmol/L
Toxic	>80–100 µg/mL	>55–69 µmol/L
Vanillylmandelic acid (VMA), urine (4-hydroxy-3-methoxymandelic acid)	1.4–6.5 mg/24 h	7–33 µmol/d
Viscosity, serum	1.4–1.8 times water	Same
Vitamin A, serum	30–80 µg/dL	1.05–2.8 µmol/L
Vitamin B$_{12}$, serum	100–700 pg/mL	74–516 pmol/L
Vitamin E, serum		
Normal	5–18 µg/mL	11.6–46.4 µmol/L
Therapeutic	30–50 µg/mL	69.6–116 µmol/L
Zinc, serum	70–150 µg/mL	10.7–22.9 µmol/L